NEUROLOGICAL ANATOMY

In Relation to

Clinical Medicine

NEW YORK

OXFORD UNIVERSITY PRESS

LONDON 1969 TORONTO

NEUROLOGICAL ANATOMY

In Relation to Clinical Medicine

SECOND EDITION

A. Brodal, M.D.

Professor of Anatomy, University of Oslo, Norway
Formerly Assistant of the University Neurological
and Psychiatric Clinics in Oslo

Copyright © 1969 by Oxford University Press, Inc.

Library of Congress Catalog Card Number: 69–17759

The first edition of the book was published
by The Clarendon Press, Oxford, in 1948.

Second printing, 1972

Printed in the United States of America

Preface

Of all the natural phenomena to which science can turn
its attention, none exceeds in its fascination the working
of the human brain. Here, in a bare two-handsful of
living tissue, we find an ordered complexity sufficient
to embody and preserve the record of a lifetime of
the richest human experience. We find a regulator and
co-ordinator of the hundreds of separate muscle systems
of the human body that is capable of all the delicacy
and precision shown by the concert pianist and the surgeon.
Most mysterious of all, we find ·in this small sample of
the material universe the organ (in some sense) of our
own awareness, including our awareness of that
universe, and so of the brain itself.

D. MacKay (1967)

Some twenty years have passed since the first edition of this book
appeared. During this time there has been a steadily increasing activity
in all fields of neurological research, which has furnished us with a
wealth of new information on the structure and function of the nervous
system. As a consequence of our increased knowledge, many points of
view have had to be modified. Some traditional concepts have had to
be discarded; new ones have been created. For example, there is no

longer any justification for retaining the traditional concept of the "extra-pyramidal motor system," as will be discussed in Chapter 4. On the other hand, the neurological literature has been enriched with concepts such as the "ascending reticular activating system," "the limbic system," and others. In order to proceed in research we obviously have to create concepts as tools in the formulation of working hypotheses. However, we are often inclined to forget the limited validity of such concepts, particularly when a concept is verbalized in a simple and catching fashion. This tendency of the human mind has been aptly characterized and ridiculed by Goethe:

> Denn eben wo Begriffe fehlen,
> da stellt ein Wort zur rechten Zeit sich ein.
> Mit Worten lässt sich trefflich streiten
> mit Worten ein System bereiten.*

The neurological literature furnishes numerous examples of the truth of this dictum. Much confusion and unnecessary disputes have arisen because a sufficiently clear distinction has not been made between facts and hypotheses, between observations and interpretations. There is little doubt that many concepts which are at present accepted and in general use will in the future have to be considerably modified or even abandoned. The speed with which new information is forthcoming makes it more important than it was some decades ago to keep incessantly in mind the provisional tenability of current concepts. This, however, is not as easy as it may sound.

The author has felt this very strongly in the preparation of a second edition of this book. Largely due to the accumulation of new data our views are today on many points quite different from those accepted twenty years ago. It has therefore been necessary to rewrite entirely several chapters and sections of the first edition. For the same reason it has been difficult to decide what to include in the text, and to make clear what may be considered as established and what is still hypothetical. The main criterion in the selection of data to be presented has been to retain the original aim of the book: to bridge the gap between basic neurological sciences and clinical neurology, with particular reference to correlations between the structure of the nervous system and its

---

* For just where fails the comprehension,
  A word steps promptly in as deputy.
  With words 't is excellent disputing;
  Systems to words 't is easy suiting.

  Goethe: *Faust,* First Part, Scene IV.
  Translated by Bayard Taylor. Strahan & Co.,
  Publishers, London, 1871.

functions as revealed in man under normal and pathological conditions.

Like the first edition, the present does not pretend to be a systematic textbook on neurological anatomy, nor is it a textbook of clinical neurology. Some subjects are discussed in considerable detail, others are treated only briefly, and still others are not dealt with at all. Attempts have been made to include anatomical data which may be of interest from a clinical point of view. However, certain subjects are selected for more comprehensive consideration, in order to convey an impression of contemporary problems in the field of neurological research, even if the subjects are not of immediate practical interest. Results of neurophysiological research have been incorporated in so far as they can be correlated with structural features and can be understood by a writer who is not a neurophysiologist. More specific neurophysiological problems are not considered. The extensive new data in neurochemistry and neuropharmacology will be mentioned only to a limited extent. This is due to two circumstances. In the first place the author's knowledge of these subjects is too limited to permit a fuller treatment. Second, at the present state of research, data from these fields can only in few instances be definitely correlated with structural features. Likewise, most of the attempts made by workers in the field of neurocommunication to prepare models or theories of the brain or parts of it are not considered. Interesting as they may be, most of the models and theories are still of rather limited interest from the clinician's point of view.

With the enormous literature in the neurological sciences of today it is virtually impossible to give references to all relevant publications, nor would this be practical. In the selection of references to original publications, preference has in general been given to recent papers (in them interested readers will find references to previous publications). Furthermore, attempts have been made to give credit to authors who have been the first to report a new observation. Finally, where reviews or monographs are available, these are mentioned. However, the selection of references will of necessity be to some extent arbitrary, and it cannot be avoided that some papers which ought rightly to have been included are left out.

The changes in our views and new data have made it necessary to include a number of new illustrations, while about half of the old ones have been dropped.

The author has been fortunate in having the opportunity to consult several colleagues concerning special subjects on which they have first-hand knowledge. Dr. Jan Jansen, Emeritus Professor of Anatomy, Dr. Jan Jansen, Jr., Associate Professor of Neurophysiology, Dr. B. Kaada, Professor of Neurophysiology, and Dr. K. K. Osen, Assistant Professor of Anatomy, all in the University of Oslo, have read selected parts of the manuscript. Dr. K. Kristiansen, Professor of Neurosurgery, Oslo City Hospital, University of Oslo, and Dr. B. Vandvik, University Lecturer in Neurology, University of Oslo, have considered especially the clinical questions treated in the book. The author is greatly indebted to all these friends and colleagues for advice and constructive criticism. However, the responsibility for errors and omissions which are to be found in the text rests entirely with the author.

The expert technical assistance given by the artist of the Anatomical Institute, Mrs. Inger Grøholt, and the photographers Mr. E. Risnes and Miss Berit Ausen is gratefully acknowledged. The author wants to thank especially Miss Oddlaug Gorset for typing the manuscript and for secretarial assistance and Dr. E. Rinvik, Assistant Professor of Anatomy, for help with the checking of references and other bibliographical work. The conscientious scrutiny of the English of the manuscript by Miss Harlean Richardson is greatly appreciated.

Financial support in connection with the preparation of the manuscript given by the University of Oslo and the Oslo University Press is gratefully acknowledged. The author would also like to thank the editors of journals and many colleagues in various countries who have given permission to reproduce illustrations from their publications.

It is a pleasure to extend thanks to Oxford University Press and to Executive Editor Mr. W. C. Halpin for an agreeable collaboration and for the efforts to make this a better book.

Finally, I would like to thank my wife for a lifelong enduring patience and forbearance during my preoccupation with the present and other works, and for encouragement and valuable criticisms.

A. BRODAL

OSLO
May 1968

From the Preface to the First Edition

THIS BOOK was issued in the Norwegian language in 1943 by Johan Grundt Tanum, Publisher. When in 1946 a new edition was in preparation, it was decided to publish it in English, since a textbook on neuro-anatomy of a similar scope is not yet available in the English language. This decision was reinforced by the fact that the book had proved very acceptable in the Scandinavian countries.

The original plan of the volume has been maintained in the English edition, that is, to correlate the clinical symptoms appearing in disorders of the nervous system with the anatomical lesions producing them, or, in other words, to explain how lesions of different structures will result in symptoms of a definite pattern. This correlation is the main aim of the work. Consequently most of those anatomical details which are irrelevant for the clinical neurologist have been omitted. Readers in need of detailed anatomical knowledge should consult one of the special text-books of neuroanatomy. As the functions of the nervous system are a matter of prime interest to the neurologist, some physiological data have also been included, which facilitate and amplify the information which can be gained from a consideration of the anatomical features alone. The results of recent research in the fields of neuroanatomy and to some extent neurophysiology have been included as far as it was deemed appropriate.

p.t. OXFORD, *May 1947*   A. B.

ix

From the Preface
to the Norwegian Edition

IN NEUROLOGY a knowledge of the anatomical basis is perhaps of greater importance than in any other field of medicine, when a clear conception of the symptomatology is to be achieved and a correct diagnosis to be made. The teaching of clinical neurology may be undertaken in two ways. If it is only directed to acquaint the student with certain major syndromes so that he is in a position to recognize them, anatomical knowledge may perhaps be dispensed with. If, on the other hand, its aim is to teach the student to base his diagnosis in each individual case on an exact analysis of the symptomatology, to determine the site and nature of the lesion as accurately as possible, then an anatomical foundation is indispensable. Only if the student possesses a basis of that kind will he be able, to a certain extent at least, to understand the numerous deviations from the so-called typical pictures of the various diseases.

In this book stress is laid on the anatomical features of the nervous system which are of practical relevance, and an attempt is made to correlate clinical symptoms with the anatomy and physiology of the nervous system. I have, however, not attempted to give a complete review of the entire field of this correlation. Some readers will probably feel that much has been left out, while others will find that there are many things which might have been omitted.

Where problems which are still under discussion have been included in the text, this is for two reasons. Partly because some of them may in the near future become of practical importance, and partly so as to prevent the student from believing that there is but one opinion on every point. This, of course, demands much more independent thinking on the part of the student, more critical evaluation, and a greater amount of logical reasoning. However, there can be little doubt that an impetus to study in this manner is desirable. The more the student and the physician know about diverging opinions, and the more aware they become of the fact that the clinical features are frequently by no means as simple and definitely established as they are often presented to them, the better they will be able to reach a correct conclusion and evaluate accurately the findings in individual cases. They will also be less inclined to indulge in a sterile faith in the authorities. It is my hope that this book will help the reader not only to widen his knowledge of the functions of the nervous system, but also to inoculate into him a certain degree of sound scepticism towards many of the medical doctrines, which have revealed themselves as being founded on very loose ground.

ALF BRODAL

ANATOMICAL INSTITUTE,
UNIVERSITY OF OSLO, NORWAY
March 1943

Contents

x i i i

CONTENTS

Contents

Contents

xvii

Contents

CONTENTS

NEUROLOGICAL ANATOMY

In Relation to

Clinical Medicine

1

Introduction, Methods, Correlations

BEFORE dealing with different parts of the nervous system certain generalizations with regard to its anatomy must be considered, since this will facilitate an understanding of the material dealt with in this book. It is necessary first of all to look briefly at the methods we have at our disposal for the investigation of the anatomy of the nervous system and especially its fiber connections.

Structure and function. Anatomy is one of the fundamental branches of medicine, but anatomy alone, without relation to function, is a somewhat barren study, for it is function which primarily interests us in medicine. Some knowledge of the structure of organs and organisms is a necessary prerequisite for the understanding of their function. In fact, a knowledge of structure will often yield information on functions which have not been elucidated by other data. It is now recognized almost as an axiom that where structural differences are found there are also functional differences and vice versa. To take a simple example from the nervous system, one can, as is well known, differentiate between the somatic and visceral efferent nuclei in the brain stem. On some occasions it is not clear that there are structural differences, but this may be due to the inability of our present methods to bring more subtle differences to light.

3

In neurology a knowledge of structural features is perhaps more important for an understanding of function under normal and pathological conditions than in any other branch of medicine. Symptoms produced by diseases of the nervous system can be multifarious and involve different functions and components of functions, according to which different structures are affected. By clinical examinations we attempt to analyze the functional conditions and to understand the extent to which normal functions have been altered. The better our knowledge of the anatomy of the nervous system, the more easily we can infer from these functional disturbances and symptoms which structures are affected. However, the *topographical diagnosis,* the determination of the site of the lesion, is not, as one would first imagine, of importance only in those cases in which surgical procedures may be applied. It may also be of great importance in the *etiological diagnosis,* the determination of the nature and perhaps the cause of the lesion. Some diseases of the nervous system affect selectively, and in some cases exclusively, certain anatomical and functional units, while in other cases the localization of the lesion is quite irregular.

The determination of the site of the lesion is therefore an important link in understanding the nature of the disease. The better and more detailed our knowledge of the anatomy of the nervous system, the better equipped we are to interpret the clinical findings and the closer we can come to an exact diagnosis. Details of the clinical phenomena which at first may seem meaningless and unintelligible can, with a widened knowledge of the structural foundation, become intelligible and give valuable information.

Methods of studying the structure of the nervous system. The older anatomists who studied the nervous system depended on dissection and macroscopic findings, and by these primitive methods succeeded in demonstrating certain fundamental features, but it was not until the development of microscopic anatomy that any considerable clarity was achieved. It is surprising to realize that microscopic study of animal and human organisms did not begin until 1840. The German anatomist Schwann demonstrated about this time that animal organisms, like plants, are built up of cells. During the past century the cell theory has, as we know, gone through a striking development. The discovery (about 1850) that animal cells could be stained after first being fixed, i.e. killed by coagulation of the cell albumen, and that the different parts of the cells absorbed stains to various degrees, was another epoch-making event. The first stains to be used, first and foremost carmine, gave rather unsatisfactory pictures, however, when compared with present-day standards. Only with the introduction of hematoxylin (about 1890) was it

4

really possible to undertake a finer structural analysis of cells. Numerous other methods then followed. *Weigert* devised a method for selective *staining of myelin sheaths,* and another for glial tissue. The introduction by *Golgi* of his method of impregnating nerve cells with silver nitrate opened new possibilities for study of the finer structure of the nervous system. The *Nissl* method, introduced about 1890, is also of decisive importance. It is based on the staining with basic aniline dyes of specimens which are fixed in alcohol and remains the routine method in investigations of the cytology of the nervous system. About the same time *Marchi's method of demonstrating degenerating myelin sheaths* was developed, and numerous other methods subsequently evolved. Of particular importance is the development of *silver impregnation methods* which permit one to trace the degenerating unmyelinated axons and terminals. These methods will be considered more fully below.

A number of *histochemical methods* have been devised by which various chemical constituents in the nerve cells can be determined and the occurrence of certain enzymes, for example cholinesterases, can be demonstrated. The *use of radioactive isotopes* in morphological studies has created possibilities for studying details in the development of the various nuclei of the nervous system and in addition has given information on metabolic processes in nerve cells and glial cells. However, the most important new research tool for the morphologist has been the *electron microscope.* In the ten to fifteen years it has been in use, a wealth of new data on the finest structural details of nerve cells and fibers and glial cells has been revealed which has immensely increased our understanding of the nervous system.

If we examine the history of microscopic anatomy retrospectively (and the same applies to all branches of science) we see that as the maximum scope of old methods is exhausted new improved methods of investigation make possible continued progress. Some of these new methods will be briefly reviewed below, particularly those which can be used for the study of anatomical data of primary concern to the neurologist in analyzing symptoms in clinical cases.

The study of normal preparations. Many features of the fiber connections of the nervous system have been elucidated by the study of normal preparations in which the fibers are followed microscopically, partly by staining of the myelin sheaths and partly by *impregnation of the cell body and processes with silver and gold salts.* The latter methods have given useful information, especially about the lower, simply constructed organisms, but in many such cases it is impossible to state definitely where the fibers end. One of these methods, the *Golgi method,* has in recent years experienced a renaissance. This is largely a consequence of progress

5

made in modern electrophysiology of the nervous system, where it is often of importance to know the distribution of axon collaterals and of dendrites in order to evaluate one's findings. With the Golgi method only random cells are impregnated; but this is the only means of visualizing the course and type of all processes of a cell. Fig. 1-1 shows an example taken from the vestibular nuclei.

The so-called *myelogenetic method,* introduced by Flechsig, makes use of the fact that the different fiber systems are myelinated at different times in embryonic life and during the first period after birth. This method is scarcely used today.

FIG. 1–1 Drawing of a Golgi preparation from the lateral vestibular nucleus in the cat illustrating the various sizes of cells and orientation of dendrites in the four main vestibular nuclei as seen in a horizontal section (cf. inset above). *S, L, M,* and *D*: superior, lateral, medial and descending vestibular nuclei. From Hauglie-Hanssen (1968).

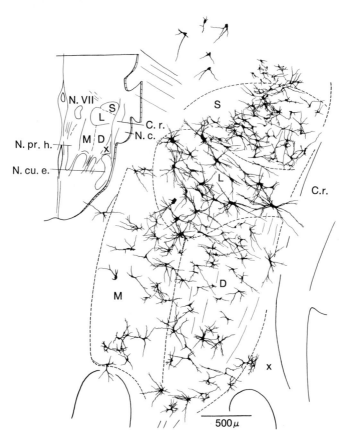

The study of pathological conditions in humans and experimental investigations on animals. By far the greatest part of our present-day knowledge of the fiber connections has been attained by the study of pathological conditions of the "degenerations" which occur after lesions in the nervous system. Cases from human pathology with lesions in different sites may be used for study, but it is the study of experimentally produced lesions in animals which has proved to be the more fruitful. In experimental investigations one usually has the enormous advantage of being able to decide the site of the lesion oneself and to vary the test conditions at will, while in human cases this is, of course, impossible. Furthermore, in human pathology the lesions are often large and diffuse and involve several different regions so that definite conclusions cannot be drawn. On the other hand, many small lesions suitable for study are undoubtedly present in humans, but being so small these lesions often do not give rise to symptoms and are therefore not investigated. There is *no essential difference between experimentally produced lesions and those which occur in human cases*. The secondary changes which accompany the lesions are also similar, and the methods used in the study of them are the same. One must, of course, exercise care in applying to human beings the results achieved by experiments on animals.

Gudden's method, secondary atrophy in newborn animals. The so-called *Gudden's method* was at one time the only method which could be used experimentally. About 1870 the German anatomist B. Gudden discovered that if one injured, for example, the cerebral cortex of a newborn rabbit and then examined the brain after 7 to 8 weeks or somewhat longer, the fiber systems which originated in the part of the cortex concerned had completely disappeared, having been resorbed, and the nuclei to which the affected tracts sent their fibers were diminished and atrophied. With this method he succeeded in demonstrating a number of fiber connections.

Originally Gudden was of the opinion that this atrophy, which he found after lesions in newborn animals, affected only the fiber systems that originated in the injured or destroyed parts. He therefore assumed that this indicated the direction of the fibers as well, and the direction of conduction in the tract concerned. Soon thereafter it was realized that this was not the case (von Monakow, about 1880). The fiber tracts which terminated in the injured or destroyed regions also degenerated. After a lesion of the cerebral cortex there also appeared atrophy and wasting of the fibers that terminate there and of their nuclei of origin, e.g. certain thalamic nuclei.

Secondary atrophy in grown animals and human beings. It is characteristic that such a marked wasting as is observed in newborn animals does not appear in fully grown animals. Some atrophy and decrease in volume of the affected systems do occur here too, but not until a much later date and to a lesser degree. This secondary atrophy in fully grown animals can, therefore, also be used for the study of fiber connections, but it is a somewhat coarse method. In such cases, as a rule, myelin sheath preparations are used, where the healthy, myelinated systems are stained a bluish color, while the affected systems, in which not only the axons but also the myelin sheaths have disintegrated, are pale. After old hemiplegias with hemorrhage into the internal capsule, one will thus find in myelin sheath preparations of transverse sections of the spinal cord the affected pyramidal tract as two pale areas in the remaining bluish-black stained white matter (Fig. 1-2). The coarser features of the fiber connections are thus brought to light, but this method is, of course, not suitable for detailed studies.

The difference just mentioned, between mature and newborn individuals, appears not only in animals but also in humans. It is a well-known fact that a cerebral injury to a newborn baby or a very young child causes bigger and more visible secondary changes in the brain than the same injury to an adult. A hemorrhage into the internal capsule, for example, which in adults causes essentially only a slight reduction in volume of the pyramidal tract, as a rule in the newborn baby

FIG. 1–2 Photograph of a myelin sheath stained preparation of the thoracic spinal cord from a patient who had a cerebral hemorrhage several years before he died. The light areas (b) in the lateral and ventral corticospinal tracts are due to the disappearance of the myelin sheath around the degenerated nerve fibers of the tracts.

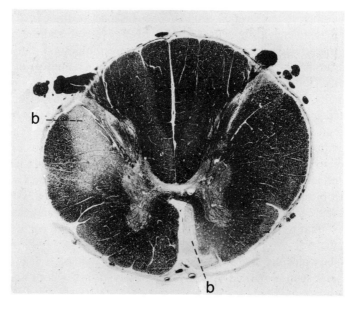

leads to retardation of growth of the whole side of the brain concerned and the contralateral cerebellar hemisphere. The reason for this striking difference is not known, but it has been thought to be due to differences in metabolic activity.

Most of the methods of investigation mentioned so far are based on the examination of large numbers of altered cells or fibers. This means that a considerably widespread injury is necessary and a great number of neurons has to be damaged. Owing to this fact detailed studies cannot be made with these methods.

The neuron theory.   At this stage a short summary of the neuron theory is appropriate. The neuron theory is in reality nothing more than the cell theory applied to nervous tissue. This concept, introduced about 1890, was strongly supported by His and Ramon y Cajal and had the endorsement of the most prominent anatomists and neurologists in the latter part of the last century—Forel, Koelliker, von Monakow, Waldeyer, and others. The most important assertion of the neuron theory is that nerve tissue, like other tissues, is built up of individual cells which are genetic, anatomical, functional, and trophic units. The neuron, a nerve cell with its processes, is the structural unit of nervous tissue, and the neurons are the only elements in the nervous system that conduct nervous impulses. The other types of cells, e.g. the different glial types, the ependyma and epithelium in the cholorid plexus, as well as the connective tissue cells, serve other functions. The neuron theory is the central point in the whole of our present-day interpretation of the nervous system and has proved very useful as a working hypothesis. This conception of the finer anatomy of the nervous system has made intelligible the development of the system as well as the function of nervous tissue.

For several decades the proponents of the neuron theory were opposed by other researchers (often called "reticularists") who, largely on the basis of silver-impregnated material, maintained that there is a continuity between nerve cells by means of fine fibrils, while according to the neuron theory the termination of an axon on a cell is a mere contact. The pros and cons of the neuron theory were carefully evaluated by Cajal in a monograph which appeared after his death and was translated into English about twenty years later (Cajal, 1954). The controversy was definitely settled in favor of the neuron theory by electron microscopic studies. Although there are many different morphological varieties of nerve terminals by which the final branches of an axon or its collaterals may establish contact with other nerve cells or their dendrites, there is always a clear separation between the elements belonging to the two neurons. Fig. 1-3 shows an example of the most common type of contact between a terminal swelling (terminal bouton, end foot, bouton terminal) of an axon and a nerve cell as seen in the electron microscope.

9

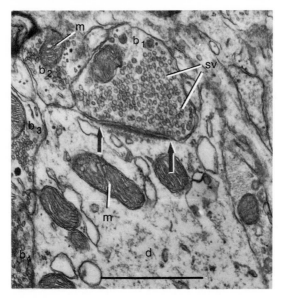

FIG. 1-3 Electron micrograph showing synaptic contact of a terminal bouton (*b₁*) with a thin dendrite (*d*). Note membrane thickenings (*between arrows*) and subsynaptic condensation of material in the dendrite. To the left three other boutons (*b₂, b₃,* and *b₄*) in contact with the dendrite, but the synaptic complexes are not included in the section. *m:* mitochondria; *sv:* synaptic vesicles. Scale line 1 *μ.*

There is a cleft of approximately 200Å (Å = Ångström unit: 1/10,000 of a micron) between the bouton and the nerve cell. At certain places along the area of contact, specializations are seen (arrows in Fig. 1-3). These indicate the areas where transmission of impulses from the bouton to the cell is believed to occur and thus represent the sites of *synapses*. Because of their importance for the understanding of nervous function the synapses will be considered separately below.

It should be emphasized that not only is the neuron a structural unit; it also, in most cases, behaves as a "trophic unit," as defined by the neuron theory. This is very obvious in lesions involving neurons and, as will be seen, this fundamental fact makes possible the study of fiber connections in the nervous system in a precise manner.

The synapse. The term "synapse" was coined by Sherrington in 1897, referring to the site of contact between two neurons where transmission of the nervous impulse occurs, i.e. as a functional term implying, however, that there is a structural basis for the phenomenon of impulse transmission. In light microscopic preparations a variety of types of end-

1 0

ings of nerve fibers has been observed. The most common type of presynaptic structure is the *terminal bouton,* referred to above, which appears as a small spherule or bulb at the end of axonal branches and collaterals (see Fig. 1-6). Such boutons may be found on the surface of cell bodies (perikarya or soma), on dendrites, and on axons. Accordingly, one speaks of *axo-somatic, axo-dendritic,* and *axo-axonic synapses.* The boutons vary in size, being commonly $0,5$-3μ in diameter. By special staining methods it can be shown that, at least in certain places, the entire surface of the cell body and its dendrites is densely beset with boutons (Fig. 1-4). (Such methods, based on the staining of mitochondria, have been described by Armstrong, Richardson, and Young, 1956, and Rasmussen, 1957. Other types of presynaptic structures, especially large, complex endings, have been described. These and many other varieties of contacts seen in the light microscope have commonly been interpreted as the morphological basis of synaptic transmission of nervous impulses. The electron microscope has, however, made it clear that a contact between two nerve cells seen in sections prepared with classical methods does not necessarily represent a synapse. On the other hand, in spite of some morphological variety between endings making synaptic contacts, the sites of synaptic contact, as shown by the electron microscope, have certain criteria in common.

A prototype of a synaptic contact is shown in Fig. 1-3. The pre-

FIG. 1–4   A multipolar nerve cell from the reticular formation of the cat, impregnated according to a special silver method. The cell body and the dendrites are densely beset with dark particles representing terminal boutons. Courtesy of Dr. Grant L. Rasmussen.

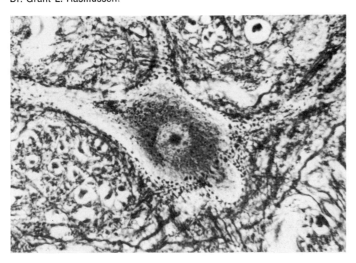

synaptic terminal, the *bouton,* is richly provided with mitochondria (indicating presumably a high rate of oxidative phosphorylation). Especially at the place of contact with the postsynaptic structure (cell body or dendrite) the bouton contains a number of small vesicles, 300–600Å in diameter, the so-called *synaptic vesicles.* In certain boutons special vesicles with a "dense core" are seen and are generally assumed to be related to biogenic amines. Sometimes "complex vesicles" and fine filaments are seen as well. At the site of contact the membranes of the presynaptic and postsynaptic structures show specializations in the form of electron dense condensations of material. In the *synaptic cleft* between these two regions, usually 150 to 250Å wide, there is often a condensation. In some synapses, for example in the cerebral cortex, this material appears as a series of fine filaments bridging the synaptic cleft. Organelles of different kinds have also been described beneath the postsynaptic membrane thickening (see Gray and Guillery, 1966; De Robertis, 1967, for some recent data).

A number of variations of the prototype of synapse described above have been encountered. Some are shown in Fig. 1-5. A bouton may be attached to a cell body or a dendrite (Fig. 1-5A). On the dendrite, boutons often establish synaptic contact with the spines (Fig. 1-5B) often found on dendrites of nerve cells. These spines were recognized by early workers in Golgi preparations, but by many they were previously thought

FIG. 1–5 Diagram of different types of synaptic contact as seen in electron micrographs. (Cf. text.) Abbreviations: *d:* dendrite; *gl:* glial cell; *m:* mitochondrion; *sp.a:* spine apparatus; *sv:* synaptic vesicles. To the right (G) an example of a complex synapse, showing some of the elements in a cerebellar glomerulus. A mossy fiber ending (*Mf*) establishes synaptic contact with dendritic branches of several granule cells (*Gr*). Collaterals of Golgi cells (*Go*) end on the latter dendrites. Diagram G adapted from Szentágothai (1965[a]).

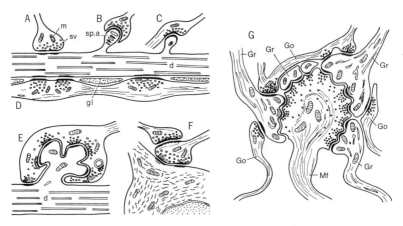

to be artifacts. The bouton may cover the entire spine. In certain cells, for example the pyramidal neurons of the hippocampus, a very large excrescence from the dendritic stem splits into several spinelike tips, and the whole structure is enclosed by a single large bouton (Fig. 1-5E) with a number of synaptic complexes between bouton and spine. The terminal branches of a dendrite may protrude into the bouton. An axon running along a dendrite and lying in close apposition to it may show several sites of synaptic contact, so-called *boutons en passage* (Fig. 1-5D). A passing fiber may contact a spine (Fig. 1-5C). In all these types of synapses, synaptic vesicles occur in the presynaptic element.

On the postsynaptic side various specializations have been described. One of these, a "spine apparatus" (see Fig. 1-5B), appears as a series of alternating, parallel-oriented plates of dense material and elongated vesicles in the spines (Gray, 1959). Or there may be no postsynaptic thickening but a flattened "subsynaptic sac" (Gray) or a "subsynaptic web" (De Robertis). On the basis of certain differences in the structure of the presynaptic and postsynaptic thickenings and the dimensions of the cleft, a distinction has been made between synapses of type 1 and type 2 (Gray, 1959). Other variations have been described as well. In certain regions complex synaptic arrangements are found, for example, in the so-called glomeruli. Fig. 1-5G shows a diagram of a cerebellar glomerulus, to be described in Chapter 5. The morphological basis of presynaptic inhibition is assumed to be a contact of one bouton and another as shown in Fig. 1-5F.

Often a particular synaptic variant is found only in certain regions or nuclei. However, it is currently generally accepted that places of contacts, provided with synaptic vesicles and membrane specializations, are the actual sites where chemically mediated impulse transmission occurs.

The transmitter substance, which is an essential link in the process, is assumed to be bound to the synaptic vesicles. On arrival of an impulse at the bouton, the transmitter presumably passes the presynaptic membrane and enters the postsynaptic cleft, to be bound to a receptor substance at the postsynaptic membrane. The permeability of this membrane is then altered with consequent depolarization if the impulse has an excitatory action on the postsynaptic structure, or hyperpolarization of the membrane with a raising of the threshold of excitability if the action is inhibitory. The transmitter is then rapidly destroyed by enzymatic action, and the cell is ready to receive another impulse. In spite of the fact that a number of pharmacologically active substances are present in nervous tissue, so far only acetylcholine appears to have been definitely established as a transmitter substance. There is fairly good evidence that noradrenaline and hydroxytryptamine may be as well (Gray and Whittaker, 1962), and that GABA (gamma-amino-butyric acid) is an inhibitory transmitter (see Elliot, 1965).

13

In spite of intensive research in this field in recent years, there are still many unsolved problems. Obviously, even on the ultrastructural level, the organization of the nervous system is extremely complex and generalizations may be misleading. As a case in point it may be recalled that synapses operating by *electrical transmission* (appearing as "tight junctions"), known for some time to exist in invertebrates, appear to be present also in some vertebrates (see Gray, 1966; Hinojosa and Robertson, 1967).

Almost every nucleus appears to have its own individuality with regard to cell types, synaptic pattern, etc. In spite of the great advances which have recently been made in all fields of neurological research, we are still very far from a complete understanding of the finer organization of the nervous system.

The basis of experimental studies of fiber connections. As indicated in a preceding section, the neuron behaves as a "trophic unit." Essentially the methods used to study fiber connections are based on this fact. If an axon is transected its peripheral parts, including its terminal ramifications and boutons, and the myelin sheath undergo degeneration. As a common denominator for these changes the term *"anterograde degeneration"* is often used, "anterograde" referring to the direction of impulse conduction in the axon. However, the parts of the neuron proximal to the site of transection are affected as well. These changes, called *"retrograde,"* involve the proximal part of the axon, the perikaryon and its dendrites. Fig. 1-6 illustrates the main features of this process. It further shows that the neuron receiving its afferent input from a damaged axon may be affected. These changes are called *transneuronal.* The histological methods which can be used for the demonstration of these changes differ, depending on which element one wants to study. It is, for example, usually not possible in the same section to obtain reliable information on both the retrograde changes in the perikaryon and the changes in the terminal boutons. When taken together, however, the various methods make possible a rather detailed mapping of the connections of the nervous system. These methods and their use and potentialities will be outlined below.

Marchi's method. Impregnation of degenerating myelin sheaths. The changes which appear in the part of the nerve fiber which is separated from the perikaryon are often collectively referred to as *Wallerian degeneration.* The degeneration also affects the myelin sheaths of transected fibers. The degenerating myelin sheaths can be demonstrated by certain stains, for example with the so-called *Marchi* method, introduced by the Italian Marchi, about 1890, and still used. The method is based on the fact that degenerating myelin becomes impregnated by an osmic acid solution when it has previously been treated with a mordant, e.g. potas-

1 4

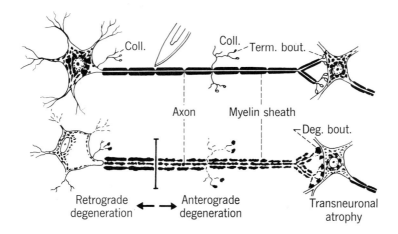

FIG. 1–6 Diagrammatic representation of the changes in the neuron which follow transection of its axon. Above, the normal situation; below, the changes as they appear some days after the lesion, central to the cut (retrograde degeneration) and peripheral to it (anterograde degeneration). Below to the right the transneuronal changes are indicated. (See text for description.)

sium bichromate. This differential reaction to osmic acid must be regarded as an expression of chemical changes in the lipids which form an essential part of the myelin sheath. These changes require some time for development, and as a rule reach their maximum 10 to 20 days after injury. The degenerating myelin sheaths appear as black dots or somewhat longer cylindrical particles (Fig. 1-7). The normal myelinated fibers are stained light yellow and provide a favorable background. Gradually the lipid globules are converted to fatty acids which no longer reduce osmic acid but which can then be stained with other fat-coloring substances: sudan black and red, and others. Finally they are completely resorbed.

The Marchi method can only be used to advantage within a definite period of time after the injury (see above). In later stages the black-colored granules are fewer and more dispersed, but they can usually be shown in sufficiently large quantities for the study of the course of the fibers up to 7 to 8 weeks after the lesion and even longer. In experiments with animals degeneration products can be seen at the end of one year (Glees, 1943), and Marion Smith (1951) has shown that the Marchi method may also be used with human material for tracing degenerating fibers at intervals up to 13 months after division of the fiber tracts.[1] It

[1] According to Marion Smith (1956a; see also Smith, Strich, and Sharp, 1956) the Marchi method can be used with advantage on human material fixed in forma-

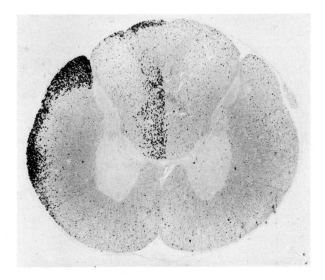

FIG. 1–7 A Marchi section from the 2nd cervical segment of a cat in which 15 days previously the lateral funiculus had been transected in the lumbar cord. Degenerating ascending fibers, interrupted by the lesion, are seen as black particles in the lateral funiculus. The degeneration in the ipsilateral dorsal funiculus is due to damage inflicted on dorsal roots at the level of operation.

should be noted that the optimal time for the use of the Marchi method varies with fiber systems and animal species. Since the myelin sheaths of the terminal parts of the axonal branches are very fine, the black globules and granules which appear there will be finer and more dispersed than along the actual course of the fiber. The sites of termination of degenerating myelinated fibers can, therefore, be determined fairly accurately with the Marchi method.

All methods of investigation are hampered by certain sources of error, and the Marchi method is no exception. So-called pseudodegenerations occur in certain cases, but as the name implies they are only apparent degenerations. (For a detailed study of the artifacts occurring with the Marchi method, see M. Smith, 1956b.) Used critically the Marchi method is, however, very useful and has given much valuable information about a number of connections in the nervous system.

lin. In the beginning the degeneration products of the myelin sheaths are extracellular, but from approximately 10 weeks after a lesion an increasing amount of the material is intracellular, i.e. taken up by scavenger cells. On formalin-fixed material the Marchi method gives better results in cases with long survival periods than in cases where death ensues within a few weeks after the lesion.

Changes in axons and terminal branches of transected nerve fibers. Anterograde degeneration.   As stated above, most terminal axonal branches end by means of globule-shaped swellings called *terminal boutons*. With silver impregnation methods the terminal boutons may appear as ringlike figures of different sizes or as solid globules, depending on the method used (see Fig. 1-4). When the distal part of a transected axon disintegrates, its terminal boutons will also degenerate. They usually swell, become irregular, and show an increased argyrophilia (see Fig. 1-6). These processes occur in the course of a few days. Consequently, it should be possible to determine exactly where the fibers of a transected tract terminate by mapping the distribution of degenerating boutons and the finest terminal axonal branches. However, in such studies it is important to consider that there are wide variations among normal boutons with regard to their appearance in silver-impregnated sections, and that there are variations between regions or nuclei, and even within subdivisions of one nucleus, as, for example, in the inferior olive (Blackstad, Brodal, and Walberg, 1951; Walberg, 1960). Furthermore, the speed of degeneration is not the same for all fiber tracts or for fibers of different calibers. Negative results may be misleading because of an inappropriate survival time.

Several methods are available for the study of degenerating boutons and fibers. With some of them (e.g. the method of Glees, 1946), normal as well as degenerating fibers and boutons are impregnated. This makes it difficult and very laborious to distinguish the degenerating particles, especially when they are few. However, extremely fine degenerating fibers can be identified (see Fig. 1-8C). In recent years the silver impregnation method worked out by Nauta and Gygax (1954) and modified by Nauta (1957) has been much used. In successful preparations only degenerating axons and branches are impregnated. These black degenerating structures contrast clearly with the yellow tone of the normal structures, which provide a favorable background. (For a recent account of the importance of certain steps in the preparation procedure, see Eager and Barnett, 1966.) A nucleus or part of a nucleus which is the site of termination of a transected fiber bundle can often be distinguished very clearly even when examined at low power of the microscope (Fig. 1-8A). This method is also very well suited for tracing the course of bundles of degenerating fibers, particularly when sections are cut in the plane of the fibers. Where the degenerating fibers branch and terminate, rows of fine black particles indicate the site of terminal branches. Quite often such fibers are seen almost to encircle a perikaryon (Fig. 1-8B) or to run along the proximal dendrites, which can usually be seen.

It is important to be aware of the fact that the various silver impreg-

1 7

nation methods differ in respect to the impregnation of degenerating fibers and of terminals (see Heimer, 1967, for a survey). For this reason negative findings may not be decisive. Disputes have occasionally arisen over divergent findings made by different authors, because one or both of them has not been aware of the differences referred to above.

It was originally assumed that the Nauta method did not demonstrate degenerating boutons. However, comparative studies with the methods

FIG. 1–8 Photomicrographs from sections treated according to the silver impregnation methods of Nauta (1957) and Glees (1946).

A: From a transverse Nauta-impregnated section through the lateral (*L*) and medial (*M*) vestibular nuclei in a cat, 10 days after transection of the vestibular nerve (*N VIII*). x 20. The terminal areas (*arrows*) are clearly indicated by the presence of darkly stained degenerating fibers. From Walberg, Bowsher and Brodal (1958).

B: From a Nauta-impregnated section of the spinal cord of a cat 6 days after a lesion of the contralateral primary sensorimotor cortex. Degenerating fibers and small fragments, some of which are presumably terminal boutons, are found close to the cell bodies. x 330. From Nyberg-Hansen and Brodal (1963).

C. From a Glees-impregnated section of the spinal trigeminal nucleus in the cat 5 days after a lesion of the frontoparietal cerebral cortex. Extremely fine degenerating fibers, some of them indicated by arrows. x 530. From Brodal, Szabo, and Torvik (1956).

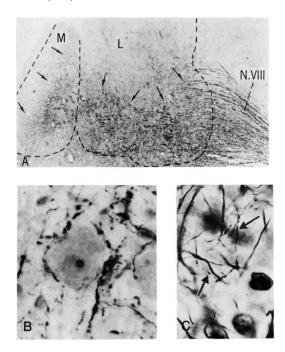

of Glees and Nauta have shown that this is not so (e.g. Walberg, 1964), although it is usually impossible to decide whether a particular black body represents a degenerating bouton or is a fragment of a fine degenerating fiber. Electron microscopic studies of material impregnated in accordance with the Nauta method have proved unequivocally that degenerating terminal boutons can be made visible with the Nauta method (Guillery and Ralston, 1964; Lund and Westrum, 1966).

Silver impregnation methods have been used by some workers on human material and with satisfactory results. (The greatest difficulty is to obtain well-fixed material.) As to the time parameters, degenerative changes in transected fibers and in boutons are usually seen as early as 4 days after the lesion, but it should be remembered that in human material the optimal periods may be different from those in animals.

When critically used, silver impregnation methods give information on many details of interest. For example, in a nucleus containing cells of different sizes or types, one may find that chiefly one type of cell is contacted by a contingent of afferent fibers. Furthermore, it may be seen that transected afferent fibers make contact with perikarya or dendrites or with both. (Usually only thick dendrites can be identified in the light microscope.) Obviously, the silver impregnation methods may be used not only following transections of axons but also when the perikarya of axons are destroyed by lesions of a nucleus.

As stated above, the final proof that contacts observed under the light microscope represent true sites of synapses can only be obtained in electron microscopic studies, since with the silver impregnation methods it is impossible to decide whether a black particle found attached to a cell is a bouton. Furthermore, a thin glial sheet, not visible in the light microscope, may be interposed between the bouton and the cell or its dendrite. It is fortunate, therefore, that degenerating nerve fibers and terminal boutons can be identified with the electron microscopic (Gray and Hamlyn, 1962; Colonnier and Gray, 1962; and others). In most places where they have been studied, degenerating boutons appear in the electron micrographs as shown in Fig. 1-9. The bouton appears to be somewhat reduced in size, its matrix has a finely granular appearance, and the mitochondria show fragmentation with loss of structural details. The synaptic vesicles are closely packed. These changes give the degenerating bouton an electron dense appearance. At early stages the sites of synaptic contacts can still be recognized (arrows in Fig. 1-9). These early changes may be apparent in boutons of many fiber systems 2 to 5 days after the axons have been cut, and the boutons may disappear rather rapidly (see for example Mugnaini, Walberg, and Brodal, 1967). In other instances degenerating boutons may be identified in electron micrographs for con-

1 9

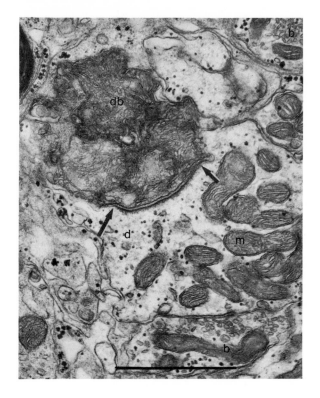

FIG. 1–9 Electron micrograph showing a degenerating bouton (*db*) in the lateral vestibular nucleus of the cat 3 days after transection of the vestibular nerve. The bouton is dark and heavily changed (cf. Fig. 1–3), but its site of synaptic contact (*between arrows*) with a dendrite (*d*) is still visible. *b:* normal boutons; *m:* mitochondria. Scale line 1 μ.

siderable periods after the lesion (e.g. 112 days in the inferior olive, Walberg, 1965a).

Electron microscopic studies of degenerating boutons open up new possibilites for establishing the synaptic relationships of fiber systems in great detail. Not only can it be determined whether or not a contact between two elements is a synapse, but information can also be obtained on other problems which cannot be solved with the light microscope. For example, it is possible to determine whether or not there are synaptic contacts with the finest dendritic terminals. It is essential in such studies that one know exactly where to look for the alterations. Therefore, a precise determination with silver impregnation methods of the area in which the fiber bundle under study terminates is a necessary prerequisite (see Alksne, Blackstad, Walberg, and White, 1966).

20

It will appear from what has been said above that the neuroanatomist of today has at his disposal powerful tools for precise studies of the distribution and modes of ending of fiber tracts in the central nervous system. Likewise, he has methods at his disposal for studying the origin of fibers, by utilizing the retrograde cellular changes.

Changes in the perikaryon and the central part of the axon after this has been cut. Retrograde changes. Originally it was erroneously assumed that no significant changes occur in the *central part of the axon* after this has been cut. The changes in the myelin sheaths are not very conspicuous, and the changes in the axon have been particularly difficult to clarify and the subject of much dispute.

Thus it has been maintained that the retrograde changes in the axon do not extend farther toward the center than to the next proximal node of Ranvier, and it has been assumed that the proximal part of the axon undergoes only a slow atrophy. Recent studies, however, indicate that this is not so. Cowan, Adamson, and Powell (1961) found that in the pigeon retrograde degeneration of the axon begins close to the perikaryon and spreads centrifugally. The same conclusion was reached by Grant and Aldskogius (1967) in a study with kittens. The degenerative changes in the central part of a transected axon may be visualized with the Nauta method. Even the dendrites are affected (Cerf and Chacko, 1958; Grant and Aldskogius, 1967). The changes in the central part of the axon require a somewhat longer period of time to develop than the anterograde degeneration in the distal part (see Powell and Cowan, 1964). (This is of practical importance, as the choice of a too long survival period in studies of efferent fiber connections may give erroneous results because of simultaneous impregnation of fibers degenerating in the retrograde direction.)

The changes that appear in the *perikaryon of a cell* after an injury to its axon are of great value in studying connections of the nervous system. Our first accurate knowledge of these changes came from Nissl. At the end of the nineteenth century Nissl undertook a systematic study of the structure of the nerve cells and of the nerve cell pictures found in various diseases of the central nervous system and thus laid the foundation of our present-day knowledge of structural changes in the nerve cells.

Retrograde cellular changes in peripheral motor neurons. Nissl (1892) found that after division or excision of a nerve, characteristic structural changes appeared in the cells of origin of its motor fibers. In rabbits in which he evulsed the facial nerve, the cells of the facial nucleus showed a tigrolysis which began centrally and in the course of a few days extended throughout the cytoplasm, leaving only a brim of fine tigroid granules in the periphery. The central parts of the cytoplasm acquired a "milky" appearance. The nucleus was displaced to the periphery, opposite the axon hillock and often was somewhat flattened. The cells appeared more round than usual, apparently because of some swelling. These changes are fully developed after 7 to 10 days, when the changed

2 1

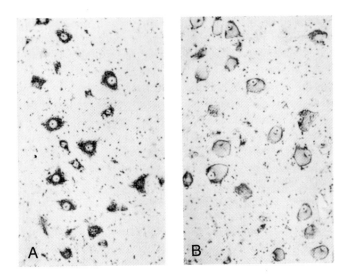

FIG. 1–10 Photomicrographs of motor ventral horn cells in the adult monkey. *A:* normal; *B:* 6 days following transection of axons. All cells present typical acute retrograde changes. x 68. From Bodian (1947).

cells can clearly be distinguished from the normal ones. Nissl called this stage *primäre Reizung* (primary irritation). Corresponding changes are seen in the motoneurons of the spinal cord following transection of their axons (Fig. 1-10). The discovery of these cell changes by Nissl (in 1892) meant that one had a new means of determining the source of origin of fibers in the peripheral nerves.

Nissl did not carry his study of cell changes beyond the stage of *primäre Reizung.* When, about 1900, several authors began a renewed study of the cell changes Nissl had described, they made the interesting discovery that the facial cells after having reached the *primäre Reizung* stage could behave somewhat differently (Fig. 1-11). Either they underwent an increasing swelling and disintegrated or a restoration took place in the following manner: the tigroid substance reappeared, first in the central parts of the cell; the cell then became smaller and took its normal contour again and the nucleus resumed its central position. After a considerable time, however, these restored cells could be attacked by a slow atrophy with an increasing diminution and darker color. It appears from later studies that this occurs when the axon of a regenerating cell does not establish functional contact with the muscle.[2]

---

[2] According to Bodian (1947) regeneration in the ventral motor horn cells of the monkey begins about two weeks after the injury and is nearly complete at 80 days, but complete regeneration may take up to six months.

22

These retrograde cell changes which are seen in the cell's perikaryon after an injury to its axon appear not only in the motor cells in the ventral horns of the spinal cord and in the motor cranial nerve nuclei, but are also seen in the cells of spinal and cranial nerve ganglia. In these instances the cell changes appear distinctly only after division of the peripheral branch, while division of the central branch which goes to the central nervous system does not produce clear-cut changes. Similar changes can also be observed in cells of the nuclei in the central nervous system which do not send their axons out of it.

Early retrograde cell changes in other types of neurons. Originally it was believed that *primäre Reizung* as Nissl had described it in the facial nerve cells appeared in the same manner in all other types of neurons, but it has since been shown that this is not the case. On the contrary, the *early changes after division of the axon can vary considerably*. Following transection of their axon, the cells of some nuclei do not swell but become smaller. The nucleus is not always peripherally displaced. Another difference between peripheral and central neurons appears at a later period. *In central connections some of the affected cells disintegrate acutely and none of them are restored*. Those which do not disintegrate undergo a slowly progressing atrophy, and after some months the atrophy may be extreme. There are variations among nuclei and among species with regard to the cellular changes and their time course, and one cannot, therefore, expect to find the typical picture of *primäre Reizung* in all neuron systems. For example, in the facial nucleus of the mouse a peripheral chromatolysis may be seen 12 hours after section of the nerve (Cammermeyer, 1963), while in the human spinal cord some cells showing the classic condition of *primäre Reizung* may be seen as late as 10

Fig. 1–11 A diagram of the usual course of the retrograde cell changes in peripheral motor neurons. To the left a normal cell. From the stage of the fully developed retrograde changes the cell may disintegrate (*above*) or recover, but then frequently the cell atrophies later on. (Cf. text.)

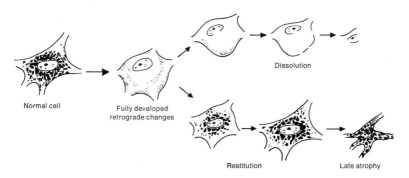

Normal cell

Fully developed retrograde changes

Dissolution

Restitution

Late atrophy

months following a chordotomy (Marion C. Smith, personal communication). It is often difficult to distinguish between less characteristic reactions and normal variations. Sometimes shrunken, dark cells have been interpreted as affected by acute retrograde changes, but it has been conclusively shown that this cell conditon arises as an artifact (Cammermeyer, 1960, 1962). However, where the *early* changes are clear-cut and typical they can be used in the study of fiber connections if one is careful in interpreting the findings.

Many studies have been made to clarify the processes going on in the cell during the acute retrograde changes. For example, there appears to be an increased activity of acid phosphatase in the perikaryon (Bodian and Mellors, 1944; LaVelle, Liu, and LaVelle, 1954), while there is a decrease in the activity of cytochrome oxidase (Howe and Mellors, 1945) and of succinic dehydrogenase (Howe and Flexner, 1947). Changes in the content of true acetylcholinesterase have been described (Friede, 1959). Some electron microscopic studies have also been made. Among recent studies those of Andres (1961), Pannese (1963), Bodian (1964), and Mackey et al. (1964) should be mentioned. The results of histochemical as well as electron microscopic studies are not all concordant as to details. This may presumably be due, at least in part, to the fact that different animal species and different cell types have been used.

Late retrograde cell changes. Retrograde atrophy. Because of the variety in pictures of the early retrograde changes and the uncertainty resulting from this, another procedure has been used to a great extent, namely, the examination of the *late retrograde changes, often called retrograde atrophy.* The animal is allowed to live for a longer time after the lesion is made, for weeks or months. Then, as mentioned above, as a rule, most of the cells whose axons are severed have degenerated so that the number of cells is reduced, and most of the remaining nerve cells will be atrophied. Often there is proliferation of glial cells. In many instances the parts which are affected in this manner stand out from the surrounding normal regions very distinctly, and it is possible to map out the affected areas fairly accurately. (Fig. 1-12 shows an example.)

Retrograde cell changes in very young animals. Modified Gudden method. By making use of the late retrograde cell atrophy, less equivocal changes may sometimes be obtained than by studying the early cell changes. In some cases, however, neither the early nor the late changes give sufficiently clear-cut pictures. This is the case with the inferior olive. A systematic investigation of the retrograde changes in the inferior olive following lesions of the cerebellum (Brodal, 1939) made it clear that the cells of the olive in very young rabbits and cats (8–15 days old at operation) behave in a manner different from those in adult animals. In the course of 4–8 days the cells show characteristic retrograde degenera-

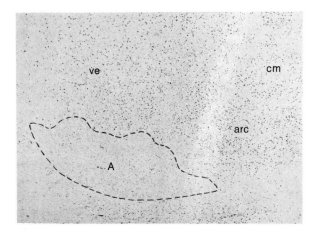

FIG. 1–12 Photomicrograph of a Nissl preparation showing retrograde loss of cells and cellular atrophy in a limited part (A) of the thalamus in the monkey, following extirpation of a cortical area. From Le Gros Clark (1937).

tion (while in the adult the changes are equivocal). Furthermore, after a few days more, all the cells disintegrate completely. The area of the olivary band which sends its fibers to the ablated part of the cerebellum then stands out as a zone free of nerve cells, with some increase in the glial cells (Fig. 1-13). Corresponding observations have been made in the pontine nuclei.

In subsequent years, this procedure, which has been called a *modified Gudden method* (Brodal, 1939, 1940a), has been used with advantage in our laboratory in studying the origin of a number of fiber connections. Usually the acute changes are clearer than in adult animals. Fig. 1-14 shows cells undergoing acute retrograde changes in the red nucleus of the kitten following a lesion of the spinal cord. In very young animals the nerve cells are apparently more susceptible to damage to their axon than the nerve cells in adult animals. Systematic studies of the pattern of retrograde changes in the cells of the facial nucleus of the hamster at prenatal and various postnatal stages have been made by LaVelle and LaVelle (1958, 1959). Also compatible with this view is the recent demonstration that in very young kittens not only the perikaryon but also the central part of the axon and even the dendrites of the affected nerve cells degenerate rapidly (Grant and Aldskogius, 1967). This discovery may prove useful for solving certain neuroanatomical problems.

When using the modified Gudden method it is important to be aware that the time parameters vary between species and between fiber systems. At a certain stage

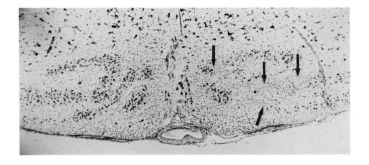

FIG. 1–13 Photomicrograph from a Nissl-stained section through the inferior olive of a rabbit in which a lesion of the cerebellar cortex was made when the animal was 11 days old. (Sacrificed 8 days later.) The complete disappearance of the nerve cells in circumscribed parts of the contralateral olive is visible (*between the arrows*). (Cf. text.) From Brodal (1940b).

of maturation the cells change their mode of reaction to the adult pattern. Consequently, if the animal is only a little too old, the advantages of the susceptibility of the young cells are lost. It is especially fortunate that with this method retrograde changes can usually be identified, not only in large cells but also in small ones (Fig. 1-14). This has made it clear that the efferent fibers of many nuclei come from cells of different sizes. For example, the vestibulospinal tract is made up of axons from small as well as giant cells in the nucleus of Deiters (Pompeiano and Brodal, 1957a). The drawbacks of the method are that the very young animals are relatively less resistant to operative procedures than adult ones, that dimensions are smaller, and that stereotaxic coordinates are difficult to establish.

Transneuronal changes. All the cell and fiber changes which we have so far discussed can be explained by the neuron theory. There are, however, other changes occurring in the nerve cells which are not easily explained. In certain cases, after a fiber system is severed, changes appear in the cells to which its fibers conduct their impulses. The neurons themselves are not directly injured, but are affected nevertheless. Since the deleterious effect of the lesion is transmitted over a synapse, the cell changes are called *transneuronal* or *transsynaptic* (Fig. 1-15). These are seen most clearly in the cells of the lateral geniculate body (Fig. 1-15) after a lesion of the retina. (The ganglion cells in the retina send their axons to the lateral geniculate body where they terminate on its cells and dendrites.) In human pathology atrophy of the pontine nuclei following long standing lesions of the cerebral cortex or cerebral peduncle (with damage to the corticopontine fibers) has been frequently observed and interpreted as being transneuronal. In other instances the changes observed have been less clear-cut. However, when more accurate methods are used, in which cell size, nuclear size, and nucleolar size are measured and counts of cells are made (Cook, Walker, and Barr, 1951), it has been possible to identify transneuronal changes in a series of nuclei following damage to their main afferent systems. As a rule the changes develop rather slowly. For example, following destruction of the cochlea in cats changes were first noticed in the cochlear nuclei after 60 days (Powell and Erulkar, 1962). However, the time required for such changes to occur varies with the species. Changes in the lateral geniculate body following transection of the optic nerve appear much more rapidly in the monkey (Glees and Le Gros Clark, 1941; Matthews, Cowan, and Powell, 1960) than in the cat and rabbit (Cook, Walker, and Barr, 1951). The cellular changes consist in a moderate shrinkage of the cell, the nucleus, and nucleolus, with some reduction in the Nissl substance. Eventually the cells may disappear completely. Just as is the case with retrograde cellular changes, the transneuronal changes occur more rapidly in young animals than in adult ones (Torvik, 1956a; Matthews and Powell, 1962). The same appears to be the case in man.

It appears that the transneuronal changes are essentially an atrophy of disuse. It is to be expected, therefore, that their intensity in any nucleus will depend on the degree of functional deafferentation. Cells which receive afferent inputs from many sources may, therefore, suffer relatively little if one afferent contingent is cut. This seems to be true in general, but as elsewhere one has to take into account variations in the morphology and function of the various nuclei, the age at which the damage is made, and species differences. So far the method of transneuronal atrophy has been relatively little used in the study of fiber connections, but in certain situations it may prove to be of some value for this purpose.

Physiological methods of tracing fiber connections.   It is clear from

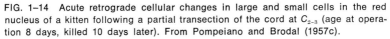

FIG. 1–14   Acute retrograde cellular changes in large and small cells in the red nucleus of a kitten following a partial transection of the cord at C_{2-3} (age at operation 8 days, killed 10 days later). From Pompeiano and Brodal (1957c).

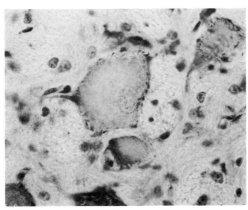

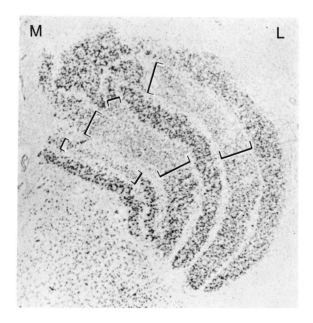

FIG. 1–15 Photomicrograph of a Nissl preparation showing transneuronal disappearance of the nerve cells in 3 of the laminae of the lateral geniculate body of a monkey after a lesion of the retina. From Le Gros Clark and Penman (1934).

the preceding account that a number of anatomical methods are at our disposal for studying fiber connections of the nervous system. However, information concerning these fiber connections can also be obtained from physiological studies. Thus the effects observed when various parts of the nervous system are stimulated may be examined and conclusions drawn concerning the pathways followed by the impulses, particularly when comparisons are made with results in similar experiments in which certain fiber tracts have been transected.

A more direct study of fiber connections has been made possible by the development of electrophysiological techniques. By means of an amplifier-cathode-ray oscillograph the action potentials arising during activity of nervous structures can be recorded, and the influence of artificial (e.g. electrical) or natural stimulation (e.g. of receptors of sense organs) on the electrical activity of the terminal area of a certain fiber system can be studied. This *method of recording evoked potentials* has given important information with regard to several fiber connections, and it will be frequently referred to in the following chapters. The method has an advantage in that it may be applied in many cases where it is difficult or impossible to place lesions which will give unequivocal evidence when anatomical methods are employed. It should, however, be stressed that anatomical control is necessary to make sure that the electrodes have been properly placed. It should also be realized that it is usually difficult or even impossible to decide whether the impulses recorded have traversed one synapse or more on their way from the point of stimulation to the site where they are recorded.

In recent years improvements in electrophysiological techniques have made it possible to record by means of microelectrodes the action potentials of single fibers or cells (single unit recordings). Important information has been obtained in this way.

The scope and application of the methods. Mention was made above of the fact that the same anatomical methods are applied in the study of fiber connections in experimental animals and in cases derived from human pathology. Attention was also directed to the frequently very extensive lesions met with in human material, which make such cases of limited value. Another circumstance which often reduces the value of human material for study of fiber connections is that the time interval which has elapsed from the development of the lesion until the death of the patient does not permit use of the method which would have been appropriate for the particular problem.

The most reliable and exact information concerning the fiber connections of the nervous system has come from experimental investigations. In animal studies the investigator himself can determine the conditions of the experiments, and he may reproduce series of more or less exactly similar cases. Especially in regard to details of the fiber connections, most of our knowledge is obtained by such studies. During the last twenty years a great many experimental investigations of fiber connections have been performed, and much new light has been thrown on hitherto obscure relationships between various parts of the nervous system. It should again be emphasized that great care must be taken when findings in animals are to be applied to man. This holds true particularly when the experiments have been performed on lower animals. However, monkeys have in recent years been rather extensively employed as experimental animals, and in some cases even apes, which are closely related to man in many respects. The correspondence between the experimental findings in animals and the data obtained from studies of human beings is very close in many instances. Examples of this will be mentioned later.

Even a cursory examination of neurological periodicals of recent years will show that experimental investigations make up the bulk of the papers published. This is a reflection of the fact that what is needed at present is a more accurate knowledge of the details of structure and function of the nervous system, not least a more minute mapping out of the vast number of different fiber systems, their exact origins, their detailed patterns of organization, their modes of ending, and their functional qualities. This goal can only be reached by extensive experimental investigations, although additional information from research along other lines may contribute to the ultimate verification of the results derived from experiments. In order to clarify details, extensive series of experiments usually have to be performed. Recent achievements from other fields of neurology (such as data obtained in clinical and biochemical studies) also have to be considered in the planning, performance, and interpretation of the experiments. Due attention must be paid to special features, such as cytoarchitecture (e.g. when making lesions in the cerebral cortex), chemoarchitecture, phylogenesis, and ontogenesis. The amount of exact knowledge derived from recent studies is enormous and has made modern neuroanatomy an altogether different subject from the old, mainly morphological, descriptive anatomy. There is reason to assume that in the years to come the new research tools will make it possible to increase considerably our understanding of the complex functions of the nervous system. This will undoubtedly have consequences for the diagnosis and treatment of disorders of the nervous system.

2

The Somatic Afferent Pathways

THE DESIGNATION "somatic afferent pathways" comprises several fiber systems and nuclei, partly differing in regard to anatomical features, partly also in regard to function. The term chosen as a heading of this chapter, it is admitted, is not unequivocal, and in order to avoid misunderstandings some preliminary remarks are necessary, delimiting more exactly what is inherent in the concept as used here.

The different sensory modalities. Most parts of the human body are equipped with some sort of receptors, although, as is well known, normally most impulses from the viscera are not consciously perceived. However, impulses from the viscera (often called interoceptive) play an important part in visceral function, being necessary for the manifold visceral reflexes. These visceral afferent impulses, and the fiber tracts they traverse, will be treated in another chapter. Here our interest will be focused on the pathways followed by somatic afferent impulses arising in the skin, muscles, ligaments and joints, and fascia, more precisely called *general somatic afferent,* in contrast to the special somatic afferent impulses originating in some of the sense organs (eye, ear). The general somatic impulses can further be differentiated into *exteroceptive* and *proprioceptive.* The former arise from receptors developed from the integument, and mediate sensations of touch, light pressure, cold, warmth, and cutaneous pain and some more complex sensations; the adequate stimuli being changes in the environment. The latter are mediated by receptors developed in the muscles, fascia, ligaments, and joints, i.e. the deeper somatic structures and their adequate stimuli are changes taking place within the body.[1] Only the exteroceptive and some proprioceptive impulses, their receptors, the tracts they use, and their relay and terminal stations, will be considered in the present chapter. Common to the sensory modalities to be treated in this chapter is that they *reach the level of consciousness* and are perceived by the individual, giving him information of changes occurring in the external world in immediate contact with the body (exteroceptive) and of the changes in the deeper somatic structures (proprioceptive). Also some impulses presumably originating from visceral receptors, such as those producing sensations of hunger, thirst, feeling of well-being, and others, are, however, consciously perceived but will not be considered in this connection. The pathways for sensory impulses passing to the cerebellum are also omitted (cf. Chapter 5 as concerns these). The muscle spindles and tendon organs, belonging to the proprioceptors, are treated in connection with the peripheral motor neurons in Chapter 3.

Our knowledge of the pathways followed by impulses aroused by the stimulation of the different types of receptors has not been obtained solely by anatomical investigations. Only through a combination of anatomical investigations with clinical observations and animal experiments has it been possible to approach the solution of the many problems in the mechanisms of the sensory apparatus. Even if considerable advances have been made, there are still many open questions.

The receptors.   Different types of sensory receptors have long been known to exist, in the skin as well as in the deeper structures, and their functional significance has been inferred partly from purely morphological data, partly also from physiological investigations. Starting with the formulation by Johannes Müller in 1840 of his "law of specific irritability," the opinion was held by many that receptors of different types give rise to sensations peculiar to each of them, regardless of the sort of stimulus applied to them. Furthermore, it was generally accepted that each type of receptor is specifically adapted to react to a definite kind of stimulus, which represents, physiologically speaking, the "normal" stimulus for that type of receptor. In other words, its threshold is low for the appropriate sort of stimuli, high for other types. Recent research shows that these conceptions are in need of some revision (see Davies, 1961; Melzack and Wall, 1962; Calne and Pallis, 1966), as will be clear from other data to follow.

[1] A special category of proprioceptive impulses, namely those originating in the vestibular part of the inner ear, is discussed in the chapters on the cerebellum and on the VIIIth cranial nerve.

The Somatic Afferent Pathways

One of the problems in the study of *cutaneous sensation,* as well as of sensation as a whole, has been to elucidate correlations between the different structural types of receptors and the various kinds of sensations which are perceived. When attempting to analyze this correlation, several difficulties are met with. These are partly purely technical, but other circumstances have frequently caused confusion, such as the failure to realize that what is perceived by the mind in normal life is not the stimulus of a single receptor or frequently not only a single type of receptor. What the individual experiences is a complex impression resulting from a spatial and temporal summation of stimuli of different kinds. This applies especially to sensations usually described as *discriminative:* the capacity to recognize differences of the objects in contact with the skin, such as their size, form, texture, surface characteristics, &c. Another source of confusion may be the choosing of less appropriate test methods.

As concerns the morphology of cutaneous receptors, some brief data will be sufficient. The receptors are commonly subdivided into *free or unencapsulated nerve endings and encapsulated endings.*[2] Free nerve endings are present nearly everywhere in the body. In the skin all over the body free nerve endings are found emerging from subepithelial nerve nets to the deeper layers of the stratum germinativum, where they terminate with arborizations between the epithelial cells (Fig. 2-1A). In the connective tissue of the subcutis and the corium many fine terminal nerve fibers are also found. The nerve fibers encircling the hair follicles are fine and form a dense network on their surface, although they are derived from myelinated fibers.

A somewhat specialized type of free endings is the so-called *disc of Merkel.* The nerve fiber, after having branched several times, ends eventually in concave, flattened, disc-like formations, each in close contact with a single enlarged epithelial cell of a special structure (Fig. 2-1B). These discs occur in man, inter alia, in the skin on the lips and external genitals, but are scarce in hairy skin.

The *encapsulated nerve endings* are enclosed within a covering of connective tissue. Most elaborate are the *Pacinian corpuscles* (Fig. 2-1C). They may attain a size of 1 to 4 mm in length and may thus be visible to the naked eye as white, egg-shaped bodies. They are covered by a capsule of connective tissue rich in fibrils, arranged in concentric lamellae. This encloses a protoplasmic bulb, consisting of a large number of cyto-

[2] For accounts of morphological and functional aspects of cutaneous receptors see the Ciba Foundation Symposium: "Touch, Heat, and Pain," 1966, and the Brown University Symposium: "Cutaneous Innervation," 1960. An extensive account of all aspects of cutaneous sensation can be found in the monograph by Sinclair (1967).

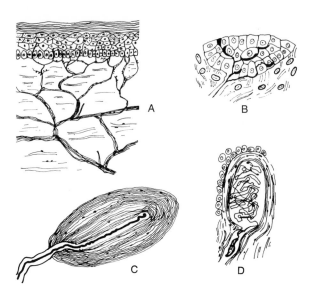

FIG. 2–1 Drawings of different types of sensory endings. *A:* free nerve endings in the skin; *B:* Merkel's disc; *C:* Pacinian corpuscle; *D:* Meissner's encapsulated ending. The nerve fibers are visible. (Cf. text.)

plasmic lamellae, separated by fluid spaces. In the center is a single terminal nerve fiber, running through the corpuscle. This nerve fiber belongs to those of large caliber, and loses its myelin sheath when entering the corpuscle. In the skin the Pacinian corpuscles are found in the subcutaneous layer, especially abundant on the tips of the fingers and toes, the palms, and soles. (Corpuscles of the Pacinian type are also found in ligaments, periosteum, and in the peritoneum, mesenteries, pancreas, and other viscera.)

Between this elaborate type of encapsulated nerve ending and the free nerve endings several transitional types exist, making any classification arbitrary. Fairly characteristic are the *corpuscles of Meissner,* found in the dermal papillae (Fig. 2-1D). They are elongated or ovoid, with their longitudinal axis perpendicular to the surface. Structurally they possess a thin connective tissue sheath, and flattened cells of an epitheloid type are found in the interior, subdividing it into transversely arranged, incompletely separated small chambers. Between these cells the entering nerve fibers wind, forming a network. There may be 2 to 6 fibers derived from axons of the thick myelinated type. Meissner corpuscles are especially numerous on the hairless volar surface of the fingers, toes, hands, and feet.

Several other types of receptors have been described, particularly in various animals. Among those said to occur in man are the corpuscles or bulbs of Krause, and the corpuscles of Ruffini and Golgi-Mazzoni. These organs were described by the older anatomists as having a rudimentary capsule. Most authors no longer consider these corpuscles as specific types of receptors, since there appear to be all kinds of transitions from encapsulated to free sensory endings.

The morphological diversity of the nerve endings has naturally made it seem reasonable to allot to each of them a special function. The well-known fact that cutaneous sensibility is punctuate in nature makes it a likely assumption that the position of the various types of end organs is the factor determining the place and number of cold, warm, touch, and pain spots, the four sensory modalities regarded by most investigators as being the primary qualities of cutaneous sensibility.

Following a study by Woollard (1935) continued investigations by Woollard and Weddell appeared to support this conception. These investigations were performed on normal individuals and on patients with nerve lesions, as well as on animals. After mapping out and marking cold spots, touch spots, etc., the corresponding areas were subsequently studied with regard to the presence of nerve fibers and endings, especially with the use of intravital methylene-blue staining. It was found that *each physiologically determined spot usually includes more than one terminal corpuscle.* Thus the touch spots contain two or three Meissner corpuscles in the dermal papillae. On the finger pads they are most densely placed, approximately ten groups per mm². (Weddell, 1941a). Furthermore the fibers covering the hair follicles are important touch receptors in the hairy parts of the skin. In the ear of the rabbit a single nerve fiber was seen to supply some 300 hairs (Weddell, 1941b). The receptors for warmth were assumed to be end bulbs resembling the Ruffini type, usually situated deep in the corium. The receptors for cold were thought to be the Krause endings. However, continued studies have made it necessary to modify this conception. Thus in regions of the body, e.g. the ear, which are sensitive to touch, cold, warmth, and pain, only two types of nerve endings occur, namely fibers ending freely and nerve fibers encircling the hairs (Sinclair, Weddell, and Zander, 1952; Hagen, Knoche, Sinclair, and Weddell, 1953). The lack of organized endings in such regions thus makes it clear that, for example, the end bulbs of Krause and Ruffini are not essential for the recognition of cold and warmth, respectively.

It appears from recent observations that conditions are far more complex than previously assumed. In the following the cutaneous receptors, the joint receptors, and the receptors for vibratory sensibility will be considered. The cutaneous receptors are generally subdivided into *mechanoreceptors, thermoreceptors,* and *pain receptors* or *nociceptors.*

Mechanoreceptors are characterized functionally by having low thresholds to mechanical stimulation of the skin. There are different kinds of mechanoreceptors. The fibers coming from the nerve plexuses surrounding the hairs respond to slight movements of a hair and adapt rapidly (see Iggo, 1966). The potentials lead off from an afferent fiber stop when the movement of the hair ceases. The receptive field, i.e. the skin area from which the fiber can be excited, is smallest on the distal parts of the body, for example the dorsum of the fingers. There are also, however, slowly adapting touch receptors in the skin. By single unit recordings some receptors (type I) have been found to show a persistent discharge for 5 minutes or longer if the mechanical effect on the skin is continued. These receptors appear to be Merkel's discs (Iggo, 1962a). Another type of slowly adapting receptor (type II) has a resting discharge which increases when a mechanical stimulus is applied to the skin. These receptors, which differ also in other respects from the first type, for example concerning the receptive fields, are found in the dermis, but their histological identification is not certain. They may be Meissner's corpuscles, which are generally believed to be tactile receptors (see Cauna, 1954; Iggo, 1962b).[3]

Thus at least three particular types of receptors appear to be definitely concerned in responses to what are usually called tactile stimuli. There is, however, reason to believe that free nerve endings may also be involved. Thus the cornea contains only free nerve endings, although it responds to tactile stimuli as well as to pain (Lele and Weddell, 1956). Furthermore, the response of tactile receptors may be influenced by changes in temperature, and receptor units have been observed which respond to temperature as well as mechanical stimuli (see Iggo, 1962b).

Particular *thermoreceptors* have so far not been identified structurally. Sensations of warmth and cold are not related to the absolute temperature of the skin as everybody knows from personal experience (e.g. lukewarm water may feel cold or warm according to the temperature of the hand when it is put into the water). The sensations of warmth and cold appear to depend on the transfer of heat to and from the skin, respectively (Lele, Weddell, and Williams, 1954). This is in agreement with the results of recent neurophysiological studies. Thus single afferent fibers have been found which respond to local application of either cold or warmth stimuli. These units often show a spontaneous discharge, which in the case of a "cold" fiber increases when the skin temperature is lowered, and ceases when the temperature is raised. The "warmth" fibers behave in the opposite way. The adequate stimulus thus is a *change* in temperature, not the absolute temperature. The temperature range for

[3] An interesting observation has been made in human studies (Hensel and Boman, 1960): the mechanical stimulus for a threshold stimulation which is conciously perceived is of the same order as that required for setting up a single impulse in a single fiber.

maximum discharge is between 38 and 43°C for the "warmth" fibers, between 16 and 27° for the "cold" fibers (Hensel, Iggo, and Witt, 1960; and others). A change of skin temperature of about 0.2°C is sufficient to cause a considerable change in the discharge of "cold" or "warmth" fibers. This corresponds with the thresholds of temperature sense in man, an observation of some interest since most studies on the temperature receptor units have been made in experimental animals. On recording from single fibers in the superficial branch of the radial nerve in man, "cold" fibers have been identified which behave as those studied in animals (Hensel and Boman, 1960).

The problems related to *pain receptors* and the perception of pain have attracted much interest, presumably on account of their clinical importance. Several difficulties arise in studies of this subject, particularly that of producing painful stimuli without concomitant excitation of receptors for other stimuli. In spite of much work and much speculation little is definitely known as yet. (For an historical account of changing views, see Keele, 1957.) It appears to be generally accepted that the pain receptors are fine, freely ending fibers in the skin and other organs. Some support for the idea that sensations of pain are mediated by thin nerve fibers is gained from studies of blocking of transmission in nerves. Thus the well-known fact that local application of cocaine blocks the transmission of pain impulses, before those of tactile sensation, has been interpreted as being due to a greater susceptibility of the thin fibers to this drug. On the other hand, mechanical compression and ischemia cause the tactile sensibility to disappear long before pain. In this instance the thicker fibers are supposed to suffer first. However, as pointed out by Melzack and Wall (1962), partial nerve block produces many changes in addition to the elimination of fibers of particular diameters (see also Glasgow and Sinclair, 1962). Subjectively there are many varieties of pain, a further indication of the complexities involved. However, it is generally agreed that as concerns pain from the skin a distinction can be made between two types. One type is aroused by superficial penetration with a fine sharp needle, is abrupt in onset, hurts little, may be accurately localized, and disappears when the stimulus ceases. The other is felt when the needle is pressed deeper into the skin, is perceived after a short latent period, is more intense and diffuse, and has a tendency to outlast the stimulus. Both types of pain, often referred to as "pricking" and "stinging," "fast" and "slow" or "first" and "second" pain, respectively, can be elicited from most parts of the body. There appears to be general agreement that sensations of pain may be mediated by two groups of fibers, thin myelinated ones (group A δ fibers) with a diameter of $8-11\mu$ and unmyelinated (C) fibers with diameters of $3-5,5\mu$ (see Zotterman, 1959). It is likewise held that the former, on account of their larger diameter, mediate the sensation of "fast" pain, the latter of "slow" pain. For a recent study on "slow" pain, see Sinclair and Stokes (1964).

However, there is little doubt that many C fibers are activated by other kinds of stimuli than painful ones, and correspondingly the A group is not related to pain only. As everyone knows from personal experience pain may be aroused by many kinds of stimuli to the skin: mechanical, thermal, or chemical. Most pain-producing stimuli appear to cause some tissue destruction. It is not known whether there is a common factor involved under all these circumstances, but from attempts to produce pain by application of various substances there appears to be some evidence that liberation of plasma kinins may be involved (see Keele, 1966). The *sensation of itching* is believed by several authors to be mediated by the "pain fibers" of the C group, because among other reasons, in clinical cases it is often seen that loss of touch sensibility does not prevent itching, but in an area insensitive to pain, itching does not occur (see Arthur and Shelley, 1959; Rothman, 1960). There appear to be itch spots as well as touch and temperature spots. While injection of histamine in the skin is known to produce itching, liberation of histamine does not appear to be the essential factor in the producton of itch (see Arthur and Shelley, 1959).

The *Pacinian corpuscles,* referred to above, are found in the subcutaneous tissue, as well as in many other places. In some respects they may therefore be grouped with cutaneous receptors. Since they are supplied by a single nerve fiber and, furthermore, can be readily identified on account of their size, they have proved useful for studies of certain general features of the function of receptors, especially because they may be isolated with their nerve fiber and examined *in vitro*. While these corpuscles have in the course of time been assumed to be receptors for a variety of stimuli, it appears now to be established that they essentially record *vibration*. When a steady pressure is applied to a Pacinian corpuscle it responds with a rapidly adapting discharge (Gray and Matthews, 1951, and others). However, when it is rhythmically stimulated with vibratory stimuli the action potentials recorded from its afferent fiber follow the frequency of the stimulus from about 50 to 800 cycles per second (Hunt, 1961). This range corresponds well with the stimulus frequencies which are consciously perceived as vibration in man. It is a further point of interest that the Pacinian corpuscles, like most receptors, show regressive changes with advancing age (Cauna and Mannen, 1958) since vibratory sensibility is likewise reduced. The afferent fibers conduct quite rapidly (in accordance with the relative thickness of the myelinated fibers supplying the corpuscles, some 9 to 16μ). The functional importance of these vibration receptors is not yet entirely clear.

In clinical neurology examinations of "vibratory sensibility" are often performed routinely by means of tuning forks, or in later years with special instruments (pallesthesiometers). The almost universal occurrence of Pacinian corpuscles explains that vibratory sensibility has been assumed to be mediated by cutaneous as well as deep receptors. In summing up available data on vibratory sensibility, Calne and Pallis (1966) in a critical review conclude that the anatomical, physiological, and clinicopathological bases for current views concerning vibratory sensibility "prove to be a tangle of truths, half-truths, and untruths."

It remains to consider *"joint sensibility."* As is well known, we are able to recognize even very small movements of joints (for example, if a joint is moved passively while the subject closes his eyes). If the joint capsules are anesthetized this is no longer possible (see Provins, 1958). As would therefore be expected, the joints are amply innervated. However, "articular neurology" has until recently attracted little interest. Most studies have been made in animals, particularly on the knee joint of the cat (Gardner, 1944, 1967; Skoglund, 1956; Freeman and Wyke, 1967; and others). A recent monograph (Poláček, 1966) gives an exhaustive account of joint innervation in man as well as in several mammals and birds.

The joints are in part supplied by separate nerve branches, in part by branches from nerves supplying adjacent muscles. Recent studies of the anatomy and physiology of the endings of these nerve fibers agree in the main points. Several morphological types of receptor endings have been found in the joint capsules and in relation to them. On account of similarities with structures found in other tissues they have often been referred to as Ruffini endings, Pacinian corpuscles, etc. However, it is advisable to avoid such analogies which may be misleading, and instead, to use neutral designations for the various types, as done by Freeman and Wyke (1967). The latter authors group the joint receptor endings in four categories. Each type appears to have its particular functional properties.

The *type I receptors* are ovoid corpuscles with a thin connective tissue capsule and are supplied by a small myelinated fiber (5 to 8μ) which arborizes within the capsule. (These endings have been likened to the Ruffini endings.) Type I receptors occur almost exclusively in the fibrous joint capsule (a few in the extrinsic ligaments) and act as slowly adapting mechanoreceptors (stretch receptors). They respond with a sustained discharge to continuous stimulation, the impulse frequency depending on the position of the joint. Each receptor is effective within a certain range of the angle of movement in the joint. The changing frequencies of the impulses from these receptors thus signal the direction of movement and also the speed, since they are sensitive to small movements (Skoglund, 1956).

Another type of receptor, called *type II,* is about twice as large as type I and is supplied by a somewhat thicker myelinated fiber (8 to 12μ) which usually ends as a single terminal within a rather thick laminated capsule. These receptors (which resemble the Pacinian corpuscles) occur only in the fibrous joint capsule and have been shown to be rapidly adapting mechanoreceptors. They are very sensitive to rapid movements in any position of the joint. They, therefore, serve as "acceleration receptors" (Skoglund, 1956).

The *receptors of type III* are the largest ones. Each is supplied by a thick myelinated fiber which branches profusely. These receptors (which resemble the Golgi organs) do not occur in the joint capsule but only in extrinsic and intrinsic ligaments. They adapt very slowly and have a high threshold. They appear to record the position of the joint.

The *type IV receptor* of Freeman and Wyke (1967) is represented by plexuses of fine unmyelinated fibers which occur in the fibrous capsule, the ligaments, the subsynovial capsule, and fat pads. These fibers are interpreted as pain receptors. In addition to these four types of afferent endings the joints receive sympathetic vasomotor fibers. These degenerate following extirpation of the appropriate sympathetic ganglia (Samuel, 1952).

It appears from these recent studies that the joints are supplied with several receptors, each of which plays a particular role in informing the central nervous system about the position and movements of any joint at any moment. This information is carried to the cerebral cortex, presumably chiefly via the dorsal column—medial lemniscus. However, information from the joints is also of importance in the regulation of motor impulses to the muscles, where it must co-operate with afferent impulses from muscle spindles and tendon organs (see Ch. 3). Most studies of the innervation of joints have been performed in experimental animals, relatively few in man. Even if there may be differences between joints and between species (see Poláček, 1966) there are, however, reasons to assume that conditions are essentially the same in man as in the cat.

The preceding simplified account of receptors which respond to various kinds of stimuli to skin, joint, and deeper tissues (Pacinian corpuscles) makes it clear that only to a certain extent are we justified in allotting a particular morphological type of receptor to a particular type of stimulus. However, to maintain, as has been done by Weddell and others, that there is no specificity among the receptors, and that sensory perception depends only on spatial and temporal patterns of nerve impulses, is obviously to go too far, as pointed out by Melzack and Wall (1962) among others, although such factors are certainly of great importance in the coding of information. The latter authors rightly emphasize the confusion which has arisen in premature attempts to correlate anatomical, physiological, and psychological observations. Furthermore, it is often overlooked that the selection of sensory "modalities" to be studied is to a large extent arbitrary. As Calne and Pallis (1966, p. 737) phrase it: "Though many sensations may readily be placed into broad categories labelled touch, pain, warmth, and cold, the vocabulary of even the most articulate is clearly inadequate to describe the innumerable gradations of sensation which fail to fall into these convenient but quite arbitrary taxonomical pigeon-holes."

The Somatic Afferent Pathways

In spite of many morphological and functional differences between the receptors considered in this chapter, it does appear quite likely that they have certain basic characteristics in common, for example with regard to the elements which are involved in the transfer of energy from the non-nervous to the nervous elements. Particular attention has been directed to the membranes at these sites. (For some data on these subjects see the Ciba Symposium on "Touch, Heat and Pain," 1966.)

Much still remains to be done before we will understand how the many more or less specific receptors provide us with that precise information, both with regard to the qualities of stimuli and their spatial localization, which enables us to be aware of even subtle changes in the environment and in our body. The problems concerned in the central transmission of this information to the "highest levels" are no less complex.

Reference should be made here to a theory which has been much debated, namely *Head's theory of protopathic and epicritic sensibility*. Experiments in nerve division which were performed by Head and Rivers on themselves formed the basis for the theory. Following the division of a cutaneous nerve of the forearm they found an area of completely abolished superficial sensibility, surrounded by a narrower zone, where pain sensibility was preserved and extreme grades of temperature were recognized, whereas touch, discrimination, and the perception of slighter differences of temperature were abolished (the intermediate zone). Furthermore, the pain elicited from this zone was abnormally intense, irradiating, and could not be accurately localized. In order to explain this a dual innervation was postulated, consisting of a *protopathic* system of primitive character, subserving pain and extreme temperature differences, yielding ungraded, diffuse impressions of an all or none type, and an *epicritic* system concerned in the mediation of smaller temperature changes, touch, and especially discrimination of all types. The epicritic system was believed to be a phylogenetically younger acquisition. The intermediate zone, as well as some phenomena observed during nerve regeneration, was assumed to be due to a wider distribution of the protopathic system fibers in the peripheral nerves.

The fact that an intermediate zone is regularly found between the normal parts of the skin and the totally anesthetic area is agreed upon by all observers. This has been emphasized, for example, by Wollard, Weddell, and Harpman (1940), who in the forearm of human beings, by anesthetizing the lateral and medial cutaneous nerves on successive days, found that the adjacent margins for anesthesia to touch of the two nerves coincided, whereas the area anesthetic to pain was approximately 1cm smaller for each nerve at the border of contact, owing to overlap in the distribution of pain fibers. However, Head's and Rivers's opinion that tactile sensibility is entirely lacking in this zone has not been uniformly verified by other investigators. For example, Trotter and Davies (1909) concluded

4 1

from similar experiments to those performed by Head and Rivers that the intermediate zone was not anesthetic to touch, but only hypoesthetic, the hypoesthesia increasing gradually when passing from the normal skin to the anesthetic area. Likewise they maintained that the changes in pain and temperature perception in the intermediate zone may be explained as due to a hypoesthesia to these qualities, and the same applies to two-point discrimination. They found it unnecessary to resort to Head's hypothesis to explain these phenomena as well as those observed during regeneration.

In a critical review Walshe (1942a) analyzed the implications of Head's theory, and pointed to the many difficulties which oppose its acceptance. However, in spite of much evidence against the theory, it still seems to have its proponents.

The afferent sensory fibers. The impulses from the receptors travel centrally through the afferent sensory fibers, having their perikarya in the spinal ganglia. The fibers found in the peripheral nerves are of varying caliber, ranging from very fine unmyelinated to thick fibers.[4] The larger afferent fibers belong to the large spinal ganglion cells, the finest unmyelinated to the smallest. In general, pure cutaneous nerves and branches are richer in fine unmyelinated fibers than are the motor or mixed nerve trunks. For example, in the deep branch of the ulnar nerve in man the proportion of unmyelinated to myelinated fibers is $0.69:1$, whereas the corresponding proportion in the superficial branch is $2.12:1$ (Ranson, Droegemueller, Davenport, and Fisher, 1935). The fibers supplying the Pacinian corpuscles, some of the joint receptors as well as the Meissner corpuscles, the muscle spindles, and tendon organs are relatively thick and myelinated, whereas the fibers in the epidermis and subepidermal layer of the dermis are mostly very fine, in keeping with the fiber distribution in the deep and superficial nerves. It has been advocated that fibers of particular sizes are related to the various kinds of receptors. This question has been tackled chiefly by recording the potentials set up in nerve fibers following stimulation of different types, since the velocity with which an impulse is conducted in a nerve fiber is related to the diameter of the fiber; the thicker the fiber the faster the conduction velocity (see Gasser, 1935). In large myelinated fibers the impulses are propagated with a speed of some 75 to 100m per second; in the finest unmyelinated fibers the velocity is only 1.5–0.3 meters per second.[5] From

---

[4] In all peripheral nerves, fibers of sympathetic origin are also present, and in mixed and motor nerves motor fibers are found in addition.

[5] According to their conduction velocity the nerve fibers are subdivided into three groups A, B, and C. The myelinated A fibers fall into four groups, partly overlapping, α, β, γ and δ with decreasing conduction velocities and diameters. The B group covers myelinated efferent autonomic fibers, the C group unmyelinated fibers. In myelinated fibers the conduction velocity as measured in meters per

a number of such studies it appears that there is no clear correlation between fiber size and sensory modalities perceived (see Melzack and Wall, 1962; Iggo, 1966). Thus the responses not only to painful but to tactile and temperature stimuli as well appear to be transmitted centrally by fibers of different diameters. Furthermore, potentials have been recorded from single fibers in response to stimuli of different kinds. Since there are differences among animal species with regard to receptors and their afferent nerves and variations between bodily regions, general conclusions are difficult. It appears, however, that certain types of receptors which can be fairly well defined, for example the Pacinian corpuscles and the joint receptors, have fibers within a relatively limited range of the fiber spectrum.

The dorsal roots. The somatic afferent fibers, discussed above, which convey impulses from skin, muscles, tendons, etc., enter the spinal cord in the dorsal or posterior roots and have their pseudo-unipolar perikarya in the spinal ganglia. The corresponding fibers from the face pass through the trigeminal nerve and have their cell bodies in the semilunar ganglion (cf. Ch. 7). The fibers composing the dorsal roots are of a highly variable thickness, ranging from heavy fibers with a thick myelin sheath, up to 20μ in diameter, to very fine, unmyelinated fibers of a diameter even less than 2μ. The total number of fibers in each dorsal root is considerably larger than that in the corresponding ventral root. (For data on the fiber spectra in the various dorsal roots of man see Rexed, 1944). It appears that fibers coming from different regions of the territory supplied by one dorsal root (a dermatome, see below) are not systematically arranged within the root. However, microelectrode recordings indicate that fibers which converge on a particular cell in the gray matter are grouped together in "microbundles" (Wall, 1960).

The fibers in the dorsal roots enter the spinal cord in the dorsolateral sulcus as a series of slender bundles. It is customary to distinguish here between two groups of fibers. Those in the smaller *lateral group* are of the thin type, mainly unmyelinated..Shortly after their entrance into the spinal cord, they dichotomize into an ascending and a descending branch, both equipped with collaterals distributed in a ventral direction and reaching the gray matter of the dorsal or posterior horn into which both branches also soon terminate. The ascending and descending branches do not extend for more than one or two segments of the spinal cord. Some of the thinnest are contained in a distinct, easily recognizable area, the

---

second is approximately the figure obtained when the diameter of the fiber is multiplied by 6 (Hursh, 1939). However, there appear to be some species and other differences (see McLeod and Wray, 1967, for some data and references).

zona terminalis, the *tract of Lissauer,* or dorsolateral fasciculus (Fig. 2–7).

The fibers composing the *medial group* are larger and thicker, and most of them are myelinated. They enter the white matter closely medial to the dorsal horn and, like the fibers in the lateral group, they dichotomize in the medullary substance into an ascending and a descending branch.[6] Some of the ascending fibers are very long and can be followed in the cranial direction to the caudal part of the medulla oblongata, where they terminate in the nuclei of the posterior funiculi, *nucleus gracilis,* and *nucleus cuneatus.* These fibers give off only scanty collaterals during their course, predominantly near their origin. Other fibers in the medial group have only short ascending and descending branches, richly endowed with collaterals. These enter the gray matter of the dorsal horn, ultimately establishing synaptic contact with nerve cells in its different groups.

Some features of the organization of the spinal cord. Termination of dorsal root fibers.   The structure of the gray matter of the cord as seen in transverse sections is not identical all over. Various cell groups stand out fairly distinctly; for example, groups of multipolar cells in the ventral horn and (in segments Th_1–L_2) the column of Clarke at the medial aspect of the dorsal horn (Figs. 2-7 and 3-1), while other groups are less clearly outlined. By making use of thick Nissl-stained sections Rexed (1952, 1954) has shown that on the basis of its cytoarchitecture the gray matter of the spinal cord of the cat can be subdivided into ten, largely horizontal, zones or laminae (Fig. 2-2). Most of these are present throughout the cord, although with minor variations between levels. In fiber-stained preparations most of the zones likewise have their characteristic features (see Nyberg-Hansen and Brodal, 1963, for some data). The assumption that the zonal subdivision of the spinal gray matter reflects functional properties is borne out by a number of data, physiological as well as anatomical. For example, the fiber systems descending to the cord from the cerebral cortex and nuclei in the brain stem end preferentially in particular zones (see Ch. 4). Other data will be mentioned later in this and other chapters. Apart from bearing witness to a detailed functional and structural differentiation in the gray matter, Rexed's (1952, 1954) studies have provided us with an exact and much needed reference map which permits precise statements as to points studied, anatomically and physiologically, in the spinal gray matter.[7]

[6] The fundamental discovery that dorsal root fibers dichotomize in an ascending and a descending branch was first made by the Norwegian explorer Fridtjof Nansen (1886) in myxine (hagfish).

[7] A corresponding map for man has not yet been made. It appears likely that the principal organization will turn out to be as in the cat.

The Somatic Afferent Pathways

From a functional point of view the neurons of the gray matter may be subdivided into three kinds. One kind, found in lamina IX (see Fig. 2-2) and the intermediolateral cell column (see Fig. 3-1 and 11-1), sends axons out of the cord into the ventral roots. Another type of cells gives off long ascending axons to supraspinal levels. A third kind consists of cells whose axons remain in the cord. These cells may be referred to as *internuncial* or *association cells*. They are extremely numerous and presumably by far outnumber those of the two other types. In the ventral horn as a whole there appear to be (in the cat) at least seven interneurons to one motoneuron (Aitken and Bridger, 1961). The topography of the internuncial cells has not yet been worked out in detail. (Some features of functional interest will be described in Ch. 3.) However, the great number of internuncial cells provides convincing evidence of a complex organization of impulse pathways in the gray matter of the cord, as does the fact that dendrites of nerve cells in the cord may extend for considerable distances from the perikaryon (Aitken and Bridger, 1961; Sprague and Ha, 1964; Szentágothai, 1967; Testa, 1964; Scheibel and Scheibel, 1966a; and others). This and other data argue against correlating the various laminae too specifically with particular functions.

Many axons of internuncial cells remain in their own segment of the cord, and are concerned in the transmission of incoming impulses to cells of the other two types at the same level. It is important to realize, however, that many cells give off collaterals which extend up or down for several segments (see Ch. 3) and thus establish an extensive network of interconnections between neighboring segments and provide possibilities for interaction between these. Some of these axons of internuncial cells course within the gray matter. Others, however, enter the white matter,

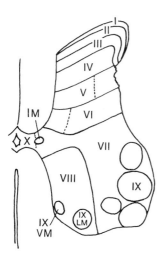

FIG. 2–2 Diagram of a transverse section through the 6th cervical segment of the spinal cord of the cat illustrating the cytoarchitectonic subdivision of the gray matter into approximately horizontally arranged laminae (I to X) according to Rexed (1954). *LM* and *VM:* lateromedial and ventromedial groups of motoneurons.

45

descend or ascend in this for various distances and then enter the gray matter again. Most of these intersegmental fibers are found close to the gray matter, where they make up the massive *fasciculi proprii* (sometimes called propriospinal fibers) (see Fig. 2-8). An impression of their abundance is obtained when in an experimental animal a couple of seg· ments of the cord are isolated by transverse lesions above and below the segments, and the corresponding dorsal roots are cut. After some time the dorsal root fibers and the ascending and descending long fibers passing through the segments will then have degenerated, and the remaining fibers should all represent segmental interconnections. Such fibers occur in all three funiculi of the cord (see Tower, Bodian, and Howe, 1941; Anderson, 1963). It should be especially noted that the tract of Lissauer, or dorsolateral fasciculus, situated peripherally to the dorsal horn and lateral to the entering dorsal root fibers (Fig. 2-7), contains a large number of thin fibers which are intrinsic, i.e. they originate in the gray matter of the cord and re-enter this after having coursed in the tract for one or two segments. In the cat some 75 per cent of all fibers of Lissauer's tract are of this type (Earle, 1952; see also Szentágothai, 1964a). An exhaustive review of the fasciculi proprii in man has been given by Nathan and Smith (1959).

In addition to connections between neighboring segments, axons of cells on one side cross the midline, making possible a co-operation between the right and left halves of the cord. Axons of such cells, which are particularly abundant in lamina VIII, pass in the ventral and dorsal commissures.

As mentioned above some dorsal root fibers turn cranially on entering the cord and ascend in the dorsal columns. These can be followed quite easily as a separate fiber system (see below). The distribution of the other, larger, contingent of root fibers which enters the gray matter directly has been studied in Golgi preparations and experimentally with the Marchi and silver impregnation methods. Particularly the latter studies have given valuable information. Unfortunately, it is not possible to decide by anatomical methods whether fibers coming from different kinds of receptors, such as muscle spindles or Pacinian corpuscles, have different sites of termination, since these contingents cannot be transected separately in the dorsal roots, and transection of peripheral branches of the nerves does not result in changes in the fibers central to the ganglion which can be detected with our present methods. Nevertheless, the sites of termination give valuable clues, particularly when considered in relation to physiological observations.

As seen in Fig. 2-3 some dorsal root fibers pass through the gray matter and end on the large ventral motor horn cells in lamina IX. In silver

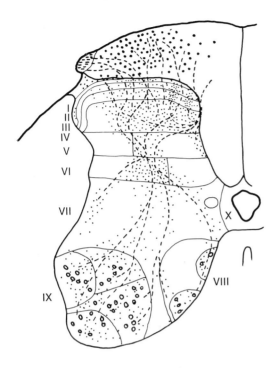

FIG. 2–3 Drawing from the 6th lumbar segment in the spinal cord of the cat to show the sites of termination of degenerating fibers 5 days following transection of the ipsilateral root of L_6 as seen in Nauta preparations. Degenerating fibers in the dorsal column are indicated by coarse dots, those in the tract of Lissauer by inter-mediate-sized dots. Small dots indicate sites of termination. Fibers of passage are shown as dashed lines. The laminae of Rexed are indicated. (Cf. text.) From Sprague and Ha (1964).

impregnation studies contacts have been seen on the somata as well as on proximal dendrites, confirming Cajal's classical Golgi observations, as will be further discussed in Chapter 3. Collaterals of dorsal root fibers have further been found to contact cells of the column of Clarke (Szentágothai and Albert, 1955; Liu, 1956; Grant and Rexed, 1958; and others). Other root fibers and collaterals end in the dorsal horn and the "intermediate zone." According to Sprague (1958) and Sprague and Ha (1964) in the lumbar cord there are terminations in all laminae (Fig. 2-3), but especially in laminae IV and VI, in the latter mainly centrally. In the brachial cord Sterling and Kuypers (1967a) have made largely corresponding findings, but stress the scarcity of endings in the lateral parts of laminae V and VI. The terminal branches show a tendency to run in the same direction as the dendrites of the cells in the particular

4 7

laminae.* Sensory afferents appear to a large extent to end on internuncial cells, as well as on cells giving rise to ascending fibers (see below). However, following dorsal root section very little or no degeneration has been found in the substantia gelatinosa, Rexed's lamina II (apart from degenerating fibers passing through it to deeper layers of the gray). This intriguing observation may find a reasonable explanation in the light of some recent studies: the substantia gelatinosa appears to play a special role in the processing of sensory information, and is not, as formerly believed, the site of the first synapse in the "pain pathway."

In the course of time different opinions have been held on the substantia gelatinosa. According to the recent Golgi and experimental studies of Szentágothai (1964a) and the experimental (silver impregnation and electron microscopic) investigations of Ralston (1965; see also Pearson, 1952) the main features in the organization of the substantia gelatinosa may be summarized as follows: the small cells of the substantia gelatinosa give off fine, largely unmyelinated, axons which either ascend or descend for a short distance (a couple of segments) within lamina II itself or return to it after having passed for a short distance in the lateral part of the zona terminalis (see above). The scanty marginal cells (Rexed's lamina I) and cells in lamina III and IV, which receive collaterals of primary sensory fibers, send axons back to the substantia gelatinosa and may influence it. Apparently, this part of the gray matter cannot act on other regions by way of axons of its own cells. However, the substantia gelatinosa contains a rich plexus of dorsally directed and profusely branching dendrites of cells in deeper layers (chiefly III and IV), oriented radially (Pearson, 1952; and others) and densely beset with terminal boutons (Ralston, 1965). The latter apparently belong to the fine axons of cells in the substantia gelatinosa (Szentágothai, 1964a). In this way the substantia gelatinosa may influence cells in deeper layers by acting on their dendrites. The cells in the deeper layers in addition to primary sensory fibers receive fibers descending in the spinal cord (thus corticospinal fibers from the primary sensory cortex end in lamina IV; see Nyberg-Hansen and Brodal, 1963). It therefore seems plausible that "the substantia gelatinosa might be considered as a system controlling or modulating synaptic transmission from primary sensory neurons to secondary systems on one hand and from supraspinal systems on spinal ones on the other" (Szentágothai, 1964a, p. 230). A new theory on the functional organization of the substantia gelatinosa has been proposed by Melzack and Wall (1965). Note (added in proof): Ample terminations of primary afferents have recently been demonstrated (Heimer and Wall, 1968).

As referred to above, recent physiological studies have produced evidence for the view that there are functional differences between the laminae in the dorsal horn. Wall (1967) studied units in laminae IV to VI following application of cutaneous and joint stimuli and found that units in all three laminae respond to cutaneous stimuli, but only those in

* A detailed Golgi study of the orientation and distribution of dorsal root afferents and of dendritic fields in the gray matter of the cord has recently been published by Scheibel and Scheibel (1968).

lamina VI are sensitive to movements. This is in agreement with the observations of some previous students (see Wall, 1967, for references) that cutaneous afferents are distributed more dorsally in the dorsal horn than proprioceptive ones. Furthermore, there appears to be a medio-laterally arranged somatotopic pattern within lamina IV, but the cells, which have small receptive fields, respond to different cutaneous stimuli, such as hair movement, touch, and cooling of the skin. It was concluded that the cells in lamina V were activated mainly via axons of cells in lamina IV. These findings thus agree with the anatomical data, as do also some other physiological studies (see Sprague and Ha, 1964, for some data and references). It appears, however, that the situation is rather complex, and that no lamina can be related to a particular sensory "modality."

The segmental sensory innervation. The dermatomes. Before following the pathways for impulses entering in the dorsal roots in their further routes within the central nervous system, a particular aspect of the peripheral distribution of the sensory fibers will be dealt with. In the peripheral distribution the originally segmental origin of the body is revealed, in the same manner as for the fibers of the ventral roots (see Ch. 3). Each dorsal root is composed of sensory fibers from those regions of the skin, muscles, connective tissue in ligaments, fascia, tendons, and joints, from bones, and also viscera which are developed from the same body segment (somite) as the corresponding segment of the spinal cord. (It should be noted that, strictly speaking, segments cannot be distinguished within the spinal cord. A spinal cord segment is by definition that part of the cord which gives rise to those root fibers which unite to form a pair of spinal nerves.) The main features of the segmental innervation have been made clear by careful dissection, in following the fibers from the roots in their course in the plexuses and further in the peripheral nerves (Bolk and others). This is most easily performed in the case of the cutaneous fibers. *The segmental innervation of the skin, the dermatomes,* may, however, be studied more exactly by other methods. For example, a continuous number of dorsal roots may be cut, leaving intact only a single root in the midst of the area. The peripheral distribution of fibers from this root will then be apparent as a zone of retained sensibility within a larger anesthetic area. By this "method of remaining sensibility" Sherrington proved experimentally in monkeys that neighboring dermatomes overlap to a greater or lesser extent. This method has been applied also in man, most extensively by Foerster in cases where several dorsal roots have had to be sectioned on account of pain, for example, from neuromas following amputations. A third method, introduced by Dusser de Barenne, utilizes local application of strychnine to

4 9

one or more dorsal roots, resulting in a hypersensitivity in the area of distribution. The distribution of the herpetic vesicles in cases of herpes zoster and the sensory disturbances in clinical cases with lesions of the dorsal roots or of the spinal cord have also given valuable information for the study of the distribution of the dermatomes. Finally, the distribution of the vasodilatation following irritation of the dorsal roots may be utilized (antidromic impulses, cf. Ch. 11), and local anesthesia of dorsal root ganglia may be used as an experimental procedure in healthy subjects. This has been done by Keegan and Garrett (1948) whose diagrams of the dermatomes, reproduced in Figs. 2-4 and 2-5, are based on a large series of cases of dorsal root compression by herniated discs.[8]

The maps of the dermatomes in man worked out by different methods are not concordant in all respects. However, the main principles are identical. Thus there is a *considerable degree of overlapping between neighboring dermatomes* (not shown in Figs. 2-4 and 2-5). For example, the 4th thoracic dermatome is covered in its upper half by the 3rd, in its lower half by the 5th thoracic dermatome. A practical consequence of this arrangement is that even a complete lesion of a single dorsal root will, as a rule, not be followed by a sensory loss, at least not definitely. This statement, however, requires certain qualifications. Considerable individual variations exist with regard to details in the areas occupied by different dermatomes. Still more important is the fact that *the borders of the dermatomes are not exactly the same for touch as for pain and temperature. The dermatomes are somewhat more extensive in regard to touch than to pain and temperature,* i.e. the "touch" fibers belonging to a dorsal root overlap to a greater extent with those from the neighboring roots than do the fibers conveying sensations of pain and temperature. This will be seen from Fig. 2-6, showing the findings in one of Foerster's cases. Thus a careful investigation of cutaneous sensibility in cases where a single dorsal root has been interrupted will frequently reveal a limited zone of hypalgesia, or more rarely even of analgesia, whereas there may be no loss of the sense of touch. It is on this account especially important to test pain sensibility very carefully in searching for monosegmental sensory loss, e.g. in suspected cases of a herniated intervertebral disc.

[8] In contrast to the dermatome charts of many other authors, the diagrams of Keegan and Garrett show the dermatomes as continuous zones extending from the spine to the distal parts of the limbs. They show only one axial line (the line where non-neighboring dermatomes meet), the ventral one, while some authors have advocated the presence of a dorsal axial line as well. The paper of Keegan and Garrett (1948) should be consulted for particulars and for an historical account on the dermatomes.

5 0

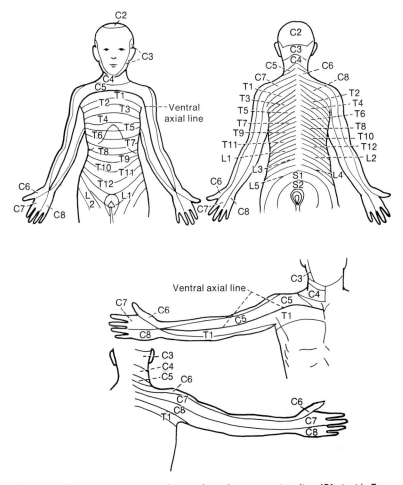

FIG. 2–4 The dermatomes on the trunk and upper extremity. (Cf. text.) From Keegan and Garrett (1948).

Where a sensory loss of the segmental, dermatomal type is encountered, it is of course of interest to determine the level of the lesion as exactly as possible, and usually one will resort to a comparison with diagrams such as those presented in Figs. 2-4 and 2-5. However, certain principal features in the dermatomal arrangement ought to be remembered, in order to enable the examiner to decide at least approximately which dorsal roots are involved in the lesion. From Figs. 2-4 and 2-5 it will be seen that, broadly speaking, the skin of the lateral (radial) side of the arm, forearm, and hand with the thumb belongs to the 5th and

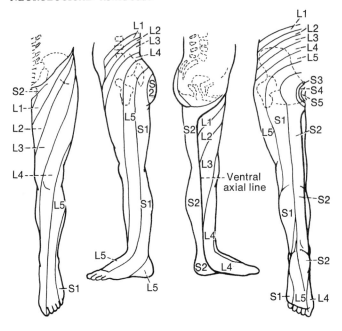

FIG. 2–5 The dermatomes on the lower extremity. From Keegan and Garrett (1948).

6th cervical dermatomes, the medial (ulnar) side to the 8th cervical-1st thoracic dermatomes. The nipple is located in the region of the 4th to 5th thoracic dermatomes, the umbilicus in the 9th to 10th. The inguinal sulcus falls within the 1st lumbar dermatome, the anterior aspect of the thigh and the knee is covered by the 3rd to 4th lumbar, whereas the heel is found in the area of the 5th lumbar and 2nd sacral dermatome, and the posterior aspect of the thigh and upper calf belongs to the 1st to 2nd sacral dermatomes. The anogenital region is supplied by fibers from the 3rd to 5th sacral roots. (For a recent clinical study on the segmental sensory innervation, see Hansen and Schliack, 1962.)

The segmental distribution discussed above refers to the exteroceptive fibers. But the visceral afferent, as well as the proprioceptive and other afferent fibers, are also segmentally distributed. There is still some uncertainty about certain details in this arrangement, but some principal features are known. Concerning the visceral afferent fibers the reader is referred to Chapter 11. With regard to *the proprioceptive fibers* some data is worth mentioning. As the afferent fibers from the muscles follow the motor fibers, the segmental distribution of muscle sensibility will not agree fully with the segmental cutaneous pattern. (The segmental motor

52

innervation of muscle is treated in Ch. 3.) With respect to the skeleton and the joints it is generally assumed that the segmental distribution is even more different from the dermatomes than is the muscular innervation. Probably the segmental areas of the skeleton of the limbs have retained more of their original pattern, partly extending as narrow longitudinal zones through the entire length of the extremity. It is probable that the deep pains, usually dull and difficult to localize, which occur in many cases of damage to the dorsal roots, may be due to irritation of the afferent fibers from the bones and joints. These pains also have a tendency to irradiate upward or downward in the limbs.

In the dorsal roots the different kinds of sensory fibers treated above are intermingled, and an interruption of a dorsal root consequently will affect all sensory modalities. Upon entering the spinal cord, however, the fibers separate, and the impulses conveyed by them take different courses. This circumstance favors the analysis of lesions of the sensory systems, facilitating as it does in many instances an exact focal diagnosis.

As referred to above, most dorsal root fibers enter the gray matter. The cells within this which give off long ascending axons transmitting impulses to the brain stem and thalamus are commonly spoken of as "secondary sensory neurons," even if presumably many of them are not secondary. The tracts into which the long ascending fibers are grouped are named according to their destination as spinocerebellar, spinoreticular, spinovestibular, spinotectal, spino-olivary, etc. Most of them will be considered in other chapters. Here we are concerned primarily with those ascending pathways which appear to be essential for the transmission of sensory impulses which reach the level of consciousness. One such pathway is the spinothalamic tract. Even more important is, however, the pathway established by the axons of *primary* sensory neurons which, as

FIG. 2–6 The 6th cervical dermatone (C_6) after resection of the dorsal roots of neighboring segments of the cord (C_4, C_5, C_7, C_8, Th_1 and Th_2). Sensibility to pain and temperature is abolished in the area limited by the broken line. In the stippled area tactile sensibility is also lacking. (Cf. text.) From Foerster (1936a).

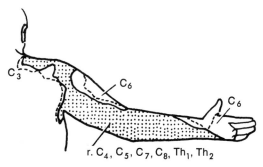

53

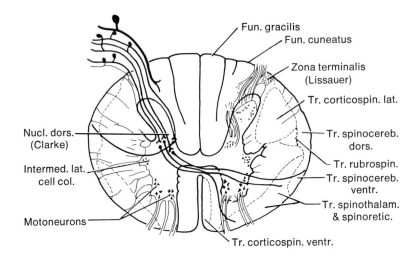

FIG. 2–7 Diagram of the spinal cord. The main ascending tracts and the course of the afferent fibers are indicated. Note that not all tracts are included and that the borders between adjacent tracts are not sharp.

mentioned previously, ascend in the dorsal funiculi. In the following discussion the latter will be considered first. Figure 2-7 is a simplified diagram showing some of the ascending spinal pathways. At the spinal level there is no clear segregation between "secondary sensory" fibers passing to different end stations, for example, the thalamus and the reticular formation.

The fibers in the dorsal funiculi and the medial lemniscus. The large myelinated dorsal root fibers, which ascend to terminate in the nuclei of the dorsal funiculi in the medulla oblongata (see Fig. 7-3), make up a considerable part of the medial group of the dorsal root fibers. At their entrance these fibers are situated immediately medial to the dorsal horn. During their ascending course, however, they are steadily pushed in a more medial direction, because the fibers entering at succeeding rostral levels intrude between the ascending fibers and the dorsal horn. As a consequence of this the fibers occupying the most medial part of the medial funiculus gracilis in the upper cervical region will belong to the sacral dorsal roots, then follow the fibers from the lumbar dorsal roots; i.e. the fibers from the lower extremity are found most medially. The fibers belonging to the upper extremity are found most laterally in the funiculus cuneatus, close to the dorsal horn; the fibers from the upper cervical roots are found more laterally than those from the lower roots. Of the thoracic fibers approximately the lower six occupy the lateral

54

part of the funiculus gracilis, the upper six the medial part of the funiculus cuneatus.[9] This arrangement is illustrated in Fig. 2-8.

The segmental disposition of the fibers of the dorsal funiculi has been established by experimental investigations and studies of human pathological cases. Even if there appears to be some degree of overlapping between fibers from adjacent roots (Walker and Weaver, 1942), *the ascending fibers of the dorsal funiculus are somatotopically organized* (Fig. 2-8), reflecting in their arrangement the original segmental pattern of the organism. *The fibers terminate in the nuclei of the dorsal funiculi, following the same principle,* as shown in the monkey (Ferraro and Barrera, 1935b; Walker and Weaver, 1942) and in the cat (Glees, Livingston, and Soler, 1951; Hand, 1966) and as confirmed in single unit recordings by Gordon and Paine (1960), Kruger, Siminoff, and Witkowsky (1961), and others.

From clinical experiences it has long been known that the *impulses ascending in the fibers of the dorsal columns mediate sensations of touch, deep pressure, vibratory sense, and sense of position of joints and are particularly important for sensory discrimination* (see below).[10] In

[9] Some of the fibers from the cervical and 4th to 5th upper thoracic roots terminate in the external cuneate nucleus, from which their impulses are conveyed to the cerebellum, as mentioned in Chapter 5.

[10] Cook and Browder (1965) report some cases of dorsal chordotomy, i.e. section of the dorsal columns, in which almost no permanent loss was found in these sensory qualities. However, they had no anatomical control of the lesions. Calne and Pallis (1966) maintain that the dorsal columns may not be the only pathway involved in the central transmission of impulses arising on response to vibratory stimuli.

FIG. 2–8 A diagram of the spinal cord showing the segmental arrangement of nerve fibers within some major tracts. On the left side are indicated the "sensory modalities" which appear to be mediated along the two main ascending pathways. Note the broad zone close to the gray matter occupied by propriospinal fibers. *C:* cervical; *L:* lumbar; *S:* sacral; *Th:* thoracic.

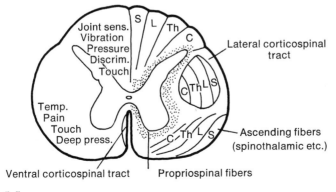

physiological experiments single unit potentials have been recorded in the dorsal column nuclei following tactile stimulation, especially movements of the hairs, stimulation of joint receptors, and sinusoidal vibrations (Kruger, Siminoff, and Witkowsky, 1961; Perl, Whitlock, and Gentry, 1962; and others). It has further been shown that the receptive area for touch, i.e. the cutaneous field which influences a single cell, varies in size in different regions of the body. The receptive field is smallest in the digits and peripheral parts of the extremities (Kruger et al., 1961; Perl et al., 1962 and others). According to Uddenberg (1968) there is (in the cat) a differential distribution within the dorsal funiculus of fibers coming from different receptors. Fibers transmitting impulses from hair receptors are found superficially, while impulses from touch and vibration receptors ascend in the deep part of the funiculi. A corresponding differential distribution is found in the dorsal column nuclei (see below).

Fibers coming from the cerebral cortex and following the pyramidal tract have been shown in experimental studies to end in the nuclei gracilis and cuneatus (Walberg, 1957a; Chambers and Liu, 1957, in the cat; Kuypers, 1958b, in the monkey and chimpanzee; Kuypers and Lawrence, 1967, in the monkey). This projection is somatotopically arranged; fibers from the forelimb area of the sensorimotor cerebral cortex end in the contralateral cuneate nucleus, those from the hindlimb area in the nucleus gracilis. The second somatosensory region likewise projects in the same manner to these nuclei (Levitt et al., 1964). These corticofugal connections to the dorsal column nuclei were assumed to be able to modify impulse transmission in the nuclei, an assumption which physiological studies (see below) have proved to be correct. The dorsal column nuclei provide a favorable situation for various experimental studies and have been quite extensively studied in recent years. Since the data obtained is of interest from a general point of view some of it will be briefly considered. (Only a limited number of the numerous papers can be quoted.)

The organization of the dorsal column nuclei has turned out to be far more complex than was generally assumed only a few years ago when it was the current belief that they were simple relay nuclei: afferents from the dorsal column establish synaptic contact with cells in the nuclei, and the cells give off their axons to the medial lemniscus. Thus to a large extent different cells in the nuclei appear to transmit impulses from particular kinds of receptors (Perl et al., 1962; Gordon and Jukes, 1964a). Most of the units activated by the afferent fibers, particularly the touch receptive ones, appear to be located chiefly at middle levels of the nuclei (Gordon and Paine, 1960; Perl et al., 1962; Andersen, Eccles, Schmidt, and Yokota, 1964b; see also Hand, 1966, for some anatomical data). It is of interest that afferent spatial, lateral, inhibition (inhibition of the "surround type," see Fig. 2-14) of cells supplied by hair receptors has been observed; i.e. a stimulus applied near to but outside the receptive field for the unit may inhibit the cell (Gordon and Paine, 1960; Perl et al., 1962; Gordon and Jukes, 1964a). In this way the spatial contrast in the incoming impulse pattern will be increased. However, afferent spatial facilitation may also occur (Gordon and Paine, 1960; Gordon and Jukes, 1964a).

A number of electrophysiological studies have demonstrated that *the sensorimotor cortex influences the transmission of impulses from the dorsal column nuclei.* This is only one of many observations (perhaps so far the most extensively studied one) which have drawn our attention to the central control exerted on receptors and sensory impulse transmission. Other examples will be mentioned later. Inhibition of the rostral transmission has been demonstrated by Magni, Melzack, Moruzzi, and Smith (1959), Towe and Jabbur (1961), and Gordon and Jukes (1964b) among others; facilitation by Towe and Jabbur (1961) and Gordon and Jukes (1964b). The effects are bilateral but chiefly contralateral, as is to be expected from the anatomical findings. Most authors agree that the inhibitory influences are mediated via the pyramidal tract fibers traced to the nuclei. According to Jabbur and Towe (1961) the facilitatory influences are likewise mediated via the pyramidal tract (while according to these authors some inhibitory influences may be relayed via the reticular formation). In a series of papers Andersen, Eccles, and collaborators have presented analyses of the synaptic mechanisms which are involved in the cortical effects.

They have found evidence that there are, in the nucleus, interneurons as well as relay neurons (Andersen, Eccles, Schmidt, and Yokota, 1964b), both of which may be influenced from the sensorimotor cortex. The inhibition produced by cortical stimulation appears to be postsynaptic by way of internuncial cells, as well as presynaptic by way of a depolarization of the terminals of the presynaptic fibers ascending from the cord (Andersen, Eccles, Schmidt, and Yokota, 1964a). Presynaptic inhibition occurs also on stimulation of sensory afferents.

The intrinsic anatomical organization of the dorsal column nuclei is not yet known in sufficient detail to permit precise correlations with all recent physiological findings. However, there are at least two types of cells in the nuclei (Cajal, 1909; Kuypers and Tuerk, 1964), differing among other things with regard to their dendritic branchings and with regard to their localization within the nuclei. The cortical afferents terminate chiefly in the ventral (deeper) parts of the nuclei, where the cells have long radiating dendrites, and electron microscopic studies (Walberg, 1966) show that they end with uniformly small boutons, largely on dendrites, while the dorsal column fibers have boutons of various sizes. The presence of axo-axonic contacts has been established in electron microscopic studies (see Walberg, 1965b, 1966).

5 7

It appears from the recent studies that the *dorsal column nuclei make possible an impulse transmission which is very specific with regard to the site of the body stimulated, presenting a very clear-cut somatotopical localization, but specific also with regard to the type of receptor involved. The activity in the nuclei is subject to control from the sensorimotor cortex.* The dorsal columns and their nuclei are thus exquisitely organized to transmit precise and detailed information from certain types of receptors to higher levels. As will be seen below, the further links of the pathway to the cortex are organized according to the same principles.

As mentioned above the axons of a great number of the cells of the nuclei gracilis and cuneatus form the *medial lemniscus* or mesial fillet ascending in the brain stem and ending in the thalamus. There is general agreement among anatomists that all fibers of the medial lemniscus cross the midline in the medulla, in man as in the monkey (Rasmussen and Peyton, 1948; Matzke, 1951; Glees, 1952; Bowsher, 1958, and others). Furthermore, the fibers do not appear to give off collaterals to the reticular formation (in contrast to the spinothalamic fibers). However, the *segmental, somatotopical organization present in the dorsal columns and their nuclei is maintained in the second link of this sensory pathway, the medial lemniscus and its terminal nucleus.* In the medulla the fibers of the medial lemniscus, after crossing, are found to occupy a triangular area dorsal to the pyramidal tract (Figs. 2-9, 7-3 and 7-6). Within this area the fibers from the gracile nucleus are situated ventrolaterally, those from the cuneate nucleus dorsomedially. Within these main subdivisions there is apparently also a finer arrangement according to the segmental pattern, as shown by the investigations of Ferraro and Barrera (1936) in the monkey and of Walker (1937) in the chimpanzee. This arrangement is also retained in the further course of the lemniscus, probably also here with a certain degree of overlapping, and the fibers from the main sensory trigeminal nucleus in the pons, which join the lemniscus, are found in the extreme dorsomedial part of its field. Conclusive evidence that the same arrangement is valid in man has apparently not been brought forward, but it appears probable that conditions are similar to those in monkeys. The segmental arrangement of the fibers of the medial lemniscus is represented diagrammatically in Fig. 2-9.

Further along the tract a certain rotation takes place, so the fibers which originally were placed ventrolaterally finally occupy the lateral position, whereas the originally dorsomedial fibers from the cuneate nucleus will be found medially. In this order the fibers enter the ventral nucleus of the thalamus, more precisely the nucleus ventralis posterior lateralis (VPL). The trigeminal fibers enter most medially, in a distinct portion of the nucleus, usually called the nucleus ventralis posterior medialis

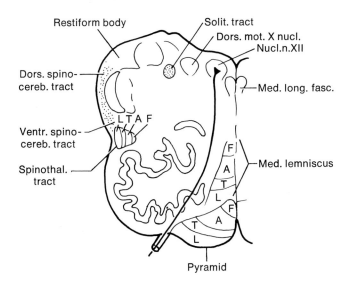

FIG. 2–9 Diagram of a section through the lower part of the medulla obiongata, indicating the somatotopical arrangement of the fibers in the medial lemniscus, the spinothalamic tract, and the corticospinal tract. *A:* arm; *F:* face; *L:* leg; *T:* trunk.

(VPM). From these thalamic regions the impulses are conveyed mainly to the somatosensory areas in the cerebral cortex. The endings of the fibers of the lemniscus and the thalamocortical projection will be described below.

The spinothalamic tract.   In addition to the dorsal column-medial lemniscus route, the spinothalamic tract represents a second pathway for sensory impulses from the body which are consciously perceived. It differs from the first system in certain respects, anatomically as well as functionally, and on the whole our knowledge of it is less.

As referred to above, a number of cells in the gray matter give off axons which ascend on both sides of the cord. Those ending in the thalamus make up the *spinothalamic tract.* (Sometimes a distinction is made between a ventral and a lateral spinothalamic tract, but this distinction is of little importance.) It should be noted that the spinothalamic tract, defined as the assembly of fibers which arise in the cord and end in the thalamus, does not occupy a well delimited region in the spinal white matter. On the contrary, *its fibers are mixed with other ascending projections from the cord* referred to above. Furthermore, some of the spinothalamic fibers give off collaterals to certain nuclear regions during their course, for example the reticular formation. These features have made it difficult to study certain aspects of the anatomy of the spinothalamic tract, for example to determine its cells of origin. It appears from Golgi studies that these are probably to be found among cells in Rexed's laminae IV to VII. Many cells here send their axons to the other side of the cord where they ascend in the ventrolateral funiculus, and it is known from the studies of the thalamic termination of the tract, that most of its fibers are crossed. However, the exact site of origin of the spinothalamic tract remains to be determined (see, however, Morin, Schwartz, and O'Leary, 1951). We do not even know if primary dorsal root afferents establish contact directly with the cells of origin of the spinothalamic fibers or whether these are acted upon via internuncial cells.

It has been known for a long time (Petrén, 1910, and others) that in man lesions of the anterolateral funiculus of the cord gave rise to loss of sensations of pain and temperature on the contralateral side of the body. Since some sensibility to touch and deep pressure remains after total interruption of the dorsal columns, it has further been concluded that the spinothalamic tract is also involved in conveying impulses perceived as touch and deep pressure. Clinical data indicates that there is an arrangement within the tract according to sensory qualities: the fibers mediating sensations of pain and temperature appear to occupy the dorsolateral part of the anterolateral funiculus, those conveying sensations of touch and deep pressure are found in the ventromedial part (see Fig. 2-8).

Physiological studies are on the whole in accord with clinical data. Thus, single units responding to touch, temperature changes, pressure, and pain-producing stimuli have been located in a lamina across the dorsal part of the dorsal horn in the cat (Wall, 1960; Wall and Cronly-Dillon, 1960). As mentioned previously these appear to be found chiefly in lamina IV (while joint movements act on cells in lamina VI; Wall, 1967). Furthermore, following transection of both medial lemnisci and one anterolateral funiculus in monkeys, leaving only one spinothalamic tract for conduction, single unit responses have been studied in the ventral posterior thalamic nucleus where the spinothalamic fibers end (see below). Units were found which were excited by displacement of hairs (touch), light mechanical distortion of the skin, distortion of muscle-fascial relations, joint rotation, pressure, heat, or stimuli of tissue damaging character (Perl and Whitlock, 1961). Usually one unit responds to only one kind of stimulus.

It appears from clinical experiences with operative section of the anterolateral funiculus that the spinothalamic fibers cross the midline shortly after their origin. Foerster (1936a) concluded that the crossing is completed in the segment above the entrance of the dorsal root fibers, since the analgesia and thermal anesthesia after the operation extend rostrally to the caudal limit of this dermatome. This view gained full support when operative section of the spinothalamic tracts for cure of otherwise intractable pain became more generally used. This operation, usually called *chordotomy,* is applied especially in cases of cancer in the pelvic organs or lower parts of the abdominal viscera. As a result of the operation the patient may be able to spend his last months of life in a tolerable condition.[11] Post-mortem findings have been reported in several cases in which the sectioned fibers have been followed by the Marchi method. From these (Foerster and Gagel, 1932; Hyndman and von Epps, 1939; Weaver and Walker, 1941; Gardener and Cuneo, 1945; and others) and from experimental studies (Morin, Schwartz, and O'Leary, 1951) it is learned that the spinothalamic tract presents a segmental lamination. The fibers crossing at a particular level are added to those coming from more caudal parts of the cord at the inner side of the tract. Thus at higher levels the longest fibers, from the sacral segments, will be found most superficially, followed inward by fibers originating at successively more rostral levels (Fig. 2-8).[12] The arrangement is not strictly a question of depth, as in addition the lowest fibers are displaced more dorsally during their upward course. Thus *the fibers in the spinothalamic tract are somatotopically arranged.* This arrangement is also of diagnostic importance, and it is of practical relevance when a chordotomy is to be performed. If the section of the anterolateral funiculus is not made sufficiently deep, the deepest, i.e. shortest, fibers will escape destruction, and the upper border of the ensuing analgesia will be found several segments below the expected level. In order to avoid failure due to a too superficial section of the tract, therefore, many neurosurgeons prefer to transect the spinothalamic tract some six segments higher than the upper border of the painful region.[13]

It appears that the somatotopical arrangement is retained during the further course of the tract in the medulla and pons, although at rostral levels the lamination has not been observed as clearly as in the spinal cord (Walker, 1940a, 1942a; Weaver, Jr. and Walker, 1941; Gardner and

[11] For surveys of the operative procedure, its indications, contra-indications, and results, see White and Sweet (1955) and Nathan (1963).

[12] It may be mentioned that fibers of the other long ascending and descending tracts in the spinal cord are organized in a similar manner, the longest fibers being situated most superficially. Besides being applicable to the fibers in the dorsal funiculi and the spinothalamic tracts, this principle is valid for the corticospinal tract, the spinocerebellar tracts, and others.

[13] The arrangement of the fibers has made it possible in some cases to produce an analgesia restricted, for example, to the chest or the upper extremity by performing a chordotomy limited to the ventral part of the anterolateral funiculus (Hyndman and von Epps, 1939; Jenkner, 1961).

Cuneo, 1945). In Fig. 2-9 the segmental arrangement in the medulla is indicated. At this level the tract occupies a rather narrow zone dorsal to the inferior olive (see also Figs. 7-3 and 7-6). Most investigators who have followed the fibers in Marchi preparations comment upon the reduction of fibers in the tract during its rostral course. Presumably this is due to the filtering off of fibers which belong to other ascending systems, and which have been cut simultaneously with the spinothalamic tract. Furthermore, the tract appears to be considerably better developed in man and chimpanzee than in the monkey and is even less massive in the cat (see Mehler, 1966a). In the cat, Marchi studies have given meager results, while silver impregnation methods have made it possible to study the tract in some detail in this animal (see below). However, in man it has been identified in Marchi preparations in the mesencephalon underneath the brachium of the inferior colliculus. Also at this level the fibers in the tract appear to be somatotopically arranged (Walker, 1942a, 1943; Morin, Schwartz, and O'Leary, 1951), at least in man and monkey, as seen in Fig. 2-10. Ventral to the spinothalamic fibers is a zone of fibers from the trigeminal nucleus, and ventral to this the medial lemniscus ascends.

From the mesencephalon the spinothalamic fibers proceed to the thalamus, where the majority end in a somatotopical manner in the nucleus ventralis posterior lateralis (VPL), in the same nucleus as the medial lemniscus fibers. The distribution is, however, not entirely restricted to this part of the thalamus, as will be discussed below. Like the medial lemniscus fibers, those of the spinothalamic tract end in a somatotopical pattern (see Fig. 2-13).

Just as the nuclei of the dorsal columns receive fibers from the cerebral cortex which may influence their activity, so *the neurons giving rise to the spinothalamic tract are subject to influences from "higher levels."* Hagbarth and Kerr (1954) demonstrated that the central transmission

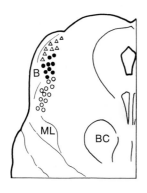

FIG. 2–10 Drawing showing the position of the spinothalamic tract and its somatotopical pattern in the mesencephalon according to Walker (1943). *Triangles:* lower extremity; *dots:* upper extremity; *circles:* face; *B:* brachium quadrigeminum inferius; *BC:* brachium conjunctivum; *ML:* medial lemniscus.

in the spinothalamic tract could be inhibited by stimulation of the sensori-motor areas of the cerebral cortex, as well as the anterior lobe of the cerebellum and the reticular formation (see also Lindblom and Ottosson, 1957). The effect was interpreted as being due to a postsynaptic action òn the second order sensory neurons. Later it was found that single units in the dorsal horn and sensory pathways responding to natural stimulation could be both inhibited and facilitated (Hagbarth and Fex, 1959). Furthermore, at least some of the supraspinal inhibition is pre-synaptic, as shown by Andersen, Eccles, and Sears (1964a) and Car-penter, Lundberg, and Norrsell (1963). In the latter case it is assumed that descending fibers influence the terminals of primary afferents (of cutaneous origin and Ib afferents from muscles) by axo-axonic synapses (see Fig. 1-5F). Such synapses have been found in the gray matter of the cord in electron microscopic studies by Gray (1963) without specifica-tion as to their precise site, and by Ralston (1965) in the substantia gelatinosa. Since the cells of origin of the spinothalamic fibers are not known, the anatomical basis for these phenomena is not clear in suf-ficient detail. However, a number of descending fiber systems from supraspinal regions end in those laminae of the cord where the neurons of the spinothalamic fibers are presumably to be found. The termination of descending fiber tracts in the cord is considered in Chapter 4. The cerebral cortex as well as other regions of the brain are obviously able to influence the central transmission of those impulses which reach the conscious level through the spinothalamic route. This mechanism may be involved in suppressing, for example, pain sensations under certain cir-cumstances, a phenomenon well known from daily life. Furthermore, it may contribute to an increase in contrast in sensory perception.

Although the nucleus had apparently been noted by some anatomists (for ex-ample, Ranson, Davenport, and Doles, 1932), it was only following the descrip-tion of Rexed and Brodal (1951) that the *lateral cervical nucleus* was recognized as a specific entity. It has since been rather extensively studied. The nucleus con-sists of a slender column of multipolar nerve cells situated in the lateral funiculus in segments C_1 and C_2, just ventrolateral to the dorsal horn. It is present in the cat and some other animals while it is either absent or present in another form in still other species. Ha and Morin (1964) claim that it is present but very small in man. The assumption that the nucleus sends its fibers to the cerebellum (Rexed and Brodal, 1951) has been disproved (Grant, Boivie, and Brodal, 1968). Lesions in the upper brain stem result in marked retrograde cell loss in the contralateral nucleus (Morin and Catalano, 1955). Its efferent fibers cross in the upper cervical region and ascend with those of the medial lemniscus (Busch, 1961). According to the physiological study of Landgren, Nordwall, and Wengström (1965) they end in a restricted part of the nucleus ventralis posterior lateralis (VPL) of the thala-mus (Bovie, personal communication). The only source of afferents to the lateral cervical nucleus which has so far been definitely established is the spinal cord.

While some afferents may be collaterals of fibers in the dorsal spinocerebellar tract (passing close to the nucleus), anatomical (Brodal and Rexed, 1953) as well as physiological studies (Lundberg and Oscarsson, 1960; Horrobin, 1966) indicate that most afferents belong to a particular pathway generally referred to as the *spinocervical tract.* According to physiological experiments the cells of origin of the tract appear to be situated in the dorsal horn in proximity to the dorsal root entry, apparently in Rexed's (1952, 1954) laminae IV and V (Eccles, Eccles, and Lundberg, 1960). They appear to be activated monosynaptically by sensory impulses.

The original demonstration by Rexed and Ström (1952) that this pathway mediates impulses of cutaneous origin has been confirmed and extended in subsequent studies. Touch stimuli, pressure, and, to a limited extent, joint movements activate the neurons of the lateral cervical nucleus. The receptive fields for some of the units are small while others are large (Andersson, 1962; Morin et al., 1963). Impulses mediated via this pathway have been found to reach the cerebral cortex, the somatosensory area I as well as II (Andersson, 1962). According to Oscarsson and Rosén (1966a) the pathway seems to activate also the motor cortex. In many respects the spinocortical route via the lateral cervical nucleus resembles the pathway via the dorsal column nuclei, but there are certain differences (see for example Andersson, 1962; Norrsell and Voerhove, 1962; Oscarsson and Rosén, 1966a). Trigeminal impulses have been led off from the nucleus (Wall and Taub, 1962). The functional significance of the pathway via the lateral cervical nucleus is not yet quite settled (see Horrobin, 1966; Oscarsson and Rosén, 1966, for some data), and whether a corresponding fiber system exists in man is an open question.

The thalamus and the thalamocortical projections. The third neuronal link in the long ascending somatic sensory fiber systems is made up of the neurons of those nuclei of the thalamus which receive the spinothalamic and medial lemniscus fibers, and whose axons transmit the impulses to the cerebral cortex. However, these fiber systems constitute only a restricted part of the extensive thalamocortical projection, as several of the other thalamic nuclei also project onto the cerebral cortex. It will be appropriate to consider the thalamus and its connections in general before treating this third link in the sensory systems in more detail.

Some of the pioneers of neuroanatomy (particularly Gudden, von Monakow, and Nissl) ascertained that extensive parts of the thalamus undergo atrophy after removal of the cerebral cortex, and they were also able to indicate definite nuclei which were connected with different parts of the cortex. Around the turn of the century the major ascending afferent connections to the thalamus had been described, and it was realized that this nuclear complex represents the final link in most afferent fiber systems transmitting impulses to the cerebral cortex. In the light of present-day knowledge the thalamus must be looked upon as being composed of a number of subdivisions which are functionally dissimilar, even if the functional role and the connections of many of the subdivisions are so far not known. The thalamus or parts of it will have to be considered in many chapters of this book. However, it is practical at this juncture to review briefly the thalamus as a whole, leaving special parts for discussion in subsequent chapters. Only aspects related to the somatic sensory pathways under consideration in this chapter will be dealt with in any detail here.

On dissection of the brain the two egg-shaped thalami, separated by the third ventricle, can each be subdivided into three gray masses or nuclei: the anterior, the medial, and the lateral thalamic. (The latter extends posteriorly to include the pulvinar.) They are separated by laminae of white matter which in transverse sections appear as a Y, the *internal medullary lamina.* Under the microscope it is possible to distinguish within each of the three main nuclei various subgroups which differ in their cytoarchitecture and in their myeloarchitecture as well as with regard to the fiber pattern, as seen in silver-impregnated sections, and often with regard to their glial architecture. Furthermore, several small cell groups are found within the medullary lamina, often collectively referred to as the *intralaminar nuclei.* Outside the main nuclei there are other small groups, thus a thin lamina of cells which covers almost the whole external (lateral) surface of the main body of nuclei, the *reticular thalamic nucleus,* and finally the so-called *nuclei of the midline.* The main nuclear groups as well as some of the subdivisions and their afferent fiber contingents are shown in the diagram of Fig. 2-11. On the whole, the princi-

FIG. 2–11 Diagram of a three-dimensional reconstruction of the right human thalamus seen from the dorsolateral aspect. The posterior part is separated from the rest by a cut to display some features of the internal structure. Only the rostral tip of the reticular nucleus is included. The main afferent contingents to some of the major nuclei are indicated. Abbreviations for thalamic nuclei: *A:* anterior; *CM:* centromedian; *Int. lam.:* intralaminar; *LD* and *LP:* lateralis dorsalis and posterior; *LG:* lateral geniculate body; *LM:* medial geniculate body; *MD:* dorsomedial; *MI:* midline; *P:* pulvinar; *R:* reticular; *Va:* ventralis anterior; *VL:* ventralis lateralis; *VPL* and *VPM:* ventralis posterior lateralis and medialis.

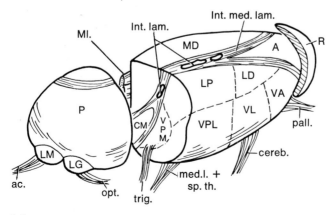

pal pattern of the thalamus appears to be the same in most animals. However, there are conspicuous differences as concerns the relative development of some of the cell groups. For example, the dorsomedial nucleus (MD), the dorsal nuclei (the nuclei lateralis dorsalis and posterior, LD and LP), the pulvinar and the centromedian nucleus (CM) are particularly well developed in primates, including man.

Several authors have proposed parcellations of the thalamic nuclei and assigned particular names to each of the subdivisions. The criteria used for definition of the subdivisions have varied. On a purely descriptive anatomical, largely cytoarchitectonic and myeloarchitectonic, basis a number of minor units can be distinguished. The most commonly accepted scheme is perhaps that suggested by Walker (1938c) and shown in Fig. 2-12 and adopted in Fig. 2-11. This is based chiefly on studies of the thalamus of the monkey and the chimpanzee. Hassler (1959) has extended this scheme for the thalamus of man and undertaken a far-reaching subdivision, distinguishing a large number of nuclei and areas. Somewhat different parcellations of the human thalamus have been made by Sheps (1945), Dekaban (1953), and Kuhlenbeck (1954). Some authors have taken into consideration embryological criteria, while still others base their subdivisions on what is known of the fiber connections or on results of physiological studies. (For a brief review of various classifications of thalamic nuclei, see Ajmone Marsan, 1965). It appears a likely assumption that when we eventually possess a sufficient knowledge of the fiber connections and the functional aspects of the various groups of the thalamus, a rational subdivision may be arrived at. However, much remains to be clarified before this goal is achieved. An essential prerequisite will be a detailed mapping of all fiber connections of the thalamic nuclei. This is, however, an extremely difficult task, since many subdivisions are very small and can scarcely ever be damaged in isolation. Furthermore, any lesion of one of these small nuclear groups is apt to interrupt fibers passing through or near to them. Physiological recordings may contribute to identifying certain connections, but again sources of error have to be considered, such as concomitant stimulation of passing fibers. There is no need to discuss minutiae of the thalamic connections here, the more so since there are still numerous open questions. Only some main features will be mentioned.

In the presentation of the thalamic nuclei it will be practical to take as the starting point the fact that a large number of them give off *fibers to the cerebral cortex* (thalamocortical fibers). These nuclei are often said to be "cortical dependent" because they show retrograde cellular changes or cell loss following ablations of various parts of the cerebral cortex (see Fig. 1-12). As first studied in detail by Le Gros Clark and

Walker most of these thalamocortical projections show a precise topical relationship between the particular thalamic nucleus and the corresponding cortical area. Among the "cortical dependent" thalamic nuclei is the *anterior thalamic nucleus,* in the gross anatomical sense (A, Fig. 2-11). It may be subdivided architectonically into three parts, all of which send their fibers to the medial surface of the cerebral hemisphere. Of the *medial group* of macroscopical anatomy only its largest subdivision, the *nucleus medialis dorsalis* (MD), sends fibers to the cortex, more precisely to various regions of the frontal lobe, chiefly at least, the orbital cortex (Fig. 2-12). Within the *lateral cell mass* certain parts give off fibers to the cortex. Proceeding in an anteroposterior direction the *inferior or ventral part* of the nucleus may be subdivided into three units (Fig. 2-11): the ventralis anterior (VA), the ventralis lateralis (VL), and the ventralis posterior. This again consists of three parts: the ventralis posterior lateralis (VPL), the ventralis posterior medialis (VPM) and the ventralis posterior inferior (VPI). These three nuclei (except apparently parts of VPI and parts of VA) all project to the cerebral cortex, the VL to the precentral, the VPL and VPM to the postcentral cortex (Fig. 2-12). As mentioned previously, VPL is the main final relay station in the spinothalamic and medial lemniscus systems, while the VPM receives fibers from the trigeminal sensory nuclei. The *dorsal part of the lateral nuclear mass* is subdivided into the nuclei lateralis (LD) and lateralis posterior (LP). The former appears to have cortical projections, at least chiefly, to the posterior part of the cingulate gyrus and probably part of the parietal cortex. The latter (LP) projects chiefly to the parietal cortex (Fig. 2-12). The pulvinar sends fibers to the parieto-temporal cortex.[14] Finally, the *lateral and medial geniculate bodies* (LG and MG), being stations in the pathways for vision and hearing, respectively, have well-defined cortical projection areas (Fig. 2-12). It is characteristic that thalamic nuclei which give off fibers to a particular part of the cerebral cortex, in general, receive afferents, *corticothalamic fibers,*

[14] Since we will return only briefly to the pulvinar in Chapter 8, it may be appropriate to record some data here. It is generally subdivided into three subnuclei. As to its cortical projections it appears that it projects to the temporal, parietal, and occipital cortex, although there are several discrepancies between authors as concerns details (see for example Le Gros Clark and Boggon, 1935; Le Gros Clark, 1936b; Le Gros Clark and Northfield, 1937; Chow, 1950; Simpson, 1952a; Locke, 1960; Akert et al., 1961). The projection appears to be fairly precise, various subnuclei having their particular projection areas in the cortex (see Chow, 1950; Simpson, 1952a). The pulvinar has been shown to receive cortical fibers from the temporal lobe (Bucy and Klüver, 1955; Whitlock and Nauta, 1956; Siqueira, 1965). Other afferent connections are insufficiently known. The pulvinar thus appears to be particularly dependent on the cerebral cortex, but little is known of its functional role.

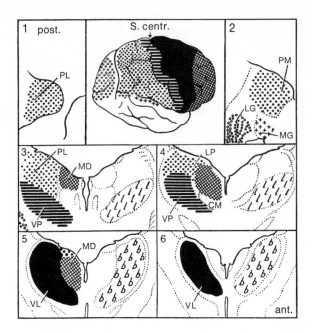

FIG. 2–12 Walker's diagram of the thalamocortical projection in the chimpanzee. 1–6: Representative sections through the thalamus, in a postero-anterior sequence. Corresponding areas of the thalamus and cerebral cortex marked with identical symbols. *LG:* lateral geniculate body; *LP:* nucleus lateralis posterior; *MD:* nucleus medialis dorsalis; *MG:* medial geniculate body; *PL* and *PM:* nucleus pulvinaris lateralis and medialis; *VL:* nucleus ventralis lateralis; *VP:* nucleus ventralis posterior; *l:* the area of termination of the fibers of the medial lemniscus and the spinothalamic tract. *b:* the area of termination of the fibers of the brachium conjunctivum. Slightly altered from Walker (1938c). Subsequent studies have necessitated certain alterations as to details in the diagram (Cf. text).

from the same cortical areas so that intimate reciprocal connections are established. The detailed arrangements within these fiber connections indicate that functional correlations between interconnected regions of cortex and thalamus must be very close.

As will be seen from the above enumeration the quantitatively largest nuclei of the thalamus together making up the bulk of its entire mass, are closely related to the cerebral cortex. For a number of the minor cell groups which have commonly been considered not to be "cortical dependent," data is accumulating which indicates that they send at least some efferents to the cortex (see Murray, 1966; Scheibel and Scheibel, 1967). It should be noted that most of the thalamic nuclei which send massive projections to specific parts of the cortex and receive fibers from corresponding cortical regions are acted upon by afferent impulses from fairly well characterized extrathalamic sources (somatic sensory, cerebellar, pallidal, hypothalamic), as will be considered in this and following chapters (see also Fig. 2-11).

In recent years it has become customary to speak of the thalamic nuclei considered so far as *"specific,"* in contrast to others which are termed *"nonspecific."* This distinction is made largely on the basis of functional, electrophysiological observations. Common to the "nonspecific" thalamic nuclei is that on electrical stimulation evoked potentials occur over wide cortical areas of the two hemispheres, appearing after a long latency and showing the phenomenon of "recruitment." These cortical responses markedly contrast with the sharply localized and rapidly occurring potentials which follow stimulation of the "specific" thalamic nuclei. Most of the "nonspecific" nuclei are situated in or near the midline or in the internal medullary lamina (see Fig. 2-11 and Fig. 6-9). The reticular thalamic nucleus (R, Fig. 2-11) is also generally considered to be "nonspecific." The "nonspecific" thalamic nuclei have been considered to form part of the morphological substratum of the "ascending activating system." Although the lumping together of certain thalamic nuclei as "nonspecific" may serve a didactic purpose, it has become more and more obvious as new anatomical and physiological data accumulate that a separation between "specific" and "nonspecific" thalamic nuclei is an oversimplification. These problems and the "nonspecific" thalamic nuclei will be considered in Chapter 6 on the reticular formation.

As will appear from the above, the thalamus is a complex of nuclei which differ with regard to their connections, and accordingly they are functionally dissimilar. In fact, one or more thalamic cell groups are related to such diverse functions as vegetative reactions, motor functions, maintenance of the conscious state and its variations, the senses of hearing and vision, and the mediation of exteroceptive and proprioceptive sensations which are perceived consciously. Only the role of the thalamus as the last subcortical station for the pathways from the spinal cord to the cortex will be considered in this chapter.

The thalamic terminations of the medial lemniscus and the spinothalamic tracts. As referred to previously it is unanimously agreed that the nucleus ventralis lateralis posterior (VPL) of the thalamus receives fibers from the medial lemniscus and the spinothalamic tract. Both fiber systems end in a somatotopical pattern within the nucleus, as illustrated diagrammatically in Fig. 2-13 which shows the distribution of the spinothalamic fibers. As is seen the fibers from the caudalmost spinal segments end most laterally; then follow in succession the terminal regions of fibers from progressively more rostral segments. A corresponding pattern is found for the fibers of the medial lemniscus. However, the medial lemniscus and the spinothalamic tract display certain differences in their distribution and in other ways which are of interest with regard to the types of peripheral stimuli which give rise to impulses in each of them.

The fibers of the *medial lemniscus* which, according to practically all students of the subject, are all crossed, behave in the simplest way. According to a number of authors their *thalamic terminal area is restricted to the VPL* (Gerebtzoff, 1939, in the rabbit; Matzke, 1951, in the cat; Le Gros Clark, 1936a; Bowsher, 1958; Mehler, Feferman, and Nauta, 1960, in the monkey; Walker, 1938a, in the chimpanzee; for previous studies see these papers).[15] In contrast, some *spinothalamic fibers* ascend on the ipsilateral side of the cord, while the majority cross the midline. Although a fair number of the fibers end in the VPL as shown in experimental anatomical studies in the rabbit (Gerebtzoff, 1939), in the cat (Getz, 1952; Anderson and Berry, 1959), in the monkey (Le Gros Clark, 1936a; Chang and Ruch, 1947; Mehler, Feferman, and Nauta, 1960; Bowsher, 1961), in the chimpanzee (Walker, 1938a) and in man (Bowsher, 1957), it appears that spinothalamic fibers in addition supply other thalamic cell groups, among these some situated posteriorly. There is still some lack of clarity concerning the latter terminations, apparently due in part to differences in nomenclature and difficulties in distinguishing particular cell groups in this region. Using silver impregnation methods Mehler, Feferman, and Nauta (1960) and Bowsher (1961) traced spinothalamic fibers, degenerating as a consequence of spinal cord lesions in the monkey, to a part of the medial geniculate body (its magnocellular part, abbreviated MGm) and to another small cell group, the so-called suprageniculate nucleus (Bowsher, 1961). These fibers are also described in the rat (Lund and Webster, 1967b). These findings are of interest

[15] Bowsher (1961) found some fibers also in the magnocellular part of the medial geniculate nucleus. MGm (see below), as did Lund and Webster (1967a) in the rat.

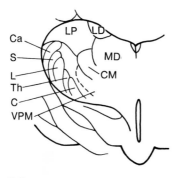

FIG. 2–13 Diagram of the somatotopical pattern of termination of spinothalamic fibers in the nucleus ventralis posterior lateralis in the tailed spider monkey. The approximate zones receiving fibers from the caudal, sacral, lumbar, thoracic and cervical segments of the cord are labeled *Ca, S, L, Th* and *C*, respectively. Redrawn from Chang and Ruch (1947). The fibers of the medial lemniscus are distributed according to the same principles.

from a functional point of view (see below and Ch. 9) as is also the demonstration by several authors of spinothalamic fibers to some of the so-called nonspecific thalamic nuclei (to be considered in Ch. 6).

Even if there is still some uncertainty about details in their terminal distribution, there is no doubt that *spinothalamic fibers are not restricted to the VPL* as are those of the medial lemniscus. Since these two fiber tracts in part mediate impulses which arise in response to different kinds of sensory stimuli, their common area of termination in the thalamus raises certain questions. For example, it may be asked whether fibers from the two pathways establish contact with the same cells, or whether the modality specificity which is to some extent evident in the fiber tracts is upheld in the further projection to the cerebral cortex. A series of physiological studies, particularly the careful single unit analyses of Mountcastle and his collaborators, have shed light on this question. It appears from these studies that *as far as the medial lemniscus is concerned the stimulus specificity as well as the place specificity is largely maintained in the VPL* (and indeed even in the sensory cortex, see below).

Thus single units of the VPL have been found to respond to only one particular type of stimulus. Of about one thousand units studied in the nucleus in the unanesthetized monkey, 42 per cent responded only to stimulation of skin receptors (gentle mechanical stimuli), 32 per cent responded to mechanical distortion of fascia or periosteum, and 26 per cent to joint movements (Poggio and Mountcastle, 1963). All units responded only to stimulation within a restricted region on the contralateral side of the body. The receptive fields are small on the fingers and toes (about 0.2cm^2), considerably larger on proximal parts of the limbs. Most of the joint units were characterized by being excited by rotation of the particular joint in one direction only. Many of them, however, signaled not only movements but also certain steady joint positions. (For various reasons the units recorded from are taken to be activated by fibers of the medial lemniscus.) An analysis of the positions within the VPL of the different types of units confirmed the somatotopical pattern described anatomically (for the termination of the medial lemniscus fibers, see Fig. 2-13) and as mapped physiologically in the monkey and other animals (Mountcastle and Henneman, 1949, 1952; Rose and Mountcastle, 1952; Gaze and Gordon, 1954; Kruger and Albe-Fessard, 1960; Poggio and Mountcastle, 1960; and others). The precise mapping of the anatomical position of the units recorded from, furthermore, enabled Poggio and Mountcastle (1963) to show some other interesting features. The distal portions of the body dispose over a much greater volume of thalamic tissue than do the proximal portions. Neurons related to deep receptors are commonly located in the dorsal part of the nucleus, while neurons activated from skin are located ventrally. It appears that neurons responding to a particular type of stimulus tend to be aggregated within small blocks of tissue. As will be seen below these arrangements conform to the pattern within the thalamocortical projection of the VPL.

The terminations of the *spinothalamic fibers* in the VPL have so far not been studied physiologically in as great detail as the medial lemniscus fibers. However, single units responding to stimuli known to give rise to impulses in the spinothalamic tract have been identified following transection of both medial lemnisci (Perl and Whitlock, 1961; Whitlock and Perl, 1961). It appears that while some of these units are modality specific and are arranged according to the known somatotopical pattern this is not so for all cells in the VPL activated by spinothalamic fibers.

In recent years *single unit recordings have been made in the thalamus of human beings,* primarily as an aid in locating the points of stereotaxically placed electrodes used in the treatment of Parkinsonism. Single units in the VPL have been found to respond to light touch, pressure, and joint movement (Albe-Fessard, Arfel and Guiot, 1963; Gaze et al., 1964; Albe-Fessard et al., 1966; Jasper and Bertrand, 1966). A somatotopical pattern corresponding to that in the monkey has been found. Responses to joint movements are obtained more anteriorly than responses to tactile stimuli (Jasper and Bertrand, 1966). On stimulation of points in the VPL by implanted electrodes, conscious patients experience highly localized sensations on the contralateral side of the body, described as tingling, pins and needles, numbness, or electricity (Ervin and Mark, 1960; Hassler, 1961), while modality specific sensations do not occur. With certain stimulus frequencies pain sensations have, however, been elicited from the basal part of the nucleus (Hassler, 1961).

As referred to above, some spinothalamic fibers end in the MGm (magnocellular part of the medial geniculate body). Others reach some of the "nonspecific" thalamic nuclei. In the former nucleus (Poggio and Mountcastle, 1960; Whitlock and Perl, 1961) as well as in the latter (Albe-Fessard and Bowsher, 1965) microelectrode recordings have disclosed the presence of units which respond to nociceptive stimuli and are activated from large and bilateral areas of the body.

It is in keeping with the known functional differences between the two large somatic sensory pathways that they appear to differ in mode of termination. The lemniscus fibers are uniformly large, appear to have a fairly straight course and to be evenly distributed throughout the VPL, while the spinothalamic fibers vary in diameter and tend to terminate in clusters (Mehler, Feferman, and Nauta, 1960; Bowsher, 1961). In Golgi studies Scheibel and Scheibel (1966e) have further demonstrated differences between the axonal ramifications of the fibers of the two tracts (Fig. 2-15). Those of the lemniscus end as regularly arranged bushy arbors (2 in the figure), each of which supplies a cone-shaped area, while the spinothalamic (as well as the reticulothalamic) fibers end in diffusely arranged networks (1 in the figure). Obviously the former mode of termination favors precise topical relations within the nucleus.

It appears from the data reviewed above that the specificity of stimulus type and of site of stimulation, characteristic to the two somatic sensory pathways to the thalamus, is largely preserved within this. Furthermore, within the thalamic relay, the VPL, lateral inhibition (see p. 57) occurs as it does at the first stations in the pathways and serves to increase sharpness in spatial localization (see Fig. 2-14 and explanation in the legend). The neurons in the VPL are subject to influences from the corresponding part of the cortex by way of corticothalamic fibers, and fibers from other thalamic nuclei and other sources may likewise be of importance. These processes are obviously very complex and not yet fully understood. It appears, however, that the VPL is concerned only, or at least predominantly with what is generally spoken of as discriminating modalities of sensation. This is further confirmed by observations of the anatomy and physiology of the final link in the main sensory pathways, the thalamocortical projection.

FIG. 2–14 A schematic drawing illustrating the role inhibition is thought to play in discrimination in the somatic afferent system. Each stimulus delivered to the skin activates a group of cells of the dorsal column nuclei, and inhibits those which surround that excited group. This pattern is repeated at each successive level of the system. When two stimuli are delivered and brought closer together the surround inhibition will delay fusion of the excited zones set up by the two stimuli, thus preserving the two peaks of activity at the cortical level, an event thought to be essential to the perception that two stimuli have been delivered. More complicated patterns of central excitation and inhibition will accompany more complicated peripheral stimuli, but the same organization should contribute to pattern and contour recognition. *DCN:* dorsal column nuclei. From Mountcastle and Powell (1959b).

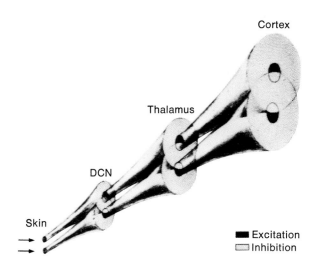

Cortex

Thalamus

DCN

Skin

■ Excitation
▭ Inhibition

The neuronal processes taking place in the VPL in its normal function are extremely complex, as appears from recent studies (see for example, Mount-castle, Poggio, and Werner, 1963; Andersen, Brooks, Eccles, and Sears, 1964; Andersen, Eccles, and Sears, 1964b). For example, postsynaptic, as well as pre-synaptic, inhibition and facilitation may occur on the arrival of impulses in afferent ascending pathways. It has been concluded from neurophysiological studies that some of these phenomena require the presence of internuncial cells in the VPL. Such cells have been described by Tömböl (1966–7), and Pappas, Cohen, and Purpura (1966) in electron micrographs from the cat's thalamus have demon-strated axo-axonal synapses (see Fig. 1-5F), assumed to be the substrate for pre-synaptic inhibition. A convincing impression of the complex intrinsic anatomical organization is obtained from the recent Golgi study of Scheibel and Scheibel (1966e), referred to above, where mention was made of the different terminal arborization patterns of the spinothalamic (and reticulothalamic) and the medial lemniscus fibers (Fig. 2-15, 1 and 2). Still another type of terminal distribution is shown by corticothalamic fibers, whose terminals occupy a coin-shaped region (Fig. 2-15,3). One of these discs encompasses a number of medial lemniscus arborizations. Other corticothalamic fibers as well as collaterals of fibers in the

FIG. 2–15 Arrangement of some of the components making up the presynaptic and postsynaptic neuropil of the *VB* nucleus. *1:* the diffuse net or matrix, generated by spinothalamic and reticular projections; *2:* the bushy arbors produced by ter-minal fibers of the medial lemniscus, arranged in an onionskin distribution around the hilus of entry; *3:* transverse discoid and more diffuse terminal patterns of cor-ticothalamic and striatothalamic reflux systems; *4:* some aspects of the postsynaptic thalamocortical units, showing the grouping of axons from adjacent neurons, the marked overlap of dendrite domains, and the relation of somata to presynaptic arbors (schematic sagittal sections). From Scheibel and Scheibel (1966e). The term *VB* (ventrobasal nucleus) used above is often employed as a common designa-tion for *VL* and *VPL*.

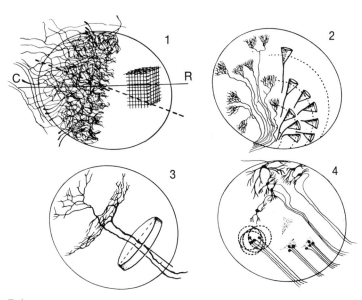

cerebral peduncle are distributed in a more diffuse manner. For further details and a discussion of some functional aspects of the findings the original paper should be consulted. Other relevant papers are found in *"The Thalamus,"* 1966.

It will appear from the above that we have considerable information on the role played by the thalamus in transmitting the somatosensory information which reaches it by way of the medial lemniscus system. Concerning the spinothalamic component much less is known, anatomically as well as functionally. Especially in physiological literature the thalamic regions outside the VPL which are related to the spinothalamic tract are often collectively referred to as the posterior group of nuclei (PO), which is not clearly circumscribed anatomically. Poggio and Mountcastle (1960), who discuss the problems raised by this situation, favor the view that the PO is related to the transmission of impulses perceived as pain, a question to which we will return in a later section when the cortical sensory areas have been considered. Figure 2-16 shows a simplified diagram of the somatosensory pathways.

The somatic sensory cortical areas. It is a matter of taste how one will define a somatic sensory cortical area. If this term is applied to all cortical areas from which potentials can be recorded following stimulation of various somatic receptors, a very extensive part of the cortex should be considered as sensory. On the other hand, one could use the term in a restricted sense, to cover only areas of the cerebral cortex which are end stations of fiber tracts which transmit responses to sensory stimuli via thalamic relays directly to the cortex. Until some years ago this definition appeared rather clear. Among such sensory cortical areas one would list, for example, the striate area, since this appeared to be the only cortical area receiving impulses from the eye via the lateral geniculate body. The cortical areas which are the sites of termination of fibers coming from those subdivisions of the thalamus where the somatosensory pathways treated in this chapter (and those from the trigeminal nuclei) terminate would likewise be covered by the definition. However, it appears that the criterion mentioned above is becoming more equivocal than was formerly assumed. For example, it appears that fibers from the lateral geniculate body do not supply the striate area only, but the two surrounding visual areas (18 and 19) as well (see Ch. 8). The cortical projections of the thalamic nuclei which receive the somatic afferent pathways are likewise less simple than formerly believed, and it seems certain that there is not only one but at least three cortical areas which are closely related to the reception of somatosensory messages, even if the final thalamocortical links are not known precisely.

From clinical and physiological observations it has been known for a long time that the postcentral gyrus in man (or the corresponding part of

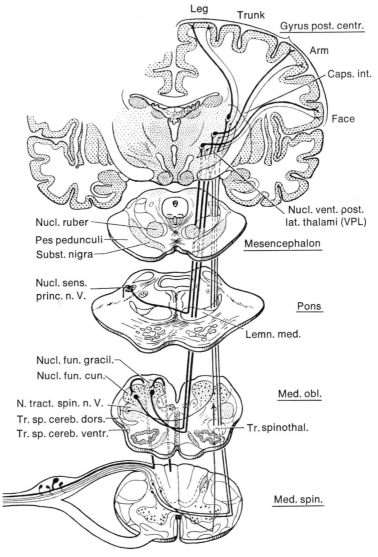

FIG. 2–16 A simplified diagram of the main features in the somatosensory pathways. Redrawn and slightly modified from Rasmussen (1932).

the brain in other species) is a main somatosensory cortical area. In 1941 Adrian demonstrated that, following peripheral somatic stimuli, responses could be picked up in the cat's brain not only in this cortical region, but, in addition, in another smaller area situated beneath the lower end of the classical sensory area. The area described by Adrian is generally referred to as the *second somatosensory area,* in contrast to the classical or *first somatosensory area.* Both areas show a somatotopical pattern. Further studies have disclosed an *additional area on the medial aspect of the cerebral hemisphere* from which somatotopically localized responses can be recorded following stimulation of peripheral nerves or dorsal roots. However, it has become evident that *none of these areas is purely sensory.* From all of them motor effects can be obtained on electrical stimulation. Among the pioneer studies in this field are those of Dusser de Barenne (1933) and Dusser de Barenne, Garol, and McGulloch (1941). It is, therefore, becoming more and more common to speak of *sensorimotor cortical areas.* Since certain parts of each area appear to be predominantly either motor or sensory, Woolsey (1964) has suggested a nomenclature which takes this into account. In the designation of an area, capital letters are used to indicate functions dominant to functions indicated by lower case letters (see Fig. 2-17). The first somatosensory area (in the post-central gyrus) is labeled Sm I; the second somatic (sensorimotor) area

FIG. 2–17 Diagram of the brain of the monkey showing the general arrangement of localization patterns within the first and second sensorimotor (*Sm I* and *Sm II*), the first motosensory (*Ms I*) and the supplementary motor (*Ms II*) regions. Question marks suggest possible incomplete information for caudal borders of *Sm I.* From Woolsey (1964).

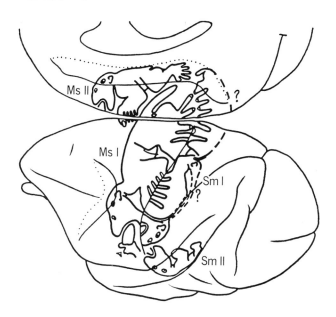

is called Sm II. The third sensory area is labeled Ms II, since it appears chiefly to be related to motor functions.[16] The precentral area, often spoken of as the "motor" area (see Ch. 4) is designated Ms I, since it is also concerned in sensory functions. In the following the easier terms, "first" and "second" somatosensory areas (S I and S II), will be employed, but it should be recalled that these areas are not purely sensory. Even if some of the areas listed above are as yet not known sufficiently to be of use in the evaluation of sensory disturbances in clinical neurology, the available data indicates that conditions in man are essentially the same as in the experimental animals. It should, however, be emphasized that extensive parts of the cortex outside these areas are involved in the elaborate processes which take place in the brain when somatosensory stimuli are perceived.

The first somatic sensory area, S I or Sm I, is fairly well known. Cytoarchitectonically it consists of three longitudinal zones in the postcentral gyrus (Brodmann's areas 3, 1, 2, area retrocentralis, see Fig. 12-2). In man this area anteriorly reaches the depth of the central sulcus (area 3 appears to extend to the operculum) and covers the entire postcentral gyrus to the postcentral sulcus.[17] On the medial surface of the hemisphere it is found in the paracentral lobule. The entire region is distinguished by a distinct lamination with prominent well-developed granular layers (2nd and 4th layers) whereas the 5th layer is faintly developed (Fig. 8-7b). This is a feature typical of cortical areas predominantly receptive in function (cf. Ch. 12). Anatomically the cortical areas 3, 1, and 2 have been shown in several animal species to receive their thalamic afferents from the ventral posterior thalamic nucleus, VPL and VPM, see Fig.

[16] Ms II is often spoken of as the supplementary motor area (see Ch. 4). According to Blomquist and Lorenzini's (1965) studies in the squirrel monkey, a *supplementary sensory* area is found caudal to the extension of Sm I on the medial aspect of the hemisphere. There would thus be altogether five sensory areas (see also Penfield and Jasper, 1954).

[17] The same subdivision into areas 3, 1, and 2 is found in the monkey and the cat. Particularly in the latter animal there has been some dispute as to the anterior border of the first somatosensory area. Some physiologists have maintained that the border between the "motor" and the "sensory" cortex corresponds to a "dimple" which is found rather constantly in the posterior sigmoid gyrus in the cat. This shallow sulcus is then taken to correspond to the central sulcus in monkey and man. The cytoarchitectonic studies of Hassler and Muhs-Clement (1964) support this notion. However, with regard to the amount of corticofugal fibers descending to certain nuclei in the brain stem, the border between an anterior, amply projecting and a posterior, relatively sparsely projecting, region appears to correspond to the cruciate sulcus (for some data see P. Brodal, 1968a; Rinvik, 1968a). This problem is of some practical importance for the interpretation of anatomical and physiological observations on this part of the cortex in the cat.

78

2-11, (Polyak, 1932; Le Gros Clark and Boggon, 1935; Le Gros Clark, 1937; Walker, 1934, 1936, 1938b; Chow and Pribram, 1956; Pubols, 1968), where the medial lemniscus and most of the fibers of the spinothalamic tract terminate. Following a restricted lesion in this part of the cortex a sharply circumscribed patch of retrograde cell loss occurs in the nucleus posterior ventralis. The conclusion that this suggests the existence of a very sharply localized pattern within this part of the thalamocortical projection has been fully substantiated in further studies. Likewise the existence of a clear somatotopical arrangement within the projection has been established. The most detailed and informative study so far is that of Welker and Johnson (1965) in the raccoon. Their combined anatomical and electrophysiological study demonstrates a remarkable degree of precision in this part of the thalamocortical projection. The main principles of the projection are shown in Fig. 2-18 and Fig. 5-9. It will be seen that regions of the VPL which receive "hindlimb" fibers project onto the upper part of the cortex of the central region, near the medial surface, while those regions which receive "forelimb" fibers project more laterally and lower. Fibers from the VPM, receiving secondary trigeminal fibers (Ch. 7), reach the lowest part of the central cortical region. This indicates that *there is within the first sensory area a somatotopical pattern, with the hindlimb represented uppermost, the face lowermost.* More precise information has been obtained in clinical and experimental physiological studies.

The somatotopical pattern in the *postcentral gyrus in man* has been studied particularly by recording the sensations which a patient experiences when this part of the cortex is electrically stimulated during expo-

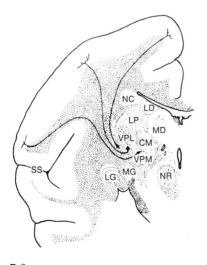

FIG. 2–18 Diagram showing the somatotopical pattern in the projection from the ventral posterior nucleus of the thalamus (*VPL* and *VPM*) onto the postcentral cortex in the macaque monkey. *NC:* caudate nucleus; *NR:* red nucleus; *SS:* Sylvian fissure. Other abbreviations as in Fig. 2–11. From Walker (1938a).

sure for brain surgery. Extensive studies have been published by Foerster (1936a) and Penfield and his collaborators (see Penfield and Boldrey, 1937; Penfield and Rasmussen, 1950; Penfield and Jasper, 1954). Most frequently the patients describe sensations as itching, tickling, tingling, numbness, or a feeling of pressure. With weak currents these sensations are sharply localized, for instance to one of the fingers. In this manner it has been established that in the postcentral gyrus in man the calf and foot are "represented" on the medial surface of the hemisphere, then follow the foci for thigh, abdomen, thorax, shoulder, arm, forearm, hand, digits, and then the face region (Fig. 2-19). Lowest on the medial surface the foci for the bladder, rectum, and genital organs are found. Electrical stimulation at this place produces sensations in the corresponding organs.[18] Occasionally the sensations provoked by electrical stimulation of the cortex also appear in the corresponding region on the homolateral

[18] Erickson (1945) has reported a case of nymphomania, due to a hemangioma in the sagittal sulcus, and concluded that the nymphomania was due to irritation of the sensory focus for the genital organs. After removal of the tumor the nymphomania, as well as the accompanying motor seizures, disappeared.

FIG. 2–19 Diagram showing the relative size of the parts of the central cortex from which sensations localized to different parts of the body can be elicited on electrical stimulation in man. From Penfield and Rasmussen (1950).

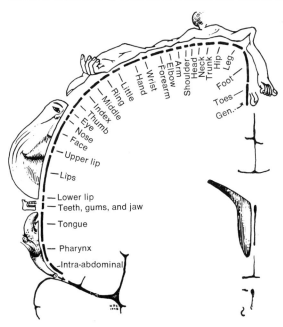

side of the body. This most readily and frequently happens as concerns the face, especially the oral region. In the larynx, pharynx, rectum, and genitalia the sensations appear to occur bilaterally. Bilateral sensations are more difficult to produce in the extremities, especially their distal parts. As referred to above, localized sensations following irritation of the cerebral cortex are not strictly limited to the areas 3, 1, and 2 in the post-central gyrus. Identical sensations may arise from irritation of the posterior part of the precentral cortex (Penfield and Boldrey, 1937, and others).

Figure 2-19 illustrates *another important feature in the somatic sensory area I: the different parts of the body are "represented" in territories of very different sizes.* Thus the "face area" is large, the "hand area" likewise, while the proximal parts of the limbs occupy relatively small territories. As will be recalled, the same principle is valid for the "representation" of various bodily regions in the VPL. Thus the amount of tissue within the sensory cortex which is allotted to a particular region of the body is related to the importance of that region in somatic sensation and not to its absolute size. In Fig. 2-17 it is seen that in the monkey the distal parts of the extremities are "represented" more anteriorly, closer to the central sulcus than are the proximal parts and the trunk. The same appears to be the case in man, but is not seen in Fig. 2-19.

A number of experimental studies in animals have given results concordant with those in man. Woolsey, Marshall, and Bard have demonstrated a discrete localization in the postcentral gyrus in the monkey (1942) and chimpanzee (1943). Leading off from the cortex they have mapped out the areas responding when different parts of the skin are stimulated. The somatic receiving area determined in this way is found to correspond well with the histologically delimited areas 3, 1, and 2. The pattern of "representation" corresponds to that found in studies of human cases. Corresponding results were obtained in Adrian's (1941) studies in the rabbit, cat, dog, and monkey. The results of these pioneer studies have subsequently been confirmed by others, for example Woolsey and Fairman (1946), Mountcastle and Henneman (1952), Benjamin and Welker (1957), Celesia (1963), and Blomquist and Lorenzini (1965). A particularly discrete localization has been described in the raccoon (Welker and Seidenstein, 1959) which has an unusually well-developed cutaneous digital sensibility. Several authors have found responses to peripheral nerve stimulation or to natural somatic stimulations in front of the areas 3, 1, and 2, in the agranular "motor" cortex (Malis, Pribram, and Kruger, 1953; Benjamin and Welker, 1957; Woolsey and collaborators, see Woolsey, 1964; Albe-Fessard and Liebeskind, 1966;

and others). These responses are preserved even if the sensory cortex is ablated.

The latter findings, as well as corresponding findings in man, raise questions of details in the thalamocortical projections to the first somatosensory area. A precise anatomical correlation between thalamic areas projecting onto the post-central "sensory" cortex and the site of termination of the fibers of the medial lemniscus does not, so far, appear to have been made. The question is further complicated by the fact that the same thalamic regions appear to project to S II as well as to S I (see below). Since the corticothalamic projection from the central region is far more differentiated than previously assumed (Rinvik, 1968a), it seems a likely assumption that the thalamocortical projection to the central gyri is equally complexly organized anatomically. Meticulous anatomical studies are needed to decide this.

Recent studies have brought forward further data of great interest for the understanding of the function of the first somatosensory area. The three subdivisions of the first somatosensory cortex (areas 3, 1, and 2) have been shown by Le Gros Clark and Powell (1953) to receive their afferents from particular regions of the VPL, although the separation between the three contingents is not quite sharp. These observations lend support to the assumption that the cytoarchitectonic differentiation within the first somatosensory area reflects functional properties, as has indeed been confirmed in physiological studies (Mountcastle and Powell, 1959a; Powell and Mountcastle, 1959b). In single unit analyses in the monkey over 90 per cent of the neurons in area 2 were found to be related to receptors of the deep tissues of the body, particularly of the joints, while the large majority of those of area 3 are activated only by cutaneous stimuli. Area 1 occupies an intermediate position. This functional gradient corresponds to a gradient in the cytoarchitecture across the region (Powell and Mountcastle, 1959a). The modality specificity appears to be present throughout vertically oriented columns of cells extending through all layers of the cortex. These columns are supposed to be capable of integrated activity of a rather complex order, which is independent of lateral spread of activity within the gray matter (Powell and Mountcastle, 1959b, and earlier papers). (A similar arrangement has been found in the visual cortex, see Ch. 8.)

It follows from these observations that *there is in the first somato-sensory area a functional differentiation within zones arranged approxi-mately across its length.* This pattern fits in with studies of the somato-topical projection, at least as far as the monkey is concerned, since it appears that the dermatomes are related to (mutually somewhat over-lapping) transversely running zones (Woolsey, Marshall, and Bard, 1942; Powell and Mountcastle, 1959b). Thus the afferent fibers of a dorsal root, comprising the full modality spectrum, appear to be "represented" in a narrow anterior-posterior band of the cortex (Powell and Mount-castle, 1959b). (Whether this "spectrum" includes thermal and painful stimuli appears, however, as yet uncertain. See also below.) Impulses arising from various kinds of receptors are transmitted to specific units within the zones in the cortex. The specificity of the cortical neurons is especially well illustrated by Mountcastle and Powell's (1959a) observations of joint receptors in the cortex. Just as in the thalamus (see above) there are cortical units which respond to movements of a particular joint in one direction only. Furthermore, when the joint is kept in a steady position, the unit goes on discharging for a long time (several seconds). When the movement is continued in the excitatory direction the rate of discharge increases. Obviously the sensory cortex thus gets very precise information on the position and movements of the joints, and it appears that this information (together with that resulting from deformation of fascia) is the basis of what is usually referred to as "position sense." This agrees with conclusions reached in clinical and clinico-experimental studies (Stopford, 1921; Provins, 1958; and others) about the importance of an intact innervation of the joints for the position sense. Whether muscle receptors contribute substantially to the appreciation of position appears not to be quite settled (Mountcastle and Powell, 1959a; see also below). The information arriving from the cutaneous receptors to the first somatic sensory cortex appears to be quite specific as well, since there are in the cat (Mountcastle, 1957), as well as in the monkey (Powell and Mountcastle, 1959b), rapidly adapting units which respond to the displacement of hairs and slowly adapting ones which are excited by pressure of the skin.

It appears that *the messages arising in various kinds of receptors and passing via the great somatosensory pathways to the ventral posterior lateral thalamic nucleus (VPL) are relayed in a very faithful manner to the first somatosensory area, so that the sensory cortex gets precise information about the kind of stimuli affecting the body at any time and about the site where they are applied.* It should be noted that at least most of the information reaching the first somatosensory cortical area, and discussed above, appears to be mediated via the dorsal column—medial lemniscus system, and accordingly it is transmitted to the contralateral cerebral hemisphere. The role played by the spinothalamic tract is less well known (see also below).

The information described above has been obtained in animal studies. There is every reason to believe, however, that conditions are similar in man, in so far as can be concluded from studies of evoked potentials from the exposed cortex in conscious human beings following stimulation of skin or peripheral nerves (see Jasper, Lende, and Rasmussen, 1960;

Kelly et al., 1965; Libet et al., 1967). Among additional data obtained the following may be mentioned: a stimulus to the skin or a sensory nerve may give rise to cortical potentials at a lower threshold of stimulation than that necessary to evoke a subjective sensation (Libet et al., 1967).[19]

Reference was made above to the fact that evoked potentials on stimulation of peripheral nerves can be recorded from the "motor" area 4 as well as the sensory areas (3, 1, and 2). The stimuli giving rise to these potentials are not completely known, but it appears that impulses from muscles are most important. In the cat, Oscarsson and Rosén (1966a) found responses from Group 1A spindle afferents, while Albe-Fessard and Liebeskind (1966), in the monkey, did not identify the receptors responsible. There is some degree of somatotopical representation, which is bilateral, and there are some differences between the responses in the "motor" and "sensory" areas. The pathways utilized are not known, but they do not appear to pass via the cerebellum or the "sensory" cortex (see Albe-Fessard and Liebeskind, 1966). It appears from these and other studies that *with regard to its sensory functions the "motor" part of the first sensorimotor region differs from the "sensory" part.* It is presumably particularly involved in the (probably subconscious) action of the cortex on motor functions (cf. the termination of the pathways from the cerebellum in the precentral region, to be described in Ch. 5). The sensory part is closely related to conscious sensory experiences. Numerous studies have been devoted to these problems, but much still remains to be done, both anatomically and physiologically. These problems will not be discussed here, except for mentioning that there is a collaboration between the two parts of the first sensorimotor cortex, in part mediated by way of association fibers (see below), that some convergence of impulses from various sources occurs in both areas, most marked in the "motor" area, and that lateral inhibition (see Fig. 2-14) serves to increase contrast. Finally, the role played in these complex mechanisms by the presence of ample corticothalamic connections should be emphasized. These are topically organized in a pattern which, in general, appears to mirror that of the thalamocortical projection, so that the cortical area of the hand in S I, for example, gives off fibers to the "hand area" in the VPL. The pattern of this projection has recently been studied in some detail by Rinvik (1968a).

The conclusion, drawn on the basis of the studies mentioned on the

[19] Some authors have attempted to study the responses by recording somato-sensory-evoked cortical potentials from the human scalp by means of a computer averaging technique. However, there are difficulties in avoiding confusion with myogenic potentials (see Cracco and Bickford, 1968).

preceding pages, that the first somatosensory area is essential for sensory discrimination, is supported by results of animal experiments. According to Orbach and Chow (1959), ablation of the postcentral gyrus in monkeys results in marked disturbances in tactile form and roughness discrimination. Other data may be found in the paper of Semmes and Mishkin (1965). Corresponding observations have been made in clinical cases. Obviously the latter, to be discussed below, can give more precise and specific information on this subject than can studies in animals.

The second somatosensory area, S II (or Sm II), is less completely known than the first. In all animals studied it occupies a smaller region of the cortex than the latter. In the cat it is found in the anterior ectosylvian gyrus, in the monkey it lies largely on the upper bank of the Sylvian fissure adjacent to the insula (Fig. 2-17). Its position in man is rather similar to that in the monkey. In all animal species studied a somatotopical pattern has been determined by studying the evoked potentials set up on peripheral stimulation (Woolsey and Fairman, 1946; Knighton, 1950; Benjamin and Welker, 1957; Welker and Seidenstein, 1959; Celesia, 1963; and others), but the localization appears to be less discrete than in S I. The face is represented rostrally, the hindleg most caudally (Fig. 2-17). Presumably the same pattern is present in man (Penfield and Rasmussen, 1950). Responses are bilateral, but the contralateral ones are more marked. Single units have been identified which react specifically to touch and vibration. Stimulation of Pacinian corpuscles gives rise to potentials more marked in S II than in S I (McIntyre, 1962). Even stimulation of a single corpuscle may be recorded in S II (McIntyre et al., 1967). Gentle movements of joints do not evoke responses (Andersson, 1962). It appears that impulses from muscles as well as from deep tissues (periosteum, fascia, etc.) reach area S II, as well as S I (Mountcastle, Covian, and Harrison, 1952; Landgren and Wolsk, 1966). According to Andersson (1962), in the cat the afferent impulses are mediated, at least chiefly, via the medial lemniscus and the ascending pathway from the lateral cervical nucleus (see p. 63ff). The transmission through the two pathways differs in some respects. While many units in S II are modality specific, others react to stimulation of skin as well as of deep structures, and several units have large receptive fields (Carreras and Andersson, 1963). As mentioned previously S II projects in a somatotopical pattern onto the dorsal column nuclei.

In man electrical stimulation of the second somatosensory area gives rise to sensations which resemble those occurring on stimulation of the first somatosensory area (Penfield and Jasper, 1954; Penfield and Faulk, Jr., 1955). Feelings of tingling, numbness, and warmth are usually referred to a particular region on the contralateral side of the body, but may be felt bilaterally. (Penfield and Faulk quite often observed abdominal and epigastric sensations, and there was a concomitant change in gastric motility.) Since the area is partly hidden in the fissure of Sylvius it is not easily accessible.

The thalamic relay for the sensory impulses reaching S II has so far not been precisely outlined. According to Macchi et al. (1959), S II receives thalamic efferents from VPL and VPM, as does S I, and they believe that certain areas of the nuclei project onto both cortical areas.

Guillery et al. (1966) support this opinion with some reservations. Stimulation of the ventral posterior nucleus (with histological verifications of the points of stimulation) produced localized responses in S II (as well as in S I), but the bilateral responses occurring in S II, following peripheral stimulation, are not explained by a projection via the VPL to S II, since this is purely ipsilateral. As stated by Guillery et al. (1966), it may be that more posterior parts (elements in the PO group of nuclei, see p. 75) also contribute to the projection onto S II, as suggested by Knighton's (1950) findings. However, in the opossum, Diamond and Utley (1963) did not find retrograde changes in PO following lesions of S I and S II. It should be noted that the study of these projections is difficult, in part because the S II is rather small and lesions may easily extend beyond its territory, but particularly because the retrograde changes in this part of the thalamus may be equivocal. Like S I, also S II projects back to the thalamus. According to Rinvik's (1968b) experimental studies in the cat, its corticothalamic projection in addition to a somatotopically organized component to the VPL and VPM comprises a correspondingly organized component passing to PO (as well as a smaller number of fibers to other thalamic nuclei). These findings indirectly support the assumption that the PO may actually possess a projection onto S II.

On the whole, S II appears to be less specifically organized than the first somatosensory area, S I. Functional deficits following ablation of S II have been found by some authors and denied by others. Orbach and Chow (1959) conclude from experiments in monkeys that S II is concerned in tactile form and roughness discrimination.

The sensory function of the supplementary motor area (Ms II of Woolsey) is relatively little known. Some observations have been mentioned above. According to Penfield's experience, stimulation of this region in conscious man gives rise to sensations in the head and abdomen and a sense of palpitation. Most often the patient describes it as a general sensation (Penfield and Jasper, 1954). There is some evidence that also in man the "sensory" part of the supplementary area is situated posteriorly to the "motor."

What is known so far of the somatosensory cortical areas makes it clear that they are not functionally equivalent. Presumably each of them has its specific tasks. Even if they all appear to be cortical receiving stations for somatosensory responses, they differ with regard to the types of stimuli which activate them, as well as in certain features of their organization. However, *they all appear to be relatively elementary links in the neural mechanisms which are related to somatosensory perception.* Disturbances in such functions are best studied in man, and clinical studies show that sensory perception may suffer even if the somatosensory areas are intact (see, for example, Weinstein et al., 1958). This is the case also in the monkey and chimpanzee (Ruch, Fulton, and German, 1938; Bates and Ettlinger, 1960; and others). The part of the cortex which appears to be specially important for sensory perception and discrimination is the *superior parietal lobule,* which in Brodmann's map (Fig. 12-2) corresponds to his areas 5 and 7 (Foerster calls Brodmann's area 7 area 5b). The cortex of these areas has a well developed layer IV, and there are many large pyramidal cells in the "efferent" layers III and V (see Ch. 12). According to Foerster (1936a), on *stimulation of the cortex in his area 5* localized sensations do not occur. Sensations are of the same type as on stimulation of the postcentral gyrus, but they are more or less diffusely projected on the entire contralateral half of the body. Furthermore, stronger currents are required, and the sensations show a greater tendency to occur bilaterally. According to these findings there appears to be no topical representation of somatic sensibility in this region.

It must be assumed that many other cortical regions in addition to area 5 are essential for the proper perception and interpretation of the large variety of sensory stimuli which reach the cerebral cortex. Furthermore, an integration of somatosensory information with optic, acoustic, and other messages will be of importance. In spite of some physiological studies on functional interrelations between various cortical areas, and their importance for processes such as perception, the question of how the brain handles all this information is still largely in the realm of speculation, and the available data gives no clues of practical value in clinical neurology. Other problems concern the collaboration between the two hemispheres in sensation and the relation between "sensory" and "motor" performances. Some clues may be gotten from a study of commissural and associational connections, to be discussed in Chapter 12. With reference to the somatosensory areas some recent findings are of interest. It has been demonstrated that in the cat there are ample interconnections between only certain parts of S I and S II, namely those related to the face, trunk, and the proximal limbs, while the distal limb areas do not have such interconnections (Ebner and Myers, 1965; Jones, 1967; Pandya and Vignolo, 1968; Jones and Powell, 1968b).

Furthermore, there are commissural connections between parts related to the face in S I and in the opposite S II and vice versa (Jones, 1967). According to Jones, with exception of the "motor" area, no other ipsilateral cortical area sends fibers to the somatic sensory areas. Corresponding findings were made in the monkey, and it was, furthermore, found that both S I and S II send a small number of fibers to the supplementary motor area. Largely corresponding findings are reported by Pandya and Vignolo (1968). The various bodily subdivisions within a sensory area are mutually interconnected. These findings indicate that there must be a much closer collaboration going on between the various sensory areas in the two hemispheres as concerns the face, trunk, and proximal parts of the extremities, than for the hand and foot.

The pathways for pain. On account of its practical importance, it is deemed appropriate to consider the problem of central pain transmission separately. It may at once be stated, however, that knowledge on this subject is rather sparse. In the following some of this information will be considered, while only few of the many hypothetical conceptions of the matter will be mentioned.

It may be right to emphasize a few facts at the outset. In the first place, pain is a subjective experience which requires the presence of consciousness. Subjectively, pain may be of many kinds. The appreciation of pain, the evaluation of its intensity, is subject to considerable variations from time to time in the same individual, depending on psychological and other factors; pain tends to increase if attention is directed to it, to decrease when attention is diverted from it.

A variety of stimuli, mechanical, thermal, chemical, and others, may produce pain. As discussed in the beginning of this chapter, the receptors for cutaneous pain are generally assumed to be free nerve endings. However, it is scarcely right to assume that sensations of pain can be elicited only on stimulation of free endings, and free nerve endings are certainly engaged in the reception of other types of stimuli. There is no particular fiber type in the peripheral nerves related to the transmission of impulses perceived subjectively as pain, but there is some evidence that a distinction may be made between two major groups conveying "fast" and "slow" pain, respectively. There is rather good evidence that in the spinal cord the substantia gelatinosa is particularly closely related to the transmission of painful impulses, but its role in this process is not clear. It may be considered as fairly certain that most of the fibers which transmit the painful impulses rostrally in the cord are found in the ventrolateral funiculus (cf. chordotomies), even if there may be other subsidiary pathways.

When we try to follow the paths taken beyond the spinal cord by impulses which give rise to the conscious appreciation of pain, we meet with perhaps greater problems than those concerning the preceding links in the "pain pathways." All too often one has been inclined to think of only the spinothalamic tract in this connection (perhaps on account of the results of chordotomies) and to forget that in the ventrolateral funiculus the spinothalamic fibers run intermingled with many others, among them spinoreticular and spinotectal fibers, which will be interrupted in chordotomies. If "pain impulses" ascend in the ventrolateral funiculus, they might, therefore, as well continue in these tracts as in the spinothalamic. Whether they do or do not has to be decided by physiological experiments and by clinicopathological studies. Both approaches meet with difficulties. For example, it is scarcely possible to be sure in experimental animals that one produces pure pain-eliciting stimuli. In human material reliable information can only be expected from cases with small and discrete lesions (which are rare) and in which a precise clinical examination has been made during life. With regard to neurophysiological observations it should be recalled that what concerns us here is the *conscious appreciation of pain.* Animal experiments in which abolition of reflexes elicitable on pain-producing stimuli has followed destruction of certain regions of the brain are accordingly of limited interest.

One of the most debated questions has been *whether the appreciation of pain involves the cerebral cortex,* more particularly, the postcentral gyrus. There is an extensive literature on this subject which goes back to the end of the nineteenth century. In spite of this, the problem is not solved. (For a brief review, see Marshall, 1951.) On electrical stimulation of the postcentral gyrus in conscious human beings, the patients very rarely report feeling pain. For example, in Penfield and Boldrey's (1937) large material only 11 of more than 800 responses to electrical stimulation of the postcentral gyrus were described as pain. Correspondingly, in the monkey, Mountcastle and Powell (1959b) found a few units in the first somatosensory area, which responded only to nociceptive stimuli. Following cortical ablations in man most authors have observed that the patient has retained his sensibility to painful stimuli. Others have found a reduction in pain sensibility or an elimination of pre-existing pain, for example phantom limb pain. As emphasized by Lewin and Phillips (1952), who described three cases of the latter type, such observations do not prove that the sensory cortex is involved in the conscious appreciation of pain, and they carefully state that "all we may conclude is that in these patients spontaneous pain is associated with activation of the sensory cortex." In a critical study of 18 patients with cortical wounds, Marshall (1951) reached a similar conclusion. He found impairment of pain and temperature sensibility in 11 of these patients. In two cases there was impairment of temperature sensibility but preservation of pain sensibility. Even if thus the cerebral cortex, presumably especially the postcentral gyrus, may be engaged in the appreciation of pain under certain conditions, it does not seem to be essential. However, there is considerable evidence that the *thalamus* is an important structure. This is evidenced by clinical as well as experimental observations.

Single units responding to stimuli which are presumably pain-producing (tissue destructive) were found by Poggio and Mountcastle (1960) and Whitlock and Perl (1961) in the posterior group (PO, see p. 75). Poggio and Mountcastle report that nearly 60 per cent of the PO neurons could be activated only by noxious stimuli and from large parts of the body.[20] Albe-Fessard and Bowsher (1965) found similar units in some of the nonspecific thalamic nuclei, including the centro-median nucleus. Although the termination of spinothalamic fibers in the CM is disputed (see Ch. 6) they supply the other thalamic regions where nociceptive neurons have been found. However, pain impulses appear to reach other regions of the brain as well. Thus following stimulation of the tooth pulp in cats (a procedure which is assumed to produce pain as it does in man) potentials were found in the n. parafascicularis and the periaqueductal gray by Kerr, Haugen, and Melzack (1955; see also Melzack and Haugen, 1957). There is some evidence that noxious stimuli give rise to potentials in the optic tectum (the colliculi), and nociceptive impulses have been shown to be particularly potent in influencing the ascending activating system, presumably by way of spinoreticular fibers (see Ch. 6).

Fiber connections from the reticular formation ascend to particularly the "nonspecific" (but also to some extent the specific) thalamic nuclei (see Ch. 6) as well as to the superior colliculus and the periaqueductal gray. The colliculi, particularly the superior (see Tarlov and Moore, 1966), project to the central gray and to certain thalamic nuclei, among them the PO complex (see also Altman and Carpenter, 1961). When taken together these and other anatomical and physiological observations strongly suggest that "pain impulses" may ascend along other routes than the spinothalamic tract. Clinical data supports this view. In order to relieve unbearable pain, transection of the spinothalamic tract in the mesencephalon (mesencephalic tractotomy) has been performed. Selective sections according to the somatotopical pattern (see Fig. 2-10) have resulted in analgesia in restricted parts of the body (Walker, 1942b, 1943). More recently, neurosurgeons have used a stereotactic approach (mesencephalotomy). There has often been immediale relief of pain

---

[20] Since such units are not likely to provide information concerning the location of the stimulus, Poggio and Mountcastle suggest as a possibility that simultaneous stimulation of mechanoreceptors may be responsible for the localization of the stimulus, an assumption which receives some support from observations in humans having suffered interruption of the lemniscal system. In these patients the capacity to localize a painful stimulus is poor.

and a more or less complete hemianalgesia or hypalgesia on the opposite side of the body and face. However, after some time spontaneous pain and pain sensibility appear often to return to some extent. This has been observed even if the lesion, in addition to the spinothalamic tract, has included part of the medial lemniscus (Torvik, 1959). Since the spino-tectal fibers ascend close to the spinothalamic in the mesencephalon, the two tracts are likely to be interrupted together. Searching for pathways which may be responsible for transmitting pain impulses following mesen-cephalic tractotomies or stereotactic mesencephalotomies, several authors have suggested a spino-reticulo-thalamic route as the most likely. Bow-sher (1957) is even inclined to associate this pathway with diffuse slow pain, the spinothalamic tract with fast, localized pain. The fact that the spinothalamic and reticulothalamic fibers in part end in the same thalamic nuclei (see Ch. 6) introduces further problems.

As referred to above, there is physiological evidence that noxious stimuli give rise to potentials in the PO group of the thalamus. One would expect, therefore, that this part of the thalamus might be especially closely related to pain perception in man. However, the evidence on this point is meager. In recent years some information has been obtained from stimulations of thalamic points during stereotactic operations for the relief of thalamic pain and from the results of stereotactic destruction of parts of the thalamus.

Cooper (1965a) reports that relatively large lesions within the specific nuclei which project to somesthetic cortex "do not produce appreciable lasting objective sensory deficit on the contralateral side of the body." On the other hand, other authors (Hassler and Riechert, 1959; Bettag and Yoshida, 1960; Mark, Ervin, and Hackett, 1960; and others) have obtained relief of spontaneous pain, with or without concomitant analgesia or hypalgesia, following stereotactic destruction of the posterior part of the nucleus ventralis posterior. Only in relatively few cases has post-mortem control of the lesions been made and, as a rule, the lesions have extended somewhat more rostrally than to the region presumably corresponding to the PO group (as evidenced by the ensuing sensory loss of other qualities than pain, sometimes somatotopically localized). Mark, Ervin, and Yakovlev (1963) have undertaken a correlation of anatomical sites of the lesions with clinical and experimental findings in stereotactic-thalamotomy. They conclude that lesions restricted to the "sensory relay nuclei" of the thalamus result in profound sensory loss with little pain relief. In cases where good pain relief with little sensory loss had been obtained the lesions included the parafascicular and intralaminar nuclei. (Lesions of the dorsomedial and anterior thalamic nuclei were followed by a pronounced change in affect, see also below.) Hassler and Riechert (1959) found loss predominantly of pain and temperature sensibility following destruc-tion of the basal parts of what appears to correspond to VPL (Hassler's small-celled V.c.pc.). On stimulation of this region the patients reported pain sensa-tions. However, Hassler (1960, 1966a) concludes that this is not the only thalamic nucleus related to pain. Other attempts to locate the thalamic structures involved in pain perception have aimed at determining the site of the lesion in cases of spontaneous "thalamic pain." In some cases of this kind a circumscribed lesion of vascular origin has been found in the caudalmost part of the VPL (Hoffmann, 1933; Garcin and Lapresle, 1954; and others). It is an apparent paradox that a destruction of this part, presumably involved in transmission (and integration?) of pain sensations gives rise to pain. Several theoretical explanations have been set forth (see, for example, Hassler, 1966a), but a satisfactory theory is still lacking.

The only conclusion which can apparently be drawn, so far, concerning the thalamus and pain is that in addition to the PO group, and presumably to some extent the VPL, other thalamic regions are probably involved, perhaps particularly some of the "nonspecific" nuclei. Central "pain transmission" does not appear to be a function of the spinothalamic tract only, but is apparently taken care of by several other fiber connections as well, not least, perhaps, the spino-reticulo-thalamic pathway. The central processes related to pain perception appear to be extremely complex. It may indeed be misleading to consider "pain sensibility" as a sensory quality of a similar kind as, for example, tactile and joint sensibility.[21] This is suggested especially by the fact that pain sensations are far more closely linked with emotion than any other sensations, a well-known experience from daily life. Objective evidence for this close correlation comes from experimental as well as clinical experience. Of particular interest are observations of patients subjected to so-called prefrontal leucotomy (see Ch. 12) since, following this operation, a pre-existing pain may still be present, but it does not hurt any more, it is not of concern to the patient. Similar effects have been described following cingulumotomy (Foltz and White, 1962). (In this connection it may be recalled that the cingulate gyrus receives thalamic afferents from the anterior thalamic nucleus, the frontal cortex from the dorsomedial nucleus.) Some aspects of visceral pain will be considered in Chapter 11.

Examination of somatic sensibility. Before describing the clinical symptoms resulting from lesions of the somatic sensory system, some remarks on the examination of sensory changes are appropriate. A complete examination of sensibility, aiming at a thorough mapping out of losses or changes of the different sensory modalities, is usually a tiresome and lengthy procedure for the patient (as well as for the examiner), and it ought on this account to be performed in several steps, if possible, the

---

[21] The problems of pain have been discussed at length in a number of publications, and theories abound. Among some relevant references the following may be mentioned: Lewis, 1942; "Pain," (vol. 23, *Ass. Res. Nerv. Ment. Dis.*), 1943; White and Sweet, 1955; Keele, 1957; Noordenbos, 1959. A recent theory (Albe-Fessard and Delacour, 1968), based on anatomical and physiological observations, appears to give a rational explanation of some features concerning central pain mechanisms. (See also Albe-Fessard, 1968).

first examination aiming only at a rough orientation. As the examination requires the co-operation of the patient, the results may be severely invalidated if the patient is tired. Without the friendly co-operation of the patient nothing can be achieved. Furthermore, it is of supreme importance for the reliability of the results obtained that the patient is of a normal level of intelligence, as clearly his mental equipment to a large extent determines his capacity not only of analyzing his sensations but also of describing them properly. In mentally defective persons even the most thorough examination of the sensory functions will be futile, not least on account of their great suggestibility.

It is important to realize that, in the examination of sensory functions, *what is registered are the subjective sensations which the patient experiences.* They are the result, not only of the stimulation of one or more types of receptors, but also of the analysis and integration of the impressions perceived, a process which must be assumed to take place at higher levels of the central nervous system, presumably first and foremost in the cerebral cortex. Saying, for example, as is often done, that the dorsal columns convey impulses of vibratory sense, joint sensibility, and two-point discrimination does not imply that each of these modalities is mediated by its separate receptors and fiber systems.[22] On the contrary, it is extremely probable, and for certain modalities practically certain, that the sensations experienced result from a simultaneous stimulation of several types of receptors, and that just this simultaneous stimulation is responsible for the complex character of the sensation. A loss of a certain type of sensibility on this account cannot always be interpreted as indicating a lesion of a definite part of the anatomical substratum.

As will be further elucidated below, more refined methods of examination may reveal changes of sensibility which are not detected by the usually applied routine methods. By grading the intensity of the stimuli, information can be obtained of altered threshold values of the receptors, and reduction of the territory to which the stimulus is applied may disguise slighter reductions of sensibility, otherwise not detected and not observed by the patient himself. The more refined the methods applied, the more complex the matter of sensibility appears to be, as has been seen from the data presented in preceding sections of this chapter.

These preliminary considerations ought to be borne in mind when the symptoms produced by lesions of the somatic sensory "systems" are

---

[22] Walshe (1942a) has emphasized this very clearly as follows: "There is no such *thing* as localization or discrimination, there are only things localized or discriminated, and we cannot conceive of an impulse that allows us to localize or to separate without making us aware of the thing localized or separated."

considered. The following description will be limited to the central parts of these "systems." The symptoms following lesions of the visceral sensory "system" are treated in Chapter 11.

Symptoms following lesions of the dorsal roots. The pathological processes affecting the *dorsal roots* may, like damage to many other parts of the nervous system, give rise to irritative symptoms as well as to deficiency phenomena.

Irritative symptoms may appear when the dorsal roots are the subject of traction, compression, or other mechanical influences, when they are the seat of inflammatory changes, or when their blood supply is interfered with. Most frequently the irritation betrays itself as pain, "radicular pain," "root pain," a pain which is more or less exactly limited to the dermatome belonging to the affected root, eventually also to the deeper structures supplied by the root. Affections of the thoracic roots therefore manifest themselves typically as girdle pains. They may vary in intensity, sometimes reaching intolerable height. If the irritation is slight the pain may occasionally be limited only to certain minor areas within the dermatome, the so-called *maximal points of Head,* e.g. to the inguinal sulcus and the trochanter major in lesions of the first lumbar dorsal root.

A special type of root pain is the *lancinating pain,* found in some cases of tabes dorsalis. It is characterized by occurring in fits, varying in intensity and irradiation in the zone of distribution of the affected roots. The *tabetic crises,* which appear to be related to the lancinating pain, appear as periodically recurring, often excessive pains, usually localized by the patient to one of the inner organs. They are frequently accompanied by motor or secretory irritative symptoms. Most usual, perhaps, are the gastric crises, where the pain is felt in the epigastrium, and is accompanied by a pronounced hyperesthesia of the skin in this region. It is generally believed that these tabetic crises are also due to an irritation of the dorsal roots, but in this case predominantly the visceral afferent fibers are affected, in the case of the gastric crises the 6th–9th thoracic dorsal roots which supply the stomach. Consequently the hyperesthetic dermatomes are those belonging to these roots. (The visceral afferent impulses are discussed more fully in Ch. 11.)

Radicular pain, however, does not necessarily accompany lesions of the dorsal roots. Occasionally the pain appears to be entirely absent in such cases, but frequently when it is absent other irritative phenomena occur, which may eventually also be present together with pain. Not infrequently *paresthesias* are met with: sensations of numbness, pricking, tingling, or other peculiar sensations. Naturally these paresthesias will occur only as long as some of these root fibers remain intact. They are localized, as well as the *hyperesthetic areas* which also may occur, to the dermatomes supplied by the affected roots. On this account they may be a valuable guide in the diagnosis of the level of intraspinal morbid processes.

If the pathological process of the dorsal roots progresses, the fibers in the root will be more or less damaged, and finally their conductive capacity will be entirely lost.[23]

The deficiency symptoms in lesions of the dorsal roots will consequently be a diminished sensibility, a hypo-esthesia, or a complete loss of sensibility, *an anesthesia,* and the distribution of these changes will correspond to the dermatomes of the affected roots, i.e. they will be *characterized by a segmental upper and lower limit.* Since the fibers conveying impulses of the various types are intermingled in the dorsal roots, *as a rule this sensory loss will comprise all sensory modalities,* superficial (cutaneous) as well as deep. However, aberrations are not infrequently encountered, in so far as the different modalities are affected to different degrees. This is usually explained by assuming that the different types of fibers display different resistance toward deleterious influences. The fibers conveying touch are said to be more resistant than those transmitting impulses of pain and temperature. In recent years *intrathectal injections of phenol* have been employed as a therapeutical measure, primarily in order to interrupt the central conduction of pain impulses. The method is based on the assumption that the phenol solution when it infiltrates the roots destroys chiefly thin fibers, among these the "pain" fibers. Experimental electrophysiological studies appeared to lend some support for this assumption (Nathan and Sears, 1960), but pathological anatomical findings have not corroborated it (see Nathan, Sears, and Smith, 1965; Hansebout and Cosgrove, 1966). It is possible to apply the phenol solution fairly precisely in the vicinity of a particular root, and also to deposit it near to ventral roots. The latter procedure has been used to counteract spasticity in paraplegic patients, on the assumption that the phenol will chiefly affect the γ-fibers. However, α-fibers are also affected (see Koppang, 1962; Pedersen and Juul-Jensen, 1965, for some data on results).

More important than "dissociations" of this type, however, is the fact, previously mentioned, that the dermatomes vary in regard to different qualities. *The dermatomes of touch extend over a somewhat larger territory than those of pain and temperature* (cf. Fig. 2-6).

As already mentioned, on this account, *interruption of one dorsal root will usually give no definite sensory loss,* although careful examination may reveal a limited zone of analgesia or hypalgesia, because of the

[23] It is worthy of notice, however, that pain may be present even when the fibers in a dorsal root are completely interrupted. This "anesthesia dolorosa," with a segmental sensory loss and concomitant radicular pain, is assumed to arise when the fibers are interrupted, but the pathological process, e.g. a tumor, still exerts some irritation on the proximal stump of the root.

somewhat more restricted overlap of the "pain" fibers. But it is important to remember that the *absence of a segmental sensory loss does not exclude the possibility of a lesion to a single dorsal root.* Using refined methods, however, in such instances some minor sensory changes can usually be detected.

When a segmental sensory symptom is present it is important to remember that within the spinal canal the nerve roots (except the upper cervical roots) follow a descending course on their way to the intervertebral foramen. The more caudal the root, the longer is the distance between its point of exit from the cord to its intervertebral foramen. This is shown in Fig. 3-8, and, as explained more fully in Chapter 3, if overlooked, may give rise to diagnostic errors.

A segmental sensory loss, produced by a lesion of one or more dorsal roots, may be encountered in different pathological processes. The most typical instances are perhaps encountered in *intraspinal tumors,* for example, neurinomas originating from one of the dorsal roots, or where a protruded intervertebral disc affects the root. In the latter case the region of impaired sensibility is most frequently localized to the 5th lumbar or 1st sacral dermatome. As a rule, an exact analysis of the distribution of the sensory loss or impairment will make it possible to decide whether it is of the radicular type or is due to a peripheral nerve lesion. The most important clue is given by the distribution of the sensory changes. Signs of motor impairment may, however, be present in both cases, but usually these are more prominent where peripheral nerves are affected. If a single mixed nerve is damaged, the motor and sensory disturbances will be confined to the structures supplied by it. The motor impairment in lesions of the dorsal roots may be due to a simultaneous affection of the ventral roots as well, caused, for example, by pressure of the tumor. In this case the paresis or paralysis will also be segmentally distributed (cf. Ch. 3). Or the disturbed motor functions may be due to affection of the long descending motor pathways, producing a mono- or hemiplegia according to the intensity and level of the lesion (cf. below). Finally, autonomic disturbances may be present or may be ascertained by special tests, such as the sweat test (cf. Ch. 11).

On account of their practical importance the symptoms occurring in cases of *intraspinal protrusion or herniation of an intervertebral disc* will be briefly considered. This condition is due to degenerative processes of one or more intervertebral discs. The result is that the nucleus pulposus is pushed in a dorsal direction, with or without a defect in the annulus fibrosus. In some cases a *thickening of the ligamentum flavum* (between the vertebral laminae) gives rise to similar symptoms. A thickening of the ligamentum flavum is occasionally found together with a herniated disc. The degenerative process in itself may also produce similar symptoms (osteochondrosis columnae).[24]

In the majority of cases the lumbar discs are affected, and among these again the discs between the 4th and 5th lumbar and between the latter and the 1st sacral vertebrae are most commonly those producing clinical symptoms. The symptoms can be explained on the basis of the conditions arising in the spinal canal when a protrusion is present and will differ according to whether it takes place laterally or near the midline. The localization of the symptoms will depend on which root or roots are affected. It is not unusual that more than one root is involved. The oblique course of the lumbar roots in the spinal canal (see Fig. 3-8) explains that when more than one root is affected the roots leaving the canal at lower levels than the one primarily affected will be involved. This is seen in Fig. 2-20, where a lateral protrusion originating from the disc between the 4th and 5th vertebrae presses on the 5th root but, in addition, also affects the 1st sacral root. A median prolapse is apt to affect the roots of both sides, and, if large, will give gross symptoms due to its pressure on the cauda equina. Extensive damage to the lumbar and sacral roots may be observed, making the differential diagnosis against an intraspinal tumor difficult.

[24] In autopsy studies of the human cord it is not uncommon to find meningeal changes in the lumbar and sacral nerve roots, in the form of arachnoidal proliferations, often combined with cyst formations (see Rexed and Wennström, 1959). These changes are most often found in elderly persons, and are commonly multiple. It is not clear to what extent they may give symptoms of "back-ache" or sciatica. Beatty, Sugar, and Fox (1968) report findings in a series of patients in whom clinical symptoms of lumbar and sacral root compression appeared to be due to a folding of the posterior longitudinal ligament. The cause of this may be a degeneration of a disc.

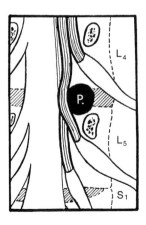

FIG. 2–20 A diagram illustrating the pressure exerted by a protruded 4th intervertebral disc. Originating laterally, the protrusion (*P*) affects the 5th lumbar root but in addition affects the 1st sacral root. Redrawn from Spurling and Grantham (1940).

The first sign of pressure of a protruded intervertebral disc usually comes from the dorsal root affected. This is manifested as pain and is frequently preceded by transient attacks of low back pain. Not infrequently the symptoms begin acutely, when the patient lifts a heavy weight while he is bending forward. In ventroflexion of the back the nucleus pulposus is pushed dorsally, and the degenerated annulus may give way or rupture. The *pain* is more or less clearly localized in the area of distribution of the affected root, and in affections of the 5th lumbar and 1st sacral clinically appears as sciatica. (It should be stressed, however, that "sciatica" may be due to several pathological conditions other than protrusion of an intervertebral disc, since the fibers proceeding from the roots into the nerve may be affected also in the pelvis and the thigh.) The pain is usually assumed to be a consequence of pressure on the nerve fibers of the root (see, however, below). Characteristic are the exacerbations following increase of intracranial pressure, such as occurs in sneezing, coughing, and straining. Compression of the jugular veins also usually augments the pain for the same reason. Raising of the straight leg (Lasègue's sign) increases the pain or is painful when spontaneous pain is absent, in severe cases even when the leg is raised only 20° or even less. This phenomenon has been explained as being due to stretching of the nerve fibers (when the ankle is dorsiflexed the pain is still more exaggerated). It is commonly assumed that reflex spasm of the muscles at the back of the thigh is also responsible for some of the pain. Most patients are in less pain when lying than sitting (usually, however, sitting with a more or less extended hip). This has been explained by the assumption that pressure on the vertebral discs is less in the lying position than when the spine is kept erect, and thus allows the protrusion to recede somewhat. When the patient is standing a *scoliosis* is regularly seen, most often with the tilt to the side opposite the protrusion. This, as well as the common flattening of the *lumbar lordosis,* may be explained on the same basis: a slight movement of the spine to the opposite side and a slight ventroflexion may relieve the protruding force and the pressure on the root. However, in other instances the tilt is to the side of the protrusion, and other explanations must be sought. The slackening of the root passing over the protrusion (see below) during the movement to this side may be of relevance. The mechanical situation in the spinal canal in cases of protruded discs may obviously be different among patients, depending on the site and size of the protrusion, its consistency, the degree of degeneration and flattening of the disc, concomitant alterations in the vertebral joints, and other factors.

If one root only is affected, a hypoesthesia will frequently not be discovered, except by testing very carefully for sensibility to pain (cf.

9 8

above). The *hypalgesia,* if present, is limited to the affected dermatome. Thus in lesions of the 5th lumbar root it will be mainly found on the lateral aspect of the calf, sometimes extending toward the dorsum of the 1st toe; in lesions of the 1st sacral root the area is found on the heel, extending beneath the lateral malleolus on the lateral aspect of the foot (cf. Fig. 2-5 on the dermatomes). The *ankle-jerk* is weakened or abolished if the 1st sacral root is affected. (The knee-jerk is usually influenced by lesions of the 3rd or 4th lumbar roots.) In some cases *paresthesias* occur, of the same segmental distribution as the pain and hypalgesia.

If the ventral roots are affected, a *motor impairment* will ensue. When one root only is damaged a pareses may be inconspicuous, but like the sensory changes, its distribution will be segmental and may aid in the diagnosis. When the protrusion is larger, there will occasionally be changes in the cerebrospinal fluid at levels beneath the lesion, but on the whole the purely clinical signs are the most important for diagnosis. Myelography may verify the exact site of the protrusion, but several neurosurgeons have stressed that it is usually possible to determine this by aid of the clinical examination alone, if a careful analysis is made of the segmental distribution of the sensory, motor, and reflex changes.

It should be remembered that although protrusion of intervertebral discs is by far the most common in the lower lumbar spine, it may occur in any intervertebral disc. Particularly those originating from the lower cervical discs should be borne in mind since they give rise to symptoms which may be interpreted as due to other affections. In the rather rare protrusions of thoracic discs, symptoms are often uncharacteristic. However, these protrusions are particularly apt to result in compression of the cord and, therefore, may require immediate operative treatment (see Kite, Whitfield, and Campbell, 1957).

As referred to above, it is commonly said that the symptoms from the spinal nerve roots in intervertebral disc protrusions are due to pressure on the roots. This view appears, however, not to be entirely correct, according to a study of Breig (1960). It has been believed that the spinal cord and the dura move up and down in the vertebral canal as the spine is bent forward or backward. Breig found no evidence of this. In an extensive study on autopsy material he demonstrated that in ventroflexion the cord is straight, and so are the dura and the roots (see Fig. 2-21, to the left). On dorsiflexion when the vertebral canal is shortened the spinal cord also shortens, with a consequent folding of the dura, most marked dorsally (Fig. 2-21, to the right). The nerve roots are slackened as well. Microscopic studies showed that while the longitudinal nerve fibers of the cord are straight in ventroflexion, they assume a wavy course when the cord is shortened in dorsiflexion. As might be expected, this shorten-

99

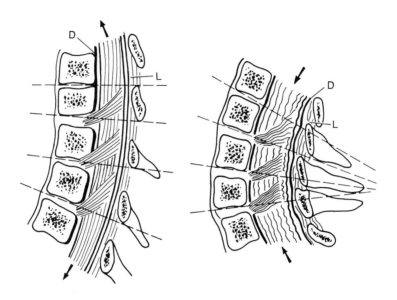

FIG. 2–21 Diagrammatic representation of the change in form of the lower cervical spine and of the concomitant changes in the cord and nerve roots occurring on bending of the spine. In ventroflexion (to the left) the cord, dura (*D*), nerve roots, and ligamenta flava (*L*) are straight. In dorsiflexion of the spine (to the right) all structures are shortened, especially the most dorsally situated ones. (Cf. text.) Redrawn from Breig (1960).

ing is compensated by an increase in the transverse direction; the cross area of all levels of the cord is larger in dorsiflexion than in ventroflexion. On lateral movements of the body the cord is shortened on the side to which the bending takes place, and straight on the other. Obviously mutual rearrangements take place between the elements of the soft tissues of the cord during movements.

These findings have important bearing on diagnostic and therapeutic problems, as dealt with in some detail by Breig (1960). Thus in exposing the cord during operative interventions, the risk of traumatization is reduced if the cord is slack, i.e. the spine is dorsiflexed. With regard to the symptoms from the roots occurring in protrusion of an intervertebral disc, it appears that the protrusion does not necessarily have to compress the root, but when the nerve "rides" on the protrusion a movement which causes stretching of the root may produce pain because the root is not free to stretch normally. Since the roots are solidly fixed in the intervertebral foramina the appearance of pain on Lasègue's test may in part be due to the ventroflexion of the spine which ensues when the leg is raised with concomitant stretching of the roots. The pain on coughing and sneezing may likewise be explained in part by the straightening of the back which takes place. The observations of Breig have a bearing also on other types of diseases involving the cord, as discussed by the author.

It is of some interest that the spinal dura is only innervated (from the meningeal rami) on its ventral aspect (Edgar and Nundy, 1966). This explains why piercing the dura on lumbar puncture is not painful. Fine unmyelinated nerve fibers have been found in the annulus fibrosus (Roofe, 1940). A recurrent branch from the 2nd lumbar nerve descends on the dorsal aspect of the vertebrae, in the posterior longitudinal ligament, and can be followed to the level of the 5th lumbar vertebra. Irritation of this branch may explain the common occurrence of low back pain in protrusions of lumbar discs.

Symptoms following lesions of the dorsal horn and of the central gray matter of the cord. A *segmental sensory disturbance can be caused* not only by affections of the dorsal roots but *also by lesions of the dorsal horns.* This is a consequence of the anatomical arrangement whereby many of the afferent fibers from the spinal ganglia are distributed to the cells in the dorsal horns in the segment in which they enter the cord. Irritative symptoms may appear, most frequently as pain of radicular distribution, or a radicular sensory loss may be found. "Dorsal horn pains," however, occur less frequently than "dorsal root pains." Presumably symptoms of this kind, indicating a damage to the dorsal horns, arise most frequently in syringomyelia or hematomyelia. However, there is a *characteristic difference between the symptoms following lesions of the dorsal roots and dorsal horns. In the latter case the classical dissociated sensory loss may be found where the sensibility to temperature and pain is abolished or weakened, whereas the sense of touch appears to be intact when tested with routine methods.* In lesions of the dorsal roots, as previously mentioned, all sensory modalities are affected. The explanation of the different symptomatology in the two types of lesions is to be found in the anatomical arrangement of the sensory fibers (Figs. 2-3 and 2-7). The fibers conveying impulses of temperature and pain are among those which enter the dorsal horn of the gray matter to terminate on its cells in the same or neighboring segments from which the spinothalamic tract takes its origin. Consequently a lesion of the dorsal horn will affect these fibers and eventually interrupt them. On the other hand, the medial group of fibers entering the cord and ascending to the nuclei of the dorsal funiculus will escape destruction as long as the lesion is confined to the gray matter. As these fibers mediate sensations of touch this sensory quality will not be affected. *Likewise the deep sensibility (joint sense, vibratory sensibility) will be preserved.* Furthermore, the sense of discrimination, the ability to distinguish qualities like smooth-

1 0 1

ness, roughness, and others, is not affected. Also, in this respect, a dorsal horn lesion differs from a dorsal root lesion.

A lesion of the central parts of the gray matter of the spinal cord will produce the same symptoms as a dorsal horn lesion. In this instance the crossing fibers from the cells of the dorsal horn forming the spinothalamic tracts will be interrupted, whereas the long ascending fibers of the dorsal funiculi will remain untouched. However, the symptoms will obviously, as a rule, occur bilaterally.

In summary, *a sensory loss with a segmental or approximately segmental upper and lower border points to a lesion of the dorsal roots, of the dorsal horn, or in the central part of the gray matter. If the sensory loss is of the dissociated type it indicates that the morbid process is located in the dorsal horn or in the central gray matter.* Most frequently this is seen in syringomyelia.

Now it is of course evident that a lesion affecting a dorsal horn or the central gray matter of the cord will often be of large dimensions, be it a syringomyelia, a hematomyelia, or an intramedullary tumor. The pathological process will frequently tend to invade the surrounding parts of the cord, ventrally the ventral horns, or to both sides the white matter. As all experience shows, the pathological processes arising in the gray matter of the cord are to a certain extent inclined to confine themselves first and foremost to it. This is, for example, often the case in syringomyelia. The process most frequently starts from the central parts of the gray matter, and later on extends in a dorsal direction to affect the dorsal horns, but also ventrally to the ventral horns. *Pari passu* with the progressing destruction of the anterior horn cells, a paresis and finally a paralysis will develop, affecting the muscles supplied by the diseased segments of the cord. (As described in Ch. 3 this paresis is of the peripheral type, characterized by atrophy, loss of tone, and weakened or abolished myotatic reflexes.) Syringomyelia, as mentioned, shows a predilection for starting in the upper thoracic and lower cervical segments; later on it extends rostrally and also caudally. The first clinical signs therefore are, as a rule, segmental sensory disturbances, usually followed soon after by motor disturbances, from the ulnar fingers and the ulnar side of the hand and forearm. With the progression of the anatomical changes the clinical symptoms spread to the radial side of the hand, frequently also the forearm and arm and eventually the thorax. A similar development of the symptoms is often displayed also by intramedullary tumors, which, likewise, most frequently start in the lower part of the cervical cord.

Sensory symptoms following lesions of the anterolateral funiculi of the spinal cord. Other types of sensory disturbances will ensue if the long ascending sensory paths in the cord are damaged. The symptoms

102

are different in lesions of the dorsal funiculi and of the anterolateral funiculi. We may begin by considering the latter, and confine ourselves to the sensory symptoms. The motor symptoms, which are frequent companions of the sensory, will be briefly treated below in connection with a discussion of transverse lesions of the cord.

From what has already been said it is evident that *a destruction of the anterolateral funiculus of the spinal cord will be followed by a loss of pain and temperature sense on the contralateral side of the body at all levels caudal to the site of the lesion,* as the tracts conveying pain and temperature sensations are made up of axons crossing the median line, arising from cells in the dorsal horn (cf. Figs. 2-3 and 2-7). Furthermore, as the crossing is completed over a distance of not more than two segments, the upper border of the sensory loss will correspond approximately to the lower border of the dermatome belonging to the lowest preserved segment of the cord. However, this will be true only under the presupposition that the lesion is deep enough to reach nearly to the gray matter of the cord, thus interrupting *all* fibers of the spinothalamic tract at the level in question. *If the lesion is limited to the more superficial parts of the tract, a more restricted sensory loss will ensue,* and its upper limit will be found several segments farther caudally, the more so the more superficial the lesion. This is a natural consequence of the anatomical arrangement of the fibers already described, the longest fibers, derived from the caudal levels, being situated most superficially (see Fig. 2-8). This is a point of considerable clinical importance, since ignorance of this condition may lead to a false segmental diagnosis.

To give an example: A patient complains of radicular pain at the level of the right nipple (corresponding to the 4th–5th thoracic dermatomes). He presents a hypo-esthetic belt at this level with affection of all sensory modalities. In addition, however, the examination reveals a hypo-esthesia to pain and temperature from the inguinal sulcus (1st lumbar dermatome) and downwards on the other, left, side. These symptoms may be due to a developing intraspinal tumor, e.g., a neurofibroma, arising from the right 4th or 5th thoracic dorsal root. This tumor causes the radicular pain, and by destruction of the fibers of the roots is responsible for the hypo-esthetic belt. But the tumor has also exerted pressure on the lateral side of the cord and has damaged the most superficially situated fibers at this place, which convey impulses of pain and temperature from the lumbar and sacral segments of the other side. If the tumor is allowed to continue its growth, the hypo-esthesia to pain and temperature will gradually ascend and include the succeeding lower thoracic dermatomes. Of course in such a case, motor disturbances are also quite frequently found, e.g. paresis of the leg on the side of the lesion, and symptoms due to affection of the dorsal funiculus.

It is customary to say that lesions of the anterolateral funiculi produce loss of pain and temperature sensibility, whereas touch sensibility is pre-

served. However, if in these cases the superficial tactile sensibility is examined by refined methods, this usually also presents some reduction. (The same applies to lesions of the dorsal horns and the central gray matter.) This and other findings demonstrate that the anterolateral funiculi also contain fibers subserving touch sensibility. Their amount appears to present some individual variation. Furthermore, as previously mentioned, clinical experience teaches that the fibers within the anterolateral column are not only arranged according to their segmental origin, but also to a certain extent, according to sensory qualities. The fibers conveying impulses of deep pressure sense and superficial touch appear to be gathered predominantly in the ventral parts, whereas those mediating impulses of pain are found more dorsolaterally and the fibers for temperature sense in the dorsalmost part of the tract, closely ventral to the corticospinal tract. This is indicated diagrammatically in Fig. 2-8.

A few individuals have what is called "congenital insensitivity to pain." Postmortem examinations of the central nervous system and nerves performed in a few such cases have been negative. However, Swanson, Buchan, and Alvord (1965) found in a boy having presented insensitivity to pain and defective temperature sensibility, an absence of small cells in the dorsal root ganglia, lack of small fibers in the dorsal roots, and absence of the tract of Lissauer.

Valuable information concerning these problems has been gained during recent years by operative section of the anterolateral funiculi, *chordotomy,* already referred to. It is found that sections which include the entire anterolateral funiculus on one side are followed by a slight reduction of the sensibility to touch also, whereas this is not the case if the ventral parts of the funiculus are spared. Furthermore, a slight reduction of temperature and pain sensibility has been ascertained on the operated side also. This agrees well with the anatomical finding that some of the axons from cells of the dorsal horns do not cross but ascend in the homolateral anterolateral funiculus. Some of the pain and temperature impulses thus evidently traverse the cord without crossing. Another observation is in accord with this. Following a successful unilateral chordotomy, the patient is usually free from pain for some time if the pain has been unilateral. After a varying interval of time, however, some pain usually recurs, and the pain sensibility reappears to a certain degree. The common interpretation of this phenomenon is that the normally subsidiary homolateral pain fibers gradually take over some of the functions previously performed by the crossing ones, and a practical consequence is that even with unilateral pain a bilateral chordotomy will give better results than a unilateral one, and is recommended. However, even following a bilateral chordotomy a certain degree of pain and temperature sensibility may reappear.

104

Foerster (1936a) assumed this to be due to scanty fibers in the extreme dorsal part of the anterolateral funiculus which may escape destruction, or to some pain-conducting fibers in the dorsal funiculi (cf. below). The possibility also exists that some pain impulses may ascend in the sympathetic trunk, for even after a complete transverse lesion of the cord some pain sensibility may be present. These "aberrant" pathways for pain and temperature sensations appear to be better developed from the lower sacral segments. At least this may be an explanation of the fact that, in lesions of the spinal cord these dermatomes, i.e., of the anogenital region, are frequently either entirely spared or less severely affected than the more rostral segmental areas. This applies to bilateral, but especially to unilateral, lesions of the cord. A possibility also to be taken into consideration where the lesion is not complete is that fibers from the lower sacral segments may be uncrossed to a larger extent than those from more rostral segments (cf. the nearly always bilateral sensations on stimulation of the anogenital area in the first somatosensory cortical area).

It may happen that following a unilateral chordotomy the patient experiences pain in a part of the body where it had not been felt before, most often the same place on the opposite side of the body. Nathan (1963) assumes that this is due to a reference of the original pain: "Impulses arising from the neoplasm are blocked in the opposite spinothalamic tract, but they reach the neurological substratum of consciousness by other pathways." In a review of the results of chordotomy in 104 patients, Nathan (1963) found that the results were not as good as may appear from many reports. In a fair number of cases there are sensory disturbances, as reappearance of pain and occurrence of dysesthesisas. Furthermore, other complications are common, some of them being indeed unavoidable, since it is impossible to transect only the spinothalamic fibers. Thus some disturbances in micturition and defecation regularly occur, due to the course with the spinothalamic tract of afferent fibers from sacral segments, and because the descending fibers to the sacral cord related to the bladder and rectum (Nathan and Smith, 1958) will be interrupted by the operation. Motor disturbances may also appear.

In any consideration of the results of chordotomy the complexities in the anatomical and functional organization of the nervous system should be borne in mind. In the first place, it is obvious that section of the anterolateral funiculus interrupts other ascending as well as descending fiber tracts than those mediating pain. Secondly, the spinothalamic tract is certainly not the only pathway along which impulses arising on stimulation of pain receptors may be conveyed centrally. As mentioned previously, it may well be that the interruption of spinoreticular fibers is as important as the section of the spinothalamic tract, since pain stimuli are potent activators of the reticular formation (see Ch. 6).

Sensory symptoms following lesions of the dorsal funiculi. Whereas the anterolateral funiculi are engaged in the transmission of pain, temperature, and, furthermore, superficial touch and deep pressure, the other large ascending sensory system, that of the dorsal funiculi, transmits primarily different types of superficial tactile sensibility and deep sensibility, namely the proprioceptive impulses which reach consciousness. Since these tracts ascend in the spinal cord without crossing, *the symptoms ensuing on lesions of the dorsal funiculi will always appear on the side of the lesion* (in contradistinction to those following damage to the anterolateral funiculi). The results of recent anatomical and physiological studies, described in a previous section of this chapter, are on the whole in good accord with the conclusions drawn from findings in clinical studies of patients, correlated with post-mortem anatomical examinations.

It has long been known that a morbid process limited to the dorsal funiculi will give no clear-cut loss of the simple sensibility of cutaneous touch, and it is sometimes stated that *the sense of touch as well as of pain and temperature is preserved in lesions of the dorsal funiculi.* However, concerning the touch sensibility, certain qualifications have to be made. Even if a patient with his dorsal funiculi severely damaged is able to perceive very slight cutaneous touch stimuli, a more detailed examination, including a determination of the amount of "touch spots" and threshold values, usually reveals some reduction of touch sensibility. Conditions are similar to those prevailing in the system of the anterolateral funiculi. It appears that if one of the two systems subserving touch sensibility suffers, the other cannot sufficiently take over the function of both. However, this reduction is so moderate that it is of no practical relevance. Clinically important, however, is that *lesions of the dorsal funiculi produce defects in the sense of discrimination.* The capacity of differentiating two simultaneously applied touch stimuli is reduced. Examining, for example, with Weber's test, it will be found that the distance between two points which can be appreciated as separate is enlarged. The capacity of recognizing figures and letters drawn on the skin is lessened, and the patient is only able to indicate approximately which point of the body is touched. In lesions of the gracile nucleus, for example, the patient cannot tell which toe is being touched. It is, furthermore, difficult or impossible for him to decide if the object with which he is being touched is rough or smooth, hard or soft.

These observations are in complete accord with physiological studies which have demonstrated a high degree of stimulus, as well as place, specificity in the dorsal column nuclei, as described in some detail above. As we have seen, the same is true for the further links of this pathway to the cerebral cortex. The different aspects of the discrimination itself are probably purely cortical processes, based on a synthesis and integration of impressions gained from several types of receptors. It seems far-fetched and illogical to postulate the existence of special paths for discrimination.[25]

[25] As already referred to, Cook and Browder (1965), in some patients sub-

In clinical studies of dorsal column affections *vibratory sensibility* is diminished or even abolished, in agreement with the physiological observations of units in the dorsal column nuclei responding to vibratory stimuli. It appears from clinical studies that pain and temperature sense also have a certain connection with the dorsal funiculi. In lesions of these a reduction of the threshold values and the number of pain spots has been noted (Foerster, 1936a), and the type of painful stimuli applied is not recognized, due probably to reduced discriminatory abilities. Direct irritation of the dorsal funiculi is painful. This data, compared with the results of studies of the sensibility in lesions of the anterolateral funiculi, tends to show that although the two large ascending exteroceptive sensory fiber systems are functionally mainly different, both of them appear to a certain degree to be concerned not only with tactile sensibility but also with pain and temperature sensations. However, these observations in clinical cases may be opposed on the grounds that a concomitant affection of dorsal roots may explain the disturbances in pain and temperature sensation.

The dorsal funiculi, as we have seen, are not only pathways for important components of the exteroceptive sensibility from the body surface, but they are also *engaged in the transmission of proprioceptive impulses from joints and ligaments.* On this account lesions of the dorsal funiculi are accompanied by *disturbances of coordination,* which from a clinical point of view are more conspicuous than are the more subtle disturbances of exteroceptive sensory function described above. Thus the typical *ataxia* occurring in tabetic patients is explained as being due to the degeneration of the dorsal funiculi, which is a fairly constant feature of the anatomical picture of this disease.[26] The basis for the ataxia has

---

jected to sections of the dorsal columns, did not find marked changes in the perception of those sensory modalities which are generally taken to be mediated via the dorsal columns.

[26] However, the dorsal funiculi are not exclusively involved in the degeneration in tabes dorsalis. The pathological process is essentially an inflammation of the dorsal roots (a "posterior radiculitis"), and this causes a degeneration not only of the long ascending tracts in the dorsal funiculi, but also of the short fibers which enter the dorsal horns as well. Anatomically the latter is, however, not very conspicuous, at least not in myelin sheath preparations which clearly show the changes in the dorsal funiculi. As described previously (Ch. 1) the methods for study of myelin sheaths were known long before more modern neurohistological technique was developed, and the old thesis of the degeneration of the dorsal funiculi as the anatomical substratum of tabes has shown a peculiar tendency to dominate the minds of neurologists. It is, however, important to realize that the symptoms arising from the diseased spinal cord in tabes are not all due to the degeneration of the dorsal funiculi, even if these usually form a conspicuous feature of the clinical picture of tabes dorsalis.

been assumed to be the loss of proprioceptive impulses, this loss being the consequence of the lesion of the dorsal funiculi. This is confirmed by the physiological demonstration that impulses arising in the joints, at least to a great extent, ascend in the dorsal funiculi (see p. 56). Clinically this is manifested as follows: *If his eyes are closed the tabetic patient is unable to tell in which position his joints and limbs are moved,* and if the limbs or parts of them are moved passively, he does not recognize whether the movement consists of flexion or extension (joint sense, position sense). If the cuneate funiculus is degenerated, the upper limbs will also be affected, and it will be difficult or impossible for the patient to estimate the weight of objects. Furthermore, he has not the normal capacity for recognizing the size and form of objects with his eyes closed (astereognosia), partly at least because he cannot properly perceive the numerous small movements, especially of the fingers, which are necessary for this purpose. In addition, the reduction of the cutaneous discriminative sense is of importance in this connection.

The so-called dorsal funiculi ataxia is revealed in a reduced capacity to perform movements smoothly and precisely. The movements become unsteady, of uneven range; the patient points now too far, now too near. It appears as if the patient tries to compensate for his loss in coordination with a surplus of muscular power. The gait is unsteady and jerky. Frequently these disturbances of coordination are more prominent if the movements are performed with the eyes closed, vision thus making up partly for the reduction in proprioceptive impulses. This is brought out also by the fact, readily observed, that the patient is able to stand in a stable position, but if he is asked to stand with his feet side by side and with eyes closed, he will usually lose his balance (Romberg's sign).

Animal experiments confirm that the integrity of the dorsal columns is essential for the proper execution of movements. Destruction of the dorsal columns in monkeys is followed by various disturbances of behavior, as most recently described by Gilman and Denny-Brown (1966).

Lesions of the somatic sensory tracts in the medulla oblongata, pons, and mesencephalon. Even a superficial knowledge of the structure of the brain stem will suffice to make clear that the clinical pictures resulting from lesions involving the somatic sensory systems in the brain stem will be far more complex than in the cord. In the brain stem the long ascending tracts are to a great extent intermingled between cellular masses and fiber bundles belonging to other neuronal systems, partly related to the cranial nerves. The symptoms following lesions of these structures are considered in Chapter 7. Many lesions of the brain stem are immediately fatal, because they involve regions which are essential in the regulation of cardiovascular functions and respiration, and there may be disturbances of consciousness (discussed in Ch. 6). The following remarks will be restricted chiefly to symptoms following lesions of the somatosensory pathways.

A lesion affecting *the lateral part of the medulla oblongata* may interrupt the spinothalamic tract (see Figs. 2-9 and 7-6), and thus give origin to a loss of pain and temperature sensibility on the opposite side of the body, whereas the sense of touch, discrimination, vibration, and deep sensibility will be intact if the medial lemniscus has escaped. (See Soffin, Feldman, and Bender, 1968, for a recent study.) Since secondary trigeminal fibers join this tract, the analgesia following a lesion at a somewhat higher level in the medulla oblongata or in the pons will also include the face on the same side as the body, and there results a complete *hemi-analgesia and hemi-thermanesthesia*.[27] It is worthy of notice, however, that a superficial lesion may give an incomplete picture, due to involvement only of the longer fibers which are placed superficially. Thus, for example, an analgesia from the mammary papilla downward may well be due to a lesion in the medulla oblongata.

A lesion of the brain stem will, however, only in rare cases be limited to the spinothalamic tract. Frequently the spinal trigeminal tract and its nucleus will be included (see Fig. 2-9), producing an additional thermanesthesia and analgesia in the face on the side of the lesion (*hemi-anesthesia alternans*). The extension of the process in a rostral direction will decide whether the crossed trigeminal area is intact or not. Symptoms indicating damage of the vagus nuclei or fibers may also appear, as homolateral paresis of the soft palate or of the laryngeal muscles, accompanying the hemi-analgesia or hemi-hypalgesia. If the lesions injure the spinocerebellar tracts and the inferior olive there will be disturbances of coordination, as will also be the case when the dorsally placed restiform body is affected. In extensive lesions of the lateral part of the medulla oblongata the pyramidal tract may also be encroached upon, leading to some motor impairment. The most usual cause of lesions in this part of the brain stem is a vascular disorder in the territory of the posterior inferior cerebellar artery or the vertebral artery (thrombosis, embolism, or hemorrhage). In such cases all the symptoms mentioned above may be present, and in addition a Horner's syndrome on the side of the lesion may be found, evidencing damage to the descending sympathetic fibers (cf. Ch. 11).

A lesion affecting the *medial parts of the medulla oblongata* will give symptoms of a somewhat different type. A unilateral lesion of the medial

---

[27] There is still some uncertainty concerning the exact course of secondary trigeminal fibers (cf. Ch. 7), and some variations in the clinical picture of lesions similar to those treated here are not clearly understood.

lemniscus will be followed by an impairment or loss of deep sensibility (deep pressure, joint, and vibratory sensibility), and reduced or abolished sense of discrimination on the entire contralateral half of the body if the lesion is situated above the crossing of the fibers. If the lesion is situated in the pons, the trigeminal area in the face on the contralateral side will usually be included (cf. Fig. 2-16). However, the lemnisci of both sides will frequently be affected simultaneously on account of their close proximity. On this account the *symptoms mentioned are nearly always bilateral,* but often of a different distribution on the two sides. A frequent accompaniment to the sensory disturbances will be a paralysis or *paresis of the tongue of the peripheral type* on the side of the lesion, with atrophy of the tongue muscles, since the hypoglossal nerve passes immediately lateral to the medial lemniscus (Fig. 7-6). If the lesion extends farther in a ventral direction the pyramidal tract and other descending tracts will be encroached upon, and in addition there appears a *hemiplegia on the side opposite the hypoglossal lesion.* If the pathological process invades the pyramidal tract from the dorsal side, a consideration of the arrangement of the fibers (cf. Fig. 2-9) will explain that a paresis of one or both upper extremities may appear, while the lower extremities are affected slightly or not at all. Symptoms indicating a lesion in the median region of the medulla oblongata are usually due to syringobulbia or an interference with the blood supply of the anterior spinal artery.

These few remarks will suffice to give an impression of the variation and complexity of the symptoms which may follow lesions of the medulla oblongata. Still, the description is far from complete. With a knowledge of the anatomical structure of the medulla it will as a rule be possible to determine the site of the lesion fairly exactly. However, it is important to remember that, owing to the segmental arrangement of the fibers in the long ascending and descending tracts traversing the brain stem, *there frequently will not be a complete unilateral sensory or motor impairment.* Monoplegias and circumscribed regions of sensory loss are not rare, and a great variety of combinations of motor dysfunction (central and peripheral) and sensory defects may be encountered. Another point is also of practical importance: *the regions presenting sensory and motor impairment are often only indistinctly outlined.* As with lesions in other regions, this is no wonder, as frequently the regions totally injured are surrounded by areas which are only more or less impaired in their function on account of pressure or edema.

Above, only the deficiency symptoms occurring in lesions of the medulla oblongata have been referred to. Without doubt these are the most important, but *symptoms of irritation of the sensory tracts* may also occur, manifesting themselves usually as paresthesias of various types. Not infrequently a peculiar form of irritative sensory symptoms occurs in lesions of the medulla oblongata. These so-called *hyperpathias* are pains of an unusual character. The intensity of the pain bears no relation to the strength of the stimulus. The slightest superficial touch may be felt as severe pain. The pain shows a tendency to irradiate in regions of the body not being stimulated, and usually lasts long after the stimulus has ceased. Similar hyperpathias may occur in lesions of the sensory system in other places, especially the thalamus (cf. below) and they may occasionally be observed in lesions of the spinal cord and, in rare instances, even of the peripheral nerves. Their genesis is not clearly understood.

Lesions affecting the sensory tracts in the pons and mesencephalon will give similar symptoms to those in the medulla oblongata. However, the accompanying symptoms may be of a somewhat different type on account of their spatial relationship to other tracts and nuclei (cf. Figs. 7-14, 7-18, and 4-4). No detailed description of the different possibilities will be given here. It should, however, be pointed out that the *most important landmark in the diagnosis of the level of lesions of the brain stem is an eventual affection of one or more of the cranial nerves.* A simultaneously developed facial paralysis or paresis of the peripheral type (affecting upper and lower territories) points to a lesion in the middle or lower part of the pons. If the pyramidal tract is involved, there appears a hemiplegia or hemiparesis on the opposite side (facial paralysis with crossed hemiparesis: Millard Gübler's syndrome). Other possible combinations are with an abducens paralysis or a trigeminal paralysis. In pontine lesions usually the pontocerebellar system will be affected, with consequent disturbances of coordination. However, an exact focal diagnosis in pontine lesions is somewhat more difficult than in the medulla oblongata, since the function of several structures is less well known.

The same applies to lesions in the *mesencephalon.* An accompanying unilateral *oculomotor paresis* or paralysis is indicative of a lesion at the level of the superior colliculus, a paralysis of the trochlear nerve of a lesion near the inferior colliculus. Lesions in the mesencephalon are frequently accompanied by *disturbances of coordination and hyperkinesias,* tremor, or athetotic and choreatic movements. The basis of these has usually been assumed to be lesions of the brachium conjunctivum, the red nucleus, or the substantia nigra. Actually, however, our knowledge is very limited concerning the symptoms which can be referred to the individual structures in this part of the brain stem. The number of anatomically controlled cases is small. These questions will be touched on in Chapter 4.

Symptoms following lesions of the thalamus. As described previously, the medial lemniscus and most of the fibers of the spinothalamic tract terminate in the nucleus ventralis posterior (VPL). However, since the thalamic nuclei are relatively small, it is to be expected that lesions affecting only one of them will be very rare. Because several large fiber systems pass in the immediate neighborhood of the thalamus, thalamic lesions will frequently be accompanied by symptoms from other structures. Most important of these are the large tracts passing in the internal capsule close to the thalamus, the corticospinal fibers and corticofugal fibers to nuclei in the brain stem (see Ch. 4). More posteriorly are the fibers to the cortex from the lateral and medial geniculate bodies (optic and acoustic radiations). Tumors especially are apt to involve neighboring structures. Among 24 patients with thalamic tumors McKissock and Paine (1958) found only 5 who had sensory impairment. The sensory modalities involved varied.

A *destruction of the entire thalamic area receiving the sensory fiber systems would be expected to result in an impairment or loss of somatic sensibility in the opposite half of the body.* In many of the cases of this kind described in the literature, deep sensibility and discriminating sense are found to be severely impaired, the sense of touch and temperature less so, while the perception of pain is only slightly affected (Head and Holmes, 1911–12; and others). Whether this may be explained by circumscribed affections of particular regions of the thalamus alloted to specific sensory modalities is unknown, and autopsy findings in such cases are scarce. In part the differences may be explained by different numbers of uncrossed fibers in the two large somatosensory pathways, since the qualities most severely affected are those mediated by the lemniscus, which is completely crossed.

Concerning the presence of a *somatotopical localization within the thalamus,* the few clinical findings reported are in good accord with experimentally established data. Some cases have been described in which smaller lesions within the nuclei of the thalamus have been followed by a sensory impairment limited only to parts of the body (Garcin and Lapresle, 1954; Hassler and Riechert, 1959; and others). Most frequently these localized lesions are of vascular origin (affecting the thalamogeniculate artery), and in most instances the sensibility has been retained in the face, corresponding to a sparing of the medially situated VPM. In cases of this type the limits of hypesthesia or anesthesia of the different sensory modalities are usually not quite identical. Fisher (1965) reports the clinical findings in 26 patients presenting what he calls "pure sensory stroke." There are no pareses, visual defects, or other signs apart from a persistent or transitory numbness or mild sensory loss over one entire side of the body, or in part of the body. The symptoms, which may be transitory, but often recur, are probably due to transient ischemia caused by thrombosis. In one case, where autopsy was made, a lacuna, 7 mm in diameter, was found in the VPL.

Peculiar to thalamic lesions is that they are frequently accompanied by spontaneous pains. These "thalamic pains" are often very intense, occur in paroxysms, frequently irradiate to the entire half of the body, and are usually intractable to analgesics. The pains are usually present together with a sensory loss, but they may also occur without, usually then as an initial symptom. Frequently the pains, as with lesions in the medulla oblongata, have the character of hyperpathia (in this connection often termed dysesthesia). Even slight stimuli, normally not painful, may provoke paroxysms lasting long after the application of the stimulus has ceased. The period of latency between the stimulus and the perception of pain is prolonged. No universally accepted explanation of these pains has been given. Some are inclined to ascribe them to vasomotor disturbances in the thalamus. Others assume that a disappearance of cortical inhibition on account of the affection of thalamocortical fibers or the lack of intrathalamic association may be the cause. As mentioned when discussing the central pathways for pain, "thalamic pains" most often occur with small vascular lesions. Surgical attempts to abolish them by stereotactic thalamotomy have been in part successful.

Symptoms following lesions of the somatosensory cortical areas. From what has been discussed in previous sections it will be apparent that *circumscribed lesions of the postcentral gyrus* (Brodmann's areas 3, 1, 2) *will be followed by a localized sensory loss in part of the opposite half of the body.* Disturbances of this type have been observed in smaller lesions, traumatic, neoplastic, or other kinds. Cortical ablations to remove a neoplasm or a depressed bony fragment have yielded evidence confirming the somatotopical organization of the retrocentral area. For example, a damage to or a removal of the upper part of the gyrus with the adjacent lobulus paracentralis results in a sensory loss limited to the contralateral leg, extending farther proximally the lower the lesion reaches on the lateral surface of the cortex. In some cases the observed sensory loss has presented an approximately segmental distribution resembling lesions of the dorsal roots, but not infrequently the borders of the affected area have been more circular, producing an anesthesia of the "glove" or "stocking" type.[28]

In an acute lesion of the postcentral gyrus the anesthesia at first comprises all sensory modalities, superficial as well as deep. After some time sensibility reappears to a certain extent, as a rule, beginning with a partial return of pain sensibility. In time this may be restored to such a

[28] Anesthesia of these distributions is most frequently seen in hysteria. The differential diagnosis will as a rule not be very difficult.

degree that only highly refined methods will ascertain the slight persistent reduction. Somewhat later the appreciation of touch stimuli is partly regained and also the temperature sense is largely restored. However, *the sense of discrimination is usually permanently and severely impaired,* and is never, or only exceptionally, completely regained. Likewise *the vibratory and joint sensibility are permanently reduced or practically abolished.* This is even more true of the stereognostic sense, where the lesion includes the foci for the hand and fingers.[29] Thus in cortical lesions the sensory modalities transmitted through the dorsal funiculi and the medial lemniscus are those usually most severely and enduringly affected.

However, in the restitution following a lesion of the postcentral gyrus, there is also a *regional difference.* The different parts of the body do not regain their sensibility at the same rate. The most rapid and extensive restitution takes place for the face, especially the oral region, larynx and pharynx, and the anogenital region. The neck and trunk are in a more favorable position in this respect than are the extremities, and especially as concerns the distal parts of the latter where restitution is usually far from complete. The parallelism with the possibilities of restitution after a hemiplegia (see Ch. 4) is very close. It is reasonable to suppose that the potencies of the different parts of the body as regards restitution in lesions of the sensory cortex are dependent first and foremost on the degree of bilateral "representation" in the cortex of the parts in question. The gradient of the restitution corresponds also to the ease with which bilateral sensory symptoms may be elicited on cortical stimulation.

Little appears to be known of the sensory defects following *lesions of the second somatosensory cortical area (S II) in man.* Since the total area is small it will most often be affected together with other parts of the cortex, particularly S I, making analyses of the symptoms observed difficult. From animal experiments one might expect some affection of discriminating sensory qualities.

The symptoms following *lesions of the superior parietal lobule* with area 5 (Brodmann's areas 5 and 7) are likewise incompletely known. It appears, however, that no somatotopical localization is present in this part of the cortex, the disturbances affecting more or less the entire contralateral half of the body. The different sensory modalities are affected according to a similar principle as in lesions of the postcentral gyrus. The permanent impairment is most conspicuous for the combined sensory qualities, i.e. discrimination of various types. This has been found by

---

[29] It is difficult to decide whether this is a "primary" asterognosia or a secondary asterognosia, due to the abolition or reduction of the more simple sensory qualities. The affection of the latter presumably plays an important role.

Foerster (1936a), while Penfield and Rasmussen (1950) did not report sensory defects following excision of most of the superior parietal lobule. Foerster's observations are compatible with Ruch, Fulton, and German's (1938) experiments on monkeys and the chimpanzee, since following lesions of the posterior parietal lobe the animal's capacity for discriminating weight, as well as roughness and geometrical forms by palpation (in darkness), is permanently impaired. However, the postcentral gyrus is also of importance in this connection. In some human cases these authors found similar disturbances.

Apart from deficiency symptoms dealt with above, *irritative symptoms* may appear in lesions of the somatic sensory areas. Real pain very rarely occurs. More often the irritation is revealed clinically as paresthesias. If the irritation (caused by a tumor, a foreign body, a bone fragment, or other causes) is limited to the postcentral gyrus, the paresthesias may be localized to a limited part of the opposite half of the body. Important diagnostic hints may thus be obtained.

However, the sensory epileptical paroyxsms or *sensory Jacksonian fits* are more conspicuous and more indicative of a process in the cortex. Just as an irritative process in the precentral gyrus may elicit a motor discharge, spreading regularly, an irritation of the cortex of the postcentral gyrus may provoke a wave of sensory irritative symptoms, traveling over the body in accordance with the somatotopical organization of the retrocentral area. For example, paresthesias of different type may start in the fingers and proceed to the forearm, arm, and so on.[30] In some instances only sensory symptoms of this type will occur; in others, however, the irritation is propagated also to the precentral gyrus, first and foremost the readily excitable area 4. In this case a motor Jacksonian fit (cf. Ch. 4) will follow the sensory phenomena, with clonic twitchings of small groups of muscles, spreading regularly. It is customary to speak of the sensory symptoms in these instances as a *sensory aura,* but really they are an epileptic fit originating from the postcentral gyrus. Just as a motor Jacksonian fit is often followed by a postparoxysmal paresis, an examination of the patient immediately after a sensory Jacksonian fit may in some instances reveal a postparoxysmal sensory loss in the parts of the body which have been affected. The sensory Jacksonian fits, like the motor, are of great clinical importance, since they indicate the presence of a focal lesion of some sort or another in the first sensorimotor area. However, occasionally such fits may occur without a cortical focus.

[30] If the attack starts in the leg, and spreads to the arm, usually the proximal parts of this are affected first. This is in keeping with a reversal of the cortical representation of the cervical dermatomes described by Woolsey, Marshall, and Bard (1942).

1 1 5

In epileptic fits originating from the superior parietal lobe, a sensory aura may occur. This usually comprises the entire contralateral half of the body and as a rule soon becomes bilateral. According to Penfield and Kristiansen (1951) an epileptic discharge starting in the parietal lobe will frequently not manifest itself until it spreads forward to the post-central gyrus where it produces a somatic sensory aura.

Apart from certain types of seizures arising from foci in particular areas of the cerebral cortex, it is difficult to relate focal or generalized epileptic seizures to well-defined regions of the brain. The many varieties of epileptic seizures, their classification, and other problems of epilepsy will not be considered in the present text. For exhaustive treatments of this subject the reader is referred to the monographs of Penfield and Kristiansen (1951) and Penfield and Jasper (1954).

3

The Peripheral Motor Neuron

IN CLINICAL neurology the examination of what is commonly called "the motor system" is a fundamental part of the analysis of symptoms in disease of the nervous system. Different types of functional disorders are observed, which, when carefully examined, may give valuable information about the localization and type of the pathological process responsible for the symptoms. A distinction can be made between the peripheral motor apparatus—the peripheral motor neurons and the striated muscles of the body—and the central motor tracts and systems. The latter will be considered in the following chapter.

The motor cells of the ventral horns of the spinal cord. The peripheral motor neurons, often called *motoneurons,* have their perikarya or cell bodies in the ventral horns of the spinal cord and in the motor nuclei of some of the cranial nerves in the brain stem. The latter will be treated in more detail in Chapter 7, but principally they are of the same type as the motor cells of the ventral horns. Following the discovery of an efferent innervation of the muscle spindles it has become customary to distinguish between large and small motoneurons, commonly referred to as α (alpha) and γ (gamma) motoneurons, respectively. We will return to the latter below. Some of the alpha motoneurons are among the largest nerve cells present in the nervous system, and on this account have been more frequently used than any other cell type for the study of finer cytological changes. Like the cells of the corresponding cranial nerve nuclei, they are polygonal, multipolar, and endowed with a rich amount of tigroid granules in the cytoplasm (see Fig. 1-10A). The numerous dendrites aborize in the gray matter, mainly of the ventral horn. The axon takes a ventral course to leave the spinal cord through one of the ventral roots. The peripheral nerves then convey the axons to the muscles. (Not all peripheral nerves contain such somatic efferent motor fibers; most of them also have somatic afferent and visceral fibers.)

The motoneurons are found within the cytoarchitectonically defined lamina IX of Rexed (see Fig. 2-2). However, intermingled with them are a number of small cells. In fact, the number of these by far exceeds that of the large motoneurons. In certain groups the relation is 1:16.5 (Balthasar, 1952; see also Aitken and Bridger, 1961). It is generally held that some 30 per cent of the fibers in the ventral roots supply muscle spindles. Accordingly, the majority of the small cells in lamina IX cannot be the perikarya of fibers to the muscle spindles, a conclusion in agreement with findings made in Golgi studies which indicate that a considerable number of the nerve cells in lamina IX are internuncials. These subjects will be considered in a later section.

The motoneurons in the ventral horns of the spinal cord and the motor cranial nerve nuclei are the "final common path" (Sherrington) for all those impulses which are transmitted to the skeletal musculature of the body. They are influenced by impulses from many sources. As referred to previously, primary sensory fibers have been found to end on them. In addition they are acted upon, chiefly through internuncial cells, by fibers which descend in the spinal cord from the cerebral cortex and several nuclei in the brain stem (to be discussed in Chapter 4).

The movements which occur as the ultimate effect of the action of the motoneurons are determined by the impulses which impinge upon the motor ventral horn cells, the latter being, as it were, played upon by the different systems. The multitude of different movements which may occur normally and in conditions of disease of the nervous system are accordingly not primarily determined by the motoneurons themselves (except when these are directly involved in the pathological process). In recent years a wealth of information on the function of the motoneurons has accumulated, as well as on other aspects of motor function, including its central control. These subjects are treated fully in textbooks of neurophysiology and will therefore be considered only briefly here, with particular reference to anatomical aspects and with reference to the light they may shed on symptoms in neurological diseases.

The arrangement of the motoneurons. *The motoneurons* in lamina IX, like the cells in some of the motor nuclei of the cranial nerves, *are arranged in a characteristic manner.* In a cell-stained transverse section through the spinal cord several groups of cells can be distinguished in the ventral horns (cf. Fig. 3-1). Actually these groups belong to longitudinally arranged columns of nerve cells. The various columns are present in certain segments of the spinal cord only, as indicated in Fig. 3-1. When a peripheral nerve is cut, retrograde cell changes occur in the motoneurons which send their axons into the cut nerve, as mentioned in Chapter 1 (see Fig. 1-10B). In this way it has been determined experimentally, in several animals, which nuclear groups are concerned in the innervation of the various muscles. In the same manner, post-mortem studies of the human spinal cord in cases of amputations of limbs or nerve injuries have given information of the conditions in man. Sharrard (1955) has published a careful study on the subject based on a correlation of the distribution of paralysis in cases of poliomyelitis with the sites of cell loss in the ventral horn. One fundamental point which has been made clear by investigations of this type is that the medial cell groups supply the muscles of the trunk and neck. Accordingly, these groups (more precisely, only the ventromedial column) are developed throughout the length of the cord, as seen in Fig. 3-1. The lateral groups, on the other hand, are present mainly in the cervical and lumbar enlargements of the cord and have been shown to supply the muscles of the limbs. Within the various lateral cell groups or columns a further pattern is found: the cells which are concerned in the innervation of the distal muscles of the extremities are, as a rule, dorsal to those which send their axons to the proximal muscles. It may also be noted that the cell groups related to the distal parts of the extremities are only developed in the caudal part of the enlargements. The motoneurons are, therefore, somatotopically arranged. This pattern of *somatotopical localization* may be illustrated in a diagrammatic way,

FIG. 3–1   Diagram of the human spinal cord presenting in a transverse section the position of the different cellular columns. The letters and figures indicate the segmental distribution of the cellular columns. Redrawn from Kappers, Huber, and Crosby (1936).

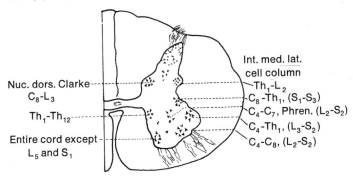

Nuc. dors. Clarke
C_8-L_3

Th_1-Th_{12}

Entire cord except
L_5 and S_1

Int. med. lat.
cell column
Th_1-L_2
C_8-Th_1, (S_1-S_3)
C_4-C_7, Phren. (L_2-S_2)
C_4-Th_1, (L_3-S_2)
C_4-C_8, (L_2-S_2)

as in Fig. 3-2. This arrangement explains why localized lesion of the ventral horn or of the motoneurons at a particular level (for example, in poliomyelitis) will result in a segmentally distributed paresis or paralysis (for example of the deltoid, supraspinatus, biceps, coracobrachialis, brachioradialis and brachialis muscles in an affection of C_{5-6}; compare Fig. 3-2 and the dermatome map of Fig. 2-4). Some investigators maintain that a still more detailed differentiation can be made, and that there is an arrangement of the cells of the various columns according to the function of the muscles which they supply (see Sterling and Kuypers, 1967b). Romanes (1953) concludes a critical evaluation of the subject by saying that apparently "the motor cell groups represent in part the morphological divisions of the muscles, but also in the majority of mammals have a topographical significance which is related to the joints moved, with occasional subdivisions representing single muscles."

The motor units.   The term "motor unit," introduced by Sherrington into the neurological vocabulary, has proved to be a very useful one. A *motor unit is an α motoneuron with its axon and the muscle fibers which it supplies.* When a motor ventral horn cell discharges, all muscle fibers belonging to the unit will contract. The size of the motor units varies widely, as a single ventral horn cell may supply from very few up to a thousand or more muscle fibers. This has been determined in ani-

FIG. 3-2   Three-dimensional representation of the gray matter in the cervical cord, showing in a diagrammatic way the somatatopical arrangement of the groups of motor ventral horn cells which supply different parts of the upper extremity. The diagram does not take into account that the distal parts of the upper extremity have a far more ample motor supply (cf. small motor units) than the proximal parts. The hand, therefore, should cover a much bigger area than shown in the diagram.

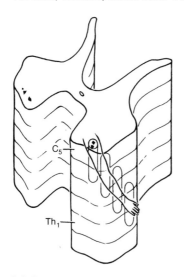

mals in the following way: After removal of the spinal ganglia of the dorsal roots which supply, for instance, one of the extremities, the experimental animal is allowed to survive until sensory fibers in the appropriate spinal nerves have degenerated. Then the number of remaining nerve fibers, which presumably are motor (some also sympathetic efferent, however), is counted in the branches supplying certain muscles and the number of muscle fibers in these muscles is also counted (Clark, 1931), and thus the number of muscle fibers per nerve fiber and, accordingly, per ventral horn cell is calculated. In some muscles, particularly such small ones as the extrinsic eye muscles and the small muscles of the hand, the motor units are small. It appears likely that in primates also the motor units are smallest in muscles which are used for finely differentiated movements, such as the small muscles of the hand, the laryngeal muscles, and the extrinsic eye muscles. This has been confirmed in some instances (Feinstein, Lindegård, Nyman, and Wohlfart, 1954). The authors counted the number of muscle fibers in several muscles and the number of fibers in the nerves to the same muscles. Assuming that some 40 per cent of the thick nerve fibers are afferent, they found the following number of muscle fibers per nerve fiber: Platysma 25, first lumbrical 108, first dorsal interossus 340, anterior tibial about 600, gastrocnemius 1600 to 1900. (For some other values, see Buchthal, 1961.) The small units have nerve fibers of a finer caliber than have the larger ones. That a single nerve fiber is able to supply a large number of muscle fibers is due to an extensive branching of the axon. This branching occurs when the nerve fiber is close to the muscle or within it (Cooper, 1929; Eccles and Sherrington, 1930). According to Sunderland and Lavarack (1953) some axons may also branch peripherally along their course.

Just how the muscle fibers which belong to the various motor units are mutually arranged within the muscle is a question of considerable interest. From physiological experiments (Cooper, 1929) it has been concluded that the muscle fibers of one unit cannot be grouped within a limited part of the muscle, but they must be assumed to be distributed throughout the length of the muscle, arranged, as it were, in series. Anatomical studies show that there is considerable overlap between fibers belonging to different units (Feindel, 1954). As to the arrangement, in cross section, of fibers which belong to one unit, anatomical findings in muscles from patients suffering from diseases in which the ventral horn cells are affected (amyotrophic lateral sclerosis, syringomyelia, poliomyelitis) give some information. As a consequence of the disintegration of some of the motoneurons the corresponding muscle fibers undergo atrophy. Muscles fibers presumably belonging to the same units, since they are in the same stage of atrophy, are usually situated rather close together, with some scattered ones around, as seen in Fig. 3-3. Frequently some "hypertrophic" fibers are also present. From electromyographic investigations it has been concluded that the muscle fibers of each unit are arranged as discrete groups of contiguous fibers (Weddell, Feinstein, and Pattle, 1944).

The occurrence of a regular arrangement of the atrophic fibers in cases of muscular atrophies due to affections of the peripheral motoneurons is of practical interest. Following the pioneer studies by Slauck (1921 and later) and Wohlfahrt and Wohlfart (1935), extensive research has confirmed that the microscopic changes in the muscles in disease of the type mentioned above (in which a damage of the motoneurons is the primary affection) differ from other types of muscular atrophy, especially the progressive muscular dystrophies, where there is no regular arrangement of atrophic fibers and commonly there is a considerable increase of fat and connective tissue in the muscles (cf. the "pseudohypertrophy" of the affected muscles in cases of infantile muscular dystrophies). There are also other differential features. However, there are a number of varieties of these diseases, which to some extent have their own particular histopathological characteristics (see Adams, Denny-Brown, and Pearson, 1962). This can be seen from examination of a small piece of an affected muscle, which may be removed by biopsy under local anesthesia. In this way it has been shown, for example, that in progressive peroneal muscular atrophy (Charcot-Marie-Tooth's disease) there is presumably a primary affection of the peripheral motor neurons (see Brodal, Bøyesen, and Frøvig, 1953), and that progressive ophthalmoplegia is to be grouped with the dystrophies (Schwarz and Liu, 1954). By using histochemical methods, further information can be obtained which may be of diagnostic value, and it is also possible to obtain biopsies from motor end plates and thus to study alterations in these (see Coërs and Woolf, 1959).

The terminal arborizations of the motor nerve fibers are found in the muscles as part of the so-called *motor end plates*. Histochemical and electron microscopic studies have clarified a number of interesting details in the structure of the motor end plates. The main features may be summarized as follows: The end plate consists of two parts: a nervous and

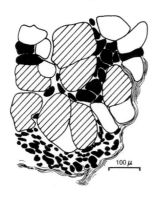

FIG. 3–3 Drawing of a primary muscle bundle from a biopsy taken from a diseased muscle in a patient suffering from progressive neuropathic peroneal muscular atrophy (Charcot-Marie-Tooth's disease). Some muscle fibers are of normal diameter (white), some are "hypertrophic" (hatched), while most fibers are atrophic (black). Note tendency to aggregation of fibers in the same degree of atrophy. From Brodal, Boyesen, and Frovig (1953).

a muscular, separated from each other by a cleft (200–300 Ångström). This *myoneuronal junction* in many respects resembles a synapse in the central nervous system. The muscular part of the end plate contains several nuclei and numerous mitochondria but lacks contractile myofibrils. The nervous part is provided with a number of grapelike swellings, much like terminal boutons. Each of these "dips into" the muscular part and contains synaptic vesicles and mitochondria. It is established that acetylcholine acts as a transmitter substance at the end plate. It enters the cleft, is bound to the muscular cell membrane and alters the ionic permeability of this. One nerve impulse produces an "end plate potential" in the muscle fiber, and when this reaches a sufficient height it gives rise to an action potential which is propagated along the fiber and elicits shortening of the myofibrils. The acetylcholine, which is liberated on the arrival of a potential in the nerve fiber, is rapidly destroyed by cholinesterase. With histochemical methods the end plates may be visualized by virtue of the presence of this enzyme. The impulse transmission at the myoneural junction may be influenced in various ways. Curare, for example, reduces the end plate potential, and eventually prevents the appearance of an action potential. Thus a paralysis of the muscle results (compare the use of curarelike substances in anesthesia to obtain muscular relaxation). The essential disturbance in myasthenia gravis is a defective transmission at the end plate (for some data, see Desmedt, 1966). The potentials recorded in electromyography are the action potentials described above.

When the nerve fiber is cut, the motor end plate, as well as the fiber, undergoes degeneration. As a rule one muscle fiber is supplied by one axon only and has a single motor end plate (see Feindel, Hinshaw, and Weddell, 1952).

The function of the motor units. Electromyography. *The motor units are the smallest functional units in the locomotor apparatus.* Variations in movements—in their range, force, and type—are ultimately determined by differences in the interaction and collaboration of motor units. Information on the function of these elementary units has been obtained particularly by the use of *electromyography,* the recording of electrical changes in the muscles during contraction. This can be done by using surface electrodes applied to the skin where a muscle is situated superficially, as for example, the dorsal interossei. When records are to be made of more deeply situated muscles, needle electrodes have to be used. These offer an advantage since one can record from a smaller total area and, accordingly, get more precise information. If the potential changes occurring in a muscle in a forceful contraction are led off, a multitude of negative and positive waves occur in the record making it extremely complicated and difficult to interpret. If, on the other hand, the muscle is made to contract only very feebly, single action potentials occur with certain intervals. Each potential is taken to reflect the activity of one motor unit. Since the potentials from different units may vary with regard to amplitude, several unit potentials can be kept apart when they are relatively few, as in a feeble contraction.

From electromyographic studies it is learned that when a contraction gradually increases in strength, more and more units appear in the record until finally an interference curve appears. It is of interest to know how different motor units collaborate during a more forceful contraction. In paretic muscles in poliomyelitis, where only some of the motor units are preserved, some features can be more easily studied than in healthy muscles (Seyffarth, 1940). However, essentially the same findings are made in both cases.

In the very beginning of the contraction there is only one motor unit visible in the electromyogram, i.e. there is only one motoneuron active in the part of the muscle examined. When the strength of the contraction increases, another unit appears in addition, then a third, a fourth, and so on. This shows that the increase in strength of a voluntary muscular contraction is, at least to a certain extent, due to the fact that more and more motoneurons discharge impulses to the muscle fibers which they supply. Furthermore, the frequency with which the different motor units discharge increases with the force of the contraction. When the strength of the contraction recedes, the frequency of the units decreases, and another characteristic phenomenon is noted: the unit which was the first to appear in the contraction is the last to disappear; and vice versa, the unit which occurred last is the first to stop discharging.

The frequency of discharge of a motor unit is an expression of the intensity of the stimuli which pass from the ventral horn cell to the muscle fibers which it supplies. According to these and other findings, the strength of a muscular contraction appears to depend partly on the number of motor units being active and partly on the intensity (frequency) with which they work.

The discovery of motor units, and of a method of recording their function, opened up new perspectives and made possible an understanding of many important problems. In clinical neurology electromyography is now routinely employed, since it gives valuable information in many cases, particularly in cases of muscular atrophies and dystrophies where it may aid in the differential diagnosis (see Buchthal, 1962, for a review). In peripheral nerve lesions electromyography may be used to decide, at an earlier stage than any other method, whether regeneration takes place satisfactorily. The appearance of motor units in a record from a paralyzed muscle must be taken as proof that some nerve fibers are acting and intact (having escaped destruction or having regenerated), even if no contraction can be seen. The electromyographic findings in completely denervated muscles will be referred to later. Electromyography has further proved to be a valuable tool in research on muscular function, for example, in studies of the muscles of mastication, laryngeal muscles, extrinsic ocular muscles, muscles of the inner ear, etc., as will be discussed later. It is able to contribute substantially in analyses of the co-operation between various muscles or parts of muscles (see, for example, Ballesteros, Buchthal, and Rosenfalck, 1965). The method has the great advantage that it can be applied to human beings, and there is an extensive literature on its application in research and in clinical diagnosis of diseases of the neuromuscular apparatus. (For references and a review see Buchthal, 1962.)

Although the electromyogram reflects the activity of the α motoneurons it can give only relatively crude and incomplete information of their function. Recent studies in various fields have greatly extended our knowledge of the motoneurons and the factors which influence their activity and co-operation. Not least new light has been shed on their behavior and control in spinal reflexes. Some of this data is of importance for clinical neurology.

The receptors in the muscles. A wealth of information on this subject is available today,[1] but in spite of this there are many unsolved problems. On several points there are still differences of opinion among specialists in the field, as evident for example from the reports from the First Nobel Symposium in Stockholm in 1965 (Muscular Afferents and Motor Control), to which the reader interested in details is referred. Here only a brief outline can be given, beginning with a presentation of the principal, well-established features. Following this, more recent data will be presented.

The skeletal musculature is provided with several types of receptors (Fig. 3-4A), which may be grouped as follows: muscle spindles, tendon organs (or Golgi organs), Vater-Pacinian corpuscles, various types of endings in the capsules of the synovial joints, and free nerve endings. Of these, only the former two will be considered here. Other types of receptors, however, situated in the skin, have been shown to influence the motoneurons as well. The Pacinian corpuscles and joint receptors have been considered in Chapter 2.

Of these receptors, the *muscle spindles* are morphologically and

---

[1] A complete bibliography of the literature on muscle receptors (Eldred, Yellin, Gadbois, and Sweeney, 1967) lists more than 1400 publications, the bulk of which have appeared since 1955.

functionally most elaborate and most complexly organized. They were rather completely described by Ruffini in the 1890's. Muscle spindles appear to be present in all muscles of the locomotor apparatus, and in many muscles supplied by motor cranial nerves as well, such as the laryngeal muscles, the muscles of mastication, the tongue and the extrinsic ocular muscles (for a review, see Cooper, 1960). The relative density of muscle spindles varies widely in different muscles. Thus, in the small human abductor pollicis brevis there are 80 spindles (Schulze, 1955–6), in the large latissimus dorsi 368 (Voss, 1956). An estimate of the number of spindles per gram of muscle weight gives the values of 29.3 and 1.4, respectively, for these two muscles. Thus, *muscles used in delicate movements are far more amply supplied with spindles than muscles used in coarse movements.*

The muscle spindles have derived their name from their shape. The principal points in their organization may be summarized as follows (see Fig. 3-4B): A spindle-shaped connective tissue capsule, some millimeters long, surrounds a few, 3-8 (in man an average of 10, Cooper, 1960), slender muscle fibers. These so-called *intrafusal fibers* are attached at their extremities to the connective tissue of the capsule and separated from this by a space filled with fluid. The *intrafusal fibers are thus arranged in parallel with the ordinary, extrafusal muscle fibers* and both are ultimately attached directly, or indirectly by way of inelastic collagen fibers, to the tendon. (See Fig. 3-4A.) When the extrafusal fibers contract, those of the spindles will be subject to a reduced tension, while a stretching of the muscle as a whole will increase the length and the tension of the intrafusal fibers. The central equatorial parts of the intrafusal muscle fibers are not contractile and harbor many nuclei. They are surrounded by spirally coursing nerve fibers, the *primary sensory* or *annulospiral ending,* made up of fine ramifications of a single relatively thick afferent fiber ($12-14\mu$ in the cat). A *secondary sensory ending* or *flower-spray ending,* coming from a thinner afferent fiber, may be present at one or both sides of the annulospiral ending (Barker, 1948). In addition the muscle spindles receive a *motor innervation.* This consists of relatively fine nerve fibers, the previously mentioned γ fibers (or fusimotor fibers), which come from the ventral horn. They terminate with small motor end plates in the distal cross-striated parts of the intrafusal fibers, which are contractile. It follows from this that a contraction of the distal parts of the intrafusal fibers in response to impulses in the γ fibers will result in a stretching of the central "sensory" part of the intrafusal fibers with a consequent stimulation of sensory endings, just as will a stretching of the entire muscle.

The *tendon organs* are much simpler than the muscle spindles. In essence, a tendon organ consists of a group of branches of a large myeli-

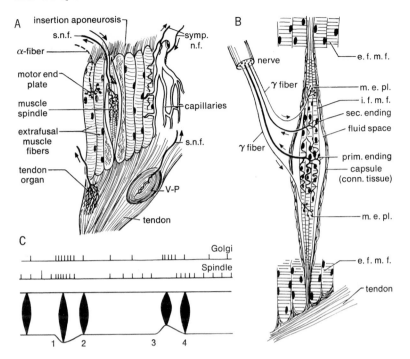

FIG. 3–4 *A:* Diagrammatic drawings of the three main receptors in skeletal muscles: a muscle spindle, a tendon organ, and a Vater-Pacinian corpuscle (*V-P*). Note that the spindle is arranged in parallel with the extrafusal muscle fibers, while the tendon organ is arranged in series with them. This has important consequences for their function.

B: Very simplified diagram of a muscle spindle to show its principal components. (Cf. text.) Abbreviations: *e.f.m.f.,* extrafusal muscle fibers; *i.f.m.f.,* intrafusal muscle fibers; *m.e.pl.,* motor end plates.

C: A diagram illustrating the response of a Golgi tendon organ and a muscle spindle ending during stretch and contraction of the muscle. The muscle is drawn below in black, between lines indicating its insertion. Action potentials are shown in upper two lines. Further explanation in text. Fig. C from Granit (1955a).

nated nerve fiber (12–18μ, Cooper, 1960) which terminate with a spray of fine endings between bundles of collagenous fibers of tendons, usually near the musculotendinous junction (Fig. 3-4A). A single fiber may supply more than one tendon organ. These are usually covered by a delicate connective tissue capsule. For the understanding of the function of the tendon organs it is essential to be aware of the fact that they are *arranged in series with the extrafusal muscle fibers.* Whether the muscle contracts or is stretched, the tendon organ will be stimulated, since in both cases the tension of the tendon organ will increase.

Physiological studies have confirmed the views on the function of muscle spindles and tendon organs which have been inferred from an analysis of their structure. By leading off from single fibers in dorsal roots which transmit sensory impulses from a muscle, action potentials can be recorded which are identified by their behavior as belonging to either muscle spindles or tendon organs. As shown in Fig. 3-4C, there is some spontaneous activity in the receptors when the muscle is at rest, most rapidly from the spindle. When the muscle is stretched (1), the frequency of afferent discharge rises in both sense organs and, after a short pause, goes back to the resting values when the stretch is released (2). When the muscle is made to contract (3) the Golgi organ again responds by increasing its firing rate on account of the pull on the tendon. The muscle spindle, however, will be unloaded during the contraction and will pause. When the contraction recedes (4) the slack spindles will again be pulled upon and consequently discharge, while the tendon organs will not respond since the tension is reduced. The *tendon organs* according to these findings are *tension recorders,* while the *muscle spindles give information about the length of the muscle.* These essential findings were made by Matthews (1933) and later confirmed by others (see Granit, 1955a, for a review).

In regard to the *efferent innervation* of the muscle spindles Leksell (1945) first succeeded in leading off action potentials from the thin fibers in the ventral roots (having a conduction velocity of 20 to 38 m.p.s.) and could show that stimulation of these γ fibers did not result in any contraction of the muscle. However, upon stimulation of the γ fibers action potentials could be recorded from the dorsal roots. These potentials were interpreted as arising from the muscle spindles, due to the stretching of the central sensory region of the intrafusal fibers produced by the shortening of the distal, contractile parts when the γ fibers were active. Leksell's (1945) findings, which have since been repeatedly confirmed, made it clear that the *muscle spindles are subject to control from the central nervous system.* The degree of stimulation of its γ fibers will regulate its sensitivity to stretch as contraction of the distal contractile parts will lengthen the central sensory part and reduce its threshold for simulation. The γ neurons are played upon by impulses from various sources, which thus may influence the activity of the spindles (see below).

From intracellular recordings Eccles, Eccles, Iggo, and Lundberg (1960) concluded that *the γ neurons lie intermingled with the motoneurons which supply the same muscle.* Anatomical demonstration of the γ neurons has been lacking until recently when Nyberg-Hansen (1965b) by means of the modified Gudden method (Brodal, 1940a) succeeded in demonstrating them. Following transection of a peripheral nerve there are, among the large motoneurons which present retrograde cellular changes, a number of small ones which display the same alterations, and accordingly must be assumed to have had their axon interrupted. However, the majority of the small cells in a particular group are not affected, in agreement with the conclusion, drawn from Golgi studies, that a considerable number of the nerve cells in lamina IX are internuncials (see below).

The very schematic account given above of the muscle spindles and their function summarizes approximately what was known about 1950. Later research has shown that the spindles are in fact far more complex, with regard to both structure and function. It has been shown that most of them contain two types of intrafusal muscle fibers (Fig. 3-5) which differ in diameter, among other things. With reference to the arrangement of their nuclei the thick fibers are called *"nuclear bag fibers,"* the thin, *"nuclear chain fibers"* (see Boyd, 1962; Cooper and Daniel, 1963, in man). Likewise, anatomical studies on the innervation of the muscle spindles have revealed a greater complexity than was previously known to exist. The primary sensory (annulospiral) endings are related to both types of muscle fibers, while the secondary (flower-spray) endings, mostly, but not always, appear to be present only on the nuclear chain fibers. Muscle spindles in man are in all essentials similar to those in the cat (Cooper and Daniel, 1963).

Early workers in the field observed some features in the response of the muscle spindles to stretch, which indicate that they might not be only length recorders. It remained for Jansen and Matthews (1962a) to demonstrate that the *potentials recorded from primary afferent fibers give information not only of the length of the muscle but also of the velocity*

FIG. 3–5 Simplified diagram of the central region of a muscle spindle, showing the two kinds of intrafusal muscle fibers and their sensory and motor innervation. There is still some doubt as to whether the "plate endings" and "trail endings" have their separate motor fibers as shown in the diagram. Slightly changed from Matthews (1964). (Cf. text.)

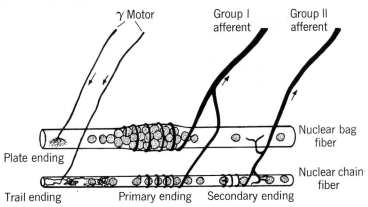

of extension. The former response is called the *static response* and is seen on maintained extension of the muscle. The *dynamic response* is the response of the receptor to actually being stretched. For various reasons the authors assume that the dynamic response originates mainly in the nuclear bag fibers while the static response is due to extension of the nuclear chain fibers, both of which are supplied by the primary endings. The secondary sensory endings appear in many respects to be functionally similar to the primary ones, but they are less sensitive to changes in length, particularly to rapid changes (see Bessou and Laporte, 1962; Matthews, 1964). They have not been as completely studied as the primary endings.

Physiological studies have further shown that *there is more than one type of γ fiber.* Jansen and Matthews (1962a, 1962b) concluded from recordings of the activity in the muscle spindles following stimulation of the efferent fusimotor fibers in decerebrated cats that the dynamic and static sensitivity of the primary endings are independently controlled. The authors' suggestion that the basis for this differential influence is the presence of two kinds of γ neurons, one acting on the nuclear bag fibers, the other on the nuclear chain fibers, has been verified by Matthews (1962). Other authors have made corresponding observations (for a review, see Matthews, 1964).[2] The secondary endings are activated chiefly by the static fusimotor fibers. Whether the two functional types of efferents correspond to different morphological types of endings is not yet clear. However, the γ fibers to the spindles are provided with two kinds of terminals. One is represented by motor end plates of the kind found in extrafusal muscles (as has been long recognized); the other terminal forms an extensive and diffuse network of fine axonal fibers and small elongated endings (see Fig. 3-5). Following Barker (1962, 1966) these are commonly referred to as "plate endings" and "trail endings," respectively. Whether the two kinds of endings belong to the γ_1 and γ_2 fibers of Boyd (1962) is disputed, nor is it settled whether the plate endings occur only on nuclear bag fibers, or the trail endings only on nuclear chain fibers. Efferent fibers which give off branches to extrafusal as well as intrafusal fibers (sometimes referred to as β fibers, or slow α fibers) have been demonstrated histologically (Adal and Barker, 1965).

[2] Further studies on the fusimotor activity in cats following transection of the spinal cord (Alnæs, Jansen, and Rudjord, 1965) and following decerebration (Jansen and Rudjord, 1965) confirm the existence of a dual fusimotor innervation and indicate that the two types of afferents are independently controlled. It appears that the activity in the dynamic system is largely dependent on sensory impulses entering in the dorsal roots, while the static system mainly depends upon activation from supraspinal regions.

There are still unsolved problems concerning the functional organization of the muscle spindles. Even the simplified account given above makes it clear, however, that the muscle spindle is an extremely complex type of receptor. The spindles inform the central nervous system of the length of the muscle as well as the speed of stretching and thus provide information which is essential for the proper activity of the spinal reflex apparatus. In addition they contribute to muscular control by sending messages to supraspinal levels, especially to the cerebellum. We will return to the muscle spindles when discussing the stretch reflexes and muscular tone.

The *tendon organs* have been less intensively studied than the muscle spindles. As mentioned above, these are arranged so as to record tension in the muscle, be this due to contraction or to extension of the muscle. It has for some time been generally held that their main task was to protect the muscle against overstretching. It appears, however, that they have a more differential function, and in fact are far more sensitive to the tension arising in the tendon on contraction of the muscle than to tension arising on stretching of the muscle. Under certain circumstances they seem to be able to respond to the contraction of even a single motor unit (Jansen and Rudjord, 1964; Houk and Henneman, 1967). This suggests that the tendon organs may be more important in the control of the motor apparatus than hitherto considered, as does also their relatively great numbers. The number of tendon organs has been determined in some muscles and has been found to be only a little below the number of muscle spindles (Swett and Eldred, 1960; Wohlfart and Henriksson, 1960). Information from the tendon organs is delivered not only to the cord, but also to central levels, especially the cerebellum.

The *Pacinian corpuscles* (discussed in Chapter 2) appear to be vibration receptors. Like the receptors of the joints (see Ch. 2), they presumably send additional information to the central nervous system, concerning what goes on during muscular contraction, and contribute to the reflex control of movements. The role of these receptors has, however, been relatively little studied so far.

The stretch reflex and the control of muscles. Even when it is isolated from the rest of the brain the spinal cord is capable of mediating a number of reflexes, somatic and autonomic. The morphological basis of a nervous reflex is generally referred to as a reflex *arc,* which, in its simplest form, consists of five links: 1) *A receptor* which reacts to the stimulus; 2) *An afferent conductor* which transmits the impulses to the "reflex center." (The afferent conductor is an afferent sensory fiber, in most cases having its cell body in a spinal or cranial nerve ganglion.); 3) A *"reflex center,"* where the afferent message from the receptor may converge with afferent impulses from other receptors, or with afferents from other sources, which may modify the effect of the afferent impulses from the receptor; 4) *An efferent conductor,* a nerve fiber going to the effector organ; 5) *An effector* which produces the reaction, and may be a muscle, a gland or a vessel, or may include several such components.

Reflexes vary enormously, from very complex ones, such as the reflex of swallowing where a number of different effectors are involved, to relatively simple ones. Here we are concerned only with *spinal reflexes,* and of these only those where the effectors are skeletal muscles, i.e. somatic reflexes. The fundamental principles governing the reflex activity of the cord were clarified by Sherrington. Many types of reflexes may be distinguished. *Flexor reflexes* are those where the response is a flexion of the limbs. The most potent stimuli are nociceptive ones, and the result is a withdrawal of the limb (withdrawal reflex). In other reflexes there is an extension of a limb; for example, in the crossed extensor reflex which may accompany a flexor reflex. There are still other more complex reflexes; for example, the scratch reflex. All of these reflexes usually involve several muscles, and the reflex response may vary according to the situation (type and site of application of stimulus, intensity of stimulus, concomitant application of other stimuli, etc.). The arcs for these reflexes are of great complexity. Quite another type of reflex is the *stretch reflex, the contraction of a single muscle in response to its being stretched.* This is an elementary reflex which occurs in all muscles. This example of a spinal reflex will be considered below; concerning spinal reflexes in general the student is referred to textbooks in neurophysiology. Due to extensive research our knowledge of the mechanism of the stretch reflexes is fairly satisfactory. These form the basis of all so-called *postural reflexes* (see Chapter 4), which, broadly speaking, aim at maintaining the correct posture of the body and adjusting it to various demands, be these due to external forces or resulting from movements performed by the organism.

When discussing the stretch reflexes and their anatomical basis, it is appropriate to start with a relatively simple model, that of the patellar reflex, routinely tested in every clinical neurological examination. In clinical terminology this and related reflexes are traditionally often referred to as "tendon reflexes" or "deep reflexes." Neither name is really appropriate, as will appear from the following. The designation *myotatic reflexes* is often used and is appropriate, but the term stretch reflex is apparently now most used.

Figure 3-6 shows the main features of a stretch reflex as deduced from experimental neurophysiological findings in the cat. As an example applicable to man we will consider the patellar reflex with reference to the diagram. A tap on the patellar tendon stretches the quadriceps (Q), both its extrafusal fibers and the muscle spindles. The latter respond by sending a train of impulses to the cord, as described in the previous section. The afferent fibers in the dorsal roots conveying these impulses (on ac-

FIG. 3–6 *A:* Diagram showing (*to the left*) the pathways involved in a stretch reflex. Impulses arising in the muscle spindles are transmitted in group *Ia* fibers. To the right are shown (*dotted*) pathways arising in the tendon organs and passing in group *Ib* fibers. Excitatory cells and synapses shown as open structures, inhibitory as black. *BST:* flexors of the knee; *m:* motor end plate; *Q:* quadriceps muscle; *sp:* muscle spindle; *t:* tendon organ. (Cf text.) Slightly modified from Eccles (1957).

B: A diagram of the proposed anatomical basis of the inhibition of motoneurons (*M*), occurring through their recurrent collaterals to Renshaw cells (*R*). Modified from Eccles (1957).

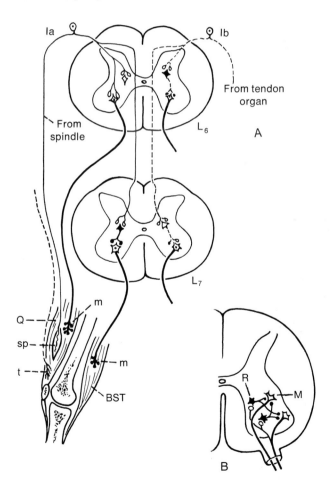

count of their large caliber belonging in physiological nomenclature to group *Ia* fibers) establish synaptic contact with motoneurons which are excited and produce a contraction of the quadriceps. In order that this may occur there must be a concomitant reduction of tension in the antagonists to the quadriceps, the flexors of the knee (Sherrington's principle of reciprocal innervation). On the basis of physiological studies by several workers (among whom may be mentioned Lloyd, Granit, and Eccles) it has been concluded that this occurs as shown in the diagram (to the left). The afferent spindle fiber gives off collaterals to a group of neurons in the "intermediate part" of the gray matter. These neurons are inhibitory and send their axons to motoneurons which innervate the antagonists. Consequently the firing rate of the motoneurons contacted is reduced, and the antagonists (BST) relax.

The pathways indicated (to the left) in Fig. 3-6 are in agreement with anatomical data. As previously noted, dorsal root fibers can be traced to the large ventral horn cells by experimental methods as well as in Golgi material (see Fig. 2-3). Whether all of these fibers are derived from muscle spindles, cannot be decided, but the fibers of a single dorsal root reach ventral horn cells situated two or more segments above or below the segment of entry (Schimert, 1939; Sterling and Kuypers, 1967a; and others). This is in agreement with the physiological observation that afferents from one muscle may activate several (usually synergistic) muscles (Eccles, Eccles, and Lundberg, 1957). Of particular interest is the demonstration of ample terminations of collaterals of such fibers (Fig. 2-3) in the medial and central parts of Rexed's laminae V and VI (see Sprague and Ha, 1964; Scheibel and Scheibel, 1966a; Sterling and Kuypers, 1967a; Szentágothai, 1967), since interneurons responding to afferent impulses from muscle spindles (as well as from tendon organs, see below) were localized by Eccles, Eccles, and Lundberg (1960) in this region. Axons of cells in this region can be traced into the ventral horn, and it appears that their axons and collaterals extend for several segments up and down the cord (Szentágothai, 1951; Scheibel and Scheibel, 1966a).

The example given above illustrates *a phasic stretch reflex,* in which the muscle spindle, by its afferent impulses, monosynaptically activates the α motoneurons to its own muscle and thus elicits a contraction of the muscle as well as causing relaxation of the antagonists. During contraction the muscle spindle will stop discharging when its length is reduced (see Fig. 3-4C), the α neurons will not be excited any more, and the muscle will again relax. However, as shown by Sherrington, the stretch reflex may also be tonic or postural.

Muscle tone.   If a normal muscle is palpated when it is resting, it

134

will be felt that it is not completely flaccid but possesses a certain degree of tension. This is also the impression gained when passive movements are made. *This normally existing condition of muscular tension is generally called muscle tone,* more properly *resting tone.* In various pathological conditions it is observed that this normal tone is changed, sometimes increased (hypertonus), in other cases reduced (hypotonus). Clinically, muscle tone is commonly examined by palpation and passive movements. However, probably two different components of muscle tone are evidenced by the two methods of examination (see below). Thus it is not uncommon to observe, for instance in capsular hemiplegias, that muscle tone is reduced when judged by palpation (the consistency of the muscles is reduced), while in passive movements it appears to be augmented, since the resistance offered to the movements is greater than normal.

There has been much debate on the problems of muscle tone, and some confusion has arisen because various definitions have been employed. While the muscle possesses some elasticity, which tends to sustain a certain tension, it has been equally clear for a long time that *most of the tension in a normal muscle is of reflex nature and maintained by afferent impulses.* It has been known since 1860 (Brondgeest) that section of the dorsal roots supplying an extremity will result in a remarkable reduction of muscle tone in the limb. Sherrington later demonstrated that it is the *proprioceptive* fibers of the afferent nerves which are involved in this phenomenon. If the skin of the entire extremity was denervated by undercutting, thus abolishing all cutaneous impulses to the cord but leaving the proprioceptive impulses from the muscles, no change in muscle tone was observed. Later studies have made it clear that the afferent impulses responsible for the maintenance of this component of muscular tone, which may properly be called *reflex tone,* arise in the muscle spindles. In the light of present knowledge it is also possible to explain why changes in muscular reflex tone may occur in lesions of the nervous system, and that it may show variations in the same individual under different circumstances.

The above example of a phasic stretch reflex illustrates one task of the muscle spindle: to activate monosynaptically the motoneurons on sudden stretching of the muscle and thus to elicit a contraction of the muscle to oppose the stretching. Sudden stretching of a muscle is a relatively simple phenomenon, but in daily life it is a rather uncommon event. It is, however, essential that the lengths of the various muscles taking part in a movement be mutually perfectly adjusted at any time. Since the muscle spindles, as described above, are length recorders, they will by reflex keep the corresponding α motoneurons in an appropriate state of

1 3 5

activity, and thus keep the muscle at a length determined by the length of the intrafusal muscle fibers. In this way the spindles regulate muscular tone by maintaining tonic stretch reflexes. The spindles form part of a *servomechanism* by signaling back to the cord information on the length of the muscle and eliciting changes in this. However, a simple system like that outlined above would not be able to take care of the fine adjustments which are necessary for the performance of movements. One of the problems is that there will be a time lag from the start of the signal from the receptor until the appropriate change in the muscle can take place. This will be the more unfortunate the more rapid the desired movements are to be. One of the ways in which this drawback could be reduced would be if the spinal cord at the same time as it received information of the changes in length of the muscle could also be informed of the speed with which the lengthening occurred. It would further be desirable that the spinal cord should have some means of adjusting the sensitivity of the spindles. As described in the previous section, recent studies have shown that both conditions are fulfilled. The γ neurons may influence the sensitivity of the spindles by altering the length of their middle, receptive segments, and the primary sensory endings have been shown to record not only changes in length of the muscle but also the speed of such changes. The reflex center in this way may "predict" the position in a future movement and adjust the extrafusal contraction accordingly. Furthermore the static and the dynamic sensitivity of the spindles can be adjusted independently by separate sets of γ fibers.

The *normal resting muscle tone is thus maintained by the tonic stretch reflex,* in contrast to the phasic stretch reflex occurring on sudden stretching of the muscle, the difference being due chiefly to the rapidity of the stretching. (The differences found between muscle tone as tested by passive movements and by palpation, referred to above, is probably explained by the fact that by moving the limb the phasic stretch reflex is elicited.)

Physiologically two types of α neurons have been distinguished, "tonic" and "phasic" (Granit, Henatsch, and Steg, 1956; and others), the tonic ones having, among other things, a lower rate of firing than the phasic ones. The axons of the former conduct more slowly than those of the latter and presumably, therefore, are thinner. The "tonic" cells are assumed to be smaller than "phasic" ones. Furthermore, the tonic fibers have been found to supply chiefly the "red" muscle fibers, the latter the "pale," more rapidly contracting fibers. The number and distribution of these types of muscle fibers vary among muscles and within the individual muscles. "Red" fibers are found chiefly in muscles which are generally used in sustained contractions, as those supporting the body (extensors of the limbs) and the diaphragm, while the "pale" fibers dominate in muscles used for rapid and forceful contractions. (As mentioned above there appear to be also some α neurons, sometimes referred to as β neurons, which supply extrafusal as well as intrafusal muscle fibers.) It is generally assumed that the *tonic* α neurons are particularly involved in the tonic function of the muscles.

Since the γ neurons may alter the sensitivity of the spindles, they are of great importance for muscle tone. An increased γ activity will "set" the spindles at a more active level, and by reflex increase the tonus of the extrafusal muscles. In this connection it is of interest that usually there is some spontaneous activity in the γ neurons as well as in the spindle afferents, i.e. they may be said to be tonically active. The spindles have been shown to activate γ neurons, but unlike their action on the α neurons, the latter action does not occur monosynaptically but by way of internuncial cells. There is thus established a circuit: receptor endings in the spindle—internuncial cells—γ efferents—contractile regions of the spindle. Even if it is still not quite clear how the γ neurons perform their task, the data so far available may suggest an explanation of spasticity and rigidity. In this connection the influences exerted on the γ and α motoneurons from supraspinal structures are of primary importance. These questions will be discussed in the following chapter, but the problem of central control of the muscle spindles is of relevance also for the subject of this chapter.

As first shown by Granit and Kaada (1952), influences from several supraspinal structures may alter the spontaneous activity of the γ neurons by means of fibers descending in the cord (see Chapter 4). This explains the well-known phenomenon that muscular tonus may change in normal persons, for example according to their mood, and this should be remembered when, in the beginning of a neurological examination of a patient, the myotatic reflexes are found to be unusually brisk.

In the execution of movements the γ innervation is of importance in determining the state of the muscles to be used as well as being active in their control, while the α neurons are responsible for the contraction itself. The collaboration of α and γ neurons in the execution of movements has been the subject of several studies, but much still remains to be clarified, and the problems are technically difficult. It has been suggested (Granit, Holmgren, and Merton, 1955) that the "motor centers" of the brain may produce movements along two routes: either by pathways acting on α motoneurons; or by pathways which act on γ motoneurons, which then, via afferents from the spindles, activate α motoneurons (the γ-loop). The latter route has been assumed to be used in "ordinary" muscular contractions, while the former is used in particularly rapid and forceful contractions. This view receives some support from the observation that in most cases where in experimental animals muscular contraction has been elicited by stimulating the cerebral cortex, the red nucleus, the vestibular nuclei, and the reticular formation, α and γ neurons have both been found to be involved. Usually the γ neurons respond a little earlier than the α motoneurons suggesting that the former have some sort of preparatory function for the latter.[3]

As referred to previously, it appears that the central nervous system is able to exert an individual control of γ_1, γ_2 and α neurons. Whether this central control is mediated by separate pathways is so far uncertain. In several instances the same structure has been found to act on γ as well as α neurons, and, at least in the cat, both actions occur via internuncial cells. However, certain fiber systems appear to excite, exclusively or at least chiefly, either flexor or extensor muscles (see Ch. 4). The co-operation between α and γ neurons has been referred to as the α-γ linkage (see Granit, 1955a), and evidence has been produced that the anterior lobe of the cerebellum is of particular relevance for this function (Granit, Holmgren, and Merton, 1955). Other data support this conclusion. Via the nuclei fastigii and interpostitus the spinal regions of the cerebellum may influence several structures which are known to act on both kinds of neurons, such as the reticular formation, the red nucleus, the vestibular nuclei, and the cerebral cortex.

Above, the problems of muscle tone and stretch reflexes have been discussed with reference to the muscle spindles alone. It should be mentioned, however, that other factors are also involved, but the role they play is less clear. Reference was made previously to the *tendon organs*. On stretching of a muscle these will be stimulated. They have a higher threshold to stretch than the spindles, and their main function has been thought to be to prevent overcontraction of the muscle and to act as a "brake," at the same time as they facilitate the antagonists. The impulses from the tendon organs pass via dorsal root fibers of somewhat smaller calibers than the muscle spindle afferents (in physiological nomenclature belonging to group 1b). These impulses (see Fig. 3-6, to the right) do not impinge directly upon motoneurons, but on interneurons, which send their axons to α motoneurons. Those reaching the α motoneurons supplying the muscle which is stretched are inhibitory, while those going to the α motoneurons supplying anatagonists are facilitatory.

In addition to impulses from the tendon organs, there is another mechanism which tends to limit the activity of the excited motoneurons, the so-called *recurrent or Renshaw inhibition*. This is illustrated in Fig. 3-6, constructed on the basis of physiological observations. When a motoneuron fires impulses, these will pass via its recurrent collaterals to cells with short axons situated in the ventral horn. These cells, called

---

[3] At variance with the above interpretation of the function of the two routes are the observations of Carli, Diete-Spiff, and Pompeiano (1967a) that stimulation of Deiters' nucleus can give activation of extrafusal fibers without concomitant activation of the γ loop. These authors (Carli, Diete-Spiff, and Pompeiano, 1967b) stress the importance of the central influences on γ neurons and are inclined to reduce the importance of passive factors acting on the spindles during muscular contraction.

Renshaw cells, have an inhibitory effect on the motoneurons. (Recently it has been shown that occasionally a facilitatory effect may occur.) Some problems relating to the anatomical identification of the Renshaw cells will be discussed in the following section.

The above account of some features of what is known of the function of the motoneurons, their role in movements and in the maintenance of muscular tonus and myotatic reflexes, shows that there are very complex problems still far from being solved.[4] Further indications of the existing complexity come from some recent data which will be briefly outlined below.

Some features of the functional organization of motoneurons. It appears from the preceding survey that the performance of even a small movement must be an extremely complicated act. It requires a harmonious collaboration of a number of motor units, distributed over several segments of the cord and supplying different muscles. The activity of all these units must be coordinated in time, as well as with regard to intensity; facilitation and inhibition of the units must be precisely timed. The complexity is well illustrated by the fact that part of a muscle may be employed in different, even opposed movements. Thus certain parts of the deltoid muscle may function as abductors in one position of the shoulder joint, as adductors in another position. No wonder we are still far from understanding these functions! Recent research has contributed in a general way to our comprehension of how the intimate collaboration between motoneurons and related cells can be achieved, but on the other hand, these studies have revealed a complexity in the minute organization which so far escapes analysis. Some of this data is of interest from the point of view of a general understanding of the nervous system and will therefore be reviewed.

The columnar and somatotopical arrangement of motoneurons is a fundamental feature of the organization of the spinal cord. However, this refers only to the cell bodies. Other data is needed if we want to understand how they are acted upon and co-operate.

As previously mentioned, dendrites of motoneurons may extend for some distance beyond the confines of lamina IX, into laminae VII and VIII. Most of the richly branching dendrites of the motoneurons are, however, arranged longitudinally within the cell column to which the cell belongs (Scheibel and Scheibel, 1966a), particularly in the columns innervating the trunk and proximal parts of the extremities (Sterling and Kuypers, 1967b). The dendrites of a single cell may overlap those of many hundreds of adjacent motoneurons. As to the dorsal root fibers supplying the motoneurons monosynaptically (muscle spindle afferents, perhaps others as well), it has been shown experimentally that a single dorsal root

---

[4] In this context it may be mentioned that apparently also the Renshaw cells are subjected to a central control (see Hasse and Van der Meulen, 1961; MacLean and Leffman, 1967).

afferent may spread its collaterals over several segments. From recent Golgi studies where longitudinal sections of the cord are used, it is learned that this spreading occurs in or near the lamina IX, where dorsal fibers course longitudinally for considerable distances (Sterling and Kuypers, 1967a). These terminations are thus oriented in the same direction as most of the dendrites of the cells on which they end, in agreement with a principle found in many nuclei. The above arrangement makes it understandable that effects from the spindles in a single muscle may activate motoneurons in several segments of the cord, as found in physiological studies. A similar principle is valid for the activation of motoneurons via internuncial cells. As referred to above, many dorsal root fibers give off a dense plexus of collaterals in the medial and central parts of laminae V–VI, and there is another in the transition between laminae VII and VIII. Many of the dorsal root fibers ending in these regions, take a longitudinal course (Sterling and Kuypers, 1967a) and thus may act on interneurons in several segments. Furthermore, a study of these interneurons (see also below) with the Golgi method (Scheibel and Scheibel, 1966a, 1966b) shows that their axonal branches and collaterals extend longitudinally for 1 to 4 segments, as concluded by Szentágothai (1951) from experimental studies.

Obviously, fibers in one dorsal root, establishing contact with interneurons, may via these influence motoneurons in several segments of the cord. A similar arrangement appears to be valid for other afferents to the motoneurons, for example the corticospinal, as described by Scheibel and Scheibel (1966b). The motoneurons are thus contacted by a great number of axons and collateral branches.

Early silver impregnation studies demonstrated that the motoneurons are amply provided with terminal boutons, but for technical reasons these could be identified only on the soma and the proximal dendrites. Bouton stains which essentially impregnate mitochondria have shown that boutons are present even on fine dendritic branches. In fact, they appear to be at least as densely placed on these as on the cell body, covering 50 to 70 per cent of the cell's entire surface area (Illis, 1964, in the cat; Gelfan and Rapisarda, 1964, in the dog). In electron microscopic studies in the monkey, Bodian (1964) likewise found boutons on all parts of the soma and dendritic tree of motoneurons, and emphasized that the density increases as one proceeds distally so that the distal branches, $0.3–1\mu$ thick, are tightly covered with boutons.[5] The total number of boutons on a single cell amounts to several thousands in the cat (see Illis, 1964, for references). Using a silver impregnation method on human autopsy material Minckler (1940) calculated that in man there are some 1475 boutons per cell, presumably much too low a figure. Even if the boutons which contact the motoneurons vary somewhat in size (from less than 2μ up to more than $4,8\mu$ in diameter in the cat, Illis, 1964) no particular distribution of boutons of different sizes has been found, although, according to Bodian (1964) large boutons may be most common on proximal dendrites. It is not known whether axons derived from dorsal root fibers differ from those of internuncial cells with regard to types or sites of contacts with the

[5] These findings are of some relevance for physiological interpretations, since there has been some dispute about the functional potency of synapses on peripheral dendrites. The ample presence of such boutons is a morphological argument in favor of the view that dendritic synapses must be active.

140

motoneurons, but physiological studies (see Terzulo and Llinás, 1966) indicate that they may. Experimental electron microscopic studies may clarify this point.

The terms *"interneurons"* or *"internuncial cells"* have been mentioned repeatedly. Traditionally these cells have been assumed to belong to the so-called Golgi II type, being characterized by an axon which breaks up into a rich tree of branches and collaterals close to the perikaryon. This concept has been used in the explanation of many physiological observations. However, recent Golgi studies have shown that such cells are rather rare. In several regions, for example the reticular formation (see Chapter 6), they have not been found.

In an exhaustive Golgi study of the spinal cord in a series of mammals, including monkey and man, Scheibel and Scheibel (1966a) found a small number of such cells only in the dorsal horn. In all other regions of the cord the cells with short branching axons always have in addition a long branch (see also Scheibel and Scheibel, 1966b). This may take a different course depending on the situation of the perikaryon. Thus many of the cells situated medially in the ventral horn send their long axonal branch across the midline, while in most other regions the long branch takes a longitudinal course and may extend through several segments. Furthermore, along their course these branches give off collaterals and thus may establish synaptic contact with a number of nerve cells. Many of these ascending or descending longer branches leave the gray matter and run in the deepest region of the white matter and thus belong to the cell category usually referred to as *propriospinal neurons* (see p. 46). These presumably serve chiefly the intersegmental co-operation within the cord. It follows from the above that while there are anatomical pathways available for the transmission of sensory impulses to the motoneurons via internuncials, these cells are not as simple, and probably not as specific, as would appear from diagrams like Fig. 3-6.

A particular type of internuncial cell which has received much attention is the so-called *Renshaw cell,* referred to above (Fig. 3-6B). According to physiological observations, most recently the single unit study of Willis and Willis (1966), most of the cells are situated in the ventral part of Rexed's lamina VII, between laminae VIII and IX (see Fig. 2-2). However, as appears from the above, cells of the type indicated as Renshaw cells in Fig. 3-6 were not found in the extensive Golgi study of Scheibel and Scheibel (1966a). All interneurons in the region of the Renshaw cells have a longer branch in addition to axonal collaterals to cells in the vicinity. The latter have some times been seen to contact motoneurons.

It cannot be entirely excluded that the physiologically identified Renshaw cells have failed to be impregnated in the study of Scheibel and Scheibel (1966a), but this does not appear a likely assumption. Admitting that no classical Golgi type II cells are present in lamina VII it may be said that: "The basic feature of the Renshaw cell hypothesis would be largely preserved, save only that the nature of the cells would be changed from short axoned Golgi type II to long axoned cells, and their positions would be shifted more laterally" (Scheibel and Scheibel, 1966a, p. 348). Szentágothai (1967, p. 12) likewise points out that "there is no real necessity to consider the Renshaw cells as true Golgi II type neurons." The Renshaw cell hypothesis further requires the termination on these cells of recurrent collaterals of the motoneuron axons. This problem can only be studied anatomically with the Golgi method. According to Scheibel and Scheibel (1966a) there may be as many as 3 to 4 such recurrent collaterals of one axon, but many motoneurons appear to lack them (see also Prestige, 1966). As to their distribution it appears from Szentágothai's (1967) study, using superimposed drawings of Golgi preparations, that the main mass of the recurrent collaterals is distributed in the region where the Renshaw cells have been identified physiologically (see also Szentágothai, 1958). On this point anatomical data thus agrees with the conclusions drawn from physiological studies.

As mentioned above physiologically a distinction can be made between "tonic" and "phasic" α motoneurons. The former are assumed to be smaller than the latter and to have thin axons. Mention has also been made of the spontaneous activity of γ motoneurons which are presumably among the smallest neurons in lamina IX. A histological study of the cell sizes in this lamina reveals transitional types, and it is not possible from the size of its perikaryon to decide whether a ventral horn cell may be a phasic or tonic α motoneuron, or whether another cell may be a relatively large γ motoneuron. Working on the assumption that there is a proportionality between the size of a perikaryon and the diameter of its axon, Henneman and his collaborators in a series of studies on the functional properties of motoneurons have presented some interesting new points of view. From their studies (see Henneman, Somjen, and Carpenter, 1965a, 1965b), in which motoneurons were excited reflexly, they conclude that the excitability of spinal motoneurons varies inversely with their size. With all types of excitatory stimuli the recruitment of the cells occurred in the order of their size (as judged from amplitudes of potentials in recordings from axons), the smaller cells being excited before the larger ones. On the other hand, "inhibility" of the motoneurons is directly related to size, the largest ones being most easily inhibited. Corresponding conclusions were drawn by Kernell (1966) from studies of spinal motoneurons in the cat with intracellular recordings.

When a muscle is made to work, this is not the result of activation of one or a few motor units, but a *"pool" of motoneurons* (Sherrington) is involved. Assuming that the synaptic input to this pool in any situation is relatively equally distributed to all of its cells, being of various sizes, the sequence of activation usually observed (γ neurons—tonic α neurons— phasic α neurons) can be explained on a morphological basis. Furthermore, the "various cells in a pool are fired rarely, moderately, or frequently according to their size" (Henneman et al., 1965a, p. 578).

142

In a further study, including histochemical investigations (adenosine tri-phosphate activity), Henneman and Olson (1965) find additional evidence in favor of the theory. Small cells appear to belong to small motor units, and the authors discuss the problems with reference to differences between red and pale muscles, and further comment on some principles which appear to govern the design of skeletal muscles. It appears that the motoneurons behave according to the same principle when activated by stimulation of supraspinal regions (Somjen, Carpenter, and Henneman, 1965). Since in the cat virtually all fibers descending to the cord end on internuncial cells (see Chapter 4) it appears that the latter are organized so as to influence the "pool" of motoneurons in a graded fashion, as do the spinal afferents. On the whole it appears from these studies, as maintained by Sherrington, that the motoneuron pool is an essential feature in the organization of the neuromuscular apparatus, and is "a mechanism which responds automatically to any input and emits an appropriately sized output." These points of view are of interest in interpreting the results of, for example, stimulation of cerebral cortical "motor" regions. They tend to emphasize the importance of the spinal mechanisms in the performance of movements, a view advocated by some authors on the basis of clinical neurological observations (see Chapter 4).

Symptoms following lesions of the peripheral motor neurons.   It follows from the preceding account that when all the motor ventral horn cells which supply a certain group of striated muscles of the body are destroyed, the corresponding muscle or part of a muscle will not be able to contract. The most clear-cut examples of such lesions are probably those met with in poliomyelitis. The virus of the disease affects first and foremost the motoneurons, those of the spinal cord as well as those of the brain stem. In cases of the latter type there will be pareses or paralyses of cranial nerves such as facial palsy, pareses of ocular muscles, etc.

In a *paralysis due to a destruction of all or practically all motoneurons supplying the muscle, not only are all voluntary movements abolished, but also no reflex contractions can be elicited.* Furthermore, since the reflex arc of the myotatic reflexes is broken, *the muscles are flaccid,* they lack their normal tonus. Their consistency is reduced, and they offer no resistance to passive movements. This flaccidity is to a certain extent characteristic of such cases, and enables one to distinguish them from paralyses due to lesions of the central motor systems (cf. Ch. 4). Another characteristic is the occurrence of a *muscular atrophy,* which is the more conspicuous the more complete the paralysis and the longer its duration. The reduced volume of the affected muscles can frequently be seen with the unaided eye, for instance when it affects the small musculi interossei of the hand. As the muscle tissue atrophies there is usually some proliferation of the intermuscular and intramuscular connective tissue.

If the peripheral motor neurons supplying a muscle are not all destroyed, only a partial paralysis, *a paresis,* will ensue, roughly proportional to the number of cells affected. By post-mortem examination of the cord, in such cases, the regions supplying the paretic muscles are found to contain a certain number of nerve cells which appear to be normal and have probably been functioning. The accompanying symptoms will be the same as in cases of paralyses, but they will be less severe. This applies to the *atrophy;* to the *muscular tonus,* which will not be abolished but only reduced; and to the myotatic *reflexes,* which may be present but weakened.[6] In such cases only the muscle fibers which belong to the affected nerve cells will atrophy (cf. above on the anatomical findings). The movements which can be performed will be more or less weak, and usually also *slower* than normally. This *retardation of movements* is to be explained by the reduced amount of innervation. In clinical cases there is a difference between the retardation of movements seen in cases of lesions of the peripheral motor neurons and in those pareses which are due to lesions of the central motor pathways. In the latter case the retardation appears to be much greater than can be accounted for by the frequently very moderate paresis. *In peripheral motoneuron lesions the retardation goes approximately parallel to the reduction of muscular strength.*

The symptoms described above, paresis, atrophy, hypotonus, abolished or weakened reflexes, and retardation, will of course occur not only in lesions of the perikarya of the motoneurons, but an interruption of their axons in the ventral roots, the plexuses, or the peripheral nerves will have similar consequences. The interruption may in some cases be only functional, without morphological destruction of the fibers. Thus intraspinal tumors may press on one or more roots, or a peripheral nerve may suffer by anoxia due to compression or circulatory disturbances.

Occasionally, in patients suffering from damage to the peripheral motor neurons, one finds so-called *fibrillary twitchings.* These are fine, rhythmical, or more often irregular twitchings of small groups of muscle fibers visible through the skin or to be felt by palpation. They become particularly evident when the appropriate part of the body is cooled. A more adequate name, now commonly used, is *fasciculations.* They can be recorded electromyographically, but their origin is not understood. It was previously commonly held that the occurrence of fasciculations indicated a primary affection of the motoneurons (for example in amyotrophic lateral sclerosis or progressive spinal muscular atrophy) and that the symptom, therefore, may help in the differential diagnosis between a

[6] When the tendon reflexes in the leg are weak or difficult to elicit, the Jendrassik maneuver may be of value. When the individual forcefully attempts to draw his interlocked hands apart, a tap on the patellar or achilles tendon may give a marked reflex response. Several studies have been devoted to the mechanism of this facilitation of the stretch reflex occurring in the Jendrassik maneuver. Somewhat different opinions have been expressed (see for example, Gassel and Diamantopoulos, 1964; Clarke, 1967).

"nuclear" lesion or a "radicular" lesion, where the disease process attacks the ventral roots. However, the diagnostic value of the symptom appears to be rather limited (see Buchthal, 1962).

In *denervated muscles,* i.e. muscles which have lost their nerve supply, another phenomenon may be observed in the electromyogram: small action potentials occurring with a high frequency. These *fibrillation potentials* appear to arise from single muscle fibers which have lost their motor innervation. The contraction of the fibers can neither be seen nor felt. The origin of the fibrillation is not quite settled, but it has been maintained that it is due to a "sensitization" of the muscular part of the end plate following denervation (compare Ch. 11, on the Autonomic Nervous System). The absence of the normal transmitter, acetylcholine, may make the muscle fiber respond to the minute amount of acetylcholine present in the circulating blood. Prostigmin, which delays the breakdown of acetylcholine, tends to increase the fibrillation in denervated muscle. The presence of fibrillation potentials in the electromyogram of a paretic or paralytic muscle may be taken as evidence that some of its nerve fibers have been interrupted, whereas the presence of true motor units indicates that some nerve fibers are intact. However, fibrillation does not necessarily indicate denervation (see Buchthal, 1962). Nevertheless, fibrillation potentials have turned out to be useful diagnostic and prognostic criteria, particularly in cases of lesions of peripheral nerves.

The clinical symptoms of lesions of the motonuerons will be of the same kind whether the perikarya or the axons are damaged. The impulses starting the contraction are prevented from reaching the muscle in either case. However, even if the *type* of symptoms is the same, their *distribution* may be different, and in many cases it will be *possible to determine the exact site of the lesion when attention is paid to the localization of pareses, atrophy, and changes of reflexes.* Since this point is of practical importance it will be dealt with in some detail.

The segmental motor innervation. Lesions of the brachial plexus. The fibers of the different spinal nerves (their ventral branches) from certain parts of the cord are intermingled in the formation of the plexuses, from which they continue in the various peripheral nerves. Consequently fibers from several segments of the cord are present in most of the peripheral nerves. In the radial nerve, for example, motor fibers from the ventral horn cells of the 5th cervical—1st thoracic segments are present. Fig. 3-7 shows the peripheral distribution of motor fibers from the 5th cervical segment. Thus the segmental arrangement of the fibers disappears during their course. However, *in the distribution of the peripheral nerves to the muscles, the segmental origin of the nerve fibers again becomes evident.* This is explained by the development of the neuromuscu-

145

lar system in ontogenesis. As will be recalled, the organism is, in the early stages of development, segmentally constructed. In the primitive metameres different parts are allotted to the future development of connective tissue and bones, of muscles, and of skin, and each of the metameres is related to one particular segment of the primitive spinal cord. Apparently the segmental pattern is completely lost during later development in most parts of the body. However, this is more apparent than real, and, particularly with regard to the peripheral innervation, it is actually retained in both the motor and the sensory innervation.

The segmental pattern of the striated muscles is clearly visible in the thorax with the intercostal muscles, and traces are seen also in the subdivision of the rectus abdominis muscle by its tendinous intersections. However, a relation to particular segments of the cord can also be demonstrated in other muscles. Most muscles receive their motor fibers from two segments of the cord, some smaller muscles only from one segment, some of the larger from three or even, in some cases, from more than

FIG. 3–7 A diagram of the brachial plexus, showing how fibers from the 5th cervical segment are distributed to various peripheral nerves. The most important muscles supplied by these fibers are indicated. From Haymaker and Woodhall (1945).

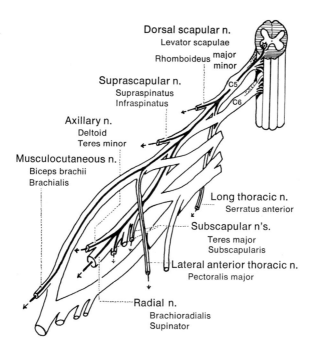

Dorsal scapular n.
Levator scapulae
Rhomboideus major
minor

Suprascapular n.
Supraspinatus
Infraspinatus

C5
C6

Axillary n.
Deltoid
Teres minor

Musculocutaneous n.
Biceps brachii
Brachialis

Long thoracic n.
Serratus anterior

Subscapular n's.
Teres major
Subscapularis

Lateral anterior thoracic n.
Pectoralis major

Radial n.
Brachioradialis
Supinator

three neighboring segments. The various muscles get their motor (and sensory) innervation from the segments of the cord which correspond to the metameres from which they were originally developed.[7] In a lesion which comprises only a few segments of the cord or a limited number of ventral roots, the affected muscles will be those which developed from the corresponding metameres. In a lesion of a peripheral nerve, all those muscles which it supplies will be affected. The segmental innervation of the various muscles need not be memorized (complete tables are found in several textbooks, e.g. Monrad-Krohn's *Clinical Examination*), but certain principal points ought to be kept in mind.

Of most practical importance is the segmental innervation of the *upper extremity*. This may be diagrammatically regarded as developing as a lateral bud from the trunk at the level of the lower cervical segments, and consequently it is these nerves (more precisely from the 5th cervical to the 1st thoracic inclusive) which supply the muscles of the arm with motor fibers. Among these nerves the fibers arising from the 5th and 6th cervical segments are concerned mainly in the innervation of muscles situated proximally and laterally, e.g. the deltoid, supraspinatus and infraspinatus, teres major and minor, and the flexors on the anterior aspect of the upper arm, the coracobrachialis, biceps, brachialis, and brachioradialis (cf. also Fig. 3-7). In a lesion of the upper parts of the cervical enlargement of the cord or the 5th and 6th ventral roots these muscles will be paralytic (in addition to some smaller muscles of the neck). As will be seen this distribution of paralysis (or paresis) does not correspond to that met with in lesions of any peripheral nerve. Some of these muscles are supplied by the axillary or circumflex nerve (the deltoid and teres minor), others by the musculocutaneous nerve (coracobrachialis, brachialis, and biceps), others by still other nerves. A paralysis of the distribution referred to above with muscular atrophy, hypotonus, and affection of the reflexes may be observed, for example, in cases of so-called *upper brachial plexus palsy* (Erb, Duchenne) which sometimes occurs in newborn babies on account of violent stretching of the plexus during delivery. (If a sensory loss is present, this will also be segmental; cf. description of the dermatomes, Ch. 2.) A similar distribution of the paresis or paralysis will be seen if the ventral roots of the 5th and 6th cervical nerves are damaged, for instance by an intraspinal tumor, or if the ventral horn cells of these segments are affected, such as may occur in poliomyelitis.

The extensors of the upper arm, triceps and anconeus, are supplied by the (6th) 7th and 8th cervical segments. The flexors and extensors on the forearm are

[7] The establishment of the segmental motor innervation has been achieved by different methods. Apart from gross dissections, the study of the retrograde changes in the ventral horn cells in cases of amputations, etc., has been utilized as mentioned in Chapter 1. Studies in cases of transverse lesions of the spinal cord have also given valuable information. Following electrical stimulation of the ventral roots during operations, the ensuing contractions of muscles may be observed and used for determining the segmental motor innervations. In recent years electromyography has been used to record the muscles activated. There appear to be considerable individual variations with regard to the segmental innervation of particular muscles, as shown for the lower limb, for example, by Thage (1964).

147

mainly taken care of by fibers from the 7th and 8th cervical segments, the small muscles of the hand by the 8th cervical and 1st thoracic segments. On this account a lesion of the lower parts of the brachial plexus or of the ventral horn cells in the lower part of the cervical enlargement of the cord will result in paralysis or paresis predominantly of the muscles of the hand and forearm. This is seen in the so-called *lower brachial plexus palsy* (Déjerine–Klumpke), which may occur in new-born babies (although less frequently than an upper brachial plexus palsy). A localization of paresis and atrophy of this distribution is most frequently observed in cases of progressive spinal muscular atrophy, in which a slowly progressing de-generation of motor ventral horn cells occurs. The disease shows a predilection for starting in the upper thoracic and lower cervical segments of the cord, and, conse-quently, quite frequently the first symptoms noted are paresis and atrophy of the small muscles of the hand (the interossei and the muscles of the hypothenar and, somewhat less pronounced, of the thenar eminences). As the pathological process proceeds upwards in the cord, the muscles of the forearm and eventually those of the upper arm and shoulder girdle also become affected. In syringomyelia the same localization is also frequently observed, indicating that the pathological process is located in the lower cervical segments. A localization of the paresis of the type mentioned above does not correspond to a lesion of any particular nerve. In an affection of the median nerve some of the flexors of the forearm will usually be involved, making flexion of the 2nd and 3rd fingers impossible, and the superficial muscles of the thenar eminence will contribute to making opposition as well as flexion of the thumb impossible or impaired. The interossei and the muscles of the hypothenar eminence, however, will not be affected. Lesions of the ulnar nerve are those most apt to cause diagnostic mistakes, since in these cases paresis and atrophy of the interossei and hypothenar muscles will be present. However, the thenar mus-cles will only be partly affected, since some of them are supplied by the median nerve (the ulnar innervating only the deep part of the flexor pollicis brevis and the adductor pollicis) and the accompanying sensory disturbance will as a rule settle the question.

In *the lower extremity* conditions are essentially similar with regard to the seg-mental motor innervation. The hip flexors (iliopsoas, rectus femoris, and sartorius muscles) and the adductors are innervated from the upper lumbar segments of the cord, mainly L_{2-3}, the gluteal muscles and those on the posterior aspect of the thigh from the (4th) 5th lumbar and 1st sacral segments, the muscles of the calf from the 5th lumbar–2nd sacral segments. The small muscles of the foot and the flexors of the toes are mainly supplied by the 1st and 2nd sacral segments (S_3 and S_4 are concerned in the innervation of the muscles of the pelvic diaphragm). Since local-ized affections of the roots of the lumbar and sacral nerves are not characteristic of certain diseases to the same extent as in the case of the cervical roots, the seg-mental innervation of the muscles of the lower extremity is of less importance than is that of the upper. However, the motor impairment may be an aid in the topo-graphical diagnosis, e.g. in cases of tumors or protrusion of intervertebral discs (cf. Ch. 2). The distribution of the segmental pareses will as a rule not coincide with those due to lesions of the peripheral nerves, although the difference is on the whole not as marked as in the upper extremity.[8]

---

[8] For an exhaustive account of the distribution of pareses following lesions of particular ventral roots, see the monograph of Hansen and Schliack (1962).

It will appear from the preceding account that an analysis of the impairment of motor function, its type as well as its distribution, may give important information in regard to the localization of a lesion. When a paralysis is found to be of the peripheral type, there is usually little difficulty in deciding whether or not it is due to a lesion of a peripheral nerve. In the latter case the determination of the exact place of the lesion, the segments of the cord affected, or the ventral roots involved is in some cases of practical importance, since this *segmental diagnosis* will determine at which place the operative measures have to be undertaken, for instance in cases of extramedullary tumors which yield themselves favorably to surgical intervention.[9]

With regard to the segmental diagnosis it is necessary to consider that the spinal nerves pursue an increasingly oblique course within the vertebral canal as they approach the caudal nerves. Whereas the upper cervical nerves pass practically in a horizontal direction from the cord to their intervertebral foramina, the lower lumbar and the sacral nerves pass obliquely downward for a long distance within the dural sac before leaving the vertebral canal. This will be seen from Fig. 3-8. The explanation is found in the so-called "ascent of the medulla spinalis" in ontogenesis, due to the fact that the growth of the spinal cord does not keep pace with that of the spine. If therefore a segmental motor impairment of the segments L_{2-4} has been ascertained, this may mean that the lesion is situated at the level of the corresponding vertebrae if the pathological process is near to the intervertebral foramina, but if the cause is an intramedullary lesion, e.g. a tumor or syringomyelia, the pathological focus will be found at the level of approximately the 11th to 12th thoracic vertebra. An intraspinal but extramedullary process, such as a tumor, a protruded intervertebral disc, or an arachnoiditis, may cause a distribution of this type when it is situated anywhere between the 11th thoracic and 4th lumbar vertebrae. It is particularly in the latter cases that an exact diagnosis of the level is of interest since surgical therapy must be considered. The final determination will be made by the examination of other features, such as signs from other ventral roots, accompanying sensory symptoms, autonomic disturbances, the conditions of the cerebrospinal fluid, myelography, and the history of the development of the symptoms.

Another point should also be stressed: since most muscles are innervated from more than one segment of the spinal cord, *a destruction of cells or fibers of only one segment will as a rule not betray itself clinically,*

[9] The condition of the reflexes may also aid in the segmental diagnosis. A list of the level of the reflex center of various reflexes is found in several textbooks, e.g. Monrad-Krohn's *Clinical Examination.*

or only when carefully sought. In this case electromyographic examinations may give valuable information, as has been mentioned above, and sensory symptoms of irritation may also afford a clue (cf. Ch. 2).

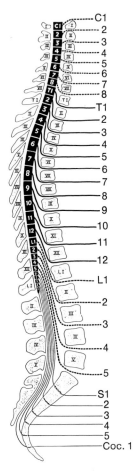

FIG. 3–8 A diagram showing the relation of the levels of the spinal cord and the spinal nerves to the corresponding vertebrae. From Haymaker and Woodhall (1945).

4

Pathways Mediating Supraspinal Influences on the Spinal Cord

THE reader will have noticed that this book does not contain chapters with the headings "Pyramidal tract" and "Extrapyramidal motor system," found in most textbooks and used also in the first edition of the present text. This deviation from current usage is rather heretical and necessitates some comments.

"Pyramidal" and "extrapyramidal" motor systems. The cerebral cortex and a number of nuclei in the brain stem are able to influence the activity of the spinal cord since they give off fibers which either descend directly to the cord or end in other nuclei which in their turn send efferent fibers to the cord. These nuclei receive afferent fibers from other sources as well (for example, from the cerebellum), and the impulse transmission from "higher levels" to the cord via these nuclei will, therefore, be subject to modifications at those places where the pathways are synaptically interrupted. Furthermore, the cerebral cortex and all nuclei projecting, directly or via intermediate stations, to the cord will receive information from this, ultimately to a large extent derived from receptors of various kinds. Some of the fiber bundles which pass from supraspinal structures directly to the cord and may influence its activity are shown in Fig. 4-1. It seems likely, a priori, that these pathways are not functionally identical, an assumption which has been amply supported by recent neurophysiological research. It must be assumed, further, that under normal conditions they co-operate in an integrated manner. An analysis of this co-operation presents considerable difficulties, and much still remains to be done in this field.

It was formerly generally thought that the task of the descending fiber systems to the cord was to act on its efferent mechanisms, determining the impulse discharges of its somatic and visceral efferent neurons. Since the 1950's it has been conclusively demonstrated that the descending fiber systems in addition have another important function, namely to regulate the transmission of sensory impulses from the periphery to the brain, as described in Chapter 2. This had indeed been hypothesized by clinical neurologists as Head, Brouwer, and others. It is, therefore, no longer adequate—and not even permissible—to talk of the descending pathways collectively as "motor" fiber systems. The untenability of such a concept is further borne out by the fact, referred to above, that the

FIG. 4–1 Diagram of fiber systems descending to the cord from supraspinal levels: the corticospinal, rubrospinal, tectospinal, interstitiospinal, pontine and medullary reticulospinal and vestibulospinal tracts. Some minor tracts, such as the solitariospinal tract, are omitted. All of these connections may influence the activity of the peripheral motor neurons.

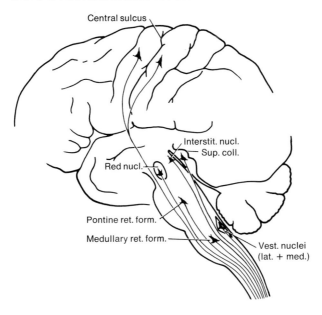

nuclei giving off fibers which influence the efferent mechanisms of the cord receive ascending fibers providing them with sensory information, necessary for their proper functioning. To deal with a "motor" function without considering its concomitant sensory phenomena is a theoretical abstraction. As Jung and Hassler (1960, p. 864) phrase it: ". . . a 'motor system' without sensory control is a fiction, not even a useful fiction."

The many new observations which have been provided by neuro-anatomical and neurophysiological research in the last two to three decades necessitate thorough revisions of many classical concepts concerning the so-called motor systems. Unfortunately, many of these concepts have got a strong hold in our minds, in part, it seems, because they are simple and for this reason easy to use in routine work (although it is admitted that they are not adequate). Furthermore, the concepts are linked with certain names, and names and designations, as is well known, have a tendency to serve as convenient labels and help us to hide our ignorance. With reference to the subject concerning us here the terms "pyramidal" and "extrapyramidal" and "upper motor neuron" are particularly relevant, and deserve brief comment.

The *pyramidal tract* by definition is all those fibers which course longitudinally in the pyramis of the medulla oblongata, regardless of their site of origin or termination. The vast majority of these fibers come from the cerebral cortex (see below), and most of them continue into the spinal cord, making up the *corticospinal tract*. However, some fibers take off in the pyramid or at higher levels to pass towards motor cranial nerve nuclei in the brain stem. Strictly speaking these are thus not pyramidal tract fibers according to the above definition. Collectively they are often referred to as the *corticobulbar tract*. Since the latter appears functionally to correspond to the corticospinal tract, the term pyramidal tract may be—and often is—used as a common term for both. Although objections may be raised against stretching the definition in this way it may be advantageous to have a common name for the two components. The term "pyramidal tract," therefore, will be used in this sense in the following, and the names corticospinal and corticobulbar tract will be used when reference is made to the particular components. The term "corticobulbar tract" is sometimes used as including also those corticofugal fibers which pass with the corticospinal fibers and end in the bulbar reticular formation and other bulbar nuclei.

Anatomically the pyramidal tract is fairly well defined. This, however, does not justify the current use of the term *"pyramidal tract syndrome"* for a certain constellation of symptoms (see below). This term implies that the symptoms are due to damage to the pyramidal tract and only to this, while what is described as the pyramidal tract syndrome is actually those motor and reflex changes which are found after a lesion of the internal capsule or certain parts of the cerebral cortex. These, however, are never true, pure lesions of the pyramidal tract, since numerous other descending fiber projections coming from the same cortical regions as the pyramidal tract fibers and passing together with them in the internal capsule will necessarily be concomitantly damaged. The only lesions which would produce a pyramidal tract syndrome are interruptions of the fibers where they are isolated, i.e. in the pyramis of the medulla, as will be further discussed in a later section. The "pyramidal tract syndrome" is, therefore, a misnomer.

The term *"extrapyramidal"* is properly an anatomical concept and strictly speaking includes everything which is not "pyramidal." However, it has been currently used with the tacit qualification that it refers to "motor systems" (the extrapyramidal motor system), implying that the name covers all descending pathways and their intercalated nuclei, apart from the pyramidal tract, which may influence motor activities. As referred to above there are a number of such pathways, and in view of the fact that several other parts of the nervous system (such as the cerebellum) are well known to influence the function of the motor apparatus, difficulties arise as to the delimitation of the concept "extrapyramidal" structures. Some authors have included in it the pontine nuclei and the intracerebellar nuclei, and particularly the basal ganglia are considered to form an integrative part of it. It is, however, not possible to delimit and define this "system" anatomically.

Clinical observations show that lesions of various regions of the brain give rise to disturbances of motor functions which differ from those of the "pyramidal tract syndrome," and consist chiefly in changes in muscular tone and involuntary movements of various kinds. These clinical pictures are often lumped together as "extrapyramidal diseases." They comprise those syndromes which are seen following lesions of the basal ganglia. Oscar and Cecile Vogt (1920) spoke of a "striate system" (including the striatum, pallidum, subthalamic nucleus, and other nuclei and tracts). As somewhat similar syndromes were found later to follow lesions of other parts of the brain as well, for example of the dentate nucleus, the concept of the "extrapyramidal system" expanded. In spite of the fact that these disorders may have some clinical features in common, it is difficult to see the advantages of considering them under a common heading, the more so since the "system" to which they are referred escapes definition. The only reason for retaining the designation "extrapyramidal diseases" would be to avoid the problems of analysing each particular syndrome on a rational basis.

Descending Supraspinal Pathways

The *"extrapyramidal system"* has in the past, by some kind of antithetic reasoning, usually been thought of as something quite separate and different from the "pyramidal system." It has for a long time been clear, however, that this distinction is untenable. It is impossible—and if it were possible, it would be artificial—to separate the function of the pyramidal tract from those of other descending fiber systems. In the intact being they must co-operate. Anatomically a separation is equally impossible. For example, as will be described below, those cortical regions which give rise to fibers in the pyramidal tract also give off fibers to a number of nuclei which project further caudally, and which are included in the "extrapyramidal system." Furthermore, there are reciprocal connections between many of these nuclei, which bear further witness of possibilities for interaction among the nuclei and with the pyramidal tract. These multitudes of connections make it clear that in almost every lesion of the brain a number of fiber connections will be involved simultaneously, making it precarious to attribute a particular clinical feature to the lesion of a particular structure. While this may be disheartening in so far as it makes it difficult to give a certain constellation of symptoms a name which refers to a specific part of the brain, the recognition of these complexities is certainly necessary if progress is to be made in the analysis of clinical disturbances of motor functions.

The expression *"upper motor neuron"* is sometimes employed, particularly it appears, in connection with symptoms attributed to damage to the pyramidal tract (upper motor neuron disease). Since there are many "upper motor neurons," the use of the term in this sense is misleading, and it might with advantage be avoided.

It is the author's firm conviction that neither theoretically nor practically is a useful purpose served by retaining the term "extrapyramidal." In the light of present day knowledge the term, as referring to structures and functions "other than pyramidal" is completely meaningless, as emphasized also by others, for example by Russel Meyers (1953) and Bucy (1957). Accordingly, the presentation to be given here will not follow the orthodox lines, perhaps to the disappointment of some students. In the following an attempt will be made to describe the essential points in the anatomy and to some extent the physiology of the pathways descending to the spinal cord which may influence the activity of the motor neurons. As will be seen, in spite of the accumulation of much new data which has increased our understanding of the subject, it is not easy to make correlations with clinical findings.

Changing views on the pyramidal tract. The pyramidal tract has got its name from the medullary pyramid where its fibers run in isolation. Its definition as generally accepted at present was mentioned above.

1 5 5

The vast majority—possibly all—of its fibers come from the cerebral cortex.

The pyramidal tract appears to be the first large fiber bundle recognized as a particular tract in the brain. It was described by Türck in 1851 as extending from the cerebral cortex to the spinal cord, and Türck also observed that in patients suffering from spastic hemiplegia a bleeding in the internal capsule is often found post-mortem. In 1870 Fritsch and Hitzig demonstrated that on electrical stimulation of the frontal lobe in dogs movements of the opposite limbs can be elicited. About the same time Hughlings Jackson (1875), on the basis of clinical observations, concluded that there must be a somatotopical "localization of movements in the brain." Around the turn of the century a number of studies were undertaken which further elaborated the pioneer observations. Thus Grünbaum and Sherrington (1902; 1903) by cortical stimulations and ablations showed the existence of a somatotopic pattern in the precentral gyrus in apes. Corresponding conclusions were drawn from clinical cases with cortical lesions. In 1909 Holmes and May reported that following transection of the pyramidal tract in the upper spinal cord in monkeys retrograde cellular changes occur only in the giant cells of Betz in Brodmann's area 4. The origin of the tract appeared now to be settled. As a result of these and other studies a notion of the pyramidal tract emerged which was generally held until about some thirty years ago: The pyramidal tract arises from the precentral gyrus and descends to the cord. Its fibers are thick and myelinated. In the spinal cord they establish contact with the peripheral motor neurons; the tract is concerned in the mediation of voluntary, particularly finely isolated discrete movements. According to this conception the pyramidal tract is rather simply organized and has a clearly defined function.

Doubts on the correctness of this simple view on the pyramidal tract had been voiced by students in various fields of neurological research when Lassek and Rasmussen in 1939 counted the fibers in the pyramid of man, where most of the corticobulbar fibers have left it. In silver impregnated sections they found about a million fibers in each pyramid. More recently DeMyer (1959) reported that the number varies between 749,000 and 1,391,000, with a mean value of 1,087,200 (21 cases). Since the number of Betz cells in Brodmann's area 4 is only some 25,000 to 30,000 (Campbell, 1905; Lassek, 1940) it appears that only between 3 and 4 per cent of the fibers in the pyramid can be axons of Betz cells, even if, as pointed out by Lassek (1941) and others, there exists no definite criterion which makes it possible to characterize a Betz cell. There are transitions to large pyramidal cells which occur in the Vth layer of area 4 as well as in neighboring areas. However, there can be no doubt that *the vast majority of pyramidal tract fibers come from other cells than the Betz cells* in the precentral gyrus. This conclusion is in agreement with observations made by some earlier authors (Wohlfahrt, 1932; Levin and Bradford, 1938). Extirpation of area 4 in the monkey results in the disappearance of only about a quarter of the fibers in the pyramid (Häggqvist, 1937; Lassek, 1942a). Further studies have shown that pyramidal tract fibers take origin from other regions of the cortex than the area 4 of Brodmann, as will be discussed later.

In the 1940's Lassek published a series of studies of the pyramidal tract, especially in man. It appears that these studies have been substantial in directing renewed interest to a fiber tract which had for a long time been considered as one of the best known and most simply organized ones in the brain. The results of anatomical, physiological, clinical, and clinicopathological studies from the last twenty-five years have necessitated a complete re-evaluation of the older concepts of the pyramidal tract. Before discussing present-day views on the pyramidal tract, its gross anatomy in man will be briefly described.

The course of the pyramidal tract. The pyramidal tract fibers descend from the cortex to the internal capsule (Fig. 4-8), where they are found collected in a relatively small area in the posterior limb. It is worth stressing their close relationship to the thalamus medial to them, and the lentiform nucleus laterally to them, as well as the presence in the internal capsule of other fibers, such as corticopontine, corticorubral, pallidothalamic, etc. Studies of the distribution of the fibers degenerating after circumscribed lesions of the "motor area" in man and experimental animals seem to show that *in the internal capsule the fibers present an arrangement according to their place of origin in the cortex and their level of termination.* (The cortical localization will be considered later.) Most anteriorly the fibers to the motor nuclei of the cranial nerves are found. Then follow in an orderly sequence those to the cervical part of the cord, supplying the muscles of the neck and arm; those to the thoracic part, innervating the muscles of the trunk; and most posteriorly those to the lumbar and sacral parts of the cord, supplying the muscles of the legs and those of the pelvis.

In Foerster's diagram of the internal capsule, reproduced in many textbooks, the pyramidal tract fibers are distributed over the entire posterior limb and the genu of the internal capsule. It appears, however, from some pathological anatomical studies (Marion Smith, 1960; Hirayama et al., 1962; Brion and Guiot, 1964, see also Marion Smith, 1967) that in man the fibers occupy only a relatively small area of the internal capsule, and that this area is found posteriorly in its posterior limb. Studies of motor responses following electrical stimulation of the

157

internal capsule in man or of deficits following small lesions of it (Guiot et al., 1959) are in agreement with this and, furthermore, indicate that the somatotopical localization is not sharp.

Concerning the gross features of the pyramidal tract in its further downward course the following may be noted. In the *cerebral peduncle* the fibers occupy the middle two-thirds, bordered laterally and medially by corticopontine fibers. There appears to be a somatotopical arrangement of the corticospinal fibers in the peduncle as maintained by Foerster (1936b) and shown in the diagram in Fig. 4-2. Barnard and Woolsey (1956) confirmed this pattern in experimental studies in the monkey and rat and, furthermore, found that corticospinal fibers from the somatic sensory area of the parietal cortex (see below) are found most laterally within the corticospinal territory in the peduncle. The fibers to the extrinsic eye muscles are probably to be sought within the area of the frontopontine tract (cf. Fig. 4-2). (For further data on the peduncle in man see Marin et al., 1962; Martinez et al., 1967.)

In the pons the fibers from the peduncle split into several bundles, which intrude between the large cellular masses of the pontine nuclei. The corticopontine fibers (to be considered in the chapter on the cerebellum) take off from it and end in the pontine nuclei. At the lower border of the pons the remaining fibers of the pyramidal tract unite and leave the pons

FIG. 4–2 Diagrammatic drawing of a section through the mesencephalon, indicating the position in the cerebral peduncle of the pyramidal tract fibers to the different parts of the body. Somewhat modified from Foerster (1936b) on the basis of findings made by other authors. (Cf. text.)

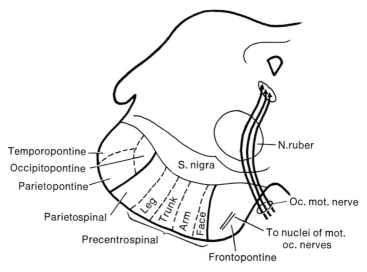

as a distinct bundle, forming the *pyramid* of the medulla oblongata. Whether the fibers retain a somatotopical arrangement during their course in the pyramid has been questioned by some but advocated by other authors. Woodburne (1939) in anatomical investigations in animals (Marchi method) verified the existence of a somatotopical arrangement, in agreement with the conception of Foerster (1936b) as illustrated in Fig. 2-9. However, Tower (1944) is inclined to deny such an arrangement, at least in the pyramids of monkeys, on the basis of the functional defects seen following partial lesions of the medullary pyramid, and Barnard and Woolsey (1956) found no localization in the cord in monkeys. (It should be emphasized that the localization is certainly not as distinct as appears from a simplified diagram such as Fig. 2-9.)

During the course of the pyramidal tract in the brain stem some fibers are given off in order to supply the motor (somatic efferent) nuclei of the cranial nerves. It is of practical relevance that some of these fibers cross the median line, others not. This means that *some of the motor cranial nerve nuclei are influenced by fibers from both cerebral hemispheres.* These conclusions are chiefly based on clinical observations. Making allowance for individual variations, it may be said that, as a rule, the hypoglossal nucleus, the nucleus of the accessory nerve, and the parts of the facial nucleus concerned with the lower part of the face appear to have purely crossed corticofugal connections. In some individuals the motor trigeminal nucleus belongs to the same group. Consequently only the corresponding muscles will be paralyzed in unilateral lesions of the corticobulbar fibers.

The *corticospinal tract* represents what is left of the pyramidal tract when it has passed the brain stem. The major part of its fibers cross in the pyramidal decussation. After having crossed, these fibers are found in the spinal cord in an area lateral to the dorsal horn as the *lateral corticospinal tract* (cf. Fig. 2-8, see also Fig. 1-2), and are presumably arranged in an orderly sequence, the shortest fibers being situated deeply, the longest most superficially. Some authors, in contrast to Foerster, maintain that in the spinal cord the somatotopical arrangement within the lateral corticospinal tract is entirely lost. The final word on this question has, however, not been said. A priori it seems reasonable that there should be some sort of somatotopical arrangement of the pyramidal fibers along their entire course, although the localization is scarcely as sharp as depicted in Foerster's diagram.

A smaller proportion of the pyramidal fibers descend uncrossed in the spinal cord, the percentage, however, varies individually. Some of the uncrossed fibers form a long recognized bundle, the *ventral corticospinal tract* in the ventral funiculus of the cord along the ventral median

159

NEUROLOGICAL ANATOMY

fissure (Fig. 2-8). This tract probably rarely descends below the thoracic part of the cord. In addition, however, *some uncrossed fibers join the crossed fibers of the lateral corticospinal tract.* The literature on the many individual variations of the human pyramidal tract has been reviewed by Nyberg-Hansen and Rinvik (1963). Some of these variations, particularly the ratio of uncrossed to crossed fibers, are of interest from a clinical point of view.

Most of our present-day insight into the anatomical and functional organization of the pyramidal tract has been derived from experimental studies of animals. However, the comparable data available for man indicates principal similarities, even if there may be some functional differences between species. Assuming that the pyramidal tract is of particular importance for the execution of delicate voluntary movements, a question to be discussed below, one might expect the number of pyramidal tract fibers to be especially large in man, as appears indeed to be the case (Lassek and Wheatley, 1945). A discussion of the function of the pyramidal tract and of the symptoms following its destruction in man will be postponed until other descending pathways from the cerebral cortex to the spinal cord have been considered.

Origin and termination of the pyramidal tract fibers. For anatomical studies of the cortical origin of the fibers of the pyramidal tract two approaches may be used. As referred to above one may look for the occurrence of retrograde cellular changes in the cerebral cortex following transection of the fibers. The difficulty here is that not all affected cells will necessarily present changes which are definite enough to permit recognition. Another procedure is to make lesions in the cerebral cortex and to trace the efferent degenerating fibers, either with the Marchi method or with silver impregnation methods which enable one to identify not only myelinated but also unmyelinated fibers. Studies of this kind are beset with other difficulties. It is almost impossible to produce lesions restricted to particular cytoarchitectonic areas of the cortex. Neighboring areas may be involved on account of vascular changes, and microscopical identification of the part destroyed or removed is difficult on account of the ensuing distortion of the tissue. Conclusions as to the origin of fibers from a particular area must, therefore, be evaluated with some caution. In spite of technical difficulties a large number of studies devoted to the origin of the fibers of the pyramidal tract have established the main points. It is obvious from these that *the area 4, the classical "motor area," is not the only source of corticospinal fibers.* In various animal species such fibers have been traced from area 6, in front of area 4 (Levin and Bradford, 1938, Russell and DeMyer, 1961, in the monkey; Minckler, Klemme, and Minckler, 1944, in man), while there appears to be no

160

conclusive evidence that the areas in front of area 6 contribute. However, the parietal cortex, particularly the "primary sensory cortex," areas 3, 1, and 2 of Brodmann, is an important source of pyramidal tract fibers in all species studied (Levin and Bradford, 1938; Peele, 1942; Barnard and Woolsey, 1956; Kuypers, 1958a, b, c; Russell and DeMyer, 1961; Nyberg-Hansen and Brodal, 1963; Liu and Chambers, 1964; and others). Furthermore, the parietal cortex above the Sylvian fissure (harboring Brodmann's areas 40 and 43, see Fig. 12-2) where the second somatosensory area (see Ch. 2 and below) has been identified, sends fibers to the spinal cord. Likewise there is a corticospinal projection from the supplementary motor region on the medial surface of the hemisphere (see Ch. 2 and below). It is possible that there are small contributions from the temporal and occipital cortices in the cat (Walberg and Brodal, 1953a) and from the temporal cortex in the monkey (Sunderland, 1940).

The fibers of the pyramidal tract are of greatly varying diameter and consequently have different conduction velocities. A large number of the fibers are thin and unmyelinated. Lassek (1942b) found that in the human pyramid, just above the decussation, 90 per cent have a diameter of only $1–4\mu$, whereas not more than 1.73 per cent are between 11 and 22μ. According to Lassek (1942b) about 60 per cent of all pyramidal fibers are myelinated in man, while DeMyer (1959), using another method, found about 94 per cent. The number of large myelinated fibers thus corresponds approximately to the estimated number of Betz cells in area 4, and it is also worthy of notice that, following extirpation of area 4, almost all large fibers disappear (Häggqvist, 1937; Russell and DeMyer, 1961). It appears indeed probable that the largest fibers in the tract are the axons of the largest pyramidal cells of the cortex, the Betz cells. The largest Betz cells are found in the lower part of area 4 (Lassek, 1941) which projects onto the lumbosacral cord, a fact supporting the general assumption that there is a relationship between the size of a nerve cell and the length of its axon.

Some students have attempted to determine the relative proportion of fibers from the various cortical regions of origin. Quantitative assessments of degenerating fibers are, however, difficult. Another approach to the problem is to count the number of normal fibers left after a sufficiently long time has passed for complete disappearance of the fibers coming from the ablated cortical area. Studying monkeys surviving for one year after ablation of various cortical areas, Russell and DeMyer (1961) conclude that in this animal 31 per cent of the descending fibers in the pyramid come from area 4, 29 per cent from area 6, and 40 per cent from the parietal lobe.

The anatomical data concerning the origin of pyramidal tract fibers agree on the whole with physiological and clinical observations (see below). They make it clear that this tract is not in all respects a uniform fiber bundle, a conclusion which is further substantiated when its terminations are considered.

By means of silver impregnation methods the *sites of termination of the corticospinal fibers* can be determined fairly precisely. Even the first studies of this kind made it clear that in the cat few, if any, of the corticospinal tract fibers establish contact with the large motoneurons. The degenerating boutons and terminal arborizations of degenerating fibers were uniformly found more dorsally, in what was usually referred to as the "intermediate zone" of the spinal gray matter and the base of the dorsal horn (Hoff and Hoff, 1934; Szentágothai-Schimert, 1941a; and others). These observations have been confirmed by Chambers and Liu (1957) and Kuypers (1958a) and agree with the results of physiological studies by Lloyd (1941) in the cat, that pyramidal tract impulses activate the motoneurons by way of internuncials. More precise information has been obtained by making use of the architectonic map of Rexed (1952, 1954). Nyberg-Hansen and Brodal (1963), using the Nauta method, found the corticospinal fibers from the "central region" in the cat to end in laminae IV to VII, chiefly laminae V to VI (Fig. 4-3), where the fibers of the lateral corticospinal tract enter the gray matter. No fibers were traced to lamina IX. Some fibers end in corresponding regions on the other side. Further, the fibers coming from the cortical region supposed by most authors to correspond to the precentral "motor" cortex in monkeys and man (for particulars see Nyberg-Hansen and Brodal, 1963), differ with regard to their distribution from those coming from the "postcentral," "sensory" cortex. The former fibers, which are on the whole thicker than those from the sensory cortex, end chiefly in lamina VI, especially laterally, and in the dorsal part of lamina VII (Fig. 4-3) while the latter terminate more dorsally, chiefly in laminae IV and V, with some overlapping onto lamina VI. These findings have been confirmed in Golgi material (Scheibel and Scheibel, 1966b) and in physiological studies (Fetz, 1968). A corresponding differential distribution appears to be present in the monkey according to Kuypers (1958b) and Liu and Chambers (1964), although these authors did not map the termination with regard to Rexed's laminae. *Even if there is some overlapping between the terminal areas of fibers from the "motor" and "sensory" cortex, they obviously have their preferential sites of termination,* an observation which is of interest for functional correlations (see below). The corticospinal fibers from the supplementary motor area end in the same regions as do those from the primary sensorimotor cortex (Nyberg-Hansen, 1969) in the cat.

Thus in the cat it appears that corticospinal fibers from the "central

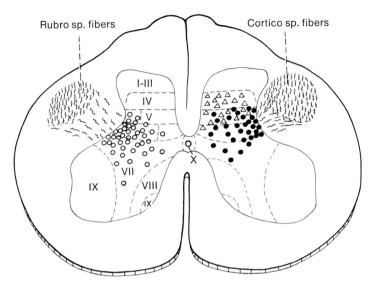

○ Sites of termination of rubro sp. fibers

● Sites of termination of cortico sp. fibers from "motor" cortex

△ Sites of termination of cortico sp. fibers from "sensory" cortex

FIG. 4–3 Diagram of a transverse section of the spinal cord of the cat at C_8 showing the location in the lateral funiculus and the sites of termination within the spinal gray matter of rubrospinal and corticospinal fibers from "motor" and "sensory" parts of the first sensorimotor region of the cerebral cortex. Note the similarities in the areas of termination of rubrospinal and corticospinal fibers from the "motor" cortex. From Nyberg-Hansen (1966a) based on experimental studies of Nyberg-Hansen and Brodal (1963, 1964).

region" can act on motoneurons only by way of internuncials,[1] as is concluded also from electrophysiological studies (Lloyd, 1941; Hern, Phillips, and Porter, 1962; and others). In the monkey, however, some corticospinal fibers have been found to end on motoneurons (Hoff and Hoff, 1934; Kupyers, 1960; Liu and Chambers, 1964), and there is physiological evidence of a monosynaptic (in addition to polysynaptic) impulse transmission from corticospinal fibers to alpha motoneurons (see Bernhard, Bohm, and Petersen, 1953; Preston and Whitlock, 1961; Landgren, Phillips, and Porter, 1962). Little is known about the situ-

[1] Since some dendrites of motoneurons extend rather far dorsally into the gray matter, at least into laminae VI and VII (Aitken and Bridger, 1961; Sprague and Ha, 1964; Scheibel and Scheibel, 1966a) these findings do not definitely exclude the possibility that contacts may be established with dendrites of motoneurons. As mentioned in Chapter 3 most of the dendrites of motoneurons take a longitudinal course.

ation in man, but some observations of Kuypers (1958c) indicate that in man some corticospinal fibers end on motoneurons.

As to *the pyramidal tract fibers influencing the somatic and special visceral efferent cranial nerve nuclei,* information is relatively scanty. However, in the cat, fibers from the central region have not been found to end in the motor cranial nerve nuclei but only in their vicinity (Walberg, 1957b; Kuypers, 1958a; Szentágothai and Rajkovits, 1958), while in the monkey and chimpanzee some fibers appear to end in the nuclei (Kuypers, 1960).

We will return to the function of the pyramidal tract at a later junction, but it is appropriate to mention here some recent electrophysiological studies which have given interesting new data. Thus it has been shown that the corticospinal fibers in general have a facilitatory action on motoneurons which supply flexor muscles, while the action on extensor motoneurons is usually inhibitory (Lundberg and Voorhoeve, 1962; Agnew, Preston, and Whitlock, 1963; Corazza, Fadiga, and Parmeggiani, 1963 and others). Furthermore, their action on the γ-neurons appears to be similar (Corazza et al., 1963). Only studies in which precautions are taken to exclude simultaneous transmission of impulses from the cerebral cortex to the cord along other pathways are conclusive in this respect. All authors appear to agree that in the cat the effect on α as well as γ neurons is mediated via internuncial cells, in agreement with the anatomical data. The internuncials involved appear to be located in laminae V–VII. Internuncial cells involved in the reflex arcs for certain somatic spinal reflexes appear to be facilitated by impulses in the corticospinal tract (Lundberg, Norsell, and Voorhoeve, 1962). For a recent study of the corticospinal influence on interneurons see Fetz (1968).

The rubrospinal tract. Recent experimental studies have shown that this pathway, coming from the red nucleus, has certain features in common with the corticospinal tract. The *nucleus ruber* or *red nucleus* (Figs. 4-2 and 4-4) has its name from being readily visible in the fresh brain by its slightly reddish color, like the red zone of the substantia nigra. It is situated in the mesencephalon at the level of the colliculi and is almost spherical. The nucleus has a high content of iron, and is covered by a sort of capsule consisting of afferent and efferent fibers. Many fibers of the oculomotor nerve traverse it (Fig. 4-4). Both in regard to fiber connections and in regard to its cellular structure the nucleus is not an entity. It is customary to distinguish between a caudal *magnocellular part,* containing large multipolar nerve cells, and a rostral *parvicellular part,* harboring small cells of various types.

This distinction appears to be derived from the situation in man, where large cells occur only in the caudalmost part of the nucleus, even if there are small cells

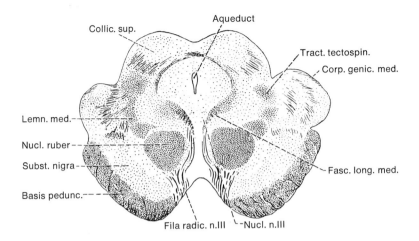

FIG. 4–4 Drawing of a transverse section through the mesencephalon. The red
nucleus is traversed by root fibers of the oculomotor nerve.

interspersed between the large ones. Within both parts several minor groups can be
distinguished. Grofová and Maršala (1959) describe four groups in the magnocellular part of the human red nucleus which altogether contains only 150 to 200
large cells. In the phylogenetic scale the relative proportion of large cells decreases.
It is unfortunate that the names "parvicellular" and "magnocellular" part have been
applied also to the red nucleus of animals because, for example in the cat, there is
an entirely gradual transition from caudal to rostral with regard to the occurrence
of large and small cells (Brodal and Gogstad, 1954). In the monkey large cells
appear to be present, although intermingled with small ones, only in the caudal
third (Kuypers and Lawrence, 1967).

The red nucleus has several efferent and afferent connections. Only a
few will be considered here, first and foremost the projection to the spinal
cord, the *rubrospinal tract* (often also called von Monakow's bundle).
Since our knowledge of the connections of the red nucleus in man is
relatively scanty, it will be appropriate to consider first the data on the
tract in animals, particularly the cat.

Following stereotactically placed lesions degenerating fibers have
been traced with the Nauta method to lumbosacral levels in the cat (Hinman and Carpenter, 1959; Nyberg-Hansen and Brodal, 1964) and in the
monkey (Orioli and Mettler, 1956; Kuypers, Fleming, and Farinholt,
1962; Poirier and Bouvier, 1966). The tract appears to be almost purely
crossed, the crossing occurring immediately after the fibers have left the
nucleus. In the cord the rubrospinal fibers are found just ventral and
somewhat lateral to those of the lateral corticospinal tract (Fig. 4-5). It
is of interest that following interruption of the rubrospinal tract in the

1 6 5

cat, small as well as large cells in the red nucleus show retrograde changes (Pompeiano and Brodal, 1957c) as seen in Fig. 1-14. In the monkey likewise small as well as large cells appear to give rise to rubrospinal fibers (Kuypers and Lawrence, 1967). This is in accordance with the presence of fibers of various diameters in the rubrospinal tract.

Of particular interest is the demonstration of a *somatotopical pattern within the projection from the red nucleus of the cat onto the cord*. This pattern emerged from a study of the distribution of cells showing retrograde changes in the red nucleus of the cat following transections of the tract at different levels (Pompeiano and Brodal, 1957c), and was further confirmed anatomically by a study of the distribution of degenerated rubrospinal fibers following lesions of different parts of the red nucleus (Nyberg-Hansen and Brodal, 1964). As seen from Fig. 4-5 fibers ending in the cervical cord take origin from the dorsomedial part of the nucleus, fibers ending in the lumbosacral cord from the ventrolateral part, from what may be referred to as a "neck and forelimb region" and a "hindlimb region," respectively, with an intermediate area representing a "trunk region." The functional validity of this pattern has been demonstrated by Pompeiano (1957) who in precollicularly decerebrated cats on liminal stimulation of the dorsomedial part of the nucleus obtained flexion of the contralateral forelimb with inhibition of extensor rigidity, while stimulation of the ventrolateral part gave corresponding results in the hindlimb (see also Maffei and Pompeiano, 1962b). The somatotopical pattern has, furthermore, been confirmed by antidromic activation of rubrospinal fibers (Tsukahara, Toyama, and Kosaka, 1964). These findings are of interest in attempts to explain certain motor disturbances in human cases, as will be discussed in a later section.

Several authors have investigated *the sites of termination of the rubrospinal fibers* in the cord (for references see Nyberg-Hansen and Brodal, 1964). Most authors found the fibers to end in the "intermediate zone" of the gray matter. When a more detailed mapping is made, using the Nauta and Glees methods, it is learned that in the cat the fibers do not enter lamina IX of Rexed, harboring the motoneurons, but are distributed to lamina V laterally, to lamina VI, and to the dorsal and central parts of lamina VII (Fig. 4-5). These sites of ending correspond largely to those of the corticospinal fibers from the "motor" cortex, a point of some interest (see Fig. 4-3).

Recent electrophysiological studies have furnished other interesting data. Thus, in agreement with Pompeiano's (1957) observations, referred to above, stimulation of the red nucleus activates contralateral flexor motoneurons, in which excitatory postsynaptic potentials can be recorded intracellularly, while contralateral ex-

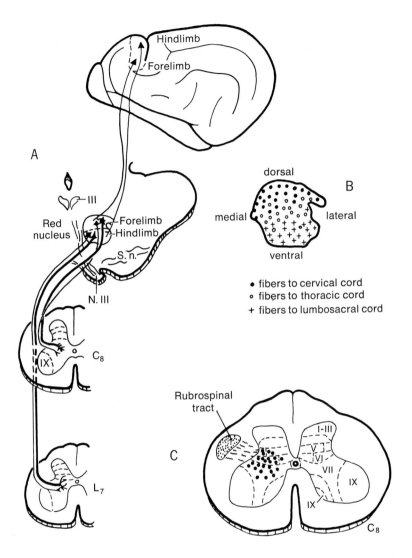

FIG. 4–5 Diagram showing the principal features in the cortico-rubro-spinal pathway as determined experimentally in the cat. *A:* The corticorubral fibers take
origin in the anterior sigmoid gyrus, the "motor cortex" (above) and end in a
somatotopical pattern in the red nucleus. The somatotopical arrangement is upheld
in the rubrospinal projection, coming from small as well as large cells in the red
nucleus. *B:* The somatotopical pattern in the red nucleus as seen in a transverse
section at middle levels of the nucleus. *C:* The sites of termination of rubrospinal
fibers are restricted to Rexed's laminae V to VII. Based on findings of Pompeiano
and Brodal (1957c), Rinvik and Walberg (1963), and Nyberg-Hansen and Brodal
(1964).

tensor motoneurons give inhibitory postsynaptic potentials (Sasaki, Namikawa, and Hashiromoto, 1960). Corresponding findings have been made by Hongo, Jankowska, and Lundberg (1965) who, furthermore, conclude that both actions occur by way of internuncial cells, as would be expected from the anatomically determined site of termination of the fibers. In fact, the physiological study of Hongo et al. (1965) indicates that the rubrospinal fibers end on internuncial cells in Rexed's lamina VI and VII. (The authors conclude that these internuncials are others than those which are excited by primary afferent impulses.) As first suggested by Granit and Holmgren (1955), the rubrospinal tract influences not only α but also γ neurons. According to Appelberg and Kosary (1963) the static γ motoneurons (see Ch. 3) of the flexor muscles are faciiltated, those of the extensor muscles inhibited.

Corresponding electrophysiological studies do not appear to have been made in the monkey, but on account of the anatomical similarities of the rubrospinal pathway in the cat and monkey, it appears likely that functional conditions are the same in the two animal species. The rubrospinal tract appears, thus, to be first and foremost a somatotopically organized fiber system involved in the excitation of α motoneurons and static γ neurons of flexor muscles. (For a review of the physiology of the red nucleus see Massion, 1967.)

It is of interest here to consider some *afferent connections to the red nucleus* which may influence its action on the spinal cord. It has been known for a long time that the red nucleus receives a considerable number of fibers from the *cerebellum*. These will be considered in the chapter on the cerebellum. Suffice it here to mention that the most important contribution comes from the nucleus interpositus anterior which again is played upon by axons of Purkinje cells in the intermediate region of the anterior lobe of the cerebellum. Of particular interest for the subject under consideration is the presence of *fibers to the red nucleus from the cerebral cortex*. The discovery of the somatotopical pattern in the red nucleus and the rubrospinal pathway (Pompeiano and Brodal, 1957c) raised the question whether a corresponding organization is present within the corticorubral projection. In experimental studies in the cat, Rinvik and Walberg (1963) were able to demonstrate that this is indeed the case (see also Mabuchi and Kusama, 1966). The fibers come chiefly from the cat's "motor" cortex (corresponding approximately to the anterior sigmoid gyrus) and pass to the ipsilateral red nucleus. Fibers from the forelimb region of this cortical area end in the dorsomedial part of the red nucleus, i.e. its forelimb region, while those from the cerebral hindlimb region end ventrolaterally (see Fig. 4-5). In addition there are some fibers from the second somatosensory area and a region which appears to represent the supplementary motor area in the cat, as well as from the gyrus proreus of the frontal lobe (Rinvik, 1965). The fibers from the supplementary motor area are distributed bilaterally.[2] The cells of the red nucleus projecting to the cord appear to be excited mono-synaptically from the cortex (Tsukahara, Toyama, and Kosaka, 1967, see also Tsukahara and Kosaka, 1968). The presence of a somatotopi-cal localization within the corticorubral projection has recently been confirmed in the monkey (Kuypers and Lawrence, 1967) as well as in the chimpanzee. In the monkey most of the fibers come from the pre-central gyrus, but smaller contingents were traced from the adjoining areas as well as from the supplementary motor cortex. There is suggestive evidence that the fibers from the latter show a somatotopical pattern similar to those from the precentral gyrus (Kuypers and Lawrence, 1967).

There is thus in the cat and apparently also in the monkey (perhaps in the chimpanzee) an indirect corticospinal pathway with a relay in the red nucleus. In its organization it shows remarkable similarities to the "precentral" component of the direct corticospinal tract. Both fiber sys-tems originate from largely the same cortical regions, contain fibers of varying calibers, and extend throughout the cord. Both show a somato-topical pattern, and their terminal regions appear—at least in the cat where they have been properly studied in this respect—to be very similar (Fig. 4-3). Both fiber systems appear to produce facilitation of flexor motoneurons (α and γ) as well as other similar effects (see Massion, 1967).

As will be shown later, these findings in animals are of some interest from a clinical point of view. It is unfortunate, therefore, that very little is known of the *corticorubral and rubrospinal tracts in man.* As to the latter, Collier and Buzzard (1901), from Marchi studies of human cases, suggested that the rubrospinal tract in man extends to sacral levels of the cord, but their evidence is not conclusive (for further references see Nathan and Smith, 1955a). The general opinion has for a long time been that the rubrospinal tract is rudimentary in man. However, there appears to be no good evidence for this. The only positive information of the tract is derived from a human case described by Stern (1936) in which retrograde cellular changes were found in the magnocellular part in both red nuclei following a total transverse lesion of the upper thoracic cord. It follows from this that the tract in man extends at least below this level. As described above there are only a few large cells in the human red nucleus, and since it has—incorrectly as we have seen—been held

[2] It is of functional interest that the corticofugal projections from the second somatosensory area differ from those from the primary sensorimotor area also with regard to their termination in other structures (pontine nuclei, thalamus, dorsal column nuclei, and others).

that the tract is composed of myelinated axons from large cells only, it has been tacitly assumed that the rubrospinal tract is rudimentary in man. However, the fact that rubrospinal fibers come from small as well as large cells in the cat and also in the monkey (see above), and that it contains a considerable number of thin fibers in these species, makes it likely that the same will turn out to be the case in man when the problem is studied with proper methods and in suitable human cases. If this suggestion proves to be correct it will have consequences for the interpretation of some clinical findings.

Corticorubral fibers in man have been described by several authors. Of more recent reports may be mentioned the study of Margareth Meyer (1949) on brains from patients subjected to frontal leucotomy and a corresponding study by Kanki and Ban (1952). At least part of the fibers appear to come from the precentral region. No details appear to be available concerning these connections in man, but it is clear that they descend in the internal capsule and in the cerebral peduncle to reach the red nucleus.

The vestibulospinal tract is another fairly well characterized pathway from the brain stem to the cord. It was well known to the classical neuroanatomists. After leaving the vestibular nuclei the fibers pass in a ventral direction before turning caudally and descending in the ipsilateral ventrolateral funiculus of the cord. As for the rubrospinal tract, most of our knowledge comes from animal experiments. The limited data available on the human tract is, however, in agreement with findings made in animals. In addition to this classical vestibulospinal tract there is another pathway from the vestibular nuclei to the cord, consisting of a smaller number of fibers which descend in the medial longitudinal fasciculus. In the cord these fibers are found bilaterally in the ventral funiculus, close to the midline, in the so-called sulcomarginal fasciculus. Following a suggestion of Nyberg-Hansen (1966a) the latter will be referred to as the *medial vestibulospinal tract,* while the former will be called the *lateral vestibulospinal tract*. Practically all studies of these pathways have been made in the cat.

When discussing the vestibulospinal connections it is essential to be aware of the fact that the vestibular nuclei are not an entity, but represent a complex of minor cell groups, each of which has its particular connections. These features will be dealt with in the chapters on the cerebellum and the cranial nerves. Here our concern is primarily with the vestibulospinal tracts.

The *lateral vestibulospinal tract* has been found by most authors (for references see Pompeiano and Brodal, 1957a) to take origin from the lateral vestibular nucleus of Deiters (Fig. 4-6) characterized by harbor-

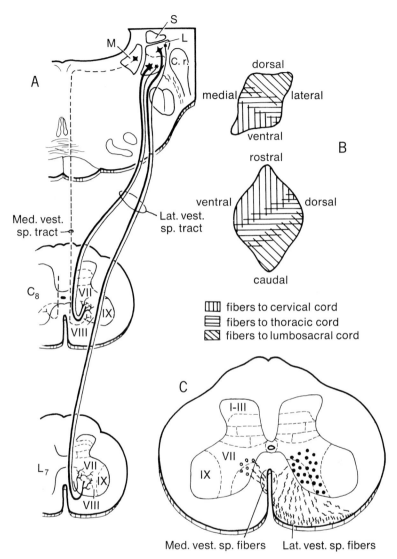

FIG. 4–6 Diagram showing the principal features in the vestibulospinal pathways as determined experimentally in the cat. *A:* The lateral vestibulospinal tract comes only from the lateral vestibular nucleus of Deiters (L) but from large as well as small cells. It is somatotopically arranged. The medial vestibulospinal tract is derived from the medial vestibular nucleus (M) and does not reach the lumbar cord. *B:* The somatotopical pattern in the lateral vestibular nucleus as seen in a transverse section (above) and in a sagittal reconstruction of the nucleus (below). *C:* The vestibulospinal tracts terminate in Rexed's laminae VII and VIII. Based on findings of Pompeiano and Brodal (1957a), Nyberg-Hansen and Mascitti (1964) and Nyberg-Hansen (1964a).

ing a fair number of giant cells or Deiters' cells. Almost all authors are agreed that the tract extends to lumbosacral levels of the cord (in man as well as in the cat and monkey). In an experimental study (Pompeiano and Brodal, 1957a) where advantage was taken of the modified Gudden method (Brodal, 1940a) it was confirmed that the tract takes origin from the lateral vestibular nucleus only. Furthermore it could be shown that its fibers are derived not only from the giant cells, but from its small cells as well, since following lesions of the tract in the cord retrograde changes are present in cells of all types in the nucleus. This fits in with the presence of thin as well as thick fibers in the tract.[3] Of particular interest was the demonstration of *a somatotopical pattern within the lateral vestibular nucleus* (Fig. 4-6). Fibers to the lumbosacral cord take origin in its dorsocaudal part, fibers to the cervical cord from its rostroventral part, with a zone of overlapping in between. Accordingly one may speak of a "neck and forelimb region," a "trunk region," and a "hindlimb region," although the borders are not sharp.

The correctness of this pattern has further been established by the study of the distribution within the cord of fibers degenerating as a consequence of lesions restricted to different regions of the nucleus (Nyberg-Hansen and Mascitti, 1964) and in electrophysiological studies by localized stimulations (Pompeiano, 1960) as well as by recordings in the nucleus following antidromic stimulation of the fibers in the tract (Ito, Hongo, Yoshida, Okada, and Obata, 1964; Wilson, Kato, Thomas, and Peterson, 1966). The localization is, however, not as distinct as might appear from the anatomical diagram (Wilson, Kato, Peterson and Wylie, 1967). In agreement with the fiber spectrum of the lateral vestibulospinal tract, the conduction velocities vary considerably, from 24 to 140 m/sec (Ito et al., 1964; Wilson et al., 1966).

The terminal site within the spinal cord of the vestibulospinal fibers differs from those of the corticospinal and rubrospinal tracts. While some previous authors had indicated a termination in the ventral horn and ventral part of the "intermediate" part of the gray matter, Nyberg-Hansen and Mascitti (1964) in a more detailed study found the lateral vestibulospinal fibers to end in lamina VIII and the ventral and central parts of lamina VII (Fig. 4-6), especially on large dendrites. Only a few fibers could be traced to lamina IX containing the motoneurons. Many of the cells in lamina VIII send their axons across the midline. This may explain the occurrence of bilateral effects on stimulation of the lateral vestibular nucleus.

It has been known for some time that the nucleus of Deiters and the

[3] It is of some practical importance that during its descent the tract shifts its position. While (in the cat) at cervical levels it is situated peripherally in the ventrolateral funiculus, it moves dorsomedially along the ventral median fissure as it descends (see Nyberg-Hansen and Mascitti, 1964).

172

lateral vestibulospinal tract increase the extensor tonus of the ipsilateral limbs (for a review see Brodal, Pompeiano, and Walberg, 1962). The increased tonus following decerebration at levels above the nucleus of Deiters (decerebrate rigidity, to be discussed later) is to a large extent due to the unopposed action of the lateral vestibular nucleus on the cord, and disappears when the nucleus is destroyed. In keeping with this, micro-electrode studies have shown that stimulation of the lateral vestibular nucleus of the cat produces excitatory postsynaptic potentials in extensor motoneurons only, while flexor motoneurons are inhibited (Lund and Pompeiano, 1965). The excitatory effect is concluded to be mediated monosynaptically. This is at variance with the lack of fibers terminating in lamina IX, but the discrepancy may perhaps be explained if a sub-stantial number of contacts are established with the peripheral parts of dendrites from motoneurons extending into laminae VIII and VII.

Like the corticospinal and rubrospinal tracts the lateral vestibulo-spinal tract acts not only on α motoneurons, but on γ neurons as well (Andersson and Gernandt, 1956; Gernandt, Iranyi, and Livingston, 1959). The action on the latter is described as being excitatory (Carli, Diete-Spiff, and Pompeiano, 1967a).[4]

While the lateral vestibular nucleus does not appear to receive fibers from the cerebral cortex it receives abundant projections from the cortex of the spinal part of the cerebellum, and from the "vestibulo-cerebellum," as well as from the fastigial nucleus. Each of these afferent fiber con-tingents has its particular area of distribution within the lateral vestibular nucleus (Fig. 7-11). These features will be considered in connection with the cerebellum. Suffice it here to emphasize the important role played by the cerebellar afferents for the function of the nucelus of Deiters.

The *other vestibulospinal pathway,* here referred to as the *medial,* is relatively modest, and less well known than the lateral tract (Fig. 4-6). It appears now to be finally established that this tract takes its origin only from the medial vestibular nucleus, according to the experimental an-atomical studies of Nyberg-Hansen (1964a), who also studied the termination of the fibers. Their terminal area is approximately the same as that of the lateral vestibulospinal tract (Fig. 4-6). The tract can only be traced to midthoracic levels. It appears, thus, that the medial vestibu-lar nucleus and its spinal tract are concerned chiefly in the mediation of

---

[4] Whether there are different fibers which mediate the effect on α and γ neurons is not known. Following vestibular stimulation the latter have been found to dis-charge at lower strength of stimulation than the α neurons. The suggestion may perhaps be ventured that this may be correlated with the fact that both large and small cells of the nucleus of Deiters send axons to the cord, and these axons have different diameters and conduction velocities.

vestibular impulses to the neck and forelimb muscles, while the lateral nucleus and tract may influence the entire body. It is of some interest that the medial and lateral nucleus appear to be supplied by primary vestibular fibers from different parts of the vestibular apparatus (see Ch. 7). Like the lateral vestibular nucleus, the medial nucleus receives fibers from the cerebellum, but it does not appear to receive fibers from the cerebral cortex (although it does receive fibers from the mesencephalon).

The *vestibulospinal tracts in man* are relatively little known (for a review see Nathan and Smith, 1955a). However, an analysis of the normal anatomy of the human vestibular nuclei (Sadjadpour and Brodal, 1968) shows that on practically all points they resemble those in the cat, and the same subdivisions can be identified. This makes it extremely likely that the fiber connections are also, in principle, identical. There is suggestive evidence from some observations by Foerster and Gagel (1932) that also in man there is a somatotopical organization within the nucleus of Deiters. Further support for this view has been provided by Løken and Brodal (1969).

Reticulospinal tracts. The presence of fibers passing from the reticular formation of the brain stem to the spinal cord was established by the classical neuroanatomists, such as Probst, Kohnstamm, and Lewandowsky (for references see Brodal, 1957). Recent physiological studies of the effects which can be elicited by stimulation of the reticular formation have fostered renewed interest in these fiber connections and their functional role.

As will be described in the chapter on the reticular formation (Ch. 6), this is not a diffuse aggregation of nerve cells and fibers. It may be subdivided into a number of more or less well-circumscribed nuclei, which in part differ with regard to their afferent and efferent fiber connections and presumably, therefore, are functionally dissimilar. As to the reticulospinal connections, these may be divided into two groups which have their particular sites of origin and differ in other respects as well. The only reliable procedure for determining the sites of origin of reticulospinal fibers with some precision is to study the spatial distribution of cells showing retrograde changes following lesions of the cord which interrupt the reticulospinal fibers, as done in the cat by Pitts (1940) and in the monkey by Bodian (1946). These authors were, however, not concerned with certain details in the projections, which became of interest following more recent research. Taking advantage of the modified Gudden method (Brodal, 1940a), Torvik and Brodal (1957) were able to demonstrate that reticulospinal fibers are derived from small as well as large cells scattered at all levels of the medullary and pontine reticular formation. However, *there are two clearly maximal areas of origin, one in the pons, another in the medulla.* Both are restricted to approximately the medial two-thirds of the reticular formation where large cells occur. These areas are indicated in Fig. 6-4, from which it is also seen that the pontine fibers descend ipsilaterally while the fibers from the medulla are crossed as well as uncrossed. Most of the medullary fibers come from the region called the nucleus reticularis gigantocellularis, while the pontine fibers are derived from the entire nucleus reticularis pontis caudalis and the caudal part of the nucleus reticularis pontis oralis. No fibers to the cord appear to come from the mesencephalic reticular formation (Nyberg-Hansen, 1965a).

The presence of changes in small as well as large cells indicates that both types send fibers to the cord, and tallies with the presence of fibers of varying diameters within the reticulospinal tracts.[5] It is estimated that more than half of the large cells of the caudal pontine reticular nucleus project onto the cord (Torvik and Brodal, 1957). Following lesions at various levels of the cord no difference in the distribution of changed cells could be ascertained. This indicates that *there is no somatotopical pattern within the reticulospinal projections.*

There has been some difference of opinion concerning the *course of the reticulospinal fibers in the cord,* in part, it appears, because authors who studied this subject by making lesions in the reticular formation and tracing degenerating fibers with the Marchi or silver impregnation methods have damaged fibers belonging to both components or fibers of other descending fiber tracts. These difficulties are significantly reduced if lesions are placed in those regions which are known to give off the majority of reticulospinal fibers. This was done by Nyberg-Hansen (1965a) in a study in the cat (Nauta method). It could then be settled that reticulospinal fibers descend to the lowermost levels of the cord, in contrast to conclusions made on the basis of retrograde cellular changes, where convincing alterations were not seen following lesions below the thoracic cord in the monkey (Bodian, 1946) and in the cat (Torvik and Brodal, 1957). Furthermore, the pontine reticulospinal fibers descend almost exclusively ipsilaterally in the ventral funiculus of the cord, in agreement with the results of several previous workers (for references see Nyberg-Hansen, 1965a). Some of the fibers cross in the anterior commissure of the cord before they terminate. The medullary fibers, however, descend bilaterally in the lateral funiculus (Fig. 4-7).

The two groups of reticulospinal fibers differ with regard to their sites of termination. Most authors have described the fibers as ending in the "intermediate zone" and the "ventral horn," for example, Kuypers, Fleming, and Farinholt (1962). Studying the terminations in greater detail Nyberg-Hansen (1965a) could establish that in the cat the pontine reticulospinal fibers terminate more ventrally than do the medullary ones

---

[5] The conduction velocity of the reticulospinal fibers has been estimated to be from 20 to 138 m/sec (Wolstencroft, 1964).

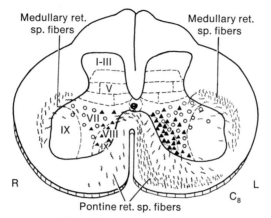

▲ Sites of termination of pontine ret. sp. fibers
• Sites of termination of medullary ret. sp. fibers

FIG. 4–7 Diagram of a transverse section of the spinal cord of the cat at C_8, showing the sites of termination and the position in the cord of reticulospinal fibers from medullary and pontine reticular formation. From Nyberg-Hansen (1965a).

(Fig. 4-7). The former end on cells of various types in Rexed's (1952, 1954) lamina VIII and adjacent parts of lamina VII, while the medullary fibers and chiefly in lamina VII with a few terminations also in laminae VIII and IX.

As to *reticulospinal tracts in man,* there are indications in the literature that they are present, but no reliable information is available (see Nathan and Smith, 1955a, for a review). The failure of Foerster and Gagel (1932) to find cell changes in the reticular formation following chordotomies is not decisive. It seems a likely assumption that the pontine and medullary reticulospinal tracts differ functionally in some respects.

Although there is some data bearing on the *function of the reticulospinal connections,* there is relatively little information concerning possible differences between the two components. This may be due in part to the fact that the correlation with anatomical data has not been of great concern to most physiologists studying the reticular formation. In addition, the anatomical arrangement of the reticulospinal projections often makes analyses of the effects of stimulations or ablations equivocal. However, it appears that the "inhibitory area" described by Magoun and Rhines (1946) covers approximately the region of origin of the medullary reticulospinal fibers (see Fig. 6-8). On the other hand, the more rostrally situated "facilitatory area" of Rhines and Magoun (1946), as usually described, appears to be situated outside (rostral and lateral to) the region giving off pontine reticulospinal fibers. (These subjects will be considered more fully in Chapter 6.) Stimulation of the medullary reticulospinal projection area gives rise to inhibitory postsynaptic potentials in α motoneurons (Jankowska, Lund, Lundberg, and Pompeiano, 1964; Llinas and Terzuolo, 1964). This effect is sufficiently strong to suppress decerebrate rigidity. It is also well established that the reticular formation influences the activity of the γ fibers (Granit and Kaada, 1952; and others). Spindle activation has been observed following stimulation of sites apparently within the facilitatory region of the reticular formation in the mesencephalon (Granit and Holmgren, 1955) or laterally in the medulla (Diete-Spiff, Carli, and Pompeiano, 1967). Whether the activity of the muscle spindles is inhibited from the medullary reticular formation appears so far not to have been settled (see, however, Shimazu, Hongo, and Kubota, 1962). Grillner, Hongo and Lund (1966b) found monosynaptic excitatory potentials in γ motoneurons on stimulation of the lower brain stem. See also Bergmans and Grillner (1968).

Obviously the reticulospinal pathways are capable of influencing α as well as γ neurons, and there is physiological evidence which supports the notion that the medullary and pontine reticulospinal pathways are functionally dissimilar (see also Ch. 6). Their different sites of termination in the cord are of interest from this point of view, as will be discussed below.

In addition to acting on motoneurons, apparently via internuncials, the reticulospinal projections, like several other descending connections, have been shown to influence the central transmission of sensory impulses (see Ch. 2). Furthermore, they may influence various reflex pathways.

In relation to the effects exerted by the reticulospinal fiber tracts on the peripheral motor apparatus it is of relevance to recall that the *reticular formation is acted upon by fibers from other regions.* As described in Chapters 2 and 6, there is a considerable influx of *ascending fibers from the cord.* Furthermore, there are *cerebellar afferents* from the fastigial nucleus (see Ch. 5). Of most immediate concern in the present chapter are the *corticoreticular connections.* As described in Chapter 6, the majority of these fibers is derived from the central "sensorimotor" region. They descend in the internal capsule and cerebral peduncle and are distributed bilaterally in the reticular formation. It is of interest that the largest proportion of corticoreticular fibers end in the two regions of the reticular formation which give off reticulospinal fibers (see Fig. 6-4), since this makes clear that *there are impulse pathways from the cerebral cortex, particularly its primary sensorimotor region, to the spinal cord via the reticular formation.* There are also corticoreticular fibers to the mesencephalic reticular formation (which, as mentioned above, does not give off fibers to the spinal cord).

Other descending tracts to the spinal cord. In addition to fibers in the corticospinal, rubrospinal, vestibulospinal, and reticulospinal tracts, the spinal cord receives fibers descending directly from other masses of gray matter. Most of these pathways are quantitatively less important than those mentioned, and their functional importance is less well known. They will, therefore, be treated rather briefly.

The tectospinal tract comes from the superior colliculus (Fig. 4-1). Its fibers cross ventral to the periaqueductal gray and descend in the brain stem, just ventral to the medial longitudinal fasciculus. In the cord the fibers travel medially in the ventral funiculus. Divergent opinions have been held concerning the origin and termination of this tract (for a review see Nyberg-Hansen, 1964b). However, it appears now to be established that the fibers come only from the superior colliculus, and that the majority end in the upper cervical segments. Only a few reach the cervical segments (Nyberg-Hansen, 1964b). They terminate chiefly in Rexed's laminae VII and VI, while some end in lamina VIII through which they enter. The tectospinal fibers thus exert their action on motoneurons via interneurons. The superior colliculus is considered as an important optic reflex center, and electrical stimulation of it gives rise to movements of the eyes and appropriate movements of the head, in agreement with the anatomical data. The superior colliculus is influenced by the cerebral cortex, particularly from the occipital lobe (see Ch. 7).

The interstitiospinal tract (Fig. 4-1) is another pathway to the spinal cord which has received relatively little attention in clinical neurology, although it has been described and discussed by many neuroanatomists. A review of the relevant literature has been given by Nyberg-Hansen (1966b) who in an experimental study in the cat confirmed the conclusion of most authors that the tract originates from the interstitial nucleus of Cajal in the rostral mesencephalon. The nucleus is situated just ventral to the periaqueductal gray (see Fig. 7-12) and separated from this by the medial longitudinal fasciculus. The fibers of the interstitiospinal tract descend to the cord in the latter bundle, chiefly ipsilaterally. They can be traced to sacral levels of the cord and terminate chiefly in lamina VIII and the adjoining part of lamina VII, but not in lamina IX. Their terminal area thus coincides approximately with that of the vestibulospinal fibers (see Fig. 4-6).

The interstitial nucleus of Cajal receives afferents from various sources, among them the vestibular nuclei (see Chapter 7). Several authors have advocated that it receives fibers from the cerebral cortex (see Pompeiano and Walberg, 1957, for references).

The interstitiospinal fibers are presumably involved in the rotation around the longitudinal axis of the head and body which can be observed following electrical stimulation in the region of the nucleus, and the nucleus probably is an important link in mediating effects on the neck and body musculature in response to optic and vestibular impulses (see Hyde and Eason, 1959). The nucleus may also be of importance for certain central effects on the autonomic nervous system (see Nyberg-Hansen, 1966b).

The solitariospinal tract is a minor projection to the spinal cord which takes origin from the nucleus of the solitary tract (see Torvik, 1957b), and presumably is of importance in activating the spinal cord in response to visceral impulses entering in the vagus and glossopharyngeal nerves. The nucleus receives fibers from the cerebral cortex (see Ch. 7).

Fibers from the raphe nuclei to the spinal cord should finally be mentioned. Studying the retrograde changes in the nuclei of the raphe complex following lesions of the spinal cord it was concluded that spinal fibers come from certain of the nuclei, particularly the nucleus raphe magnus (Brodal, Taber, and Walberg, 1960). The fibers do not appear to pass beyond the thoracic cord. However, this conservative estimate may be due to the strict criteria employed in the evaluation of the cell changes. Recently the spinal projections of the raphe have received considerable attention in physiological studies, following the demonstration by Dahlström and Fuxe (1964) that there is a mono-amine positive pathway from the raphe complex to the spinal cord. These parts of the raphe receive afferents from the spinal cord, the fastigial nucleus, and the cerebral cortex, chiefly its primary sensorimotor region (Brodal, Walberg, and Taber, 1960). Little is so far known of the functional importance of the nuclei of the raphe, which are rather small and difficult to keep apart from the adjoining reticular formation in stimulation experiments. The similarities in the anatomical organization of the raphe nuclei and the reticular formation suggest that there may be some functional similarities as well (see Taber, Brodal, and Walberg, 1960).

The olivospinal tract, mentioned in many textbooks, is probably non-existent. At least no evidence is available from experimental studies. In man a triangular zone found in the ventral funiculus at upper cervical levels and having a light hue in myelin-stained preparations (Helweg's Dreikantenbahn, triangular bundle of Helweg) has been claimed to be an olivospinal tract, but this appears to be entirely conjectural.

The basal ganglia and some related nuclei. It is apparent from the above that there are a number of fiber bundles which descend to the cord from higher levels and thus must be able to influence its activity. The cerebral cortex may influence the cord directly via the corticospinal tract, but in addition indirectly by fibers passing from the cortex to some nuclei which send fibers to the cord (red nucleus, parts of the reticular formation, superior colliculus, nucleus of the solitary tract, some of the raphe nuclei). Furthermore, there are other, more circuitous routes, by which the cortex may play a role in acting on the spinal cord, for example by

179

connections from the cerebral cortex to the cerebellum and from this to the vestibular nuclei and reticular formation (to be considered in the chapter on the cerebellum). Other pathways are, however, also available, namely some passing via the basal ganglia. Since the basal ganglia and their connections have attracted much interest, and since they make up a large and characteristic part of the brain, they will be considered in some detail. While they were previously thought to represent important links in pathways leading from the cerebral cortex to the cord, and thus to be primarily "motor" in function, recent research has necessitated revisions of this concept.

In the course of time the term *"basal ganglia"* has carried different connotations. The old anatomists used it as a common denominator for all the large nuclei in the interior of the brain, including the thalamus. When the development of the brain became better known, the thalamus was excluded, while, for instance, the amygdaloid nucleus was included. There is still no generally accepted definition of what one should include in the concept "basal ganglia" although all authors consider the caudate nucleus and the lentiform nucleus with its two divisions, the putamen, and globus pallidus as representing the main mass. The claustrum is usually included, while the amygdaloid nucleus, on account of its largely different connections and functions, is often excluded. It is common to consider the subthalamic nucleus and the substantia nigra in conjunction with the basal ganglia. This will be done also in the following account. The term *striate body* or *corpus striatum* is often used as almost synonymous with the basal ganglia and covers the claustrum, caudate, putamen, and globus pallidus. The name refers to the appearance in myelin-sheath-stained sections, where a number of myelinated fiber bundles traverse the cellular masses and give them a striated appearance. In the following a brief account of some of the main features of these nuclei will be given, before their connections are described.

The large gray nuclear masses of the *corpus striatum* are situated in the medullary layer of the hemisphere and subdivided by fiber strands into different portions (Figs. 4-8 and 4-9). Most laterally, beneath the insula, the *claustrum* forms a thin sheet of gray substance. It is separated laterally from the cortex by a thin medullary layer, the capsula extrema, and medially from the putamen by the capsula externa (Fig. 4-8). The claustrum appears to be derived from the cerebral cortex of the insular region, and developmentally it, therefore, does not belong to the striate body in a restricted sense. The striate body proper, the caudate-lentiform nuclei, presents some features worth mentioning. *Both in regard to phylogenetic development and finer structure the caudate nucleus and the putamen are similar, whereas they both differ from the globus pallidus.* The

180

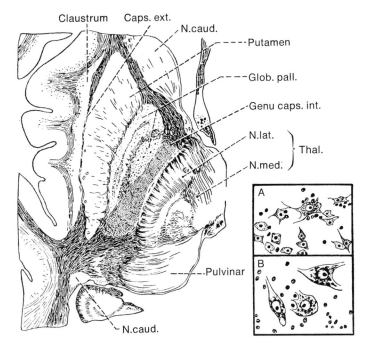

FIG. 4–8 Drawing of a horizontal section through the human brain, showing the corpus striatum (myelin sheath staining). Redrawn from Ranson (1943). Below to the right representative cells from the striatum (*A*) and the pallidum (*B*). Redrawn from Foix and Nicolesco (1925).

latter, or *pallidum* as it is often called, forms the medial part of the lentiform nucleus and takes its name from its pale color compared with the putamen and caudate nucleus. It can be subdivided into an outer or anterior-lateral segment and an inner or posterior-medial (Fig. 4-8).[6] The pallidum is phylogenetically older than the two latter nuclei, and is developed from the basal plate of the primitive neural tube (in the diencephalon).

The *caudate nucleus* and the *putamen,* on the other hand, which appear later in phylogenesis, are derived from the telencephalon and increase in size corresponding to the development of the cerebral cortex to a greater extent than does the pallidum. In lower animals the putamen and the caudate nucleus are not clearly separated by any internal capsule, since this fiber mass becomes conspicuous only with the more progressive

[6] There seems to be general agreement that the inner segment of the pallidum in monkey and man is represented in carnivores by the entopeduncular nucleus (see Fox et al., 1966).

development of the cerebral cortex. Particularly in man the internal capsule is rich in corticofugal (e.g. pyramidal) and corticopetal fibers. It is, however, bridged by strands of cells connecting the nucleus caudatus and the putamen. The pallidum represents the so-called *palaeostriatum;* the putamen and the caudate nucleus together constitute the *neostriatum.* (The amygdaloid nucleus is the archistriatum.)

Subdivision in this manner is justified by the cytological structure of the palaeostriatum and neostriatum, respectively (Figs. 4-8A and B). The pallidum is composed of large, mainly spindle-shaped cells situated rather far apart, while the striatum is distinguished by densely lying small polymorph cells with interspersed larger multipolar cells. Caudally the pallidum is continuous with the rostral part of the substantia nigra (its red zone). The pallidum, just as the substantia nigra and the nucleus ruber, contains a rich amount of iron which can be identified histochemically. Also, the capillary bed is different, being very dense in the striatum, but not in the pallidum (Alexander, 1942a). The structural differences described above between the pallidum and the striatum correspond to functional differences, evidenced, inter alia, by the symptoms following diseases in these nuclei (cf. below).

The *subthalamic nucleus* or body of Luys is situated in the basal part of the diencephalon at the transition to the mesencephalon. This is an approximately ovoid nucleus, which caudally and ventrally is continuous with the substantia nigra (see Fig. 4-9). This nucleus is relatively larger in man than in other mammals and is composed of multipolar medium-sized cells.

FIG. 4–9 Drawing of a myelin sheath stained frontal section through the human brain, showing the basal ganglia.

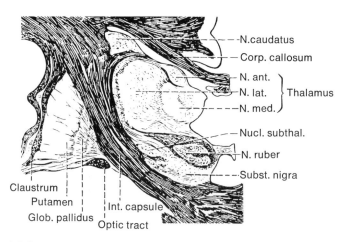

The *substantia nigra,* particularly well developed in man (Figs. 4-4, 4-9), is seen on macroscopic inspection of the transected mesencephalon as a darkly colored arched stripe in the cerebral peduncle on each side. The dark color is due to the presence in its large, multipolar nerve cells of abundant pigment granules (melanin) dispersed in the cytoplasm. Ventral to this dark zone the substantia nigra consists of a broader zone, composed of somewhat smaller and more scattered nerve cells, which partly penetrate the bundles in the pes pedunculi ventrally. This part of the substantia nigra (the red zone of Spatz) can also be discerned with the naked eye ventral to the dark zone. Like the pallidum and the red nucleus, it contains a certain amount of iron, particularly in the glial cells. The cells are very similar to those composing the pallidum, and it has already been mentioned that the two nuclei are continuous at the rostral end of the substantia nigra. In addition to the similarities mentioned between the two nuclei, they often display corresponding changes in pathological conditions.

Fiber connections of the basal ganglia and related nuclei. Concerning this subject our knowledge is still rather incomplete. One reason for this is that these nuclei are difficult to examine by experimental methods, as they lie buried in the interior of the brain. It is very difficult to place a lesion in one of these structures without inflicting some damage to others and to adjacent or passing fiber tracts. Some of the various fiber connections which have been described are probably only by-passing fibers.

Human material seldom gives satisfactory results. Even if the lesions may be limited to the deeper parts of the brain without injuring superficial structures, they are, as a rule, so large that they involve different, frequently heterogeneous, nuclei. Studies of normal material are not decisive as concerns the direction of fiber tracts, and can only give crude information. Nevertheless, the introduction of silver impregnation methods for experimental studies (see Ch. 1) and the use of stereotactical placement of restricted lesions have made it possible to obtain much additional and rather precise information on many of the fiber connections of the basal ganglia and related nuclei. As usual it has turned out that there are more connections than previously assumed and, furthermore, that the relations between nuclei are more specific than was formerly believed. The account given below is restricted to the major points.

In a general way it may be said that the basal ganglia receive numerous fibers from the cerebral cortex. Some of their efferents descend to lower levels in the brain from which connections are established to the spinal cord. However, in addition they send efferent fibers to other parts of the brain, such as the thalamus, and they receive "ascending" connections. Some of the main connections are shown in Fig. 4-10.

 Cortical projections to the striate body have been a matter of some dispute. While some authors using the Marchi method, for example Mettler (1945), found fibers from all four lobes of the cerebrum to the caudate and the putamen, other authors doubted the existence of such fibers. However, with silver impregnation methods these fibers, many of which appear to be unmyelinated, can be demonstrated (Glees, 1944). From the systematic experimental study in the rabbit by Carman, Cowan, and Powell (1963) it appears that *all parts of the cerebral cortex give off efferent fibers to the caudate and putamen* (together representing the neostriatum). The same is the case in the rat and the cat (Webster, 1961, 1965). Furthermore, the *corticostriate projection is topically organized*

FIG. 4–10 Diagram of some of the fiber connections of the basal ganglia. In the left half of the figure are shown some "closed circuits" of connections. Several connections, for example efferent projections to the inferior olive and ascending afferents from the spinal cord, reticular formation and cerebellum, are not included. (Cf. text.)

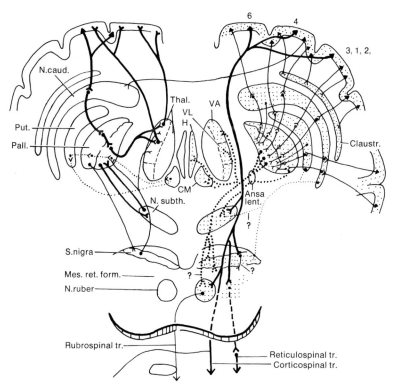

in both anteroposterior and mediolateral dimensions. Anterior lesions result in degeneration in the anterior parts of the nuclei, posterior lesions give degeneration in the posterior parts. The frontal cortex, for example, projects onto the head of the caudate nucleus and the rostral part of the putamen. Each part of the cerebral cortex thus has its particular projection area in the caudate–putamen. (The cortex on the dorsomedial margin of the hemisphere, in contrast to the rest, projects only to the caudate nucleus.) Most of the cortical projection is ipsilateral. Only the region of the primary sensorimotor cortex has bilateral connections (Carman, Cowan, Powell, and Webster, 1965). The contralateral projection is established by fibers which cross in the corpus callosum and reach the caudal part of the head of the caudate nucleus via the fasciculus subcallosus (which passes along the dorsolateral aspect of the caudate) and the putamen via the external capsule.

It is not known whether the corticostriate fibers are axons of separate cortical cells or collaterals of other corticofugal, for example, corticospinal, fibers. It is obvious from the recent findings, however, that the *neostriatum must be functionally dependent on the cortex and influenced by it in a topical manner.* There is so far no good evidence that the striate body sends fibers back to the cerebral cortex (see Burandt, French, and Akert, 1961). The majority of the efferents from the neostriatum appear to pass to the pallidum (see below). While fibers from the cortex to the pallidum are denied by most students (see, however, Meyer (1949), in man) the *cerebral cortex sends fibers to the claustrum, the subthalamic nucleus, and the substantia nigra.*

The *claustrum* (Fig. 4-8) is a morphologically well-characterized lamina of gray matter separated from the cortex of the insula by the capsula extrema. Nothing definite appears to be known of its function, and only recently have we got some information on its fiber connections. While Berke (1960), who reviews the subject, did not obtain decisive results with the Marchi method in the monkey, authors using silver impregnation methods have succeeded in demonstrating a projection from the cerebral cortex. According to Carman, Cowan, and Powell (1964) and Druga (1968) the projection is very similar to the corticostriate projection in so far as all parts of the cerebral cortex project in an orderly topical pattern onto the claustrum. Its efferent connections are unknown.

Cortical fibers to the subthalamic nucleus or *corpus Luysii* (Fig. 4-10) have been observed by some authors, for example Mettler (1945, from Brodmann's area 6 in the monkey) and De Vito and Smith (1964, from the "prefrontal lobe" in the monkey). Evidence for their presence in man has been given by Meyer (1949). It appears that corticofugal fibers end also in the cellular region rostral and dorsal to the nucleus

1 8 5

subthalamicus, called the *zona incerta*. These connections deserve further studies.

Cortical fibers to the substantia nigra have been claimed by many authors on the basis of Marchi studies and human pathological cases and have been described as coming from various cortical regions. According to recent experimental studies in the cat with the Nauta and Glees methods (Rinvik, 1966), the corticonigral projection appears to be rather modest. Many fibers coursing through the nucleus and ending in the red nucleus and the reticular formation have probably been mistaken as ending in the substantia nigra by authors who used the Marchi method. The predominantly ipsilateral projection descends in the internal capsule and cerebral peduncle and comes from the primary and second sensorimotor cortices, the supplementary motor area and the gyrus proreus (in front of the primary sensorimotor region). In man some students have found fibers from the frontal cortex to the substantia nigra, while others have not seen them (for references, see Rinvik, 1966).

With regard to *descending connections from the nuclei discussed above,* our knowledge is far from complete. There are indications from some studies that the subthalamic nucleus sends fibers to the red nucleus and the mesencephalic reticular formation. However, in a recent careful study Carpenter and Strominger (1967) found that this is probably not the case. As to the *substantia nigra, most of its efferents appear to be ascending and to go to the medial segment of the pallidum* (see Carpenter and McMasters, 1964), possibly some to the striatum. Other efferents pass to the VA of the thalamus (Carpenter and Strominger, 1967). Likewise the *subthalamic nucleus gives off ascending fibers to the pallidum* (Glees and Wall, 1946; Whittier and Mettler, 1949; Carpenter and Strominger, 1967). Thus both the subthalamic nucleus and the substantia nigra have their main efferent projections in the ascending direction, and, therefore, presumably are only to a slight extent involved in transmitting impulses caudally.

The efferent pathways from the basal ganglia proper are rather complex and are not known in all details. However, there is no doubt that *most of the efferent fibers leaving the basal ganglia take their origin in the pallidum, while the striatum sends most of its efferents only to the latter.* The *projections from the putamen and caudate to the pallidum* have recently been studied systematically with silver impregnation methods in the cat by Johnson and Clemente (1959) and Voneida (1960) and in the monkey by Szabo (1962) and Nauta and Mehler (1966). Cowan and Powell (1966) studied the gliosis ensuing in the pallidum following localized lesions in the striatum. In the main, the results of these studies are concordant. They show that the *striatopallidal projection is topically organized:* each part of the striatum sends fibers to a circumscribed part of the pallidum. Axons, chiefly of fine calibers, pass from both the caudate and the putamen to the globus pallidus, where they terminate in its external as well as its internal segment (see Fig. 4-10). In view of the orderly pattern in the corticostriate projection, described above, it is apparent that *different parts of the pallidum are influenced via the striatum from particular regions of the cortex.* The architectonic differences between the two segments of the pallidum make it seem likely that they differ functionally in some way. This might be reflected in differences in the efferent projections of the two segments or in differences between afferents from other sources. (For some details see Szabo, 1962; Cowan and Powell, 1966.)

While the main efferent outflow of the striatum goes to the pallidum, *the striatum has other efferent connections as well.* Thus fibers have been traced to the *substantia nigra* from the putamen (Szabo, 1962; Nauta and Mehler, 1966) as well as from the caudate (Voneida, 1960; Szabo, 1962). Whether there are fibers to the subthalamic nucleus has been disputed (see Hassler, 1949). Finally there are fibers from the caudate nucleus to restricted parts of the inferior olive (Walberg, 1956, in the cat).

The *efferent fibers from the pallidum* form rather massive bundles which were observed by the classical nueroanatomists and labeled by them. Unfortunately, there is much confusion in the literature concerning nomenclature (see Woodburne, Crosby, and McCotter, 1946; Nauta and Mehler, 1966, for discussions). Most authors describe a fairly compact bundle, the *ansa lenticularis,* emerging from the ventral aspect of the inner segment of the pallidum and turning in a mediocaudal direction (Fig. 4-10). A branch of the bundle, taking a more dorsal course, is often referred to as the *fasciculus lenticularis,* H_2-bundle or dorsal division of the ansa (Woodburne et al., 1946). This appears to arise more dorsally than the ansa proper. A middle division of the ansa is sometimes referred to as the *subthalamic fasciculus,* passing to the nucleus of the same name.

No attempt will be made here to describe in detail the course of the various components of the ansa. Emphasis will be put on data on their sites of termination. By way of summary it may be said that *pallidal efferents have been traced to several nuclei: the thalamus, the subthalamic nucleus, the substantia nigra, the red nucleus, the mesencephalic reticular formation, the inferior olive, and the hypothalamus* (see Fig. 4-10). Nauta and Mehler (1966) recently confirmed the original statement of Ranson, Ranson, and Ranson (1941) based on Marchi studies in the monkey, that the fibers of the ansa originate only from the internal segment of the pallidum (see Fig. 4-10) with the exception of the fibers to the nucleus subthalamicus which come from the external segment. The latter projection appears to be arranged in a topical pattern (Nauta and Mehler, 1966). The pallidal fibers to the inferior olive end in certain parts of it only (Walberg, 1956). Pallidonigral fibers have been found by some (Johnson and Clemente, 1959, in the cat; Carpenter and Strominger, 1967, in the monkey), but were not observed in the monkey by Nauta and Mehler (1966). As concerns pallidal projections which via intercalated stations may affect the spinal cord, these appear to be relatively scanty. In this category come the projections to the red nucleus and to the mesencephalic reticular formation (for a review, see Nauta and Mehler, 1966).

It appears from the above that the basal ganglia are not provided with conspicuous efferent projections which would enable them to exert any marked influence on nuclei which give off fibers to the spinal cord. This indicates that *the basal ganglia can scarcely be considered as important "motor centers,"* as was previously often assumed and casts further doubts on the justification for speaking of an "extrapyramidal motor system," as discussed elsewhere (Brodal, 1963). The *basal ganglia appear to be first and foremost concerned in the collaboration between the cerebral cortex and the thalamus.* This follows from the fact that in addition to receiving well-organized projections from the cortex, they give off the bulk of their efferents to the thalamus. In recent years these *pallidothalamic connections* have attracted considerable interest in connection with surgical attempts to relieve the symptoms in parkinsonism (see below). These connections were seen by the classical neuroanatomists, but their functional importance was not generally appreciated. Recent experimental studies have given more precise information. It appears, as referred to above, that the pallidothalamic fibers are derived only from the internal pallidal segment. They make up the bulk of the ansa lenticularis and are usually described as being components of the fasciculus lenticularis, referred to above. The fibers ascending to the thalamus are often collectively called the *fasciculus thalamicus* (or field H_1). It is of relevance for surgical interventions, that these fiber bundles, when they pass medially, interdigitate with other fibers in the internal capsule. It appears that most of the fibers end in the *nucleus ventralis anterior* (VA) of the thalamus (Fig. 4-10) in experimental animals (Glees, 1945; Johnson and Clemente, 1959; Nauta and Mehler, 1966; Carpenter and Strominger, 1967) as well as in man (Hassler, 1949; see also Jung and Hassler, 1960; Martinez, 1961). According to Nauta and Mehler the medialmost magnocellular division of the VA does not receive such fibers. Corresponding results have been obtained in Golgi studies (Scheibel and Scheibel,

1966c). In addition, fibers end in the *nucleus ventralis lateralis* (VL) of
the thalamus, but the termination appears to be restricted to certain parts
of the nucleus. Both these thalamic nuclei project onto the cerebral cortex. The VA, according to studies of brains from patients subjected to
prefrontal leucotomy (Freeman and Watts, 1947; McLardy, 1950),
projects onto the frontal lobe, particularly area 6, while Angevine, Locke,
and Yakovlev (1962) conclude that it projects chiefly to the insula ("cortex anterior to the central insular sulcus"). The projection has so far not
been completely mapped in experimental studies. According to Locke
(1967) in the monkey the VA does not project to the insular cortex.
However, it is clear that the *VA is an important link in a pathway from
the pallidum to the cortex of the frontal lobe.* Additional connections
demonstrate that the VA is more than a relay in a pallidocortical pathway.

In a recent Golgi study Scheibel and Scheibel (1966c) have given an account
of the complexities in the organization of this nucleus. There are afferents ascending from the "nonspecific nuclei," and from the reticular formation. The latter end
chiefly in the same regions as do the pallidal afferents. Corticothalamic fibers represent another group of afferents recently studied experimentally in some detail by
Rinvik (1968c). There are, furthermore, efferent connections to certain of the "nonspecific" thalamic nuclei, and there is a projection from the pallidum to the nucleus
centrum medianum (Nauta and Mehler, 1966; Carpenter and Strominger, 1967),
which appears to project predominantly to the putamen (Nauta and Whitlock,
1954; Powell and Cowan, 1956). In this way there is established an impulse route
or circuit: putamen—pallidum—center median—putamen. These and other anatomical findings are of interest for the interpretation of the activation of the
cerebral cortex occurring from the ascending activating system (see Ch. 6), as is
also the observation that among the various cell types present in the VA there are
a considerable number of short-axoned cells of the Golgi II type, which presumably act as internuncials. This fits in with an observation of Powell (1952) that in
a decorticated human brain some 50% of the cells in the VA do not disintegrate.

The VL, which receives a smaller number of fibers from the pallidum,
projects on to the precentral motor region, areas 4 and 6. Its main afferent influx is provided by fibers from the dentate nucleus in the cerebellum
(see Ch. 5).

The above account of the fiber connections of the basal ganglia and
the subthalamic nucleus and the substantia nigra is far from complete.
As already mentioned, it is clear, however, that these parts of the brain
can only to a limited extent influence motor functions by descending
routes to the spinal cord. On the contrary, their main effects on motor
functions appear to be exerted on the thalamus and, via this, on the cerebral cortex. The presence of "closed circuits" between these nuclei, the
thalamus, and the cortex should be noted. Some of these "circuits" are
shown in Fig. 4-10 to the left. In view of the complex fiber connections

189

of the basal ganglia it is no wonder that it has been difficult to clarify their functional role. However, considerable progress has been made in recent years. It is deemed practical, however, to postpone a discussion of these problems until we have considered the motor cortical areas and the symptoms occurring in lesions of the basal ganglia in man.

The "motor" regions of the cerebral cortex. The term "cortical motor area" is usually employed without any definition. With strong electrical stimuli movements may be elicited from many parts of the cortex. Various factors, among these the type and depth of anesthesia, influence the excitability of the cerebral cortex and determine the results of stimulation. By varying the stimulus parameters one can obtain different motor maps on the same brain, as shown by Liddell and Phillips (1950). It cannot be stressed too often, that electrical stimulation is an entirely artificial method of exciting nervous tissue. However, it is so far the only method (in addition to local application of strychnine and certain other substances) which can be used for local stimulation of the cerebral cortex. If a cortical area is said to have a motor function on the basis of stimulation experiments, it must be required that motor responses are obtained with liminal stimuli. Furthermore, the defects following its destruction should affect motor functions, although these defects need not necessarily be detectable with ordinary methods of examination. (On the other hand, disturbances of motor function following damage to a part of the nervous system does not prove that this part has a "motor" function. Such disturbances may follow damage to definitely sensory structures, the most clear-cut example being perhaps the dorsal funiculi.) To be classified as a "motor" region a cortical area should be provided with efferent fibers which directly or via a few intercalated cell groups establish a pathway to peripheral motor neurons.[7] As will be described below, the three areas considered today as motor more or less fulfill the requirements mentioned above. However, it appears that a clear definition of what we consider a motor cortical area cannot be given. Here, as in so many other instances in biology and medicine, there are no unequivocal criteria which enable us to define our subject precisely, functionally, or structurally.

For a long time it was customary to speak of one "motor region" of the cerebral cortex, situated in the precentral gyrus in monkeys, apes, and man. This view has had to be thoroughly modified. As discussed in Ch. 2 (p. 84), the precentral "motor cortex" receives sensory information,

---

[7] It would be rather far-fetched to consider, for example, all cortical areas giving rise to corticopontine fibers (see Ch. 5) as "motor," even if the pons, via the cerebellum and the projections of the latter to brain stem nuclei, may act on motoneurons.

and motor effects can be obtained on stimulation of the "sensory," post-central gyrus. Accordingly one could speak of a *sensorimotor cortex,* of which the part in front of the central sulcus is preponderantly motor, the part behind the sulcus preponderantly sensory. (In Woolsey's nomen-clature they are labeled Ms I and Sm I, respectively, see Fig. 2-17). Fur-thermore, just as there is more than one somatosensory cortical area, as described in Chapter 2, *there are at least three somatomotor areas, the first, the second, and a supplementary.* These will be considered below.

Before the presence of the latter two areas had been established, attempts were made, particularly by Fulton and his collaborators in the 1930's to distinguish, in the precentral cortex, between a "motor" and a "premotor" area, the latter cor-responding approximately to area 6 of Brodmann (see Fig. 12-2) and being func-tionally different from the former. Ablation of the premotor cortex resulted in the appearance of the grasp reflex (see below) and its stimulation gave rise to complex movements. With the use of stronger electrical stimuli than those required for pro-ducing discrete movements from the "motor" cortex, movements could, further-more, be elicited from certain other regions of the cortex. These movements were slower and more complex than those obtained from area 4. Mainly, it appears, due to the general belief that the pyramidal tract came only from area 4, these other, less clearly delimited cortical regions were lumped together as "extrapyramidal motor areas" and were supposed to be essential in the production of coarse move-ments. These areas were particularly studied in man by the German neurosurgeon Foerster (see his account in *Handbuch der Neurologie,* 1936b) and covered exten-sive parts of the cortex of all four cerebral lobes.

In the course of time a voluminous literature has grown up on the motor functions of the cerebral cortex, and on the clinical consequences of lesions of the "motor" area, and heated debates have taken place. Not least have there been differences of opinion between experimental work-ers and clinicians. One of the most ardent spokesmen for the latter has been Sir Francis Walshe, whose eloquent writings on this subject (see, for example, Walshe, 1942b, 1943) still are fascinating reading and certainly did much to focus attention upon discrepancies between clinical and experimental observations. It would take us too far to go through the development in the views of the motor functions of the cerebral cortex. (The situation about 1944 is well summarized in *The Precentral Motor Cortex.*) In the following, reference will be made to only some of the earlier studies. Emphasis will be put on more recent observations on cortical motor function and their anatomical basis in man and in experi-mental animals. The results of the two lines of research can today be linked in a more fruitful way than was possible a few decades ago.

The first, primary, central or Rolandic, somatomotor area. This was previously considered to be represented by Brodmann's area 4, which belongs to the so-called agranular cortex (see Ch. 12, and Figs. 8-7 and 12-3). Area 4 is characterized by the presence of the giant cells of Betz in layer V, while layers II and IV are poorly developed. The formerly commonly held notion that area 4 is the sole origin of pyramidal tract fibers has turned out to be erroneous. As described in a preceding section of this chapter, the pyramidal tract receives fibers not only from cells in area 4, but almost as many from the cortex in the postcentral gyrus (areas 3, 1 and 2), as well as from the region in front of area 4, i.e. area 6.[8] Furthermore, corticorubral, corticoreticular, and other major efferent cortical projections arise from the same cortical regions. Judged on the criterion of efferent fibers the primary motor cortex will thus extend beyond the confines of area 4 frontally and will include most of the postcentral gyrus as well. This is in agreement with the results of electrical stimulation of the cortex in animals as well as in man. The same kinds of movements (see below), as can be elicited from the cortex immediately in front of the central sulcus and belonging to area 4, can be obtained from the parts of the postcentral gyrus close to the sulcus, as well as from precentral cortex belonging to area 6, although motor responses are less frequent in the postcentral than in the precentral gyrus (Clark and Ward, 1948; Woolsey et al., 1952; Welker et al., 1957; and others). Fig. 4-11 shows Penfield and Boldrey's (1937) map of their observations in man. The central or primary motor area thus is far more extensive than previously assumed. (As mentioned above, Woolsey has suggested that the precentral part may be referred to as Ms I, the postcentral as Sm I; see Fig. 2-17.)

All students appear to agree that *on application of weak electrical stimuli to the first somatomotor region (Ms I and Sm I) discrete movements may be obtained on the opposite side of the body.* This was shown as early as 1870 by Fritsch and Hitzig in the dog and has since been amply confirmed, e.g. by Grünbaum and Sherrington (1902, 1903) in monkeys and anthropoid apes, and by C. and O. Vogt (1919) in monkeys, to mention only some of the pioneers in this field. In man similar results have been obtained (Ferrier, Horsley, Foerster, Penfield, and others).[9] It was established by early workers that *there are discrete points from which each small movement is evoked.* In this manner it is possible to construct a cerebral map of the motor "foci" for the different parts of the body (Fig. 4-12). The excitable area extends onto the medial surface

---

[8] Area 6, like area 4, belongs to the agranular cortex, but unlike area 4, it lacks Betz cells. In the areas in the postcentral gyrus, the layers III and V, giving rise to long corticofugal fibers, are rather well developed.

[9] The studies in man are made in patients where the cortex has to be exposed as part of a therapeutic measure. Since this can usually be done under local anesthesia the neurosurgeon has the advantage that the patient can communicate with him and report his subjective sensations (see below).

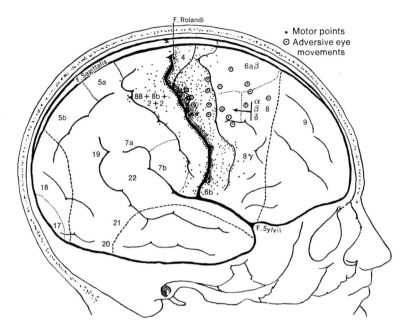

FIG. 4–11 Drawing of the right hemisphere in man showing (dots) the points from which discrete movements can be elicited on electrical stimulation. Note that points are found in the postcentral gyrus and in the entire precentral gyrus. From Penfield and Boldrey (1937).

of the hemisphere (the paracentral lobule). Lowermost, in part buried in the central sulcus, are found the foci for the face, lips, jaw, tongue, larynx, and pharynx. The foci for the distal parts of the extremities are found closer to the central sulcus than the foci for the proximal parts (Fig. 2-17). It is important to be aware that *the cortical areas allotted to the different bodily regions are of unequal size.* Generally speaking, those parts of the body which are capable of performing the most delicate movements have the largest "representation" as shown in Fig. 4-12. (Compare, for example, the cortical "representation" of the fingers with that of the abdomen.)

The movements elicited on stimulation of the primary "motor" area are always contralateral as far as the extremities are concerned (see Penfield and Jasper, 1954). However, movements of the soft palate, the laryngeal muscles, and, as a rule, the masticatory muscles always occur bilaterally. Bilateral movements of the muscles of the trunk can also be provoked quite easily, while movements of the face are usually contralateral. Muscles, which under normal circumstances as a rule are active bilaterally, appear to be influenced bilaterally on cortical stimulation.

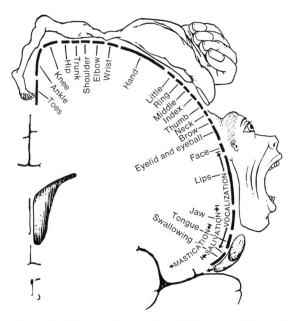

FIG. 4–12 Diagram showing the relative size of the parts of the human primary motor cortex from which movements of different parts of the body can be elicited on electrical stimulation. From Penfield and Rasmussen (1950).

These differences are probably to a large extent a functional consequence of an anatomical feature, namely a varying proportion of crossed and uncrossed corticofugal connections.

The "representation" of bodily regions in the primary motor cortex described above should not be taken to be too rigidly fixed. It may happen, for example, that when the focus for the thumb is stimulated there ensues first an isolated flexion of the thumb. After this has been repeated several times, the thumb remains immobile, but instead there occurs, on continued stimulation, a movement of the index finger. On continued stimulation this movement also ceases, and is replaced by movements of the wrist. If the stimulation is continued longer, after a while the thumb flexion reappears.[10] The problem of the *stability of the motor points* has attracted considerable interest. It is clear that the responsiveness of

[10] This was interpreted as follows by Foerster: within the cortical area representing the focus for flexion of the thumb, there must be other cellular elements, whose axons are concerned in the innervation of the muscles moving the index and even the wrist. When these elements do not make themselves apparent at the beginning of the experiment, this may mean that they have a higher threshold than those to the thumb. When the latter cells are fatigued, the other elements in the area respond. When the "thumb cells" have recovered they are again susceptible to irritation.

194

cortical cells is influenced by several factors and may show what has been referred to as "temporal fluctuations," "functional instability," etc. Nevertheless, there appears to be a rather fixed basic arrangement. Landgren, Phillips, and Porter (1962) studied this problem in monkeys by recording intracellularly from motoneurons (which in the monkey are in part activated monosynaptically by pyramidal tract fibers). They found that for many motoneurons there appears to be in the cortex a "best point," but the same motoneuron can be brought to discharge from a larger surrounding area as well. The "best point" seems to be confined within a cylindrical sector of the cortex of a diameter of about 1 mm. There is, however, overlapping between foci of different motoneurons. Corresponding findings have been reported in the cat (Asanuma and Sakata, 1967) by testing monosynaptic reflexes following intracortical stimulation. The cortical cell groups influencing (monosynaptically in the baboon) motoneurons of distal muscles are more restricted than those influencing motoneurons of proximal muscles (see Phillips, 1967). The foci for γ neurons likewise appear to be very discrete, and the foci for activation of α and γ neurons to the same muscle appear to be identical (Mortimer and Akert, 1961). As the latter authors say (p. 243, loc. cit.), this indicates that "a close tie between alpha and gamma innervation exists not only at the spinal level but at the highest level as well."

It should be emphasized that *electrical stimulation of the primary motor cortex never elicits co-ordinated purposeful movements,* as amply documented in man, particularly by Penfield and his collaborators (Penfield and Boldrey, 1937; Penfield and Rasmussen, 1950; Penfield and Jasper, 1954). When the strength of the stimulus is increased beyond that necessary to give a small isolated contraction of a single muscle, only contractions of synergic muscles with relaxation of the antagonists occur. Another interesting observation made in studies of humans is the following: If stimulation is done while the patient performs a movement which would require the co-operation of the point in case, stimulation will cause the movement to stop. The patient then often reports that he has a funny feeling, and he feels that his arm (or leg) is paralyzed.

It seems permissible to conclude from the available data that there exists a fairly rigidly fixed pattern of connections from a particular motor cortical point to the motoneurons supplying specific muscles or even parts of muscles.[11] However, *the notion that patterns of skilled move-*

[11] Bates (1960) investigated the cortical maps to electrical stimulation in patients where the cortex was exposed on two different occasions (with intervals of three months to more than three years). In general, identical results were obtained from stimulation of the same points on the two occasions. His studies further lend support to the notion of Leyton and Sherrington (1917) that there is some degree

ments are "represented" in the motor cortex is scarcely tenable. Apart from the fact that co-ordinated movements are never elicited on cortical stimulation, other observations argue against this view which for a period was held by some students. Thus the results of stimulation are the same in a child of 8 years as in a man aged 60, and the same if the man is an accomplished pianist or a manual laborer (Penfield and Jasper, 1954). This view is only in apparent contradiction to the fact that removal of the hand area of the motor cortex, for example, results in loss of skilled movements of the contralateral hand and fingers. While this shows that the performance of skilled movements requires the co-operation of the motor cortex, it does not tell us anything about its organization. When discussing the role played by the primary motor cortex in the initiation of movements, it has sometimes been likened to a clavichord, upon which impulses from other sources play. Little is known precisely of this. However, it seems likely that sensory impulses and impulses from the cerebellum, (see Ch. 5) the thalamus and hypothalamus, as well as from other parts of the cortex are involved, as has indeed been shown experimentally.

In many of the numerous physiological studies of this subject which have been undertaken, more refined methods than crude stimulations have been employed. The activity of the motor cortex has to a large extent been judged on the criterion of activity in corticospinal neurons (by recording from their axons or by studying the effect of stimulation of corticospinal fibers on motoneurons or on spinal reflexes, as mentioned above). The results obtained are extremely complex and will not be discussed here, except for mentioning that the activity of corticospinal neurons has been shown to be influenced by visual, auditory, and somatosensory stimuli, as well as by stimulation of the caudate nucleus, and "specific" and "nonspecific" thalamic nuclei (for some data, see Buser, 1966). Attempts to analyze the activity of corticospinal neurons during movements in nonanesthetized monkeys (see Evarts, 1968, and earlier) seem promising, but the interpretation of the findings is difficult.

It should be emphasized that *studies of the corticospinal neurons can give information on only a fraction of what really goes on in the motor cortex.* For example, the many other efferent projections are left out of consideration. These certainly play an important role in the influence exerted by the primary motor cortex on the peripheral motor mechanisms. (We will return to these questions and the consequences of lesions of the primary motor cortex in a later section.) Bates (1957) has ventured the suggestion that the fundamental patterns of discrete movements are actually organized largely at the spinal level. This view is based on data mentioned above as well as on others (see Bates, 1963), such as studies of the movements of which the newborn is capable. Further sup-

of individuality in the cortical "representation," since the responses differ in some respects between individuals.

port comes from the observation (Bates, 1953) that there is a close similarity between the movements in response to stimulation of the cortex and stimulation of the internal capsule after hemispherectomy. According to Bates's hypothesis the role of the cortex would be chiefly to modulate the activity of the spinal patterns of movement and to impose a degree of discreteness on them. This view is in accord with recent experimental observations which indicate that the spinal cord is capable of a considerable degree of integrated activity in the motor sphere. Bates's hypothesis raises the interesting question whether the learning of motor skills may be as much a task of the spinal cord as of the cortex.

The supplementary motor area was described in the monkey and man by Penfield and Welch (1951). It is found on the medial surface of the cerebral hemisphere, above the cingulate gyrus and extends forward from the "leg region" of the primary motor area where this continues onto the medial aspect of the hemisphere. In the monkey (see Fig. 2-17) its anteroposterior dimension is approximately 1 cm; in man it is larger. In the monkey, Penfield and Welch on *stimulation of this area* obtained movements of contralateral extremities, in a topographic pattern, movements of the hindlimb being elicited most posteriorly. Most often the responses involved distal musculature. In the monkey, as well as in man, the threshold for the stimulation is a little higher than for the precentral and postcentral regions, and bilateral responses are frequent (there are other differences in the excitability of the two motor regions as well). The results obtained by Woolsey and his collaborators (Woolsey et al., 1952) in experiments on monkeys largely correspond to those obtained by Penfield and Welch (1951; see also Penfield and Jasper, 1954) concerning a somatotopic organization within the supplementary motor area.

However, the results in man differ in some respects from those obtained in the monkey. No somatotopical pattern has so far been demonstrated, and the motor effects usually consist in inhibition of voluntary activity or in the production of synergies resulting in the assumption of characteristic postures and in the performance of complex maneuvers. In addition, vocalization has often been observed, and sometimes pupillary dilatation or acceleration of the heart rate. Some patients report sensory experiences during stimulation.[12]

The results of *ablations of the supplementary motor area* are not entirely consistent. This may in part be due to the fact that the posterior part of the supplementary area appears to fuse with the primary motor area (the hindlimb regions of both areas are closely related). Erickson and Woolsey (1951) observed a weak and short-lived grasp reflex after

[12] As mentioned in Chapter 2, there is evidence that the supplementary motor area is also sensory (Woolsey's Ms II, see Fig. 2-17).

unilateral involvement of the area in man. This has been confirmed by Penfield and Jasper (1954) who, furthermore, found that even after the passage of a year there is some slowness of movements on the opposite side, particularly of alternating movements. In the monkey they consider forced grasping a specific sign of removal of the supplementary area, as does also Travis (1955). While Coxe and Landau (1965) did not observe persistent changes following bilateral ablations of the supplementary motor area in the monkey, Travis (1955) in addition to the occurrence of transient grasp reflexes found disturbances in posture and tonus, but practically no paresis. There was increased resistance to passive movements of the limbs, with hypertonia in the flexor muscles. The spasticity demonstrated topographical localization.

The discrepancies between the observations made on the supplementary motor area in man and in the monkey are presumably due largely to methodological difficulties. There is, however, reason to assume (Travis, 1955) that "the precentral and supplementary motor areas for the most part exert different influences on the motor reflex systems." Some anatomical data supports this conclusion. Thus the efferent projections from the two motor areas differ in certain respects, even if the fibers from the supplementary motor area have been traced to the spinal cord and descend with those from the primary motor cortex (Nyberg-Hansen, 1969, in the cat). According to the electrophysiological study of Bertrand (1956) the proportion of uncrossed fibers is greater than in the corticospinal projection from the central region.

In the cat there is most probably a corresponding supplementary motor area (see Woolsey, 1958). In experimental studies on the efferent projections of this cortical region in our laboratory it has been observed that the terminal area in the spinal cord is largely the same as that of the corticospinal fibers from the anterior and posterior sigmoid gyri. Most fibers end contralaterally (Nyberg-Hansen, 1969). Furthermore, there is a topically arranged projection to the thalamus (Rinvik, 1968c), in part ipsilateral, in part contralateral (via the anterior commissure), and the fibers terminate largely in the same thalamic nuclei as do those from the primary motor area. Likewise, there is bilateral topical projection to the dorsal column nuclei and pontine nuclei, while the projections to these nuclei from the primary motor area are unilateral. These bilateral connections may be related to some of the functional phenomena observed.

While the supplementary motor area has been outlined fairly precisely in the monkey with methods of stimulation, its anatomical boundaries have not yet been defined. It appears that the posterior part of it is found within area 4 of Brodmann, where this extends onto the medial surface of the hemisphere, while its anterior region covers part of area 6. Whether this is related to some differences in connections and functions of the forelimb and hindlimb regions of the supplementary motor area is not known, but may be considered. If not, a revision of the cytoarchitecture of this part of the cortex may prove it to be more of a distinct entity than appears so far. The fact that the hindlimb region of the supplementary area touches on the hindlimb region of the primary motor cortex may explain certain discordant results of ablation studies, particularly concerning the hindlimb.

The grasp reflex and forced grasping. As the name implies, *forced grasping* is a compulsory grasping movement and is of reflex nature. This symptom was known clinically as a sign of frontal lobe affection (Adie and Critchley, 1927) some time before it was concluded from experimental investigations that it was dependent on a lesion of area 6 (Fulton, 1934; Richter and Hines, 1934). However, it now appears well established that the responsible cortical region is the supplementary motor area. An analysis of reports attributing the symptom to lesions of area 6 indicates that in the relevant cases the lesions have in fact involved the supplementary motor area (Travis, 1955). The grasp reflex is essentially similar in man and in monkeys. It is elicited when the palmar surface of the hand or fingers is gently touched, for example, by a stick. A flexion of the fingers then appears and the stick is held firmly.

According to an exhaustive study of Seyffarth and Denny-Brown (1948) the adequate stimulus for the full reaction is dual. There is an initial tactile "catching phase" followed by a proprioceptive response, the "holding phase," due to traction on the appropriate muscles. The latter phase is a heightened stretch reflex which is triggered by the tactile response. The grasp reflex is usually grouped with the postural reflexes (cf. later), since it is influenced by changes in the posture of the body. When a grasp reflex is present and the animal is lying on its side, the reflex is far more vigorous in the uppermost hand than in the other on the under side of the animal. Emotional factors, also, influence the reflex, anxiety, for example, increasing it. It appears that the reflex is entirely subcortical, and it is supposed that when it occurs this is due to loss of a normal inhibitory cortical influence.

It is well known that in *human infants a grasp reflex is normally present*. Its gradual disappearance during the first months of life has been explained by a development of cortical dominance over lower "centers." According to Pollack (1960) the infantile grasp reflexes are, however, not identical with the responses seen in adults with frontal lobe damage. It might be advisable, therefore, to reserve the term "grasp reflex" for the normal reflex in infants, and to use the term "forced grasping" for the phenomena seen in lesions of the supplementary motor area.

The motor functions of the *second somatic sensorimotor area* are less well known than those of the supplementary motor area. As mentioned in Chapter 2, this area has been labeled Sm II by Woolsey in order to emphasize that although it is mainly concerned in the reception of somatic sensory impulses, it should to a lesser degree also be considered a motor region. In pioneer studies Adrian (1941) and Woolsey (1947) obtained motor responses upon stimulation of the second somatic sensory cortical area. Furthermore, the motor effects were somatotopically organized. These findings have been confirmed by Welker et al. (1957) and others.

199

There is evidence (Penfield and Rasmussen, 1950; Penfield and Jasper, 1954) that in man there is a corresponding second sensorimotor area in the upper bank of the fissure of Sylvius, but motor deficits have not been observed following isolated ablation of this area.

Since these investigations in animals and man were carried out, subsequent studies on Sm II have almost exclusively been concerned with its role as a sensory cortical region (see Ch. 2). Little is known concerning the corticofugal projections from this area. Woolsey (1947) appears to have traced degenerating myelinated fibers from this area in the pyramidal decussation and to the upper cervical segments in animals. More recently, ample corticofugal connections from Sm II to the dorsal column nuclei and the main sensory relay nuclei of the thalamus have been described in the cat (Levitt, Carreras, Liu, and Chambers, 1964; Kusama, Otani, and Kawana, 1966; DeVito, 1967; Rinvik, 1968b). Likewise there is a somatotopical projection onto the pontine nuclei (P. Brodal, 1968b). Obviously much remains to be done before the role of Sm II in motor functions is understood.

Symptoms following lesions of supraspinal structures and pathways influencing peripheral motor neurons. This heading covers a great variety of disorders of motor functions. Since the disturbances are not caused by damage to the peripheral motor neuron, they have in common that there is no marked atrophy of the muscles, and although there may be changes in the myotatic (stretch) reflexes these will not be abolished. Nor will muscular tonus be abolished, even if changes in this are the rule, due to alterations in the normal action of supraspinal structures on the motoneurons (α and γ). We are still far from being able to understand the mechanisms at work when motor symptoms follow lesions of supraspinal structures and pathways. It is, therefore, not possible to discuss these subjects in an entirely satisfactory fashion, and a correlation of experimental findings and observations on humans can only be made to a certain extent. For this reason it is deemed practical in the following presentation first to describe the symptoms seen in humans, and then to discuss their relation to experimental observations and the attempts to explain the symptoms.

Before turning to the motor disturbances occurring in lesions at supraspinal levels it will be appropriate to devote some attention to the mechanisms in the spinal cord which ultimately mediate the supraspinal influences on the motoneurons, and to consider the consequences of lesions of the descending fiber systems within the cord.

Some features in the organization of supraspinal influences on the spinal cord. Essentially the spinal cord may be considered as a series of segments of nervous tissue charged with the nervous regulation of the corresponding segments of the body. Co-operation between the segments is secured by intersegmental connections, and the integration into patterns of reaction subserving the entire organism is chiefly taken care of by descending connections from higher levels of the nervous system. In order that this central control can function properly, ascending pathways, bringing sensory information to the cord as well as to higher levels, must be intact.

As discussed in Chapter 2, several of the long descending fiber systems have been shown to influence the ascending transmission of sensory impulses from the cord, postsynaptically, by acting on "secondary" sensory neurons, or presynaptically, by acting on the terminations of dorsal root afferents. Here we are concerned with the effects of supraspinal structures on motor functions. It seems clear from many recent studies (see below) that most of these effects are exerted not directly on the motoneurons but on the spinal reflex mechanisms. Furthermore, the spinal reflex paths can be influenced by fibers from supraspinal structures via internuncials in the cord as well as by primary afferent depolarization (presynaptic inhibition of dorsal root afferents).

In any evaluation of supraspinal influences on the cord it should be recalled that the spinal reflexes are not fixed and stereotyped, but may be modified according to the stimulus site, the intensity of the stimulus, the concomitant application of other stimuli and other factors. Furthermore, there are numerous descending pathways which may act on the spinal reflex apparatus. Since all motor reflexes (except the stretch reflex) appear to have multisynaptic reflex arcs, it follows that the internuncial cells are of particular interest, the more so since in the cat (on which most experiments have been made) all supraspinal fiber systems (except possibly the lateral vestibulospinal tract) exert their action on the motoneurons via internuncial cells. In monkeys, and presumably also in man, the corticospinal tract can influence the motoneurons monosynaptically as well (whether this is true also for other descending systems is not known). Nevertheless, it appears likely that the spinal reflexes in man are organized essentially as in the cat, even if the spinal cord seems to lose some of its autonomy in the phylogenetic ascent.

As mentioned in an earlier section of this chapter it has been shown for several supraspinal fiber systems that they act on α as well as γ neurons. In general these effects are parallel for a particular fiber system, and both (in the cat) are mediated via internuncials. Thus the corticospinal and rubrospinal tracts activate neurons supplying flexor muscles, and inhibit neurons supplying extensor muscles. Medullary reticulospinal fibers appear to have a similar action. On the other hand, vestibulospinal impulses have the opposite effect, facilitating (apparently monosynaptically) extensor motoneurons. The pontine reticulospinal fibers appear to belong to the same group. In view of this the sites of termination of the descending fiber systems within the gray matter are of interest. As seen from Figs. 4-3, 4-6, and 4-7, the fiber systems giving facilitation of flexor motoneurons end in laminae V–VI and the dorsal part of VII, while those facilitating extensor motoneurons terminate more ventrally in lamina VII and the adjoining part of lamina VIII. These morphological observations suggest that different groups of interneurons are presumably involved in the supraspinal effects on flexor and extensor motoneurons.[13] This appears indeed to be the case since physiologically interneurons which are intercalated in reflex pathways excitatory to flexor and inhibitory to extensor motoneurons are found in laminae V–VII, chiefly laterally, while interneurons mediating the opposite effect are located in lamina VIII and adjacent parts of lamina VII (see Eccles, 1964). It is further of interest that the pathways giving excitation of flexor motoneurons are found more dorsally in the ventrolateral funiculus than those exciting extensor motoneurons (see Figs. 4-3, 4-6, and 4-7). The former pathways are considered to be phylogenetically younger than the latter (see Nyberg-Hansen, 1966a).

It appears from the above that in a very simplified fashion the supraspinal pathways may be subdivided into two groups, concerned in opposite actions on the motor apparatus (flexion and extension). While both act on motoneurons via interneurons, these appear to be different for the two groups. Some recent findings of Lawrence and Kuypers (1968b) support this view. Following recovery from a prior bilateral pyramidotomy, lesions of the spinal cord were made in monkeys. The lesions involved either the lateral or the ventral funiculus. In the latter the motor impairment concerned chiefly the axial and proximal extremity movements and there was a bias towards flexion of trunk and limbs. Lesions of the lateral funiculus gave rise to impairment of independent distal extremity and hand movements and an impaired capacity to flex the extended limb.

The anatomical and physiological observations mentioned above can give no more than a simple sketch of a very complex mechanism. The different supraspinal descending pathways within each of the two main groups are certainly not functionally equivalent in all respects. Furthermore, the intrinsic anatomical organization of the spinal cord, discussed in Chapters 2 and 3 (pp. 44 and 139) is extremely complex, and provides wide possibilities for interactions between several descending sys-

[13] It is interesting to notice (Nyberg-Hansen, 1966a) that the former groups of interneurons are situated closer to the motoneuron groups supplying the distal musculature, the latter closer to the groups for the proximal limb muscles and those of the trunk (cf. Ch. 3 on the somatotopical arrangement of motoneurons).

tems and a variety of spinal afferents. In recent years the effects of supra-spinal systems on the reflex activity of the cord have been intensively studied, particularly by Lundberg and his collaborators. In spite of many interesting observations, it is scarcely possible to put them together to form a coherent picture of the functional organization of the cord. Some of the observations may be mentioned to give an idea of the complexity of the problems.

As mentioned previously, supraspinal structures may influence the reflex activity of the cord in two ways (leaving out of consideration here possible monosynaptic actions on motoneurons): the descending fibers may act on interneurons which are intercalated in most reflex arcs, inhibiting or facilitating them; or the fibers may produce depolarization of afferent fibers and in this way reduce or block the reflex response that a sensory impulse would otherwise produce. Both types of action have been demonstrated (for reviews see Lundberg, 1966; Marchiafava, 1968), and a very complex picture of the supraspinal control of reflexes is emerging. For example, the corticospinal tract has been shown to facilitate polysynaptic reflex arcs where the afferents belong to Ia, Ib, cutaneous, and so-called flexor reflex afferents (Lundberg and Voorhoeve, 1962). This effect appears to be due to facilitation of interneurons of the segmental reflex arc. Likewise, the rubrospinal tract has a facilitatory action on interneurons of reflex pathways which mediate the Ib inhibition (Hongo, Jankowska, and Lundberg, 1965). In both cases the interneurons appear to be situated in the region of the gray matter where the two pathways end (see Fig. 4-3). Facilitatory actions have further been found from the rubrospinal tract on interneurons activated from group Ia muscle afferents and belonging to reflex arcs mediating inhibitory effects on flexor and extensor motoneurons (Hongo, Jankowska, and Lundberg, 1965). The Ia inhibitory pathway from extensors to flexor motoneurons (see Fig. 3-6) can be facilitated from the vestibulo-spinal tract through a monosynaptic excitatory action on the Ia inhibitory interneurons (Grillner, Hongo, and Lund, 1966). However, interneurons may also be inhibited from supraspinal fiber systems (see Lundberg, 1966, 1967, and Marchiafava, 1968, for some data). Recently much attention has been devoted to the chemical aspects of transmissions in the spinal cord (see Lundberg, 1966). However, these will not be considered here.

From a clinical point of view those aspects of the functional organization of the cord which are related to the supraspinal control of muscular tone and myotatic reflexes are of particular interest, since changes in these functions are common in lesions of the central nervous system. Increasing knowledge of the organization of the normal stretch reflex, discussed in Chapter 3, has provided valuable clues for the understanding of the phenomena of spasticity and rigidity. A consideration of these subjects will be postponed until the clinical conditions where they occur have been dealt with.

Transverse lesions of the spinal cord and the Brown-Séquard syndrome. Spinal shock. In Chapter 2 the symptoms due to lesions of the sensory paths of the spinal cord were discussed. However, pathological processes affecting one of these fiber tracts exclusively are not very frequent. In most diseases affecting the cord the morbid changes will involve several ascending and descending tracts (the fibers of which are even partly intermingled) and the gray matter of the cord. The lesions may be of several kinds or sizes, from complete transverse lesions where all fiber tracts are interrupted, to partial transverse lesions of half of the cord or less. Frequently the lesions will have an irregular distribution, affecting, predominantly for example, the gray matter. Possessing a knowledge of the anatomical features of the cord the neurologist will be able to draw conclusions from the symptoms present concerning the approximate place of damage to the cord, its level in the cord, i.e. the segmental diagnosis, and its site in the transverse section of the cord. The number of possible combinations of lesions and consequently of symptoms is, of course, practically unlimited.

A typical clinical syndrome, the so-called *complete transverse syndrome,* is met with in cases where an acute, complete interruption of the spinal cord has occurred. (For a detailed study, see Kuhn, 1950.) Usually this is caused by traumatic injury, gunshot wounds, stab wounds, or compression fracture of the spine (in other cases inflammatory processes, myelitis, may be the cause). Immediately following the injury a complete paralysis of all muscles which get their motor innervation from segments of the cord caudal to the lesion is observed; likewise a complete anesthesia is present in the same territory, all modalities of sensation being abolished, superficial as well as deep. The paralysis is, immediately after the injury, of the flaccid type, the tendon reflexes as well as the superficial, cutaneous reflexes are absent. Nearly always there is retention of urine (of practical importance!), and as a rule peristalsis is severely impaired and no emptying of the bowels takes place. Sweat secretion is abolished below the level of the lesion, and the blood pressure suffers a temporary drop. Erection is abolished.

If death does not ensue, this *initial stage of spinal shock* gradually passes into what is usually called the *"stage of reorganization":* the spinal cord below the lesion resumes some of its functions, in spite of its lacking connections with the higher levels of the central nervous system. Usually the first signs of this are shown by the bladder and rectum. Occasionally a spontaneous emptying of the bladder occurs, eventually also of the rectum: *automatic reflex activity of bladder and rectum,* and sweat secretion reappears.[14] Somewhat later the muscles resume some of their tone, and simultaneously signs of reappearing *reflex activity of the muscles* will be noticed. Especially on painful stimuli or on cooling parts of the body below the lesion (e.g. when uncovering the patient) the so-called *re-*

---

[14] The symptoms referable to the autonomic system, including disturbances of bladder and rectum, are discussed more fully in Chapter 11.

flexes of spinal automatism appear, most frequently as a flexion of the legs in hip and knee joints, often accompanied by emptying of the bladder, eventually the rectum (Riddoch's mass reflexes). These reflexes of spinal automatism can as a rule be elicited from any part of the body below the segment of lesion, but frequently not with the same ease from all regions. By and by the lower extremities become permanently fixed in a drawn-up position, with flexion at the hips and the knees and dorsiflexion in the ankle joint, due to a tendency to shortening of the flexor muscles. The result will be a *spastic paraplegia in flexion.* Later on the tendon reflexes reappear; the patellar and achilles reflexes can be elicited. "Mass extension" of one or both lower limbs may occur in response to proprioceptive stimuli. (For some data on the reflex mechanisms see p. 201.) This "reorganization" usually requires several months. The same phenomena occur in animals following experimental transection of the cord, but in animals the "reorganization" occurs more rapidly, the more so the lower the position of the species in the evolutionary scale. It thus appears that the spinal reflex apparatus, which is responsible for these phenomena, loses more and more of its independence in phylogenetic ascent.

The occurrence of "spinal shock" following an acute transverse lesion of the cord cannot yet be adequately explained. It has been generally assumed that the shock is due to the disappearance of the normally present descending influences on the spinal gray matter, leaving its internuncial cells and the motoneurons at a lower level of excitability. From a comparison between the H-reflex [15] and the ankle jerk in patients with acute traumatic spinal cord lesions. Weaver, Landau, and Higgins (1963) conclude that a depression of fusimotor function contributes to the general hyporeflexia in spinal shock, but it is not the only factor (see also Diamantopoulos and Zander Olsen, 1967). Illis (1967) has advanced a hypothesis based on experimental observations of boutons on cells in the spinal cord following interruption of afferents. In the first two days after the transection of afferents there is a general disorganization of the "synaptic zone" of the nerve cells, affecting all of the many thousand boutons. The boutons belonging to transected afferents will disintegrate, while the neighboring ones are not irreversibly changed and recover. The places on the neuronal surface occupied by the degenerating boutons are temporarily covered by glial cells, but ultimately appear to be again contacted by boutons, which are assumed to be formed by sprouting of intact afferents (see Liu and Chambers, 1958). The disorganization of the "synaptic zone," according to Illis (1967) may account for the reduced level of excitability of the spinal cord neurons in the first

[15] The H-reflex, described by P. Hoffmann in 1918, has been used for studying certain features of the stretch reflexes in man. The H-reflex is elicited by electrical stimulation of the tibial nerve in the popliteal fossa, and the response is a contraction of the calf muscles (triceps surae). The central delay is so brief that the reflex may be assumed to have a monosynaptic reflex arc. The H-reflex is thus considered to be an electrically induced equivalent to the ankle jerk, the difference being that in the latter the muscle spindles are stimulated by the stretching of the triceps surae, while in the H-reflex the spindle afferent fibers are stimulated directly.

205

days, and the ensuing reorganization may explain the return of excitability, a process which requires some time. (For a recent study of spinal shock in the monkey see McCouch, Liu, and Chambers, 1966.)

The development of the symptoms outlined above will not always appear in its complete form. Particularly when urinary infections, leading to pyelonephritis, or decubitus ulcers (bed sores) with secondary infections and ensuing weakening of the organism, develop, the spastic paraplegia in flexion is usually replaced by a flaccid paralysis. The prognosis of a complete transverse lesion was formerly very bad. Following World War II great interest has been taken in improving the prognosis in paraplegic patients. It has been shown that if infections and the development of bed sores are prevented it is possible by physiotherapy to rehabilitate many of these patients to a useful life. The therapy aims at enabling the patient to substitute for the functions of the paralyzed muscles by using those which are intact. In the first place the muscles of the shoulder girdles are utilized. It is indeed astonishing to see to what extent patients may regain mobility in this way.

The picture outlined above refers primarily to complete transections in the thoracic or lumbar region of the cord. Naturally the symptoms will not be wholly identical if other levels of the cord are injured. Thus an injury to the upper part of the cervical region is usually instantly fatal, on account of respiratory paralysis due to involvement of the motor cells of the phrenic nerve (C_{3-4}). Even when the lesion is situated in the lower part of the cervical cord and is followed by paralysis of all four extremities, the phrenic nerve will frequently be affected secondarily (edema, circulatory disturbances). The symptomatology in lesions of the sacral region of the spinal cord is dominated by the autonomic disturbances and will be treated in the chapter on the autonomic system.

Above, only the acute, complete transverse lesion of the cord has been considered. If a complete transverse lesion develops gradually, the final result will be the same, but during its development certain clinical features appear rather regularly. In these cases the morbid changes may be of neoplastic type, an intraspinal, extramedullary or more seldom intramedullary tumor, or there may be inflammatory processes, myelitis. Diseases of the spine are another not infrequent cause of compression of the cord (tuberculous caries, metastases to the vertebrae from malignant tumors, osteomyelitis) or meningeal lesions may be responsible (pachymeningitis, arachnoiditis, epidural abscesses). The details of the symptomatology will naturally depend on the site of the changes, not only its level in the cord, but also from which side it takes its origin.

An extramedullary tumor, for example, springing from a dorsal root, will usually start with radicular pain, accompanied eventually by sensory changes (hyperesthesia) in the corresponding dermatome, but later on it will usually affect the adjacent roots and a segmental sensory loss will appear. Pressure on the cord may then elicit symptoms, indicating damage to one or more of the long fiber tracts, for example sensory loss or a paresis of the spastic type below the segments of the lesion. This paresis, of course, will affect the muscles on the side of the lesion, and frequently at the start will be most conspicuous caudally, when the most superficial fibers of the descending tracts only are affected. This paresis is usually of the spastic type, with exaggerated tendon reflexes and extensor response of the plantar reflex, and weakened or abolished abdominal reflexes. The sensory loss which may occur on account of pressure on the dorsal funiculi will likewise be found on the side of the lesion, and will involve deep pressure sense, vibratory sensibility, and the sense of discrimination, whereas the cutaneous sensibility to simple touch, pain, and temperature will be intact on this side, at least when tested with routine methods. The affection of the dorsal funiculi, furthermore, may produce ataxia on the side of the lesion, most frequently of the leg only. If in the further course of the disease the anterolateral funiculus is also affected, impairment of the sense of pain and temperature will develop in addition, but on the contralateral side, as the paths for these sensory modalities cross in the cord. In the same manner as for the motor impairment, the upper border of the sensory functional loss may be found several segments lower than the lesion, due to the segmental arrangement of the fibers in the spinothalamic tract (the longest fibers are located most superficially).

The complete picture of a lesion comprising one lateral half of the cord is the so-called Brown-Séquard syndrome. This is characterized by a homolateral spastic paralysis below the level of the lesion, with extensor response of the plantar reflex, abolished abdominal reflexes, exaggerated patellar and achilles reflexes, abolished deep sensibility and sense of discrimination in the same regions, and abolished pain and temperature sensibility in the same region of the contralateral side of the body. In addition a segmental motor loss may also be found corresponding to the level and side of the lesion. The functions of the bladder, rectum, and genital organs are usually not interfered with (bilateral innervation).

A complete Brown-Séquard syndrome is not frequently encountered, as might be anticipated. As a rule the lesion of the cord is more irregular and the symptoms consequently somewhat different. A feature which is usually found in incomplete lesions of the cord is the sparing of the sacral segments, already referred to. In this connection another matter may be briefly mentioned. In a gradually developing compression of the cord it is usually observed that the different long fiber systems are affected in a constant order. First appear symptoms indicating damage to the dorsal funiculi and descending tracts; later, disturbances of pain and temperature sense ensue as evidence of damage to the spinothalamic tract, whereas the tactile sensibility mediated through the spinothalamic tract is the last to be affected. This is often taken to indicate a gradation of vulnerability of the long fiber systems. If restitution takes place the function is regained in the inverse order. The vibratory sensibility, joint and position sense, and sense of discrimination are the last to recover.

Symptoms following lesions of the primary (central) motor area and the internal capsule in man. All efferent pathways from the primary motor area (Ms I) destined to act on the peripheral motor neurons—directly or via intercalated cell groups—descend in the internal capsule. Although this also contains other fibers which may be injured by a damage to the internal capsule but would escape involvement in a pure cortical lesion, the motor symptoms following lesions of the internal capsule or motor cortical areas are in the main similar. In order to avoid repetition they will therefore be treated together. Affections of the cortico-fugal fibers from the (primary and supplementary) motor areas in man are far more frequently due to lesions of the internal capsule than to lesions of the cortex. The symptom complex resulting from lesions of this kind has in the past usually been referred to as the "pyramidal tract syndrome." The justification for this will be discussed later, following an account of the symptoms encountered in lesions of this kind. Before dealing with such "deficiency symptoms," it is appropriate to discuss some symptoms following lesions of the primary motor cortex and which produce abnormal activity in its cells, so-called *irritative lesions.*

Previous to the discovery that the cerebral cortex is electrically excitable and that stimulation of the motor cortex yields muscular contractions, the British neurologist Hughlings Jackson had prophesied the principal points in the organization of the primary motor area. His conclusions were based on close clinical examination of patients suffering from epileptic seizures. In some of these cases he had, like other clinicians, observed that chronic contractions may start locally in a circumscribed part of the body, for example, one foot, and then may be propagated in a regular sequence to other parts, for example, from the foot to the calf, further to the thigh, the trunk, and from here they may proceed to the shoulder, upper arm, forearm, hand and fingers, and finally to the muscles of the face. This type of convulsion, in which the patient frequently remains conscious for a relatively long period, is now commonly named a *Jacksonian fit.* As a result of present knowledge it is easy to explain these convulsions as being a result of an abnormal excitation which spreads in the cerebral cortex of the motor area, in the case referred to starting from the medial aspect of the hemisphere (due, for example, to a parasagittal meningeoma), and traveling downward in the primary motor area. The muscular contractions (mostly clonic twitchings) are the result of a stimulation of the cells in the corresponding foci. *In general, a localized beginning of the convulsions in epileptic fits points to the presence of a pathological irritation somewhere in or near the primary motor area,* be it a scar, a tumor, a foreign body, a syphilitic gumma, or an infective process of another type.[16]

[16] The classification of epileptic fits has been the subject of much debate. It has been common to distinguish *symptomatic epilepsy* from *cryptogenetic, essential* or

The occurrence of Jacksonian fits thus is an indication that a localized cerebral lesion exists. *An exact determination of the starting point of the convulsions will give information on where in the motor area the focus responsible for the attacks is likely to be found.* As a rule the convulsions always start in the same muscles in the same patient. In

---

idiopathic epilepsy. In the former the site of a lesion producing the seizures can be identified, while this is not so in the other type. However, there are a number of clinical variants of cryptogenetic epilepsy. Some of them (petit mal, myoclonic petit mal, grand mal, petit mal automatism, and "psychomotor" automatism) are grouped by Penfield and Jasper (1954) as "centrencephalic seizures," since they are assumed to originate from an epileptogenic discharge in the "centrencephalic system" (see Ch. 6). The term "cerebral seizures" is applied to epileptic attacks which can not be localized as to the site of origin of the discharge. Focal seizures may originate in other parts of the cortex than the first motor area. If starting in a sensory area, the attack usually manifests itself in subjective sensations. This may represent an "aura" (somatosensory, visual, acoustic, olfactory, vertiginous, autonomic) to a motor attack. Many varieties may be distinguished. The EEG alterations are to some extent characteristic of the different kinds of epileptic seizures. These subjects will not be considered here (see Penfield and Jasper, 1954, for an exhaustive account.)

In some instances the spreading of the abnormal irritation is limited and the convulsions may be confined, for example, to the fingers and hand or to the leg (*focal epileptic fits*). In focal and Jacksonian fits loss of consciousness is usually lacking or the patient becomes unconscious only late in the fit. If the convulsions have spread considerably, general convulsions are likely to end the seizure, accompanied by loss of consciousness. After a Jacksonian fit a paresis of the muscles which have been involved in the convulsions is frequent. This *postparoxysmal paresis* usually disappears in the course of some minutes or hours. If a paresis is present before the fit, it is usually more marked immediately afterward. Occasionally a suddenly developing and vanishing local paresis may replace the convulsions.

Certain particulars concerning these convulsions ought to be added. Jackson has pointed out that these unilaterally beginning fits have a tendency to start at certain points, namely, the thumb or index finger, the angle of the mouth, and the big toe. This may be interpreted partly as a consequence of the larger area of "representation" of these parts in the motor cortex. When starting peripherally in an extremity, the convulsions are regularly propagated in a proximal direction in the limb, but if they spread to the other extremity they usually start proximally. The intensity of the convulsions at their onset shows a certain proportionality to the degree of spreading, e.g. faint contractions are more apt to be restricted than more violent ones. Some patients state that peripheral stimuli or emotional factors (frequently accompanied by hyperventilation) are apt to precipitate a convulsion. On the other hand, it is well known that some patients suffering from Jacksonian convulsions are able to prevent their development, e.g. by pressing the part in question firmly for a certain period, when they notice the start of an attack (for references see Walshe, 1943). These phenomena are most probably due to alterations in cortical excitability which may occur on sensory stimulation.

numerous cases it has been verified by operation that a pathological change has been present at the place determined as the probable site of the lesion. It is important to realize that convulsions of the Jacksonian type may be the only clear-cut symptom of organic disease of the brain. The clinical neurological examination may be entirely negative, or the only positive finding may be, for example, a doubtful inversion of the plantar reflex (extensor plantar response) or a slight asymmetry of the tendon reflexes. This is easy to understand since the pathological process, giving rise to the abnormal irritation of the motor area, may be very small, e.g. a small depressed fracture or a dislocated bone spicule after a head injury.

Certain circumstances tend to minimize the diagnostic value of Jacksonian fits. Frequently the start and spread of the attacks is not sufficiently clearly observed by the patient or his relatives, and they are not able to give any information on this point. (Thus not infrequently there may even be doubt whether the convulsions start on the left or right side.) Methods aiming at provoking the EEG changes accompanying an attack may be used for diagnostic purposes (small doses of metrazol, flicker stimulation).

Far more frequent than the "irritative" symptoms described above are the *deficiency symptoms due to lesions of the motor areas and their efferent fibers.* A destructive lesion of the primary motor area will result in impairment of voluntary movements, particularly the discrete, skilled movements. On account of the somatotopical organization a circumscribed lesion may produce a *monoplegia,* e.g. a paralysis (virtually only a paresis) of a limb or part of it. Thus a vascular disorder of the anterior cerebral artery may lead to a monoplegia affecting the contralateral toes and foot, and eventually also the leg, since the foci for these parts are found in the paracentral lobule supplied by this artery.

It might be expected that small lesions of the motor area would give rise to very circumscribed pareses, e.g. paretic flexion of the thumb. Such cases are, however, very infrequently encountered, although they have been occasionally observed, particularly following small gunshot wounds in wartime (see, for example, Aring, 1944). Their infrequent occurrence is partly due to the rarity of such small injuries, but in addition the overlapping of foci, referred to previously, must be taken into consideration. Even if, for example, the center of the focus for flexion of the thumb is destroyed, there may be enough nerve cells of this focus left to maintain its function.

Identical monoplegias, in principle, may result from damage to the *internal capsule.* Since the corticofugal fibers in the cord and the brain stem lie rather closely packed in the internal capsule, *monoplegias* will be rare. As a rule the lesion of the internal capsule will more or less destroy all these fibers, and a *hemiplegia* will be the result: a paralysis or paresis of all finer voluntary movements of the contralateral leg and arm. In addition the contralateral lower part of the face and half of the tongue will frequently be involved. The most frequent cause of a capsular hemiplegia, as is well known, is a hemorrhage, or a thrombosis commonly stated to affect one of the branches of the middle cerebral artery [17] (apoplexia cerebri).

It may be appropriate to consider somewhat more closely the *symptoms seen in cases of cerebral apoplexy.* Immediately following the interruption of the cortifugal fibers, i.e. when the hemorrhage has occurred, the face, arm, and leg on the contralateral side of the body are toneless, there is a *flaccid hemiplegia.* As a rule the patient is unconscious for some time after the bleeding has taken place, and during this time, of course, all muscles are flaccid. Even when he regains consciousness, the paralysis of the affected parts is a flaccid one. The muscles are without tonus, and if an arm or a leg is elevated and then released, it drops passively. In addition to the paralysis and the abolished or very diminished muscular tone, all reflexes are abolished on the paralyzed side, the superficial as well as the deep. This *initial stage,* frequently called *shock stage,* is, however, transient if the patient recovers. The first evidence of recovery is shown by the reflexes. As early as 5 to 10 hours after the onset of the symptoms the plantar reflex can be elicited, but the *plantar reflex is now inverted.*[18] Somewhat later, tendon (myotatic) reflexes reappear, usually after 2 to 3 days or somewhat longer in the upper extremity. At first they are weak, but later they increase, and *some time after the hemorrhage the myotatic reflexes are as a rule clearly brisker on the paralyzed side than on the intact side.* Parallel with this increase in the tendon reflexes a *change in the muscular tone* takes place (both features are evidence of the fact that the spinal cord resumes its reflex function). The muscles present an *increased resistance to passive movements.*[19] As a rule, this *spasticity* as well as the hyperreflexia are

[17] According to Alexander (1942a) this statement is too schematic. Some parts of the internal capsule, e.g. the anterior crus and the dorsal part of the posterior crus, are supplied from striate arterioles, which ultimately are derived from the middle cerebral artery in one third of all cases, whereas more frequently the anterior ones come from the anterior cerebral artery. The knee of the internal capsule is always supplied by small branches from the internal carotid. As a rule the anterior choroidal artery contributes to the supply of the posterior crus.

[18] The plantar reflex and the sign of Babinski will be discussed in a later section.

[19] However, in spite of this, the muscular tone as judged by palpation of the muscles may be lowered. Often the "clasp-knife reaction" is present. When a spastic muscle is progressively stretched the resistance increases up to a certain point at which it suddenly disappears and the muscle can be extended further without resistance. The basis of this phenomenon will be discussed later.

more pronounced in the lower than the upper extremity. It is characteristic that the spasticity seen in capsular lesions in man is not equally
distributed in flexors and extensors. In the *upper extremity* more resistance is felt when it is being extended passively, i.e. the *spasticity is more
marked in the flexors,* and the arm has a tendency to remain in a flexed
position. In the *lower extremity* it is different. The leg tends to be permanently extended since the *spasticity is greatest in the extensor muscles.*

Other features of the same kind are also present. The arm tends not only to be
flexed at the elbow, but also to be adducted at the shoulder, and pronation pre-
vails in the hand, the fingers being flexed. In the hip there is a tendency toward
adduction, in the foot and toes toward plantar flexion. This is clearly evident and
easily recognized when one regards the position of the affected limbs in a patient
who has suffered from a capsular hemiplegia.

Why the spasticity in these cases shows such a predilection in its distribution is
not known. The position of the joints in the paralytic stage does not seem to be of
particular importance. Thus if the leg of a patient suffering from capsular hemiplegia is kept in a flexed position in the early stages, the typical extension spasticity
does not develop, but spasticity appears about equally in flexors and extensors. But
as soon as the continuous flexor position is given up, the usual extensor overaction
appears (Foerster, 1936b). Nor is there any exact correspondence between the
strength of the different muscles and their liability to become spastic, even if, e.g.
in the arm, the flexors are stronger than the extensors.

In a capsular lesion, as discussed above, other fibers than the corticofugal will of course often be involved. Concomitant with the hemiplegia
there will therefore commonly be some sensory loss on the same side as
the paralysis, due to damage to somatosensory pathways having a relay
in the thalamus (cf. Ch. 2). When the lesion is situated low in the capsule the fibers of the optic radiation may be affected, resulting in homonymous visual field defects (see Ch. 8). Aphasic disturbances (cf. Ch. 12)
may also occur. A *pure motor hemiplegia* is relatively rare. Fisher and
Curry (1965) studied 50 cases of this type, in 9 of which pathological
anatomical examination could be performed. They concluded that as a
rule a pure motor hemiplegia is the result of a small vessel thrombosis in
the posterior part of the internal capsule. In other instances it may be due
to a similar lesion in the basis of the pons. Transient attacks of hemiparesis often precede the final stroke. Even if there is usually arterial
hypertension, the prognosis is good.

In most cases in which an initially complete paralysis of one side of
the body is seen following a lesion of the internal capsule *a certain capacity for performing voluntary movements reappears after some time.* Conditions are essentially similar whether there has been a lesion of the
primary motor area—perhaps more correctly the precentral gyrus—or
if there has been a damage to the internal capsule. As paradigms, the

conditions following an extirpation of the parts of the precentral gyrus related to the arm and the leg respectively, may be described. Operations of this kind are sometimes performed in order to cope with a local lesion which has given rise to Jacksonian fits. After the operation a brachial or a crural monoplegia will result, and in the course of recovery a fairly regular development can be observed.[20]

In a *crural monoplegia,* following extirpation of the paracentral lobule and adjoining part of the uppermost parts of the precentral gyrus on the convexity, there appears, in the contralateral leg, a flaccid paralysis which soon is changed into a spastic paresis, with increased myotatic reflexes and inversion of the plantar reflex (sign of Babinski). The leg is kept in an extended position, with plantar flexion in the ankle joint. After some time a certain degree of *voluntary* movement reappears in the initially paralyzed leg. However, the movements which the patient can perform are only *crude, stereotyped, and massive.* Finely differentiated, delicate movements, such as movements of one toe only, are impossible. As discussed especially by Foerster (1936b), there are, strictly speaking, only two slow complex movements which the patient is able to perform voluntarily, one consisting primarily of flexion and called the *flexor synergy* by Foerster, the other an extension movement, the *extensor synergy.*

The extensor synergy in the leg consists of extension at the knee, adduction (more frequently an abduction) of the hip, plantar flexion of the ankle, and plantar flexion of the toes. These movements always occur in combination. If the patient intends to extend his leg at the knee, for example, there occurs concomitantly a plantar flexion of the foot and toes and, as a rule, also adduction of the hip. Isolated plantar flexion of the foot cannot be performed: it can only be combined with an extension of the knee. In the flexor synergy other movements take part; there occurs abduction of the hip, a flexion of hip and knee, dorsiflexion of the foot and toes, and usually inversion of the foot. As is the case with the extensor synergy, the different components of this movement cannot be performed individually, but are forcibly linked together. An attempt at flexing the knee is followed by a dorsiflexion of foot and toes and abduction in the hip.

In the *upper extremity* conditions are similar. Following a lesion of the arm area in the precentral gyrus all fine movements are lost, for example movements of a particular finger cannot be performed. After some time, however, two complex, slow, combined movements can be voluntarily executed. One is a *flexor synergy,* consisting of abduction and usually elevation of the shoulder, flexion in the elbow, pronation and volar flexion at the wrist, and a flexion (or in other cases an extension) of the fingers. Just as in the leg, the different components cannot be isolated, but always occur in combination. The other is the *extensor synergy,* consisting of adduction of the upper arm with lowering of the shoulder, extension of the elbow and wrist, and, as a rule, pronation of the hand (as in the flexor synergy). The fingers are extended or may be flexed.

[20] Cases of this type have been described for example by Bucy (1944a). See also Aring (1944).

Thus, after a complete destruction of the primary motor area, voluntary movements are not completely abolished. However, the complex synergic movements which remain are of a limited value to the patient. Particularly the movements of the hands are not very useful, mainly on account of the compulsory pronation of the hand which accompanies every attempt at flexing the arm. This makes it difficult for the patient to grasp objects and to use them properly (for example in taking a glass of water and drinking: the glass will be turned over and emptied before it reaches the patient's mouth, because the appropriate supination cannot be performed). In the lower extremity conditions are more fortunate. The flexor and extensor synergies will enable the patient to stand and walk, even if his steps are small and hampered by the existing spasticity.

In capsular hemiplegias the same synergies are observed as following cortical ablations. However, in both cases the possibility of further improvement is not exhausted with the achievement of the combined movements, the synergies. *Some capacity for performing more differentiated delicate movements may reappear* at a later stage of the disease. However, this is frequently masked by the presence of a pronounced spasticity, which opposes the finer movements. When the improvement takes place, the patient will be able, for example, to flex the foot without concomitant movements of the entire lower extremity. Appropriate physiotherapeutic exercises may be of great importance for improvement in these patients.

The improvement described above may be explained in different ways. One possibility is that certain parts of the foci for the part in question have escaped destruction, and when the initial edema and possible circulatory disturbances at the site of the lesion have receded, these foci resume their function to a certain degree. This may be a factor in cortical lesions. When there has been damage to the internal capsule, some fibers may likewise escape destruction and only have suffered temporarily from a functional block. Another circumstance which is probably of some importance is the presence of uncrossed descending connections. Through these fibers impulses from the intact motor area may influence the motoneurons supplying the paretic muscles.

In agreement with the results obtained from stimulation of the motor area the *capacity to regain discrete movements is not equal in different parts of the body*. Thus conditions are more favorable in the leg than in the arm, and in the arm the proximal parts are better situated than the distal ones. It is a common clinical experience that the capacity to perform discrete movements of the fingers is practically never regained after lesions of the internal capsule, or of the arm region of the motor area. (This is in accord with the fact that bilateral discrete movements of the fingers are practically never obtained on stimulation of the cortex.)

Some additional observations on movements in hemiplegic patients may be mentioned (see Foerster, 1936b, for a complete account). As mentioned above the capacity to perform discrete movements is opposed by the spasticity present. Since in the lower extremity this is most developed in the extensors and the plantar flexors, an isolated plantar flexion will be more easily performed than an isolated dorsiflexion of the foot (if the plantar flexion is not previously maximal). But a dorsiflexion is possible if some of the dorsal roots supplying the plantar flexors are sectioned. The spasticity, which is of reflex nature, is then diminished and does not prevent dorsiflexion of the foot. (A tenotomy of the Achilles tendon may also reveal that an isolated dorsiflexion is possible.)

If an ordinary hemiplegic patient tries to dorsiflex the affected foot, usually a complex, slow, combined movement occurs, the "flexor synergy" as described above. This is often called the tibialis phenomenon of Strümpell and is only one of several similar observations which can be made in patients with capsular lesions. These movements have been collectively termed "co-ordinated associated movements." Another phenomenon is the following: If a hemiplegic patient is asked to dorsiflex the nonparetic foot against resistance as strongly as possible, it is often noticed that the paretic foot also performs a correspondingly pure or nearly pure dorsiflexion. This is an example of the so-called "symmetric associated movements," which clinically have been described as signs of pyramidal tract lesions and often have been interpreted as reflexes. (As is well known, normal persons are usually able to perform a forcible dorsiflexion of one foot, without concomitant dorsiflexion of the other, or at least with only a minute movement.)

A satisfactory explanation of the "associated movements" described above can not as yet be given. Foerster (1936b) considered them as resulting from an interruption of the corticospinal tract with preserved "extrapyramidal" pathways. This simple explanation can, however, no longer be upheld. It should be noted that the phenomena demonstrate that voluntary movements are not completely abolished, even if there is a severe damage of the internal capsule. Furthermore, it is of practical interest that the symmetric associated movements may be utilized in the rehabilitation of hemiplegic patients. It will be advantageous at the onset of the patient's physical exercises to let him try to perform the same movements in the intact extremity as in the paretic, and also at the very beginning, allow him to try to produce isolated movements of the paretic limb by maximal effort of the healthy one.

Symptoms in diseases of the basal ganglia and related nuclei. In this field we meet with an intricate complex of motor abnormalities, abnormal movements, and changes of muscular tone; and we are still far from comprehending clearly how and why the different symptoms appear in the various pathological conditions. Even if it is found that in some diseases there are lesions which are usually confined to one or two of the basal ganglia or associated nuclei, it is not permissible to conclude that this nucleus or these nuclei are "centers" regulating a particular phase of the motor functions. It is far more reasonable to interpret the facts in a general way as follows: The various lesions produce a disturbing effect on a normally existing finely adjusted collaboration and co-operation between various structures. If a lesion affects one of these, for example, the substantia nigra, this harmonious interaction will be disturbed in some way, yielding symptoms of one kind, while if another part is damaged, for example the pallidum, the ensuing disturbances will be of another type. Clearly this does not allow us to conclude that, for instance, the substantia nigra is a "center" for one or other of these functions. We will return in a later section to attempts at explaining the symptomatology.

A brief survey of the principal symptoms following diseases of the basal ganglia is appropriate at this juncture. The symptoms are mainly of two types, disturbances of muscular tone and involuntary movements of different kinds, frequently called "hyperkinesias." Not unusually, however, symptoms of autonomic disturbances are also present, presumably due to concomitant lesions of the hypothalamus or of fiber connections in this region. Some of the pathological conditions form rather well-defined clinical entities, and will be described.[21]

A disease with fairly constant symptoms and fairly consistent localization of pathological changes is *paralysis agitans* or *Parkinson's disease*. This is characterized by two cardinal symptoms, a *rigidity* of a definite type and a *tremor*. (For a recent account of the prevalence and natural history of Parkinson's disease, see Pollock and Hornabrook, 1966.)

The rigidity, which may be very marked, differs from the spasticity seen in lesions of the internal capsule in man. It affects all muscles approximately to the same degree, and in typical cases is of the cogwheel type. The voluntary movements suffer from a marked *retardation,* but muscular strength is well preserved. The myotatic reflexes are normal or slightly brisker than usual. There is often a *poverty in movements* (akinesia) which changes the patient's appearance. He appears rigid, the usual pendular movements of the arms in walking are reduced or lacking, and his physiognomy lacks the normal mimics (mask face). Speech is slow and monotonous, and the handwriting changes. The *tremor,* which may be absent, is usually described as a rhythmic tremor at rest, particularly prominent in the fingers, and comparable to the movements performed in pillrolling. This tremor is of quite another type than the coarse intentional tremor seen in cerebellar disease (cf. Ch. 5). The latter appears in voluntary movements, but the tremor of paralysis agitans may also sometimes be seen to increase in intentional movements, be these static or phasic.[22] It disappears during sleep, but is exaggerated on emotional tension. Frequently symptoms of autonomic disturbances are observed, such as an increased sebaceous secretion (greasy face), salivation, and vasomotor disturbances. Mental deterioration is not uncommon (see Pollock and Hornabrook, 1966).

[21] Clinically a distinction is often made between two groups of syndromes. In the *hyperkinetic-dystonic syndromes* there is an excess of motor activity. In this group Jung and Hassler (1960) place the choreic, the ballistic, the athetoid, the dystonic, and the myotonic syndromes. In the *hypokinetic-rigid syndromes* there is a reduction in spontaneous motor manifestations, as in Parkinsonism.

[22] Lance, Schwab, and Peterson (1963) discuss the differences between resting tremor and action tremor in Parkinson's disease.

2 1 6

Descending Supraspinal Pathways

The symptoms in paralysis agitans have been regarded by many as being due to a specific distribution of anatomical changes. *Changes are usually found in the pallidum and the substantia nigra* (particularly its dark zone), and are frequently regarded as senile, degenerative. There is a loss of cells, and many of those which remain are abnormal, shrunken, and pale. Slight glial increase may be present. In some cases smaller changes are also found in the striatum (particularly its large cells), presumably being of retrograde nature, since the striatal fibers passing to the pallidum will probably suffer when this is degenerating. Occasionally less marked changes in other of the basal ganglia are found. Changes in the cortex have been described by some authors. In cases where the clinical symptoms have been pronounced only unilaterally, the most clear-cut anatomical changes have usually been found in the contralateral pallidum and substantia nigra. Cases may be observed clinically where the symptoms of Parkinson's disease are limited at first only to one limb. In cases of this type some authors claim to have observed that the pallidal changes are restricted to a certain division of this nucleus. This is in agreement with recent findings of the cortico-strio-pallidal connections (see p. 184). The region representing the face is said to be found most anteriorly, followed by the representation of arm, trunk, and leg in that order posteriorly.

A clinical picture resembling that of paralysis agitans in all particulars, especially the cases without tremor, was formerly seen quite often and interpreted as representing the late stages of the *epidemic encephalitis,* or *encephalitis lethargica (v. Economo).* The condition was usually spoken of as *postencephalitic parkinsonism,* more correctly *chronic encephalitis,* since anatomical investigation often revealed clear-cut, inflammatory changes. As might be expected in a disease of inflammatory nature, the clinical symptoms, as well as the course and the distribution of the pathological changes, were more irregular than in the idiopathic Parkinson's disease. It appears that at present there are only few survivors from the epidemic of encephalitis lethargica in the 1920's, and that parkinsonism with this etiology is becoming increasingly rare (Duvoisin et al., 1963).

The pathological examination in the acute stages of epidemic encephalitis revealed inflammatory foci, with a predilection for affecting the gray matter, first and foremost the pallidum and the substantia nigra. Affection of the hypothalamus or the gray substance surrounding the aqueduct may explain the common occurrence of sleep disturbances and ocular palsies, respectively. In chronic encephalitis the pathological changes are found in the same regions as in the acute stages of the disease. An occasional flaring up of the inflammatory processes, which may be latent for long periods, explains the common fluctuations in the symptomatology, which may serve as useful guides in the differential diagnosis between paralysis agitans and chronic encephalitis. The scattered localization of the pathological foci also explains several of the concomitant symptoms which were frequent in chronic encephalitis, such as the oculogyric crises (probably due to damage to the supranuclear pathways to the eye muscle nuclei), or autonomic disturbances on account of hypothalamic foci. Changes in the cerebral cortex were assumed to be responsible for some of the changes in character and the mental deterioration which were not infrequent in chronic encephalitis, particularly when the acute stage occurred in infancy.

Both paralysis agitans and chronic encephalitis thus show a rather uniform localization of the pathological changes in the brain, both affecting predominantly the substantia nigra and the pallidum. From the point of view of correlation between anatomical structures and symptomatology, it is interesting that some other diseases occasionally involve the same nuclei and produce similar symptoms. Thus cases of "atherosclerotic parkinsonism" occur, in which, owing to cerebral atherosclerosis, predominantly the pallidum and substantia nigra present patches of cell loss and changes in the cerebral vessels. The cerebral cortex, also, is usually more or less affected. (Davison, 1942, reported eighteen cases which were thoroughly examined pathologically.) Clinically the presence of signs of atherosclerosis in other regions, the more advanced age of the patient, and the not infrequent apoplectiform onset of the symptoms may be a guide to the correct diagnosis. Syphilitic inflammation of the brain may, also, result in the same clinical picture, *luetic parkinsonism,* in this instance primarily due to vascular changes. Here again the cerebral cortex is usually affected, and clinically features of general paresis are commonly present in addition to the motor disturbances. Finally, mention should be made of the occurrence of parkinsonism in cases of *acute carbon monoxide poisoning.*

When death does not ensue in the acute stages, a varying amount of the pallidum is destroyed, and the changes found betray a vascular etiology. According to Alexander (1942a) the pallidum (and the hippocampus) are supplied by the anterior choroidal artery, and the capillary density of the pallidum is not very great. These factors may explain the vulnerability of the pallidum to vascular changes (mainly revealed as thrombosis) occurring in carbon monoxide poisoning, atherosclerosis, and tertiary syphilis. In rare cases tumors have been observed in the pallidum, producing a clinical picture of parkinsonism. Following the administration of ataraxic drugs symptoms of parkinsonism may occur. For some references see Pollock and Hornabrook (1966).

The dominant hereditary *Huntington's chorea* is characterized by involuntary muscular contractions, which usually begin at the age of forty and progress steadily. The choreatic movements may at first be limited to a small part of the body, the face, or an arm, but by and by they tend to involve all musculature of the body. The movements are jerky, irregular, uncoordinated, and changing. In more advanced cases the patient is never at rest. If the facial musculature is involved, speech and swallowing may suffer. There is no reduction of muscular power, but muscular tone is said to be diminished. This, however, is very difficult to judge on account of the incessant movements. In later stages mental changes appear, leading finally to dementia, but the mental changes do not develop parallel to the somatic alterations, and may start before the choreatic movements.[23]

The prominent pathological changes in this disease are found in the *striatum*. The nucleus caudatus and the putamen become atrophic, as can be seen in advanced cases even on macroscopical inspection of the brain. Microscopically the characteristic feature is a reduction or loss of the small nerve cells of the striatum, while the large cells are preserved or present only minor changes (see, however, Denny-Brown, 1962). There is an increase of the glial elements and a reduction of myelinated fibers in the striatum. Less marked changes may be found in the pallidum and the subthalamic nucleus, but most authors regard these as secondary to the affection of the striatum. Practically always, however, the *cerebral cortex* displays loss of cells, particularly in the frontal regions and the precentral gyrus and mostly in the deeper layers. These cortical changes are probably responsible for the mental deterioration.

A similar localization of the pathological changes as in Huntington's chorea is seen in *chorea infectiosa* or *chorea minor, Sydenham's chorea*. This disease which occurs in children, most frequently girls, usually after a preceding infection ("rheumatic" or otherwise), shows involuntary movements very similar to those observed in Huntington's chorea. They are rapid, purposeless, and irregular. Since chorea minor is a benign disease, autopsy material is rare, and often other complicating diseases have been present which are responsible for the fatal outcome and which obscure the anatomical picture. As far as can be seen from the reports in the literature, the localization of the changes, which are mainly inflammatory, is first and foremost the striatum, the small cells of which suffer predominantly. The so-called *chorea gravidarum*, which is most frequently seen in women who have suffered from chorea minor in infancy, is also inadequately investigated with respect to its pathological anatomy, but it appears to present changes similar to those in chorea minor.

Some less usual types of involuntary movements will be briefly mentioned. *Athetoid movements* are usually very characteristic and easily recognized. They appear predominantly in the fingers and toes, and are as a rule less characteristic and less marked in the proximal muscles. The slow, bizarre movements of the fingers most frequently consist of a forcible

---

[23] In rare instances Huntington's chorea occurs in children. The clinical picture then often differs from that in adults, but the pathological changes are chiefly the same (Jervis, 1963).

extension or hyperextension of the metacarpophalangeal or interphalangeal joints, eventually combined with abduction movements of the fingers
and extension of arm and hand. Like other types of involuntary movements, they increase during emotional stress.

Athetoid movements may be seen in various diseases. Thus the so-
called *"infantile cerebral paralysis"* ("cerebral palsy"), particularly
where it occurs as hemiplegia ("infantile hemiplegia"), may be accompanied by such movements. The anatomical basis of the disease is
frequently an intracranial hemorrhage following birth trauma, or it may
be a malformation or an encephalitis. In this syndrome the abnormal
movements are not a cardinal symptom, but occur in addition to other
signs of severe cerebral injury, such as hemiparesis or hemiplegia, severe
reduction of intelligence, and frequently epileptiform convulsions.[24]
Athetoid movements may also be observed in diseases of the basal ganglia
that start in adults, particularly in *chronic encephalitis,* in which, occasionally, any type of involuntary movements may occur. The so-called
"athétose double" described by O. Vogt is a rare disease in which athetoid
movements occur bilaterally in early infancy without later progression.
The anatomical changes underlying the athetosis in these cases are
characteristic. On account of the anatomical picture the disease has been
called *"status marmoratus of the striatum."* (For an account of the
pathology see Alexander, 1942b.)

In the rare cases of *torsion dystonia* in which the brain has been examined the dominating changes have usually been found in the striatum.
These changes have been regarded as responsible for the slow mass torsion movements of trunk and extremities which characterize the disease.
These may occur, it appears, as a separate disorder, but more frequently
they are part of the abnormal movements due to chronic encephalitis, or
other rare types of affections of the basal ganglia. *Hemiballismus* is another type of disorder in which large-scale involuntary movements of
arms and legs and the trunk on one side occur. In most of these cases a
more or less isolated damage to the contralateral *subthalamic nucleus*
has been found (see Whittier, 1947). Occasionally the abnormal movements are restricted to one arm or one leg (monoballism; for a review
see Carpenter and Carpenter, 1951), a finding of interest in connection
with some experimental evidence for the existence of a somatotopical organization within the subthalamic nucleus (Mettler and Stern, 1962).
However, cases of hemiballism have been described with lesions in other

---

[24] In recent years great interest has been devoted to the study of this disease
group. Modern treatment of affected children has given encouraging results. Interested readers will find information on all aspects of the condition in the journal
Developmental Medicine and Child Neurology.

locations and not in the subthalamic nucleus (Schwarz and Barrows, 1960). So-called *myoclonic twitchings* may be seen in chronic encephalitis in its acute stages. They consist of rhythmic, or more irregular, very rapid contractions in individual muscles or parts of muscles, which usually do not produce movements. The same symptom may also be found in the very rare *myoclonus-epilepsy,* where "inclusion bodies" have been found in the nerve cells, particularly in the substantia nigra, often also in the striatum and dentate nucleus. Myoclonic twitchings in the muscles of the larynx, pharynx, and the soft palate have, probably erroneously, been attributed to lesions of the inferior olive and dentate nucleus which have been observed in these cases.

A type of involuntary movement which has been the subject of much debate is the so-called *tics:* simple involuntary twitchings of smaller muscle groups which occur repeatedly in a stereotyped manner at certain intervals. They may be suppressed by voluntary effort for a while and disappear during sleep. In most cases their cause remains unknown, but sometimes stereotyped movements of this type may be an initial symptom of some affection of the basal ganglia, such as Huntington's chorea. Even if it cannot be denied that in some cases tics may be purely "functional," having no organic basis, their occasional occurrence as an initial symptom and, likewise, the fact that they may remain as the only persistent symptoms in cases of, for example, chorea minor when the patient is otherwise free from symptoms, speaks in favor of their organic origin.

Correlations between clinical observations and experimental findings in animals. On account of the practical importance of disturbances of motor functions in man and their frequent occurrence it is no wonder that much work has been devoted to understanding their functional and structural basis. As described in the preceding sections, there are certain clear differences between the motor disturbances following lesions of the central motor cortex and the internal capsule and those seen in cases where the pathological changes are found in the basal ganglia. For a time this appeared to be explicable on the assumption that there are two separate supraspinal systems influencing motor functions, the pyramidal and the "extrapyramidal." As repeatedly alluded to in this chapter this dualism can, however, no longer be upheld. For this reason, many of the interpretations and hypotheses set forth to explain results of experimental observations have turned out to be untenable and must be discarded, even if the observations themselves are essentially correct. (As a relevant example may be mentioned forced grasping, described above. Before the supplementary motor area was discovered the symptom was considered to be due to damage to the "extrapyramidal" cortical area 6.) Many observations made in the past, therefore, have to be reinterpreted in the light of present-day knowledge. Unfortunately, this is often not possible, because the observations made and the experimental conditions under which they were obtained have not been recorded in sufficient detail.

In recent years the traditional approach of studying the effects of ablation of gray masses or transections of fiber tracts or of electrical stimulation has been supplemented with refined neurophysiological studies of the "intrinsic machinery" of the nervous system with recordings from single cells and fibers. However, a correlation of data from the two fields of research is often difficult. Furthermore, findings in animals cannot always be applied to man. It is therefore not yet possible to "explain" the disorders of motor functions occurring in diseases of the central nervous system in man. In the following, an attempt will be made to discuss certain features of such disorders in the light of recent studies, in animals as well as in man. For reasons given above, observations from the older literature will not be discussed at any length. The main purpose will be to focus attention on certain points where some degree of correlation seems possible.

Decerebrate rigidity. Postural reflexes.   Decerebrate rigidity is a condition which appears when the brain stem of an animal is transected above the vestibular nuclei. It is characterized primarily by an increased muscular tone in the extensors (antigravity muscles). The animal is able to stand with rigid legs, usually the tail is a little elevated and the chin is tilted somewhat upward. The myotatic reflexes (see Ch. 3) are strongly increased. Since Sherrington first observed this phenomenon in 1898, several investigators have studied it intensely. Rademaker performed sections of the brain stem at different levels and concluded that the presence or absence of the red nucleus was a deciding factor in the development of the rigidity. However, if the transection is made caudal to the level of the vestibular nuclei, the rigidity fails to develop and all muscles are flaccid. Furthermore, destruction of the lateral vestibular nucleus on one side nearly abolishes the rigidity on the same side, produced by a preceding more rostral transection of the brain stem. Descending impulses from the reticular formation of the brain stem appear to be, in part at least, responsible for the phenomenon of decerebrate rigidity (see Brodal, Pompeiano, and Walberg, 1962, p. 109 ff., for a more complete account of the subject and Marchiafava, 1968, for some recent data). As has been mentioned, the lateral vestibular nucleus exerts a strong facilitatory action on ipsilateral extensor motoneurons (α as well as γ), and there is little doubt that a main factor in the appearance of decerebrate rigidity is the following: the vestibular excitatory action on the extensor motoneurons lacks the normally opposing actions from other regions, such as the red nucleus, which facilitate flexor motoneurons. Since the spinal parts of the cerebellum (see Ch. 5) have an inhibitory effect on the lateral vestibular nucleus of Deiters, ablation of this part of the cerebellum will increase the decerebrate rigidity and even produce opisthotonus, while stimulation reduces it. The rigidity is, however, not dependent only on descending impulses to the motoneurons. Afferent impulses from the periphery are also of importance. This was clearly demonstrated by Sherrington who found that when the dorsal roots supplying one of the extremities are sectioned, the rigidity disappears from this limb.[25] It is the interruption of afferents from the muscle spindles which is the important factor. This type of decerebrate rigidity is, therefore, often spoken of as a "γ-rigidity" (Granit, 1955a), on the assumption that the main factor is an increased excitability of the γ neurons (which via the spindle afferents produce an excitation of the α neurons). However, when a so-called anemic decerebration is made (ligation of both carotids and the basilar artery) in which half the cerebellum and a considerable part of the pons are destroyed, the animal presents an intense rigidity, even when the dorsal roots are cut. In this instance, therefore, the α neurons are able to maintain an increased muscular tonus without support from the γ neurons and spindles (α-rigidity). Even if it is possible that this distinction between α and γ-rigidity may be too strict, and that most instances of α-rigidity may include also a component of γ-rigidity (see, for example, Batini, Moruzzi, and Pompeiano, 1957), there are obviously two different ways in which an increased excitability of the α motoneurons can occur, a fact of interest for clinical problems. The mechanisms involved in the production of decerebrate rigidity are, however, far more complex than appears from the above. Animals with decerebrate rigidity have proved very useful for the study of *postural reflexes*. This is a collective designation for a large number of reflexes which aim at preserving the normal posture of the body.[26] To these belong the tonic neck and labyrinthine reflexes.

The *tonic neck reflexes* are revealed as a change in the distribution of muscular tone when the position of the head relative to the body is altered.

During movements of the head impulses arise in the sensory epithelium of the labyrinth as well as in the proprioceptors of the neck. In order to elicit the tonic neck reflexes, therefore, the labyrinths must be destroyed. If, then, in a labyrinthectomized, decerebrated animal the head is rotated to one side, the increased extensor tonus following the decerebration is further augmented on the side to

[25] Section of one vestibular nerve does not abolish the decerebrate rigidity in the ipsilateral limbs, indicating that labyrinthine impulses are not of major importance.

[26] For an exhaustive account of postural mechanisms see Roberts (1967).

which the snout is pointing, while it diminishes on the other side. If the head is tilted to one side, the tonus increases on this side, but is reduced on the other. If the head is bent forward there ensues a flexion and reduced tone of the forelimbs but extension and increased tone of the hind limbs. If the head is bent backward the opposite change appears, flexion of hindlimbs, and extension of forelimbs. Since these reflexes disappear when the dorsal roots of the upper three cervical nerves are cut, it is clear that they are initiated by impulses from the neck. The afferent impulses which elicit the changes arise in the receptors in the upper cervical joints (McCouch, Deering, and Ling, 1951).

If in a decerebrated animal the upper cervical dorsal roots are cut, or if the head is fixed so as to prevent any movement of it in relation to the body, the *tonic labyrinthine reflexes* can be elicited.

Changes of the animal's position in space are then followed by a regular alteration of tone distribution. In the supine position, with the snout elevated about 45°, the rigidity is maximal, but it is minimal if the animal is placed in the prone position with the snout tilted 45° below the horizontal axis. In intermediate positions the degree of the rigidity varies between the two extremes. These reflexes are elicited from the sensory epithelium of the utricle (and, possibly, the saccule) of the labyrinth (they disappear if the otoliths are detached from their proper place by centrifuging the animal) and they are maintained as long as the *position* is upheld. They are not to be confused with the vestibular reflexes which are provoked by *movements* in space and which are initiated from the semicircular canals (rotatory nystagmus, etc.; see Ch. 7). These tonic neck and labyrinthine reflexes are present in decerebrate animals in which the transection of the brain stem is made so far caudally that practically only the medulla oblongata is in connection with the spinal cord.

The same reflexes are present in animals in which, in addition, the mesencephalon and thalamus are in connection with the lower parts. In such animals several other postural reflexes can also be elicited.

One of them, which is dependent on the labyrinth, is the following: If a normal animal, or one in which the cerebral cortex has been removed (decortication), is blindfolded and then placed in various positions in space, it will always keep its head in the natural, horizontal position, whether the animal is placed on its side or in other positions. However, if both labyrinths are destroyed this reaction is abolished. This reflex righting of the head initiated from the labyrinth is called *the labyrinthine righting reflex,* and it serves the animal to orientate itself in space. When by means of this reflex the head has assumed its natural position, the rest of the body can be oriented after the head by means of other reflexes, initiated from the proprioceptors of the neck and of the trunk (neck righting reflexes, body righting reflexes acting upon the head, body righting reflexes acting upon the body). Other reflexes serving a similar purpose of orientation are dependent on the integrity of parts of the cortex. Thus the optic righting reflexes require an intact area striata, since they depend on vision. Hopping and placing reactions appear to be dependent on the motor cortex.

The postural reflexes are present in the normal human being and are essential for normal motor performances. In lesions of the brain stem the tonic neck and labyrinthine reflexes may appear in an exaggerated form. Furthermore, these reflexes may operate in influencing other reflexes, as mentioned previously with reference to forced grasping and the grasp reflex in infants (Pollack, 1960). They are, therefore, of clinical interest, the more so since some use may be made of these and other postural reflexes in physiotherapeutic exercises in some instances. In severe lesions of the brain stem decerebrate rigidity may be seen in man (see Ch. 6), resembling the same condition in animals. In these patients tonic neck and labyrinthine reflexes can often easily be elicited.

Spasticity and rigidity. Reference to the phenomena called spasticity and rigidity in man was made previously. The condition called spasticity is regularly seen following lesions of the internal capsule and often in lesions involving the primary motor cortex,[27] while the term rigidity is used for the changes in muscular tone occurring in parkinsonism.[28]

As described in Chapter 3, muscular tone is essentially a reflex phenomenon which may be influenced by sensory impulses (first and foremost from the muscle spindles), by impulses from other parts of the spinal cord, and by impulses from higher levels. Ultimately muscular tone thus depends on the activity of the motoneurons. When it is altered in a different way in capsular lesions than in parkinsonism this must be due to different derangements of the normal supraspinal influences on the spinal reflex apparatus of the stretch reflex (including the motoneurons). No entirely satisfactory explanation can so far be given of these differences, but some information is available concerning the changes in the reflex mechanism occurring in the two conditions. The problems are far from solved, and no exhaustive treatment of the subject will be attempted (for a review, see Jansen, 1962).

Clinical spasticity in many ways resembles the situation in decerebrate rigidity in animals. As mentioned previously, sections of dorsal roots in patients with spastic hemiplegia abolishes spasticity (Foerster, 1911) as well as the increased stretch reflexes (in severe spasticity in man patellar and ankle clonus are common). This suggests that there must be an increased activity of the γ neurons in spasticity. Further support for this view is found in the fact that procaine infiltration around the nerves to spastic muscles eliminates spasticity without impairing voluntary power

[27] According to some authors lesions restricted to area 4 in man do not result in spasticity. However, such restricted lesions are rare.

[28] It is unfortunate that the experimentally produced condition in animals which in many respects appears to correspond to spasticity in man has been termed decerebrate *rigidity*. It should be kept in mind that this is quite different from the rigidity seen in parkinsonism.

(Walshe, 1924; Rushworth, 1960). However, as mentioned previously, in a capsular hemiplegia muscle tone as judged by passive movements is regularly increased, while often little or no increase of tone is felt on palpation. These findings may be explained, on the basis of experimental studies, on the assumption that there is an increase in the phasic stretch reflex (see Ch. 3), while the tonic stretch reflex is not changed or is less changed. On rapid movements the phasic reflex is brought into play, just as when a tendon jerk is elicited. The heightened excitability of the reflex explains that much slower movements will elicit it than is the case in normal persons. If in cases of mild spasticity stretching of a muscle is performed very slowly, there is no or very little increased resistance to passive movements. Thus, the speed of the movement is important. In the light of recent studies of the complex afferent and efferent innervation of the muscle spindles (see Ch. 3) it may be surmised that chiefly the speed-sensitive primary ending is responsible for the changes, particularly since its dynamic sensitivity may be increased by the γ_1 fibers. Jansen (1962, p. 46) reaches the tentative conclusion "that the spastic states with weak static stretch reflexes are due mainly to a release of the nuclear-bag fusimotor system, and that spastic states as a whole are characterized by a greater degree of release of the bag system with only moderate increase in the activity of the nuclear-chain intrafusal fiber system." However, as stressed by Jansen (1962), spastic states may in the end turn out to be a rather heterogenous group with different degrees of release of the two intrafusal systems. It is in agreement with the above interpretation that the tendon reflexes are increased in spasticity since they represent only the dynamic component of the stretch reflexes.

To what extent conclusions concerning spasticity drawn from animal experiments can be applied to conditions in man is not quite clear. (No explanation has so far been found for the fact that in man spasticity affects chiefly flexor muscles in the arm.)

Several authors have attempted to analyze spasticity in man, most of them making use of the H-reflex (see footnote p. 205) which is considered to correspond to the stretch reflex, except for the fact that the spindle afferents and not the spindles are stimulated. Landau and Clare (1964) conclude from studies with this method that although the motoneurons are hyperactive, "in spastic hemiplegias, there is no evidence which requires the presumption that fusimotor hypertonus is of etiological significance in pathological hypertonic states." (See also Diamantopoulos and Zander Olsen, 1967.) Support for this view was found in the observation that no hyperactivity of the fusimotor system accompanies hyperactive tendon jerks in the monkey (Meltzer, Hunt, and Landau, 1963). Increased excitability of the motoneurons in spasticity has been concluded to be present in several studies (Angel and Hofmann, 1963; and others). Lance, de Gail, and Neilson (1966) made use of the observation that sustained vibratory stimuli applied to a muscle in normal man suppress phasic reflexes (tendon reflexes, H-reflex) and provoke a reflex

226

tonic contraction in the muscle stimulated. They concluded that it is not necessary to postulate the existence of two kinds of motoneurons (phasic and tonic) in
man in order to explain their results. They found vibration-induced tonic contractions diminished in hemiplegia (but they were normal in parkinsonism). Obviously
studies of the mechanisms in spasticity in man are difficult, and the methods employed are less direct than those which can be used in animals.

The *"clasp-knife reaction,"* often seen in the spastic limbs in hemiplegia (see p. 211) and also found in decerebrate rigidity in animals, can
be explained as an example of the so-called *lengthening reaction,* described by Sherrington. It is due to impulses arising in the Golgi organs
in the muscle when this is stretched. As discussed in Chapter 3, the
afferent impulses exert an inhibitory action on the agonists taking part in
the stretch reflex, while they facilitate the antagonists (see Fig. 3-6). The
Golgi organs appear, however, to have other functions than to prevent
excessive tension of the muscle.

Whether the primary disorder in spasticity is essentially a hyperactive
dynamic reaction of the muscle spindle due to facilitation of the γ_1 efferents with consequent hyperactivity of the α motoneurons, (particularly
the phasic ones), or whether there is a primary hyperexcitability of the
latter, as some authors conclude from studies in man, the changes must
be due to an altered supraspinal innervation. From this point of view it is
interesting to recall that a lesion of the internal capsule or precentral
motor cortex will interrupt the cortico-spinal and cortico-rubro-spinal
(as well as some other) pathways. The two former both have a facilitatory action on flexor motoneurons. A lesion of this kind will, however, scarcely affect the lateral vestibular nucleus to any great extent,
since this does not receive fibers from the cortex. The strong facilitatory
action exerted on the extensor α and γ motoneurons by the lateral
vestibular nucleus will then lack the normally opposing influence of the
corticospinal and cortico-rubro-spinal pathways, making it understandable that there is an excess of extensor innervation in capsular lesions,
and that spasticity affects the extensors.[29]

The similarity between the changes in stretch reflexes and muscle
tone in decerebrate rigidity and capsular lesions is intelligible from this
point of view.[30] In both cases the influence of the lateral vestibular

[29] However, we are here again faced with the paradox that in man this is not
true for the upper extremity, where the flexors are the spastic ones. One may indeed wonder whether man's assumption of the upright posture, when the forelimbs
are relieved of their body-supporting function, has been accompanied by some
hitherto unrecognized changes in the organization of the supraspinal influences of
the cord, and presumably reflected in the anatomical organization of the pathways
involved.

[30] This is obviously a very simplified scheme, since possible influences from
the reticular formation and other regions are not considered.

nucleus on the cord is retained. Those differences which are present between the two conditions may presumably be related to the fact that following decerebration even more supraspinal pathways are interrupted than in a capsular lesion, for example the tectospinal and interstitiospinal tracts.

As described in a preceding section exaggerated stretch reflexes occur also following *transverse lesions of the cord*. However, there is no pure spasticity as in a capsular lesion, or in decerebrate rigidity.[31] Flexion reflexes are also enhanced. Since in transverse lesions of the cord all descending pathways are interrupted, it is conceivable that the effects on the reflex mechanisms of the cord will differ from those in capsular hemiplegias and in decerebrate rigidity.

In paraplegic patients there is a general excessive activity of motor units, as shown by Dimitrijević and Nathan (1967a, 1967b) in extensive clinical and electromyographic studies. It is characteristic, in contrast to a spastic hemiplegia, that there is lack of normal reciprocal innervation. Certain muscles or groups of muscles are activated by every kind of stimulation (proprioceptive and exteroceptive). On eliciting stretch reflexes in a muscle there appears a recruiting of motor units after the stimulus has ceased, and this spreads to motoneurons of other muscles. The exaggerated stretch reflexes are taken to indicate that some of the spastic state is due to hypersensitivity of the spindles, an assumption which receives support from the observation that "chemical posterior rhizotomy" with phenol solution (see p. 95) has been shown to have a beneficial effect on the spasms and to reduce the spontaneous activity which is usually present in most muscles in these patients.[32] With reference to physiological studies the increased excitability of the spinal cord is explained as a consequence of the loss of tonic inhibitory descending impulses from the brain stem, some of which act on interneurons intercalated in flexion reflex arcs.

The rigidity seen in parkinsonism differs in many respects from spasticity following lesions of the internal capsule. The resistance to passive movements involves flexors as well as extensors and is almost equal throughout the range of movement. This "plastic" rigidity is independent of the speed of the movement. The tendon (myotatic) reflexes are not appreciably altered, indicating that the phasic stretch reflex is not ex-

[31] However, in slowly developing damage to the cord (myelopathies) due to diseases in the cord (intramedullary tumors, inflammations) or to pressure on the cord (extramedullary tumors, hematomas) there is often in the beginning a spastic mono-, para-, or hemiplegia, rather similar to that following a capsular lesion. No satisfactory explanation of this can be given. It may be presumed that first and foremost the dorsal parts of the lateral funiculus are affected.

[32] As mentioned earlier, Foerster used posterior rhizotomies in order to relieve exaggerated stretch reflexes in spasticity. Dimitrijević and Nathan (1967a) comment upon the fact that this operation has been so little used and advocate a more extensive therapeutic use of procedures which may cause a reduced inflow from the periphery to the spinal cord.

aggerated as in spasticity. However, since procaine infiltration of a muscle (presumably blocking the transmission in the γ efferents) abolishes rigidity in the muscle (Walshe, 1924; Rushworth, 1960), it has been concluded that rigidity is dependent on an increased sensitivity of the muscle spindles. In view of recent observations of the functional characteristics of the muscle spindles (see Ch. 3), it has been suggested (Jansen, 1962) that in rigidity there is an increased activity in the nuclear-chain intrafusal system, which augments the *static* responsiveness of the primary endings. Clinical observations (Schimazu et al., 1962) as well as other data (see Jansen, 1962) lend some support to the conclusion that exaggeration of the tonic properties of the stretch reflex is an important feature in parkinsonian rigidity.

During increasing stretch of a rigid muscle continuous lengthening reactions occur. This may be the explanation of the *"cogwheel phenomenon."* The frequency of cogwheeling is not consistently related to the rate of stretch, according to Lance, Schwab, and Peterson (1963), who suggest that the phenomenon is related to the resting or action tremor seen in some of these patients. (The tremor, often seen in parkinsonism, will be considered in a later section.)

The changes in the function of the motoneurons and muscle spindles in rigidity must ultimately be due to changed supraspinal influences on the reflex arc of the stretch reflex. However, since the nuclei which show pathological changes in parkinsonism (chiefly the globus pallidus and the substantia nigra) have only very sparse caudally directed efferents, they can scarcely influence the cord directly via descending pathways. We will return to this problem when the functions of the basal ganglia are discussed.

"Pyramidal" and "extrapyramidal" cortical motor areas?   When discussing the motor cortical areas the results of electrical stimulation of these areas were considered, while the results of ablations were only briefly mentioned, especially as concerns the primary motor cortex. It will now be appropriate to consider the symptoms seen in cortical lesions and in capsular hemiplegias in man in the light of studies in animals and man directed at clarifying their mechanism. In the description given previously of the symptoms following the two kinds of lesions they were treated together, since in most clinical cases they appear to be very much the same. The reason for this appears to be that most cortical lesions affecting the precentral motor area in man extend beyond this and will involve other neighboring areas, all of which give off efferent fibers descending in the internal capsule. Here our concern will be whether particular symptoms in these cases can be considered as consequences of a lesion of the pyramidal tract.

As mentioned previously, attempts were made in the 1930's, par-

229

ticularly by Fulton and his collaborators, to study the effects of lesions of area 4 in monkeys and chimpanzees, and to compare the resulting motor disturbances with those following lesions of the "premotor" area, and with combined lesions. The consequences of lesions of area 4 were considered to give information of the role of the pyramidal tract. Isolated sections of the tract were taken to support this view. The interpretations of the findings made are chiefly of historical interest, since data from later research has necessitated thorough revisions of the older views. Only some of the findings made in the 1930's will therefore be mentioned.

In the monkey and chimpanzee a cortical lesion restricted to area 4 results in an impairment of finely co-ordinated movements on the contralateral side. (Fulton and Kennard, 1934; and others, in the monkey; Fulton and Kennard, 1934; Tower, 1944; and others, in the chimpanzee). There is no spasticity (except for some transient involvement of the fingers) but a slight hypotonia and reduced tendon reflexes. In the chimpanzee an inverted plantar reflex (Babinski sign) occurs (Fulton and Keller, 1932). After some time the paretic muscles show some atrophy.

A lesion confined to area 6 in the chimpanzee leads to a transitory weakness in the contralateral limbs. After about a week the gross motor performances are normal. But on closer analysis it is found that there is an impairment of the capacity to perform skilled movements, which are only awkwardly carried out. This is most evident when the animals have been trained, before the operation, to solve problems which require fine muscular adjustments (Jacobsen, 1934; Fulton, Jacobsen, and Kennard, 1932). The affected muscles do not develop spasticity, but all muscles present an approximately equal degree of increased resistance to passive movements. This is present throughout the range of the movements. The increased resistance is transient if the lesion is restricted to area 6. The tendon reflexes are moderately increased, but this feature disappears in the course of a week or more. The sign of Babinski is not present, but "forced grasping" is seen.

Marion Hines (1937) described a "strip area" (area 4s) on the border between areas 4 and 6. On stimulation of this, movements elicited from area 4 were inhibited and contracted muscles relaxed. Extirpation of area 4s, according to Hines, was followed by spasticity, particularly in the proximal joints. If area 6 and area 4s were removed simultaneously a muscular hypertonus followed, which was very marked, but not of the spastic type (Hines, 1944). The tendon reflexes, however, were brisk and irradiating. Ablation of areas 4 + 4s yielded a moderate spasticity. Later, other strip-like areas similar to 4s (8s, 3s, 2s, 19s and 24s) were described and collectively called "suppressor areas," since electrical stimulation or strychninization of these regions gave rise to a decrease in the spontaneous cortical electrical activity, abolition of cortically induced movements and relaxation of muscular contractions. Further research, however, has brought forward evidence which has led to abandoning of the notion of cortical "suppressor areas." Some of the phenomena seen following stimulation of the "suppressor areas" appear to be results of what is called "spreading depression," others are interpreted as consequences of inhibition of muscle tone and inhibition of cortically induced motor after-discharges. Neither of these effects are specific for the "suppressor areas." (For early critical reviews seen Sloan and Jasper, 1950; Druckman, 1952; see also

Kaada, 1960). Reliable criteria for a cytoarchitectonic identification of the "suppressor areas" have not been produced.

As a result of the studies briefly reviewed above as well as others it was for some time generally held that lesions of the area 4 or of the pyramidal tract give rise to an impairment of discrete, co-ordinated voluntary movements and (in apes and man) the sign of Babinski but not to spasticity and increased tendon reflexes. The latter two phenomena were assumed to be due to damage to "extrapyramidal" cortical areas, especially to area 6 and area 4s, or their efferent projections. These conclusions rested on the assumption that the various cortical areas are functionally different.[33] Even if one accepts this as a working hypothesis (and there are several observations in support of its being generally true) objections may be raised against the interpretation of the findings.

Histological control of the lesions was seldom made, and even when it is made it is extremely difficult to draw definite conclusions as to which areas have been removed. There may be secondary changes which escape identification. In stimulation experiments the importance of stimulus parameters often did not receive sufficient attention, and factors influencing the cortical excitability, such as anesthesia, were insufficiently known. While several students had noted that on stimulation of the precentral gyrus movements of the fingers were most easily obtained close to the central fissure, this did not attract much interest.

As has been described, in the primary motor region the trunk and proximal limb muscles are "represented" farthest from the central sulcus (see Fig. 2-17). The effects, predominantly on proximal and distal musculature, following ablations of areas 6 and 4, respectively, may therefore be related to the pattern of cortical representation, particularly since points giving rise to movements of the trunk and proximal extremities are found definitely in front of area 4. Different effects on proximal and distal muscles with regard to muscular tone and stretch reflexes may be dependent on differences in efferent projections from the anterior (area 6) and posterior (area 4) parts. The specific efferent projections of these and adjacent cortical areas have not yet been studied systematically, but it appears that differences will be found when properly searched for (see Kuypers, 1960, for some data).

At a meeting as early as in 1950 Woolsey et al. (1952, p. 259) formulated their view on the problem as follows:

[33] Attempts have been made by some (see for example, Hassler, 1966b) to indicate more specifically the motor functions of minor subdivisions of the main areas, described by students of cortical cytoarchitecture. Area 6 was subdivided by the Vogts and Foerster into areas 6a and 6b, area 6a again being divisible into 6aα and 6aβ. Area 4 of man was subdivided by von Bonin (1944) into sub-areas 4γ, 4a and 4s. The studies and nomenclatures of the various investigators are not entirely consistent, however.

Rather than conclude that there is no possible correlation between cytoarchitecture and the pattern of localization in the precentral motor area we would suggest that one ought to expect a varying histological picture to correspond with differences in character of representation encountered in the precentral field. Near the central sulcus where the digits are best represented the finest differentiations of movement are obtained on stimulation whereas stimulation at the rostral border of the field produces the least differentiated movements. In the digital area projection from the cortex is apparently focused relatively sharply upon the spinal cord but from the rostral border of the area connections are made with many spinal levels. Variation in structure, therefore, would seem more appropriate to this arrangement than uniformity.

This view gains support from other data and obviates the necessity of postulating "extrapyramidal cortical areas," which are functionally distinct from a "pyramidal area." It is in complete agreement with recent data on the widespread cortical origin of corticospinal fibers from the central region (and from the supplementary motor and the second somatosensory area). This, as well as the different sites of termination of corticospinal fibers from precentral and postcentral regions and the results of some physiological studies leave no doubt that the *pyramidal tract is not a homogeneous fiber system, but consists of components which differ anatomically and functionally. Its origin covers regions traditionally considered as "extrapyramidal."* Our knowledge of these features is still fragmentary. In view of the importance attributed in clinical neurology to the pyramidal tract it appears worth while to see to what extent available data necessitates modifications of the traditional concepts.

"The pyramidal tract syndrome"; a misnomer. The "pyramidal tract syndrome" has been mentioned several times in the preceding text. As described (p. 211) it consists essentially of a loss of the capacity to perform co-ordinated skilled movements. This paresis is combined with spasticity of a particular distribution and exaggerated tendon reflexes. The cutaneous reflexes are abolished or diminished, and there is an inversion of the plantar reflex (sign of Babinski). The origin and course of the pyramidal fibers and the presence in the internal capsule of corticofugal fibers to many other destinations than the cord make it clear that *neither lesions of the cortex nor of the internal capsule can give rise to what may properly be called a "pyramidal tract syndrome."* This can occur only with lesions in the two situations where the pyramidal tract runs in isolation: the medullary pyramids and the central part of the cerebral peduncle (Figs. 2-9 and 4-2).[34] While isolated lesions of the

---

[34] As concerns the cerebral peduncle this statement is not quite correct, since

pyramids have been made in animals, no clear-cut case of this kind appears to have been recorded in man. Some relevant cases, all imperfect in one way or another have been discussed by Tower (1940.) More recently a case has been described by Meyer and Herndon (1962). However, transections of the cerebral peduncle have been performed in humans in order to treat involuntary movements. When considering the effects of lesions of the pyramidal tract it is essential to remember the species differences as concerns the development and size of the tract.

Following the first study of the *motor performances of monkeys with transected pyramids* by Tower (1940) few other students have undertaken similar investigations. Tower found that such animals are unable to perform discrete movements of the fingers. However, there is no spasticity but a hypotonia of the muscles and the abdominal and cremasteric reflexes are abolished or weakened. In chimpanzees (Tower, 1944) somewhat similar findings were made. Recently Lawrence and Kuypers (1968a) reported their findings in a series of monkeys. The lesions were carefully controlled histologically, and the animals were kept for several weeks. The defects were less marked than those described by Tower (1940), perhaps because Tower's lesions extended outside the pyramidal tract, and because her animals survived for short periods only. According to Lawrence and Kuypers, animals having a bilateral interruption of the pyramidal tract regain their capacity for independent use of their extremities and within three weeks can use their hands adequately to pick up morsels of food. However, the capacity for individual finger movements never returns. In cats the defects following transection of the pyramids are less marked than in the monkey, but there is an increase in muscular tone (Liddell and Phillipps, 1944). Laursen and Wiesendanger (1967) found, in cats, an increased response latency in discrimination tasks requiring motor skill.

There are several reports on *the consequences of interruption of the pyramidal tract in the cerebral peduncle,* where it occupies approximately the middle three-fifths. Neurosurgeons have performed this operation in order to relieve abnormal, involuntary movements (for references, see Bucy, Ladpli, and Ehrlich, 1966). The section is placed at the lowest level of the peduncle (cf. footnote, p. 232). Bucy (1957) and Bucy and Keplinger (1961) found that following the operation a con-

---

some corticoreticular fibers as well as corticofugal fibers to the inferior olive have not yet left the pyramidal tract proper at this level. However, the number of such fibers appears to be relatively modest (most fibers to the reticular formation appear to take off above the lower end of the peduncle). To facilitate the discussion these fibers will, therefore, not be taken into account in the following, but they should be remembered in more subtle analyses.

siderable degree of useful finger movements is retained, and there is no spastic paralysis with hyperactive tendon reflexes, even if the latter may be somewhat increased. The Babinski sign is usually present. Since it may be objected that the surgical interruption of the peduncle has not been as planned, it is of considerable interest that in one patient the lesion could be controlled at autopsy. Only some 17 per cent of the fibers in the medullary pyramid appeared to be present some years after the operation (Bucy, Keplinger, and Siqueira, 1964). In order to gain more information on the subject, corresponding experimental studies were performed in monkeys, with anatomical control of the lesions (Bucy and Keplinger, 1961; Bucy, Ladpli, and Ehrlich, 1966). It turned out that monkeys in whom a complete degeneration of the pyramid was found at autopsy had been able to walk, climb, and jump, and when time was allowed for recovery special tests showed that the animals had retained their ability to grasp and manipulate small objects even after bilateral pedunculotomies. More marked spasticity and hyperreflexia were seen only in animals where the damage involved the mesencephalic tegmentum. Walker and Richter (1966) in a corresponding study got largely corresponding results, but on the whole found greater functional impairment. They emphasize particularly the lack of spontaneous movements of the paretic limbs.

The findings reported above leave little doubt that *the classical "pyramidal tract syndrome" does not follow lesions of the pyramidal tract, and accordingly is a misnomer*. A true pyramidal tract syndrome would consist only of some impairment of skilled movements of the fingers, slight if any hypertonus and hyperreflexia, and usually the sign of Babinski (in man and chimpanzee). There are thus marked differences between this and the classical pyramidal tract syndrome. These differences must be due to additional damage inflicted on other structures besides the pyramidal tract in cases showing the classical syndrome. More specifically, pathways from the cortex and passing in the internal capsule must be affected. As pointed out by Bucy, in a pedunculotomy and even more in a pyramidectomy, most of the corticofugal fibers entering the brain stem and descending in the capsule with the pyramidal tract will not be interrupted. It seems a likely assumption therefore, that the preservation of these pathways may be essential for the retained capacity to perform rather discrete voluntary movements following a pedunculotomy and for the modest changes in reflexes and muscle tone. It is not possible to decide which of these pathways may be most important. Presumably several may play a role and may influence different functions. However, as far as the capacity to perform discrete movements is concerned, the cortico-rubro-spinal pathway seems to be the most likely candidate. Since this assumption was first ventured (Brodal, 1963, 1965a) further studies have provided supporting evidence.

As discussed in a previous section (p. 164 ff.) there are close anatomical and physiological similarities between the cortico-rubro-spinal pathway and the component of the corticospinal tract which arises in the anterior "motor" part of the primary sensorimotor cortex. Both pathways present a somatotopical localization, terminate in the same laminae of the spinal cord, and facilitate motoneurons to flexor muscles (α as well as γ). The cortico-rubro-spinal pathway might therefore be almost as well suited for inducing discrete movements as the corticospinal.[35] Physiological studies lend support to this assumption. Lewis and Brindley (1965) who studied the responses to cortical stimulation in lightly anesthetized baboons found that a bilateral pyramidotomy had little or no effect on the character of the movements elicited or their somatotopic organization in the cortex. Following operation there was, however, a reduction of the number of movements that could be obtained at any one exploration of the cortex and an increased electrical threshold. Lewis and Brindley (1965) do not suggest a pathway for these impulses. In a corresponding study following pedunculotomy in the macaque (Walker and Richter, 1966) the responses were less clear and required strong stimuli. In cats, Hongo and Jankowska (1967) on cortical stimulation following unilateral or bilateral pyramidotomy obtained effects similar to those from stimulation of the corticospinal tract (postsynaptic excitatory effects on motoneurons, mainly flexor; facilitation of spinal reflexes to motoneurons; and depolarization of presynaptic terminals of group Ib fibers). They recorded potentials in the rubrospinal tract following cortical stimulation. From findings in their animals following lesions of the spinal cord they concluded that some effects are mediated via the cortico-rubro-spinal pathway (facilitation of reflex paths and effects on primary afferents), while they assume that reticulospinal paths are involved in some of the effects. Since the latter pathways are not somatotopically organized (see p. 175) it appears that they are probably not as immediately concerned in the production of localized movements following transection of the pyramidal tract as is the cortico-rubro-spinal pathway. The recent study of Lawrence and Kuypers (1968b), mentioned above, appears to be compatible with the view set forth here.

Further studies are needed to clarify the role played by the different routes from the cortex to the spinal cord which are involved in the production of movements on cortical stimulation when the pyramidal tract is interrupted. It does, however, seem rather likely that in the role played by the primary motor cortex in the elicitation of discrete movements the corticospinal and other corticofugal pathways, especially the cortico-rubro-spinal tract, collaborate closely. For perfect voluntary movements both pathways are needed. Lesion of only one of them leads to rather moderate disturbances.

The above hypothesis is based largely on studies in animals. At-

---

[35] The main difference between them is the synaptic interruption of the former pathway in the red nucleus, where particularly cerebellar afferents may influence the corticospinal impulse transmission. For a discussion of the functional role of the red nucleus, see Massion (1967).

tempts to apply it to man will be met with the objection that man's rubrospinal tract is rudimentary. However, as discussed previously (p. 169) there is no evidence that this general assumption is correct. If the hypothesis is tenable, one would expect that a lesion of the red nucleus in man would result in impairment of discrete voluntary movements, and perhaps other changes resembling those seen in a pure lesion of the pyramidal tract. Such cases appear to be extremely rare. Usually other neighboring structures, not least the cerebral peduncle, will be involved. However, in the old literature there are a few cases which are of interest. For example Raymond and Raymond Cestan (1902), Halban and Infeld (1902), Marie and Guillain (1903), Gautier and Lereboullet (1927), and von Bogaert and Bertrand (1932) have described cases with anatomically verified circumscribed lesions of the red nucleus without involvement of the cerebral peduncle. Although the descriptions of the symptoms are far from complete and the cases are not identical in all respects it appears that lesions of the red nucleus may be followed by some degree of contralateral hemiparesis, occasionally with somewhat exaggerated tendon reflexes and weakened abdominal reflexes. Whether a sign of Babinski occurs appears doubtful.[36] Anatomical as well as clinico-anatomical studies of the cortico-rubro-spinal pathways in man are needed to decide whether the hypothesis ventured here is tenable.

The above discussion has been focused on the role of the pyramidal tract in the cortical influence on voluntary movements. There can be no doubt that in addition to the pyramidal tract other pathways are involved, even if we are not at present able to specify them.[37] The situation appears to be rather similar with regard to the other symptoms seen in the classical "pyramidal tract syndrome." Increased tendon reflexes and muscular hypotonus are not necessarily signs of injury to the pyramidal tract. As discussed previously (p. 227) the occurrence of *spasticity in capsular or central cortical lesions* may presumably be explained in a general way by an imbalance between the influence of interrupted tracts and intact supraspinal pathways (especially the lateral vestibulospinal tract). It remains to consider the weakened or abolished cutaneous reflexes and the sign of Babinski belonging to the syndrome.

The sign of Babinski is "probably the most famous sign in clinical

---

[36] Often there have in addition been symptoms from the oculomotor nerve and cerebellar symptoms.

[37] It should of course be kept in mind that the motor regions of the cortex are acted upon by impulses from many sources, which may thus be of importance for their role in the production of voluntary movements. From the point of view concerning us here it is especially relevant to remember that the cerebellum acts not only upon the motor cortical regions but also on several of the relays of cortico-fugal paths to the spinal cord, such as the red nucleus and the reticular formation.

neurology" (Nathan and Smith, 1955b, p. 250). In clinical neurology it is often taken to be the most reliable sign of damage to the pyramidal tract. Normally a plantar flexion of the big toe is elicited when striking the sole of the foot with a pin or a fairly sharp object from the heel toward the toes. Often the other toes flex as well (and adduct). A dorsiflexion of the hallux following this stimulus is named an *inverted plantar* reflex and is considered a pathological phenomenon. Often there is at the same time a fanning of the toes. When this occurs there is a fully developed "sign of Babinski." Both variants were described by the French neurologist Babinski around the turn of the century, and soon found their way into the test battery of the routine neurological examination. The clinically most decisive feature is the dorsiflexion of the great toe, and it is generally agreed that noxious stimuli are the adequate stimuli. Nathan and Smith (1955b) in a review of the development of views on the Babinski response since it was first described draw attention to the way hypotheses have been transformed gradually to a dictum: the presence of a Babinski response is evidence of a damage of the pyramidal tract. The reflex arc of the normal plantar reflex was considered to be long, involving the leg area of the primary motor region. Cases where the sign of Babinski was found in lesions of this region have been described in man. In experimental studies in chimpanzees, Fulton and Keller (1932) found support for the view.

A perusal of the neurological literature from the first decades of the present century brings to light numerous observations which do not fit the theory. From the review of Nathan and Smith (1955b) as well as of those of Lassek (1944, 1945) it appears that the Babinski sign may be present when there is no damage to the pyramidal tract, and may have been absent in cases where this tract was found affected in post-mortem examinations. In a study of the spinal cord of 38 patients subjected to chordotomy Nathan and Smith (1955b) could confirm this lack of correlation between pyramidal tract injury and the sign of Babinski. Their conclusions were vehemently challenged by Walshe (1956), who also criticizes Lassek's work as well as conclusions reached by some physiologists concerning the mechanism of the plantar reflex and the sign of Babinski. Walshe emphasizes the dangers in attempting to explain clinical phenomena on the basis of findings in animals. In recent years clinical neurophysiological observations have been made which are ,of interest for the problem and may help to clarify the matter.

In these studies the activity in the muscles of the foot and leg have been recorded electromyographically. In order that exact measurements of the reflex time can be made some authors have used electrical stimulation by electrodes applied to the skin or deep tissues. These stimuli were assumed to be noxious. In such studies it is found that *in normal subjects* the reflex response varies according to the site of stimulation. The different responses appear to be "specifically adapted to the form of the human foot and represent the adequate withdrawal movement in relation to the site of stimulation" (Kugelberg, Eklund, and Grimby, 1960). For example, noxious stimulation of the ball of the toes elicits the general flexion reflex, including dorsiflexion of the great toe, while stimuli applied to the ball and hollow of the foot evoke the normal plantar reflex: plantar flexion of the toes and flexion at the ankle, knee, and hip.[38] These findings have been extended in further studies on normal subjects by Grimby (1963a), who emphasizes the existence of individual variations in the reflex pattern as the locus of stimulation is varied, and that changes in the subject's attention and expectancy may occasionally result in deviations from the basic pattern elicited from a particular site. The earliest responses have such short latencies (as little as 55 msec for the reflexes in the short hallux flexor and extensor which are the main muscles activated and which show reciprocal innervation) that *only purely spinal reflex arcs can be involved.* (There are, however, also responses of latencies of more than 150 msec, which are generally elicited on weaker stimulation.)

The *pathological plantar response,* inversion of the plantar reflex or the sign of Babinski, has been held by clinical neurologists (see Walshe, 1956) to be an integral part of the general flexion reflex in man, homologous with the nociceptive flexion reflex studied extensively in spinal and decerebrate animals by Sherrington and others. In this a general flexion of a limb follows when a nociceptive stimulus is applied to it.

The clinical neurophysiological studies of Kugelberg, Eklund, and Grimby (1960) support this view. In patients with severe spinal cord lesions there was a pure short hallux extensor activity independent of the stimulus site. In studies of the pathological plantar response in patients, Grimby (1963b) found that the receptive field for the extensor hallux response (the ball of the feet) spreads to a larger area as a normal reflex pattern is converted into a pathological, and vice versa. This further supports the contention of Kugelberg, Eklund, and Grimby (1960) that the extensor reflex (dorsiflexion of the hallux) obtained on hallux stimulation in normal cases is fundamentally the same as that elicited on plantar stimulation in pathological cases. The individual variations in the receptive fields, mentioned above, may be a factor in explaining why the pathological plantar reflex is most easily (or only) elicited in some patients on stimulation of the

[38] It is important to be aware of the fact that dorsiflexions of the toes and ankle are physiologically flexion movements, even if the muscles producing these movements are called extensors. On the other hand, plantar flexions of the toes and ankle are in reality extensions. Thus dorsiflexion of the toes is part of a flexion reflex. Not infrequently an extensor response occurs in the other leg when a flexion reflex is elicited from the sole (see Brain and Wilkinson, 1959).

medial, in others (and more often) of the lateral aspect of the planta, a common clinical experience. Landau and Clare (1959) made corresponding findings on many points, but they maintained that in the pathological plantar reflex there is concomitant activation of the long hallux extensor (as well as the extensor digitorum longus and tibialis anterior). To these authors the extensor response is a hyperactive flexor response in which the extensor hallucis longus is included by irradiation.

It appears from these recent studies that the normal plantar reflex is a manifold phenomenon, different patterns of reflex responses having differently located receptive fields. The reflex patterns are closely correlated to the sites of the stimulus, so that the resulting response always represents the most appropriate defense reaction. The pathological response pattern (dorsiflexion of the great toe, etc.) is a normal response to stimulation of the ball of the feet. Transitional forms to the normal response occur. Under pathological conditions the reflex pattern is less adaptive to the stimulus site.[39] The essential difference between the normal and pathological response thus appears to be a question of the receptive fields.[40] The two responses are not fundamentally different phenomena. The reason for the disruption of the finely integrated patterns of the plantar reflexes, resulting in the sign of Babinski, must presumably be sought in changes in the suprasegmental control of "the discriminating capacity of the reflex mechanism as regards the strength, modality and site of the sensory stimulus" (Kugelberg, Eklund, and Grimby, 1960). For some additional data see Grimby (1965).

Thus it appears that the normal as well as the pathological plantar reflexes are spinal (even if there may be some doubt as to the late responses). When a pathological response occurs this is scarcely due to interruption of a long reflex arc passing via the motor cortex, but to interference with the supraspinal control of the spinal reflex mechanisms. The pyramidal tract may well be concerned in this control (cf. the findings of Fisher and Curry, 1965). However, it must again be stressed that in most situations where the pyramidal tract may be injured there will necessarily be damage to other fiber systems as well. This point appears to be disregarded by clinicians who attempt to defend a close relation between the pyramidal tract and the sign of Babinski (see Walshe, 1956; Brain and Wilkinson, 1959), and invalidates their con-

[39] Occasionally the dorsiflexion of the great toe is most easily elicited from the lateral side of the dorsum of the foot (Chaddock's sign).

[40] When in a hemiplegic patient presenting the sign of Babinski the peroneal nerve in the paretic leg is anesthetized, the Babinski response disappears since the dorsiflexors of the toes and ankle are paralyzed. However, the response to plantar stimulation is then a plantar flexion of the big toe. This seems compatible with the above views on the organization of the plantar reflexes (see also Landau and Clare, 1959).

clusions. It appears indeed plausible that a derangement in spinal reflex patterns resulting in a Babinski sign may be caused by damage to several descending fiber systems. It is not even necessary to postulate that there is damage to one particular pathway. Presumably lesser or partial damage to more than one tract may be effective. However, it should not be overlooked that a histologically demonstrable lesion can not be expected to be present in all instances where a Babinski response is found. In the first place the microscopical changes may not be marked enough to permit recognition. Secondly, there is no doubt that functional disturbances of the nervous system may make the normal plantar response change into an extensor response. Thus a temporary Babinski response can be found in general anesthesia (see Grimby, Kugelberg, and Löfström, 1966) in hypoglycemia, following administration of various drugs, following an epileptic seizure, following long marches, during sleep, and in various general affections of the central nervous system (see Lassek, 1944, for references). The presence of a Babinski response should therefore not too hastily be interpreted as evidence of organic damage to the brain, and especially not to the pyramidal tract. The normal variations in the reflex response should be kept in mind.[41]

Weakening or absence of abdominal reflexes and the cremasteric reflex are usually considered as parts of the "pyramidal tract syndrome." They belong to the cutaneous reflexes, where the receptors are situated in the skin. Kugelberg and Hagbarth (1958), using electromyographic recordings, concluded that the central latency was short enough to prove that the abdominal reflexes are mediated by a spinal reflex arc. (See also Teasdall and Magladery, 1959.) In addition to contraction of the abdominal muscles there occurs a reciprocal relaxation of the trunk muscles. The reflexes are considered to belong to a spinal defense mechanism, securing that the resulting movement causes withdrawal from the stimulus. It is well known that the abdominal reflexes are subject to considerable incidental and individual variations. In further studies Hagbarth and Kugelberg (1958) analyzed factors influencing the reflex, such as habituation and sensitization, and conclude that such changes depend on "cerebral events." However, nothing can be said of pathways involved in this central influence. The abdominal reflexes have not been studied as intensively as the plantar reflexes.[42] However, there does not appear to be convincing evidence that weakening or abolishment of the abdominal

[41] In infants the plantar reflexes are usually extensor until between the 9th and 24th month of life. In the beginning the receptive field extends to the abdomen or higher, but it gradually shrinks (see Brain and Wilkinson, 1959).

[42] The abdominal skin reflexes are present from birth in man, but their reflexogeneous zone is wider in infants than in later life (Harlem and Lønnum, 1957).

reflexes, often seen in central nervous lesions, particularly of the internal capsule, can be ascribed to damage of the pyramidal tract. (The reflexes may obviously be affected segmentally in lesions of dorsal or ventral roots or in segmental lesions of the gray matter of the cord.)

In conclusion it may be stated that *the "pyramidal tract syndrome" is a misleading term. The syndrome represents the consequences of lesions of many other structures in addition to the pyramidal tract, and there is no symptom or syndrome which is pathognomonic to injury of the pyramidal tract.* As a matter of fact, this is not surprising when we consider the many interconnections in the nervous system, the many tracts and gray masses, which are engaged in almost all activities in the brain. The case of the "pyramidal tract syndrome" appears to be only one of many where we must abandon the attempts to find a particular symptom or symptom constellation as the functional and clinical expression of injury to a particular structure. (The basal ganglia, to be considered below, furnish other examples.) It follows from the above that *the term "pyramidal tract syndrome" should be discarded.*

From a practical point of view it may be disheartening to have to give up traditional views—and names. It is often convenient to have a designation of a symptom complex, but the name should not be such that it implies incorrect relations to definite structures. As an alternative term which is purely descriptive, *"pure motor hemiplegia,"* as used by Fisher and Curry (1965), may be suggested to cover the changes in the motor sphere of the "pyramidal tract syndrome." Since this symptom constellation is by far most commonly seen in lesions of the internal capsule, another solution would be to speak of an "internal capsule syndrome." This has the advantage that it does not fix attention unduly on one component of the internal capsule only, but it suffers from the drawback that it may cover different symptoms according to the part of the capsule involved (for example, homonymous scotomas or hemianopsia when the posterior part, and aphasic disturbances when the anteriormost part, is included in the lesion). This again illustrates the difficulties mentioned above. It is to be feared that the ghost of the "pyramidal tract syndrome" will survive in clinical neurology for many years to come.

The role of the pyramidal tract. It is celar from the preceding account that the pyramidal tract is only one of several pathways leading from the cerebral cortex, especially its sensorimotor regions, to the spinal cord. It is further obvious that the tract is not a homogeneous system, either anatomically or functionally. However, in one respect the pyramidal tract differs from all other corticospinal routes: it is the only fiber bundle which proceeds without synaptic interruption from the cortex to the cord. From a functional point of view this means that it enables the cortex to exert a more immediate control over the spinal mechanisms than does any other route. The relative increase in the size of the pyramidal tract in the phylogenetic scale of mammals makes it clear that this direct cortical control of the segmental mechanisms of the cord (as well as of corresponding mechanisms in the brain stem) acquires an increasing importance in higher mammals, reaching its peak in man. The same tendency is demonstrated by the fact that in the monkey and chimpanzee some fibers of the "motor" component of the tract establish direct synaptic contact with α motoneurons, while in the cat all contacts are made with interneurons. Presumably this monosynaptic component is even more prominent in man, but precise information is not available on this point. With regard to the role of the "motor" component of the pyramidal tract it should be recalled that its influence on flexor motoneurons is predominantly excitatory, while extensor motoneurons are inhibited.

Speculations concerning the particular functional role of the pyramidal tract have been especially directed to its importance in the initiation of skilled voluntary movements. Even if the pyramidal tract is not alone involved in mediating cortical impulses concerned in these, it may well play a special role (regardless of whether the patterning of such movements to a large extent may be a matter of the spinal cord; see p. 196). It has been pointed out by several students that the predominant flexor activities following stimulation of corticospinal fibers (and the same applies to the rubrospinal fibers) and of the cerebral cortex may be seen in relation to the function of the antigravity muscles. As expressed by Corazza, Fadiga, and Parmeggiani (1963, p. 360)

> . . . it does not seem too far-fetched to surmise that the functional meaning of the flexor prevalence of pyramidal excitatory drive (and of the extensor prevalence of the inhibitory one) may be that of counteracting, at the beginning of a "voluntary" pattern of movements, the extensor bias which under normal conditions must obtain as a result of myotatic reflexes from antigravity muscles.

Somewhat similar views have been expressed by others, for example Agnew, Preston, and Whitlock (1963). In this connection it is worth recalling that most of our skilled motor functions engage primarily flexor muscles.

Other results of physiological studies in animals are of interest. In studies of voluntary movements in unanesthetized monkeys, Evarts (1965) found slowly conducting pyramidal neurons to be tonically active in the absence of movements, while rapidly conducting neurons fired intensely only during the movement, supporting older conclusions concerning tonic and phasic properties of the pyramidal tract. As mentioned previously its fibers act on α and γ motoneurons, and it has been suggested by several authors that the influence on the γ system is a preparatory step for the activation of α fibers occurring in rapid, phasic movements. It is of particular interest that motoneurons supplying proximal muscles are influenced by spatially extensive colonies of cortical cells while the colonies acting on distal muscles are more focal (Phillipps, 1967), indicating a more specific organization of the corticospinal influence on distal muscles. Furthermore, distal motoneurons receive a stronger monosynaptic input than do proximal motoneurons.[43]

Many studies have been devoted to the ways in which pyramidal tract neurons are brought into action (for a recent review see Marchiafava, 1968). Afferent impulses from many sources and from different kinds of receptors interact in a very complex fashion, and provide the sensory information for a necessary properly adjusted cortical influence on the motor apparatus.

In spite of many detailed studies on the pyramidal tract, it is not yet possible to formulate more than rather general concepts of its functional importance. *It appears, however, that the following may safely be concluded:* The anatomical and functional peculiarities of *the pyramidal tract* strongly suggest that it *plays a particular role in the central control and initiation of movements, presumably especially skilled voluntary movements of the hand and fingers.*[44] This role is of greater importance in primates than in other mammals, and especially great in man. This, however, should not induce us to overlook the fact that the corticospinal tract is scarcely alone in this function.

Studies on the function of the basal ganglia.   As described in a preceding section diseases of the basal ganglia and related nuclei may give rise to a variety of disturbances of motor functions. In the course of time a number of theories have been advanced to explain the relation between the site or sites of the pathological changes and the ensuing symptoms. These theories will not be considered here (for recent accounts see Jung and Hassler, 1960; Kaada, 1963). The earlier conceptions were mainly based on clinicopathological correlations. In later attempts at explanation the results of experimental studies have been taken into consideration as well, and the results of stereotactic operations on the basal ganglia and thalamus in man have given much useful information. In spite of much work, it is, however, not yet possible to formulate clear concepts of the function of these parts of the brain, even if it may be safely concluded that they to a large extent must be involved

---

[43] The recent experimental study of Buxton and Goodman (1967) of the corticospinal projection in the racoon is of interest in this connection. In this animal, which has a well-developed dexterity of the fingers, degeneration following motor cortical ablations extends into laminae IX in C_{7-8}, but not in other segments.

[44] The facial and laryngeal movements should probably be included, but they have been studied relatively little.

in what is usually referred to as "integrative processes at a relatively high level," as must indeed be assumed from a study of the complex fiber connections. This complexity makes interpretations of physiological observations on these nuclei difficult.

There are several reasons which explain that our knowledge of the subject is still relatively scanty. It is difficult to make lesions which involve one of the nuclei completely without damaging others or by-passing fiber tracts. It is also quite possible that if parts of a nucleus are preserved they may be sufficient to maintain its functions. Observations of finer differences of movements and muscle tone in experimental animals are not easily made. In physiological investigations of the effect of lesions, careful anatomical control is far too often lacking. Here, as elsewhere, when an anatomical examination is performed, considerable changes may be found apart from those intentionally made. In attempts at stimulation of the basal ganglia it appears that spread of current to neighboring structures, particularly the internal capsule, has often occurred and has given rise to faulty conclusions. Variations in stimulus parameters, in anesthesia and species differences may explain some of the discrepancies in the literature. It is further evident that until quite recently attention has been focused almost exclusively on the effects of stimulation and lesions upon rather elementary motor functions, and other effects may easily have been overlooked. Finally, there is disagreement about the mutual relationships of the various types of movements seen in patients, for example as to whether two varieties are expressions of disturbances of a common mechanism or not.

In any present-day analysis it should be kept in mind that, as emphasized in a preceding section, the basal ganglia and related nuclei give off only few fibers to lower levels. The structural organization of their fiber connections make it clear that *most of the actions of the basal ganglia must be exerted on the cerebral cortex.* Their influence on motor functions must therefore to a considerable extent involve the cortex, as has indeed been suggested by neurosurgeons (see for example, Bucy, 1944b) who noted that following ablations of the precentral cortex in man pre-existing involuntary movements disappeared.[45] There is an increasing body of physiological evidence in support of this notion.

In the following, only some of the many investigations of the function of the basal ganglia will be considered. It may be said at once that attempts to produce in animals symptoms resembling those seen in patients with diseases of these parts of the brain have not been too successful.

As concerns *lesions of the caudate nucleus, the putamen, and the globus pallidus,* it appears that convincing changes in motor performances have not been seen in lesions restricted to these nuclei in the monkey and

[45] It is a common clinical experience that if a patient with parkinsonism has a cerebral stroke involving the internal capsule his tremor disappears on the side of the ensuing hemiplegia.

2 4 4

chimpanzee (Mettler, 1942; Kennard, 1944; and others) (except for some tremor in very extensive lesions). According to Mettler (1945) extensive bilateral lesions of the globus pallidus in monkeys result in marked poverty of movements. In cats only transient symptoms were observed (Laursen, 1963). When lesions of the basal ganglia are combined with lesions of cortical areas 6 and 8 there develops, however, a spasticity, and often tremor has been recorded to appear.

More information has been obtained in studies of *stimulation of the basal ganglia,* even if, as pointed out by Laursen (1963), there has presumably often been inadvertent stimulation of fibers descending in the internal capsule (corticospinal and others). In unanesthetized cats stimulation of the *caudate nucleus* results in head turning and circling movements toward the opposite side (Stevens, Kim, and MacLean, 1961; and others). It appears from the controlled studies of Laursen (see Laursen, 1963) that the effects are not due to spread of current. According to Forman and Ward (1957) the responses from the head of the caudate show a somatotopical pattern. However, on low frequency electrical stimulation of the caudate (Akert and Andersson, 1951; Kaada, 1951), prolonged stimulation by injection of long-acting cholinergic agents in crystalline form (Stevens, Kim, and MacLean, 1961) or by injection of alumina cream (Spiegel and Szekely, 1961) the most conspicuous effect has been a cessation of spontaneous movements and a prolonged state of quietude. This effect is seen even if the frontal lobe or the "motor" cortex has been ablated (Spiegel and Szekely, 1961). The *putamen* has been less extensively studied than the caudate, but recently Hassler and Dieckmann (1967), using the method employed by Akert and Andersson (1951), report inhibition of movements (as well as an "arrest reaction" and an "empty gaze") following low frequency stimulation in the awake cat. These authors briefly mention that similar effects were evoked from the pallidum. The recent results extend some early observations of Mettler, Ades, Lipman, and Culler (1939), who performed simultaneous stimulation of the striate body and the motor cortex in cats and monkeys. When movements were elicited by stimulation of the motor cortex, simultaneous stimulation of the caudate nucleus and the putamen reduced or inhibited the movements.

More recently some students have investigated the influence of stimulation of the caudate nucleus on conditioned avoidance behavior (see Stevens, Kim, and MacLean, 1961) and on learned responses in unanesthetized animals. Learned responses appear to be inhibited, and inhibition of unit activity in the thalamus (VA and VL) and cortex (followed by bursting of units) has been found to occur concomitantly (see Buchwald and Hull, 1967).

The interpretation of these findings is so far uncertain, and it should be noted that corresponding behavioral and electrophysiological changes have been recorded following stimulation at other sites. Stimulation of parts of the striate body in (chloralosane-anesthetized) cats inhibits the evoked "nonspecific" sensory activity in the brain stem, thalamus, and cortex (see Krauthamer and Albe-Fessard, 1964). Findings of this kind as well as others have focused attention on the functional relationships between the basal ganglia and the thalamus, particularly the "nonspecific" nuclei, and on the possible role of the basal ganglia in functions more complex than simple motor acts. This is still a field chiefly for speculations.

It appears from the above that neither lesions nor stimulations of the caudate nucleus, putamen, or globus pallidus in cats and monkeys result in symptoms resembling those seen when these parts of the brain are affected by disease in humans. The role played by these structures under pathological conditions in man are apparently far from simple. However, several observations strongly suggest that in addition to the pallidum the thalamus (especially VA and VL) is concerned in the appearance of tremor and rigidity in parkinsonism. We will return to these problems later.

More satisfactory correlations between experimental and clinical observations than for the striatum and pallidum appear to be possible as concerns the substantia nigra and the subthalamic nucleus. *The substantia nigra* is often found changed in cases of parkinsonism. On the assumption that lesions of the substantia nigra may be responsible for rigidity and/or tremor seen in this disease, numerous authors have attempted to produce isolated lesions of the substatnia nigra, particularly in monkeys. It will be realized that it is extremely difficult to obtain isolated lesions of this small nucleus, lying in close relation to several other structures, among these the cerebral peduncle. Some authors have reported that static tremor resembling that seen in parkinsonism follows lesions of the substantia nigra in monkeys. However, in subsequent studies it was established that the static tremor observed in these experiments is probably due to concomitant lesions of the ventral tegmentum, situated just dorsal to the substantia nigra (see below), and several authors (most recently Carpenter and McMasters, 1964; Stern, 1966), succeeding in making more restricted lesions in the substantia nigra, failed to obtain tremor. In cases with partial or unilateral lesions usually no symptoms at all were observed. However, if bilateral and larger lesions are made there ensues a *hypokinesia* with lack of spontaneous motor activity and a tendency to assume immobile postures (Stern, 1966). Additional damage to the globus pallidus increased this tendency. Caution should be exerted in applying conclusions drawn from such observations to conditions in man, but it is of interest that according to several clinical neurologists there is no constant relation between the appearance of hypokinesia and rigidity in parkinsonism, hypokinesia being a distinct clinical feature. From this point of view it is of interest that in several cases of parkinsonism no pathological changes have been found in the substantia nigra, while this has been found altered in the absence of symptoms of parkinsonism (for references see Mettler, 1964; Stern, 1966). Markham, Brown, and Rand (1966) in stereotactic lesions of the thalamus in parkinsonism obtained good effects on tremor and rigidity, but a present or developing akenesia was not influenced. The mechanisms by which the substantia nigra influences motor function and by which its lesion produces akenesia are not known. Several hypotheses have been suggested.

Lesions of the subthalamic nucleus in man are regularly followed by hemiballismus. A corresponding dyskinesia has been produced experimentally in the monkey by stereotactic lesions of the nucleus, particularly by Carpenter and his collaborators (see Carpenter, 1961). In order to produce hyperkinesia the lesions must comprise at least 20 per cent of the mass of the nucleus, and the globus pallidus and its efferent projections must not be damaged. The dyskinesia occurs in the limbs on the side contralateral to the lesion. There is some evidence for a somatotopic pattern within the subthalamic nucleus (Carpenter and Carpenter, 1951; Mettler and Stern, 1962).

The production of dyskinesias of a choreiform-ballistic type by lesions of the subthalamic nucleus is the only instance where it has so far been possible, experimentally, to produce symptoms resembling those seen in patients with similarly placed affections. The observations made in monkeys may therefore give information of the mechanism of dyskinesias of this type in man. From this point of view it is of interest that in animals in which subthalamic dyskinesia has been experimentally produced, this can be abolished by a subsequent lesion of the pallidum. Most effective are lesions of the medial segment, presumably because they interrupt a larger number of pallidofugal fibers (see Carpenter, 1961). Likewise, lesions of the lateral thalamic nuclear group are effective, while lesions of the substantia nigra are without effect (Strominger and Carpenter, 1965). The clinical experience that ablation of the precentral cortex alleviates or abolishes dyskinesias in the contralateral limbs in man although leaving a hemiplegia, has been confirmed in monkeys having experimentally produced lesions of the subthalamic nucleus (Carpenter and Mettler, 1951). Furthermore, transections of the lateral funiculus of the spinal cord at the cervical level (interrupting, among other tracts, the corticospinal) abolish subthalamic dyskinesia, while lesions of the dorsal funiculus or the ventral part of the lateral and the ventral funiculus are without effect (Carpenter, 1961). From these observations it is concluded that the corticospinal tract is the chief pathway which ultimately transmits the impulses to the abnormal movements to the cord. The integrity of the pallidum and the lateral nuclear group of the thalamus appears to be necessary for the appearance of the subthalamic dyskinesias. It is assumed (see Carpenter, 1961; Carpenter and Strominger, 1967) that the impulses for the abnormal movements arise in these structures, and that the subthalamic nucleus normally exerts an inhibitory effect on the medial segment of the pallidum (via its efferent projection onto the latter, see Fig. 4-10). The occurrence of hemiballismus when the subthalamic nucleus is intact may be due to affections of afferent or efferent connections of the nucleus (Carpenter and Strominger, 1966). In a general way these views fit in with suggestions made concerning the role played by the basal ganglia, thalamus, and cortex in the appearance of parkinsonian tremor and rigidity. Modern neurophysiological investigations in animals and studies of patients subjected to surgical treatment for parkinsonism have given information of interest on this subject.

Surgical treatment of patients suffering from involuntary movements has a relatively short history (see for example, Meyers, 1958; Markham and Rand, 1963; Marion Smith, 1967). As mentioned previously some neurosurgeons observed good effects on tremor and other dyskinesias following ablations of the precentral cortex. Other procedures employed with success have been transection of the cerebral peduncle (discussed at some length above, p. 233) or transections of the dorsolateral funiculus in the spinal cord. In all these instances the abolition of the involuntary movements was followed by hemiparesis. As mentioned previously these results supported the notion that corticospinal pathways were involved in the production of the abnormal movements. Attempts to destroy parts of the basal ganglia by an open approach have been tried but carry considerable risks. The introduction of stereotactic methods for placing lesions in the basal ganglia by Spiegel, Wycis, Marks, and Lee (1947) and others opened up new possibilities. Several variants of the technique have been developed in which the lesions are produced by such diverse means as alcohol injections, electrolysis, radiofrequency waves, ultrasound, placing of radioisotopes, or freezing. A number of nuclei have been the goal for the lesions, most frequently the globus pallidus and, somewhat later, the lateral thalamus, especially VA and VL. Some have attempted to destroy the centromedian nuclei or the substantia nigra. Satisfactory relief has been reported following all of these procedures, although the results differ.

There are several reasons for this, such as variations among patients selected for treatment as to age and stage of the disease and differences as to the size of the

248

lesion achieved, but a main factor appears to be the difficulties inherent in the placing of the lesion precisely where it is intended without inadvertent damage to other structures. Even if certain landmarks, such as the foramen of Monroe and the anterior and posterior commissures can be found on ventriculography and can be used for comparisons with the many atlases of the human brain prepared for this purpose, the individual variations among human brains are too great to permit entirely reliable placements of the destruction in this way. In recent years the recording of potentials from microelectrodes inserted in the target area have made it possible to increase precision considerably (for example the VPL can be identified by the potential changes occurring in this on somatosensory stimulation, Albe-Fessard et al., 1964; Gaze et al., 1964). Other thalamic nuclei can also be identified (Albe-Fessard et al., 1967; Bertrand, Jasper, and Wong, 1967). Likewise, stimulation may give information, for example, of whether the electrode is situated in the internal capsule. Moderate cooling down to some $+10°C$ or somewhat less may produce a temporary inactivation of the target area (Le Beau, Dondey, and Albe-Fessard, 1962; see also Siegfried et al., 1962).

In spite of improvements in the methods for accurate placements of lesions in stereotactic surgery it is essential for an analysis of the results and for further progress to have precise information of the destructions actually made at operation. This information can only be obtained when careful post-mortem studies are performed in patients who have been clinically thoroughly examined. Relatively few studies of this kind are available, and in most of them only the site of the lesion is described. In quite a number of cases in which good results have been obtained the internal capsule has been found to be involved in the lesion. This was the caes in at least 12 of 15 patients whose brains were carefully examined by Marion Smith (1962) and in 15 of 17 operations on 12 patients studied by Nörholm and Thygstrup (1960) as well as in several others reported in the literature (see Marion Smith, 1967, for references). This is in keeping with other observations concerning the effects of cortical lesions and of lesions affecting corticospinal fibers, for example, in pedunculotomies. However, as mentioned previously, the corticospinal fibers are situated in the posterior part of the internal capsule, and they are therefore not very likely to be affected in the injury inflicted on the internal capsule in stereotactic operations aiming at the pallidum or ventrolateral thalamus (see Fig. 4-8). Only in one case of several with lesions of the internal capsule did Marion Smith (1967) find degeneration of corticospinal fibers. The favorable effects of lesions of the internal capsule (see for example, Gillingham, 1962) may therefore be due to interruption of some of the other fiber contingents passing in it. This may be important in view of the fact that lesions involving many different regions have been claimed to give satisfactory effects on rigidity as well as tremor and other dyskinesias. We will return to this question below.

The steadily growing literature on the mechanisms and the treatment

2 4 9

of dyskinesias and parkinsonian rigidity is rather confusing, and no attempt will be made to discuss these subjects exhaustively.[46] Chiefly, points which are of relevance for the anatomical basis will be considered. It will be practical to discuss separately observations bearing on parkinsonian rigidity and on dyskinesias.

As to the mechanism underlying *parkinsonian rigidity* little is known for certain. It has apparently so far not been possible to produce a corresponding state experimentally in animals by placing lesions in the brain or by stimulation. Recently studies have been made in animals given reserpine (see Steg, 1966) in whom a state of akinesia, rigidity, and tremor develops. The basis for this is assumed to be the blocking effect of this drug on the uptake of monoamines in the granules of the nerve terminals. However, electrical stimulation in animals and man have given information of some interest.

Electrical stimulation of the VL and the pallidum influences the muscle spindles. Stern and Ward (1960) found inhibition of the contralateral spindle discharge in cats. The integrity of the motor cortex was necessary for this to occur. Langfitt et al. (1963), however, also in the cat, observed complex alterations in spontaneous activity of flexor and extensor γ neurons, including reciprocal and nonreciprocal inhibition and facilitation, and concluded that the cortex is not involved in mediating the responses. According to Gilman and van der Meulen (1966), ablations of what they refer to as "pyramidal" or "extrapyramidal" cortical areas in the monkey are followed by alterations in the "tonic gamma as well as alpha mechanism." In man, Ohye et al. (1964) observed that high frequency stimulation of the VL results in nonreciprocal increase of muscle tone in the contralateral forelimb muscles, and Walter et al. (1963) report various alterations in the patients' abnormal movements on stimulation of the globus pallidus and VL. The divergent results obtained by these and other authors may perhaps in part be explained by differences in the experimental situations (anesthesia, etc.). Since there is evidence that especially the tonic stretch reflexes are increased in parkinsonism it is interesting that following stereotactic lesions of the pallidum these are reduced while the phasic responses to stretch are not influenced (Shimazu et al., 1962). Hassler (1966a) has observed that stimulation of his nucleus V.o.a. (apparently corresponding to VA) increases muscle tone in parkinsonian patients, while coagulation of this nucleus abolishes rigidity as effectively as does coagulation of the pallidum. Hassler (1966a) further reports that on stimulation of certain nuclei in the ventrobasal thalamus in conscious patients there is an acceleration of contralateral movements and of speaking, while stimulation of other regions has the opposite effect and results in an increase of muscle tone.

These and other observations indicate that the pallidum and thalamus (especially VL and VA) are able to influence the reflex apparatus of the cord (presumably chiefly the tonic stretch reflexes). The action appears to occur via the cortex (chiefly the precentral) from which impulses are

[46] For a recent account on various aspects of the problems see *Advances in Stereoencephalotomy,* III, 1967.

transmitted to the cord via corticofugal fibers descending in the internal capsule. These conclusions appear to be compatible with the results of stereotactic operations in man, since destruction of any of the above links may abolish the increased activity of the tonic stretch reflex in parkinsonism.

Dyskinesias of different kinds have been reported to be alleviated by surgical lesions of the pallidum or the ventrolateral thalamus (for example, dystonia musculorum deformans, Cooper, 1959, 1965b; hemiballismus, Martin and McCaul, 1959; intention tremor, Cooper, 1965b; Fox and Kurtzke, 1966; and others), but the bulk of observations concern *parkinsonian tremor*. This is essentially a tremor at rest (see p. 216) and differs in several respects from the tremor in lesions of the cerebellum and from "physiological tremor."

> *Physiological tremor* is the name currently used for tremor found in many persons with no demonstrable disease. This shows great individual variations and has been found by several students to have a frequency of about 10 per second. It is influenced by a number of factors, such as the part of the body tested, the position of the extremity, the amount of work by the limb prior to testing, the weight of the extremity, the patient's age, the state of consciousness, emotional state and several other factors, among these intoxication. It appears currently to be accepted that physiological tremor "is due to a slight oscillation of the length servoloop which involves the complete stretch mechanism, including gamma efferents of the spinal segmental level" (Wachs and Boshes, 1961, p. 68).

According to Wachs and Boshes (1961) the tremor observed in parkinsonism shows a lower dominant frequency than the physiological tremor, and is less affected by the position of the extremities but more influenced by emotional and other endogenous factors. By employing a special recording device these authors sometimes found tremor to be present where it could not be seen clinically, for example on the non-affected side in patients with unilateral symptoms. This corresponds to the pathological observations of Davison (1942). In patients with unilateral parkinsonism he often found bilateral changes in the pallidum and substantia nigra.

In recordings from the human thalamus during operations for Parkinson's disease a spontaneous rhythmic activity has been recorded when the patients are awake (Albe-Fessard, Arfel, and Guiot, 1963; Albe-Fessard, Guiot, Lamarre, and Arfel, 1966; Albe-Fessard et al., 1967). The thalamic units fire in bursts at the frequency of the tremor, as further confirmed in simultaneous electromyographic recordings. It has been concluded that the thalamic rhythm is not due to afferent impulses arising by the tremor movements, even if the central rhythm can be influenced from the periphery. These thalamic units were found in a region anterior

251

to but partly overlapping the VPL, apparently in VL (but also in a more dorsoposterior region, the LP). Largely corresponding observations have been made by Jasper and Bertrand (1966) and Bertrand, Jasper, and Wong (1967). Whether the rhythmic activity arises locally in the thalamus or is triggered from other structures (from the cerebellum?) can not be decided. However, it seems a likely assumption (Albe-Fessard et al., 1967) that in parkinsonism there occurs a release of a "rhythmic center" from an inhibition arising from a region which is destroyed in the disease.

Attempts to produce in animals an experimental tremor resembling that seen in parkinsonism have not been too successful.[47] Some authors maintain that, in the monkey, lesions of the ventromedial quadrants of the mesencephalon give rise to a postural tremor of this kind (see Carrea and Metttler, 1947; Poirier, 1960). It appears that tremor develops only if the substantia nigra is damaged in addition to near-by structures. In the cat corresponding lesions were not followed by tremor (Ganes, Kaada, and Nyberg-Hansen, 1966). As referred to previously, lesions restricted to the substantia nigra in the monkey do not result in tremor. Carpenter and McMasters (1964) suggest that the tremor which has been observed in monkeys following lesions of the ventromedial tegmentum is probably due to interruption of cerebellofugal fibers even if lesions of the cerebellum involving the dentate nucleus or the brachium conjunctivum below the red nucleus result in coarse intentional tremor (as well as ataxia). Carpenter (1961), who discusses this problem, focuses attention on the fact that lesions of the ventrolateral thalamus abolish cerebellar tremor in monkeys (Carpenter, Glinsmann, and Fabrega, 1958), just as intention tremor has been abolished in man by similar lesions (Cooper, 1965b; Fox and Kurtzke, 1966; and others). Experimental lesions of the pallidum appear to have some effect on cerebellar tremor and ataxia. It appears further from the experimental studies that impulses responsible for the appearance of cerebellar dyskinesias, including tremor, are transmitted to the cord by corticospinal connections, perhaps particularly the corticospinal tract. Thus, on many points there are marked similarities between the observations made in cases of cerebellar dyskinesias and those made in studies of subthalamic dyskinesias, described above. In both instances, as well as in parkinsonian tremor, it appears that impulses giving rise to dyskinesias are mediated via the ventrolateral thalamus–cortex–corticofugal fibers to the cord, and, probably except for cerebellar tremor, the pallidum should be included in these structures.

---

[47] In any comparison between experimental observations and findings in man it should be recalled that most affections giving rise to dyskinesias in man develop slowly, and are not strictly parallel to an acute severe damage.

Some authors advocate the importance of "nonspecific" thalamic nuclei as well.

Why tremors and dyskinesias result in diseases of the basal ganglia, the subthalmic nucleus, and the cerebellum is so far not clearly understood. Even if many varieties of involuntary movements appear to be mediated via the same structures and pathways it must be presumed that their basic mechanism is not identical. A number of theories have been set forth. These will not be discussed here. Suffice it to mention that in most attempts at explanation emphasis has been put on the presence of numerous closed loops within the connections of the basal ganglia and between these and other structures (see Fig. 4-10). These connections represent the basis for feedback mechanisms between various gray masses, and their importance was early stressed by Bucy (1944b). A closer scrutiny of the fiber connections reveals an abundance of mutual interrelationships which might be concerned. Any attempt to pick out destruction of links in a particular circuit as being responsible for one or another kind of dyskinesia will therefore necessarily represent a great oversimplification. Furthermore, the anatomical arrangement of the various connections thought to be involved is such that there is virtually no locus where only one fiber connection can be damaged in isolation. This has been discussed more fully by Marion Smith (1967) who draws attention to some salient points. The pallidofugal fibers running in the internal capsule have a very wide distribution both in the anteroposterior and craniocaudal planes. Furthermore, the pallidal efferents lie very close to the thalamic afferents from the cerebellum and the red nucleus, and the dentatothalamic and pallidothalamic fibers end in the same nuclei of the thalamus, even if there are probably more pallidal efferents to VA, more cerebellar and rubral efferents to the VL. In view of these and other features in the fiber connections and considering that in stereotactic operations the lesions are certainly not always as circumscribed as planned and not placed precisely where intended, it is not surprising that destructions of almost any target (pallidum, ansa lenticularis, the thalamus (VL or VA), the internal capsule, and others) have been reported to alleviate different kinds of dyskinesias. Even in the reports of cases in which the anatomical site of the lesion has been mapped it is not possible so far to correlate a specific lesion with beneficial effect on a particular kind of dyskinesia (see for example the papers of Dierssen et al., 1962; Cooper, Bergmann, and Caracalos, 1963; Markham, Brown, and Rand, 1966). It appears, however, that lesions of the pallidum are more effective in relieving rigidity, while thalamic lesions are superior in abolishing tremor. Bertrand and Martinez (1962) reported that, in a large material, tremor never responded satisfactorily to pallidal lesions, but results were very good in lesions of the ventrolateral thalamus. This and other observations may suggest that a disturbance in the impulses from the cerebellum to the thalamus may be of some importance in the production of tremor in parkinsonism and of other dyskinesias. Stereotactic destruction of the dentate nucleus in man has been tried in some cases of dyskinesias (see Zervas et al., 1967), but the results are so far not conclusive. However, whether the cerebellar impulses are of relevance or not, it is clear from the fiber connections that an appropriately placed lesion of the ventrolateral thalamus will interrupt pallidothalamic as well as dentatothalamic and rubrothalamic fibers, making thalamotomy preferable to pallidotomy as a method for alleviating dyskinesias. This indeed appears to be the experience of many neurosurgeons.

The considerations made ábove on the subject of the mechanisms and treatment of dyskinesias are rather elementary. A number of detailed physiological studies on particular aspects of the problem have not been considered. It is clear, however, that we are obviously still far from understanding the mechanisms underlying the various kinds of dyskinesias in man.[48] However, this does not prevent the empirical search for regions whose destruction will alleviate particularly one or the other type of dyskinesia. In order to attain this goal "it is essential that more evidence is obtained by the rigorous follow-up of patients who have had stereotactic operations, ensuring that the actual location of the lesions is ascertained. Further, the pathological changes due to the underlying disease must be determined in these patients. Only when many such studies have been made will we be able to put these successful, though empirical, operations on a rational basis" (Marion Smith, 1967, p. 47). A study of this kind has recently been made by Beck and Bignami (1968). It appeared too late to be considered in the above text.

[48] In recent years much interest has been devoted to studies of the biochemistry of the basal ganglia and related nuclei. The relations of biochemical changes to dyskinesias have been discussed (for a recent review see Curzon, 1967).

5

The Cerebellum

IN SPITE of numerous anatomical and physiological studies devoted to the cerebellum we do not yet properly understand its function and its co-operation with other parts of the brain. Sherrington coined the term "the head ganglion of the proprioceptive system" for the cerebellum. However, subsequent research has shown that the cerebellum is not only related to "the proprioceptive system" but to activities in other functional spheres as well. Judging from its fiber connections, the cerebellum appears to be able to influence almost any other part of the brain. It might, therefore, be surmised that in general it co-ordinates and controls almost any function in which the nervous system is involved, in much the same way as it is known to regulate muscular activity. It may be essential for the full perfection of a number of bodily functions. The cerebellum is, however, not essential to life. In fact, individuals who are born without a cerebellum do not betray themselves in daily life by any obvious defects.

Comparative anatomical aspects. Some comparative anatomical data is valuable as a basis for the understanding of cerebellar function, since it reflects a functional subdivision within the cerebellum which is also demonstrated by other methods of investigation. In the paired primordia of the cerebellum two parts can be distinguished. One of these has an intimate relation to the matrix of the vestibular nuclei, the other develops immediately rostral to this. The former is present in a rather constant form in most vertebrates. Following the designation applied to it by Larsell, who has extensively studied the comparative anatomy of the cerebellum, this part is now commonly called the *flocculonodular lobe,* since it is made up of the flocculus and the nodulus (Fig. 5-1).

The other major part of the cerebellum is separated from the flocculo-nodular lobe by a fissure, the *fissura posterolateralis.* This fissure is the first to appear, phylogenetically as well as ontogenetically. The part of the cerebellum developing rostral to this fissure is called the *corpus cerebelli* (Fig. 5-1). In contrast to the flocculonodular lobe, the corpus cerebelli increases considerably in size in the phylogenetic ascent of verte-brates. However, this increase does not involve all parts of the corpus cerebelli to an equal extent. The most rostral part, called *lobus anterior* and separated from the rest by the so-called fissura prima, shows only moderate changes (the fissura prima is not, as previously commonly maintained, the oldest fissure of the cerebellum). The most caudal parts of the corpus cerebelli, the lobuli called the *pyramis* and *uvula,* are also relatively constant in most vertebrate species. It is the middle part of the corpus cerebelli which increases markedly in size. This holds true with respect to its vermal portions, and particularly its lateral parts. These are clearly developed only in mammals, and in monkeys, apes, and man their size is so large that they entirely overshadow the other parts of the cerebellum. These lateral parts correspond roughly to what is called

FIG. 5–1 A very simplified diagram of the mammalian cerebellum. In the left half the three main subdivisions which can be recognized on a comparative anatomical basis are seen. Black: Archicerebellum, flocculonodular lobe. Hatchings: Palaeo-cerebellum, the vermis region of the anterior lobe, the pyramis, uvula, and (?) paraflocculus. White: Neocerebellum. In the right half the terminal areas of the vestibulocerebellar fibers are indicated by heavy dots, the terminal areas of the spinocerebellar pathways by light dots. (Cf. text, and Fig. 5–8).

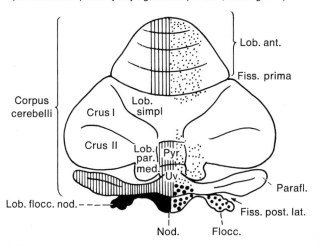

the *cerebellar hemispheres.* In the increase of the lateral parts the lobus anterior also takes part.[1]

The lateral parts of the cerebellum and the middle portion of the vermis represent the phylogenetically youngest parts of the cerebellum, and are often collectively designated as the *neocerebellum* (white in Fig. 5-1, left half). In contradistinction to this the other parts are sometimes grouped together as representing the paleocerebellum. However, the subdivision proposed by Larsell (1934, 1937) is to be preferred. According to this author the flocculonodular lobe is termed the *archicerebellum* (black in Fig. 5-1, left half), and the term *paleocerebellum* denotes the vermal part of the anterior lobe, the pyramis, uvula, and the paraflocculus (hatched in Fig. 5-1, to the left). This nomenclature will be employed here.

The subdivision of the cerebellum arrived at on the basis of comparative anatomical data, briefly outlined above, on the whole *corresponds to a subdivision made on the basis of the afferent cerebellar fiber connections.* (See, however, below.)

The archicerebellum is therefore sometimes referred to as the *vestibulocerebellum* (see Fig. 5-1), the paleocerebellum as the *spinocerebellum,* and the neocerebellum as the *pontocerebellum.* The basis for these designations, which will often be employed in this text, will be considered in a following section. Until fairly recently there has been some uncertainty concerning the homologies of some cerebellar lobules in man (especially in its posterior parts) with those of other mammals. Since most of our knowledge of the fiber conections and functional features of the various cerebellar subdivisions are derived from studies of animals, it is of interest that the main homologies appear now to be clarified, as shown in Fig. 5-2.

The paraflocculus, especially, has been the subject of much dispute. According to recent comparative anatomical studies (Scholten, 1946; Jansen, 1950, 1954) the ventral part of the mammalian paraflocculus (the ventral paraflocculus) is homologous with the tonsilla of the human cerebellum, while the dorsal paraflocculus corresponds to the lobulus biventer. The paramedian lobule, on which much experimental information is available, corresponds to the lobulus gracilis. The paraflocculus, medially connected with the uvula and pyramis, is a peculiar part of the cerebellum, being enormous in aquatic mammals (see Jansen, 1950). Little is so far known of its function. Anatomical (Walberg, 1956) and physiological (Jansen, Jr., 1957) studies indicate that it is acted upon by the periaqueductal gray via the inferior olive. There are indications, among other things from studies of its fiber connections, that the ventral and dorsal paraflocculus are functionally

[1] For reviews of the comparative anatomy, embryology, and fiber connections of the cerebellum see Dow (1942a), Larsell (1945), Jansen and Brodal (1954, 1958), and Larsell (1967).

dissimilar. It is questionable whether the entire paraflocculus should be grouped with the paleocerebellum as in Fig. 5-1.

In the following account the various cerebellar lobules will be referred to as they are found in the cat and monkey. The names applied to corresponding lobules in the human cerebellum can be seen from the diagram of Fig. 5-2. Here are also included the Roman numerals for the various lobules, suggested by Larsell (1952, 1953) and now commonly used. For example, the pyramis and uvula are labeled VIII and IX, respectively, the nodulus being lobulus X. Corresponding hemispheral parts are referred to as VIIIH etc. A detailed description of the human cerebellum can be found in the atlas of Angevine, Mancall, and Yakovlev (1961).

The cerebellar cortex. On account of its many deep sulci the cerebellar cortex covers a very large surface area. If the human cerebellar cortex is imagined unfolded the distance from its most anterior to its

FIG. 5–2 Diagram of the subdivision of the human cerebellum, based on comparative studies of the mammalian cerebellum. In the left half of the diagram the classical names of the various lobules are shown, to be compared with the names used in mammals in general in the right half. On the left is further indicated the principal subdivision of the cerebellum in the flocculonodular lobe and corpus cerebelli, the latter again being subdivided into an anterior and a posterior lobe. In the vermis the Roman numerals I to X suggested by Larsell (1952, and later) for the transverse foliation are shown. Finally the longitudinal subdivision into vermis, intermediate zone, and lateral part (cf. text) is indicated. Abbreviations for vermal lobules: *Li.:* lingula; *L.c.:* lobulus centralis; *Cu.:* culmen; *De.:* declive; *F.v.* and *T.v.:* folium and tuber vermis; *P.:* pyramis; *U.:* uvula; *N.:* nodulus. From Jansen and Brodal (1958).

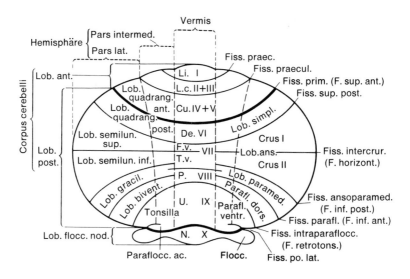

most posterior part exceeds one meter (Braitenberg and Atwood, 1958). Since most folia run transversely the lateral extent of the cortex is only about one seventh of the longitudinal.

In spite of some regional variations, the *cerebellar cortex is principally identically structured all over.*[2] (For details the reader is referred to other sources, for example, Jansen and Brodal, 1958; Fox et al., 1967; Eccles, Ito, and Szentágothai, 1967; in the two latter publications electron microscopic data is included.) Here only some major points will be mentioned with reference to the diagram of Fig. 5-3.

The cerebellar cortex has three distinct layers, the *molecular layer,* the *Purkinje cell layer,* and the *granular layer.* The latter borders on the white matter. The most conspicuous cellular elements in the cortex are the *Purkinje cells.* The axons of the large flask-shaped, regularly arranged cell bodies are given off into the white matter, while richly branched dendritic trees extend outward into the molecular layer. It is peculiar that the dendritic tree is spread out in one plane only, perpendicular to the longitudinal axis of the folium, and that each tree appears to have its own territory. Except for the initial smooth branches, the dendritic branches are densely beset with spines, which are contacted by the afferent parallel fibers (see below). The axons, which pass either to the intracerebellar nuclei or the vestibular nuclei, give off recurrent collaterals which establish contact with *Golgi cells.*

The latter are found in the *granular layer,* which is made up chiefly of an enormous number of densely packed small cells, with very scanty cytoplasm, the *granular cells.* In Golgi preparations these are seen to be provided with about four to five dendrites, radiating in various directions and ending with clawlike expansions (see Fig. 5-3). These are synaptically contacted by endings of mossy fibers (see below). The axons of the granule cells are characteristic. They ascend to the molecular layer where they bifurcate in a T-shaped manner, the two branches, called *parallel fibers,* running always along the longitudinal extent of the folia across the dendritic trees of the Purkinje cells.

Together the two branches of the parallel fibers are 1.5–3 mm long in the cat (Fox and Barnard, 1957), and even longer in man (Braitenberg and Atwood, 1958). Electron microscopic studies have shown that they establish synaptic contact with the dendritic spines of the Purkinje cells (in addition they contact stellate, basket, and Golgi cells). The number of parallel fibers passing through the dendritic tree of a single Purkinje cell has been estimated to be about 200,000 (Fox and Barnard, 1957). It follows from this arrangement that a single parallel fiber may

[2] However, there are variations as to details. The flocculonodular lobe, for example, differs from other parts with regard to the types of mossy fibers present (Brodal and Drabløs, 1963) and with regard to the Golgi cells and myelinated fibers (see also Brodal, 1967a).

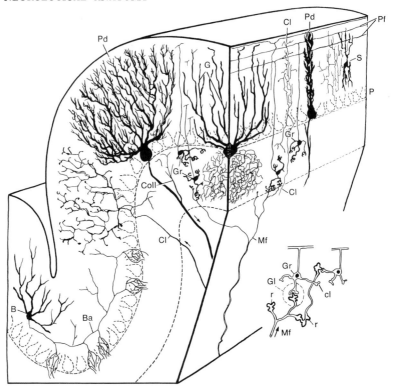

FIG. 5–3 Semidiagrammatic representation of part of a cerebellar folium to show the main elements of the cerebellar cortex and their topographical relationships and orientation. Note especialy the arrangement of the Purkinje cell dendrites (*Pd*) and basket cell axons (*Ba*) in the transverse plane of the folium and the longitudinal arrangement of the parallel fibers (*Pf*). Other abbreviations: *B*: basket cell; *Cl*: climbing fiber; *Coll*: recurrent collateral of Purkinje cell; *G*: Golgi cell; *Gr*: granule cell; *Mf*: mossy fiber; *P*: Purkinje cell; *Pd*: Purkinje cell dendrites; *Pf*: parallel fiber; *S*: stellate cell. Slightly altered from Jansen and Brodal (1958). The figure below to the right illustrates diagrammatically the relation between the rosettes (*r*) of the mossy fibers (*Mf*) with the dendritic "claws" (*cl*) of the granule cells (*Gr*) in a glomerulus (*Gl*). Other elements of the glomerulus are not shown. Adapted from Hámori and Szentágothai (1966a).

act on a large number of Purkinje cells (probably some 450) situated along a folium, and that each Purkinje cell is under the influence of a tremendous number of granule cells (see Fox, Siegesmund, and Dutta, 1964).

The other element in the granular layer, *the Golgi cell* referred to above, in some respects resembles the Purkinje cell. The Golgi cells are large and have branching dendritic trees which largely extend outward into the molecular layer, but unlike those of the Purkinje cells, these trees spread their branches in all directions (see Fig. 5-3). The dendrites are contacted by parallel fibers as well as other afferents (some dendrites remain in the granular layer and are contacted by mossy fibers). The axons of the Golgi cells are richly branched but do not leave the cerebellar cortex. They end in synaptic contact with dendrites of granule cells.

The *molecular layer* is dominated by fibers and contains relatively few nerve cells. Some of these are stellate cells, of which there are several varieties. A particular type is the so-called *basket cell*. These cells are situated just above the Purkinje cells. Their dendrites, like those of the Purkinje cells, are oriented in the transverse plane of the folium and receive collaterals of climbing fibers (see below). The characteristic feature of the basket cells is the arrangement of their axon. This passes for a considerable distance across the folium, immediately above the Purkinje cell bodies and at right angles gives off descending collaterals. These collateral branches surround the cell bodies of the Purkinje cell as a kind of basket (hence the name of the cells) and establish synaptic contact with it. The arrangement of the basket cells makes them capable of acting on a series of Purkinje cells arranged across the folium, in contrast to the parallel fibers which provide for an activation of a series of Purkinje cells along the folium. These and other peculiar geometrical arrangements are of interest in analyses of the function of the cerebellar cortex.

The *afferent fibers entering the cerebellar cortex* are of two entirely different types (see Fig. 5-3). The *climbing fibers* are thin and pass, without dividing, through the granular layer. At the level of the Purkinje cells each fiber divides into several branches, which closely follow and wind along the dendritic branches of a Purkinje cell. Synaptic contacts are established with the smooth parts of these dendrites, but electron microscopic studies have revealed contacts with spines also. While the main target of a climbing fiber is thus the dendrites of a Purkinje cell, some of their collaterals end on neighboring Purkinje cells, stellate cells, basket cells, and Golgi cells (Scheibel and Scheibel, 1954; Hámori and Szentágothai, 1966a). It appears from this anatomical arrangement that the climbing fibers must be able to exert a powerful synaptic action on the Purkinje cell, as has indeed been found to be the case (see below). The majority of the climbing fibers come from the inferior olive (Szentágothai and Rajkovits, 1959), but some may come from other nuclei in the brain stem.[3]

---

[3] It is often stated that there is a specific relation of one climbing fiber to one Purkinje cell. Whether this is so remains to be settled; likewise, whether or not all climbing fibers come from the inferior olive. In this connection it is of interest that the number of nerve cells in both olives of man is about one million

The other type of afferent cerebellar fiber, the *mossy fiber*, differs in almost all respects from the climbing fiber. The mossy fibers are relatively thick. Having entered the cerebellar cortex they branch repeatedly. One fiber may supply two or even more folia. During their course they give off abundant collaterals, which, like the final branches, end in the granular layer with a cluster of small endings, forming what is often referred to as *rosettes*. These endings interdigitate with and are in synaptic contact with the clawlike dendritic terminations of the granule cells (see Fig. 5-3). The contacting elements belong to what is usually called a *cerebellar glomerulus*.

In cell-stained sections the glomeruli appear as empty spaces among the granule cells ("cerebellar islands") since the nerve endings do not stain. There has been much diversity of opinion concerning the nature of the cerebellar glomeruli, but electron microscopic studies appear finally to have established their architecture (Gray, 1961; Hámori and Szentágothai, 1966b; Fox et al., 1967; and others). As referred to above, axons of Golgi cells likewise end in the glomerulus (see Fig. 1-5G) where they contact granule cell dendrites (and dendrites of Golgi cells are contacted by mossy terminals). Since a single mossy fiber gives off collaterals to a large number of rather widely dispersed granule cells, and these give rise to the parallel fibers, it follows that an impulse entering the cerebellar cortex in a mossy fiber may act on a rather large cortical area. On account of the arrangement of the parallel fibers, this area will be long in the direction of the folium but relatively narrow in the transverse plane.

Most afferents to the cerebellar cortex, except those from the inferior olive, appear to end as mossy fibers. However, there appear to be certain differences between mossy fibers from various sources with regard to their degree of branching within the granular layer and presumably also in other respects (for some data see Brodal, 1967a).

The above account of the main features of the structure of the cerebellar cortex shows that this is indeed a very regularly constructed part of the brain. It is a likely assumption that this regularity and the geometrical patterns among its elements are reflected functionally also. The regularity, furthermore, facilitates functional studies. In recent years much work has been devoted to the analysis of the physiology of the cerebellar cortex, particularly by Eccles and his collaborators. From a series of detailed experimental studies there has emerged a picture of the mode of working of the cerebellar cortex that will be briefly considered below. (For reviews and references, see Eccles, 1966a; Eccles,

(Moatamed, 1966; Escobar et al., 1968). This is only 1/15 of the calculated number of Purkinje cells (Braitenberg and Atwood, 1958). In the cat Escobar et al. found some 140,000 cells in both olives. The number of Purkinje cells in the cat has not yet been determined.

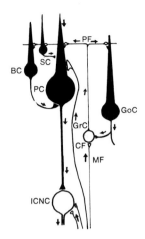

FIG. 5-4 Diagram of the most significant neuronal connections in the cerebellar cortex, according to physiological studies of Eccles and his collaborators. Cells and terminals shown in black are inhibitory. Abbreviations: *BC:* basket cell; *CF:* climbing fiber; *GoC;* Golgi cell; *GrC:* granule cell; *ICNC:* intracerebellar nuclei; *MF:* mossy fiber; *PC:* Purkinje cell; *SC:* stellate cell. (Cf. text.) From Eccles (1966[n]).

Ito, and Szentágothai, 1967.) The main conceptions are summarized in Fig. 5-4, in which the actual anatomical arrangements are represented in a diagrammatic and simplified way.

One essential point is that the climbing fiber exerts a powerful excitatory action on the Purkinje cell. Stimulation of the inferior olive elicits excitatory monosynaptic responses in the Purkinje cells. The mossy fiber impulses have been found to excite the granule cells. The parallel fibers (i.e. the axons of the granule cells) excite the Purkinje cells (by way of their contact with its dendritic spines). Thus, both mossy and climbing fiber inputs to the cortex may excite the Purkinje cells. However, the situation is far more complex, particularly as concerns the mossy fibers. The granule cell axons (parallel fibers), in addition to exciting Purkinje cells, establish synaptic contacts with dendrites of basket and Golgi cells, both of which are inhibitory. The basket cell will thus inhibit the Purkinje cell, the Golgi cell will inhibit the granule cell and will then "counteract" the excitatory effects of mossy fiber impulses on the Purkinje cells. Since the inhibitory pathways to the Purkinje cells include one synapse more than the excitatory route (see Fig. 5-4), stimulation of parallel fibers gives rise first to an excitatory postsynaptic potential (EPSP) in the Purkinje cell, followed 1–2 msecs later by an inhibitory potential (IPSP). This will tend to limit the area of cortex excited by an incoming volley. A final point deserves mention. It has been concluded (Ito and Yoshida, 1966) that the Purkinje cells have a purely inhibitory action on the cells with which they establish synaptic contact (intracerebellar nuclei, vestibular nuclei). Not all authors are convinced, however, that this is so for all Purkinje cells.

The diagram of Fig. 5-4 shows only some of the many possible circuits which may be followed by the impulses set up in the cerebellar cortex on activation of climbing and mossy fibers. Obviously, the time of arrival of afferent impulses will be of importance for the resulting activity. It should, furthermore, be recalled that the mossy fibers ending in a particular region are derived from many sources, carrying information of different kinds and of different physiological significance. Conditions are certainly extremely complex, and far more so in the living being than in the experimental animal where one or a few elements are studied separately. Nevertheless, the new data has given rise to interesting discussions of the working machinery of the cerebellar cortex and has prompted the construction of models of its principal mode of function, in which deductions based on the observations of the properties of the various elements and their geometrical arrangement have been combined. For an account of these subjects the reader is referred to Eccles (1966a) and Eccles, Ito, and Szentágothai (1967).

The intracerebellar nuclei, the corticonuclear projection, and the longitudinal zonal subdivision of the cerebellum. In man there are four distinct cellular masses in the white matter of each half of the cerebellum. Most medial is the *fastigial nucleus,* then follow more laterally two minor masses, the *globose and emboliform nuclei,* and most laterally, deep in the hemisphere, the characteristic *dentate nucleus,* appearing in sections as a wrinkled band of gray matter (see Jansen and Brodal, 1958, for particulars). In the monkey, cat, and other mammals it is common to distinguish three nuclei: a *nucleus medialis,* corresponding to the fastigial nucleus; a *nucleus interpositus,* supposed to correspond to the globose and emboliform; and finally a *nucleus lateralis,* corresponding to the dentate nucleus. Differing opinions have been held concerning the homologies of the various nuclei in man and mammals, particularly the interpositus. However, it appears to be settled that the fastigial nucleus in man represents the medial nucleus in other mammals. The dentate nucleus corresponds largely to the lateral nucleus, but the exact transition between the lateral nucleus and the nucleus interpositus has been difficult to define. The final answer will probably have to await further studies of the connections of these two nuclear groups.

Flood and Jansen (1961) conclude from a cytoarchitectonic study in the cat that part of what has often, in this animal, been considered as belonging to the lateral nucleus (for example by Snider, 1940; Jansen and Brodal, 1940, 1942) actually belongs to the interpositus. Courville and Brodal (1966) concluded that the border between these two nuclei should be placed even a little more laterally than suggested by Flood and Jansen (1961). The latter authors emphasized that the nucleus interpositus in the cat, as in most mammals, is actually two nuclei, *a nucleus interpositus anterior* and a *nucleus interpositus posterior,* a point which is further supported by studies of the intracerebellar nuclei in whales (Korneliussen and Jansen, 1965). The intracerebellar nuclei contain cells of different types, and to some extent particular cytoarchitectonic subdivisions can be recognized (see Jansen and Jansen, Jr., 1955; Flood and Jansen, 1961).

It appears that the axons of all cells in the intracerebellar nuclei pass out of the cerebellum.[4] On the whole the efferents from each nucleus have their particular destinations, as will be described in a following section, indicating that the nuclei differ functionally. Furthermore, the phylogenetic development of the intracerebellar nuclei follows the development of the cerebellar cortex. For example, it is only in primates that the dentate (lateral) is clearly the largest of the nuclei, in keeping with the marked increase in size of the cerebellar hemispheres. In fact, each of the nuclei appears to be anatomically and functionally related to a particular region of the cerebellar cortex. This becomes evident especially in the arrangement of the projection of the cerebellar cortex onto the nuclei. As mentioned above this projection is made up of the axons of the Purkinje cells. Following lesions in various parts of the cerebellar cortex the sites of terminations of the Purkinje cell axons from these parts have been studied by several authors with the Marchi method. In studies of this kind in the rabbit, cat, and monkey (Jansen and Brodal, 1940, 1942) it appeared that the cerebellum can be subdivided into three longitudinal zones (see Fig. 5-5). The vermis, in a restricted sense, sends its fibers to the fastigial nucleus, the anterior parts of the vermis to the rostral part of the nucleus, the posterior to the caudal. There is thus a fanlike arrangement within this zonal projection. In a corresponding manner, the nucleus interpositus receives its cortical afferents from a zone lateral to the vermis in the restricted sense. This zone was called the *intermediate zone* following Hayashi's (1924) developmental studies. In the caudal part of the cerebellum it covers the paramedian lobule. The *lateral zone,* comprising the hemispheres, sends its fibers to the lateral (dentate) nucleus.[5] The principal zonal arrangement is seen in the diagram of Fig. 5-6.

In recent years the corticonuclear projection has been studied in various mammals with silver impregnation methods (Eager, 1963a, 1966; Goodman, Hallett, and Welch, 1963; Walberg and Jansen, 1964; Voogd, 1964). It has been maintained that the projection may not be as precise as it appears in Figs. 5-5 and

[4] Following transection of all three cerebellar peduncles in newborn kittens, the ensuing changes in the nuclei are so marked that it is unlikely that some of the few remaining normal cells are short axoned (internuncial) cells (Jansen and Jansen, Jr., 1955; Flood and Jansen, 1966). The view that some nuclear cells give off climbing fibers to the cerebellar cortex (Carrea, Reissig, and Mettler, 1947) appears to rest on inconclusive evidence. See Eccles, Ito, and Szentágothai (1967) for further data on these nuclei.

[5] Concerning the paraflocculus, its projection onto the lateral as well as to the interpositus nucleus deserves further study, particularly since certain findings indicate that the dorsal and ventral paraflocculus differ in some respects. The parallel great development of the paraflocculus and the interpositus posterior in whales suggests that they are closely related (Korneliussen and Jansen, 1965).

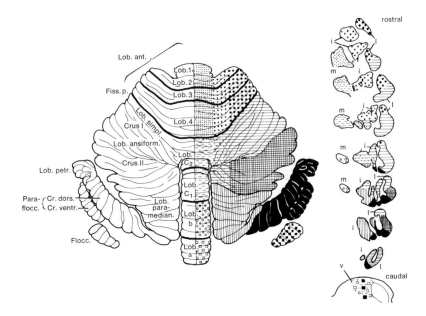

FIG. 5–5 A diagram of the corticonuclear projection in the cerebellum of the monkey based on experimental investigations. Corresponding areas of the cortex and the nuclei labelled with identical symbols. *m:* nucleus medialis s. fastigii; *i:* nucleus interpositus; *l:* nucleus lateralis s. dentatus; *v:* vestibular nuclei. The projection of the flocculonodular lobe after Dow (1936, 1938a). From Jansen and Brodal (1942).

5-6. However, when very small lesions are made, a rather discrete patch of degeneration is found in the nuclei.[6] The change in position of the lateral lobules during development may create difficulties of interpretation concerning these parts. At present it appears extremely likely that the idea of an orderly longitudinal zonal projection is in principle correct (see, however, Voogd, 1964). This view receives support from studies of cerebellar function (see below) and of the patterns of distribution of cerebellar afferents, to be discussed in the following section. These, as well as studies on the ontogenesis of the cerebellar cortex in the whale and the rat (Korneliussen, 1967, 1968), have shown that the vermal and the intermediate zones may be even further subdivided longitudinally.

The Purkinje cell axons end as a bushy network of collaterals within the nuclei, each fiber thus supplying a small area (Cajal, 1909–11).

[6] It should be recalled that in anatomical studies it is almost impossible to demonstrate these relations precisely, since the degeneration following a minimal lesion of the cortex will be too scanty to be identified. Furthermore, the anatomical spread of fibers from a small part of the cortex is likely to exceed the central area from which potentials may be picked up. (Cf. the principle of lateral inhibition, referred to in Chapter 2.)

Experimental electron microscopic studies show that the terminals end in synaptic contact with somata as well as thin and thick dendrites (Mugnaini and Walberg, 1967), a point of relevance to the claim, mentioned above, that all Purkinje axons are inhibitory.

Another subject which has a bearing on this hypothesis concerns the presence of *other afferents to the intracerebellar nuclei,* besides those from the cerebellar cortex. (If the latter are only inhibitory it must either be supposed that there are other afferents which may excite the cells or they must be "spontaneously" active, the latter assumption being unlikely.) Many authors have concluded from Marchi studies that several afferent cerebellar tracts end in or give off collaterals to the intracerebellar nuclei. It is, however, possible that the degeneration observed has been due to degenerating fibers of passage. In silver-impregnated material Grant (1962a) searched in vain for evidence of terminations of spinocerebellar fibers in the fastigial nucleus, and, following transection of the vestibular nerve, Brodal and Høivik (1964) found degeneration only in one particular small region of the lateral nucleus. Apart from the latter, fibers from the red nucleus to the nucleus interpositus (Courville and Brodal, 1966) have been demonstrated conclusively as ending in the intracerebellar nuclei. There is indirect evidence (Brodal, 1940b) that fibers from certain parts of the inferior olive may end in the intracerebellar nuclei

FIG. 5–6   A simplified diagram of the longitudinal zonal subdivision of the mammalian cerebellum based on the pattern in the corticonuclear projection. The cortical sites of origin of fibers to the various intracerebellar nuclei and the vestibular nuclei are indicated by corresponding symbols as in the nuclei. From Jansen and Brodal (1958).

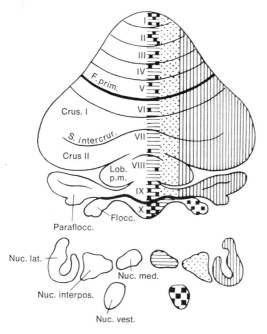

(see Fig. 5-9). Szentágothai (see Eccles, Ito, and Szentágothai, 1967) recently reports the termination of spinocerebellar and other cerebellar afferent fibers in the intracerebellar nuclei. In view of the many recent and detailed neurophysiological studies on these nuclei, there is an urgent need for more precise information of their anatomical organization.

Afferent cerebellar connections and the somatotopical localization within the cerebellum. The idea that a somatotopical localization might exist within the cerebellum was first set forth by the Dutch anatomist Bolk, in 1906, on the basis of comparative anatomical investigations in mammals. Bolk concluded that there was a parallelism between the development of certain parts of the cerebellum and particular parts of the body in respect to their muscular masses. Thus, the part of the corpus cerebelli situated immediately behind the fissura prima, called by Bolk the lobulus simplex (see Fig. 5-1), was assumed to be concerned in the co-ordination of the neck muscles, an assumption which received support from the fact that this lobule is particularly well developed in the giraffe. The extremities were "localized" to the large lateral parts of the cerebellum, the upper extremity in the anterior part (Bolk's crus I of his lobulus ansiformis), the lower extremities in the posterior part of this lobule (crus II). Bolk's hypothesis was received with enthusiasm. However, when physiological experiments were performed to test it, neither stimulation nor extirpation yielded conclusive evidence in favor of the hypothesis, and anatomical studies brought forward data which were more or less incompatible with his view.

The first convincing demonstration that there is a somatotopical localization within certain parts of the cerebellum came with the works of Adrian (1943) and Snider and Stowell (1942, 1944), in which it was shown that stimulation (natural or electrical) of nerves from various parts of the body gives rise to action potentials in specific regions of the cerebellar cortex depending on which part of the body is involved. Thus, as seen from Fig. 5-7, potentials arising in the hindlimb are found in the anterior part of the ipsilateral anterior lobe and in the caudalmost part of the paramedian lobule (bilaterally), while the forelimb is "represented" in the caudal part of the anterior lobe and rostrally in the paramedian lobule (bilaterally). Furthermore, face areas were found (see Fig. 5-7). It is to be noted that these responses were most easily obtained from skin receptors or cutaneous nerves. Finally, Snider and Stowell found that in the middle part of the vermis there is a zone (overlapping the face areas) where action potentials occur following acoustic and optic stimuli. Further studies demonstrated that the same somatotopical regions of the cerebellum could be activated by stimulation of the corresponding bodily areas in the sensorimotor region of the contralateral cerebral cortex

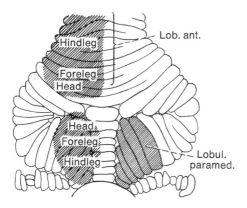

FIG. 5–7 Diagram of the surface of the cerebellar cortex of the monkey, showing (shaded) the areas in which discrete movements of hairs on the left side of the body give rise to action potentials. The somatotopical "representation" is indicated. In the middle part of the vermis and overlapping with the "head areas" is the audiovisual area. (Cf. text.) From Snider (1950).

(Adrian, 1943; Snider and Eldred, 1948, 1951, 1952; Hampson, 1949), and that stimulation of the acoustic and optic regions of the cerebral cortex give rise to potentials in the audiovisual area of the cerebellum (Snider and Eldred, 1948; Hampson, 1949; Hampson, Harrison, and Woolsey, 1952). These findings have been confirmed and amplified by other workers, and further particulars concerning the somatotopical cerebellar localization have been discovered. Some of these will be considered later. So far a somatotopical localization has been found to exist only for the vermis and the intermediate zone, corresponding to the somewhat imprecise term "spinocerebellum." There appears to be a corresponding pattern in Bolk's crus II of the neocerebellum (see Jansen, Jr., 1957; Sousa-Pinto and Brodal, 1969), while there is no evidence as concerns the flocculonodular lobe. Since a discussion of these problems presupposes a knowledge of the connections of the various parts of the cerebellum, further comment will be postponed until the connections have been dealt with.

The *afferent connections to the cerebellum* may, as stated earlier, be schematically divided into three main categories: 1) fibers from the vestibular nerve and vestibular nuclei; 2) pathways mediating impulses from the spinal cord to the cerebellum; 3) pathways transmitting impulses from the cerebral cortex and certain nuclei in "higher parts" of the central nervous system. Pathways of groups 2 and 3 are to some extent synaptically interrupted in the same brain stem nuclei.

1. The *vestibulocerebellar fibers* are in part *primary,* i.e. their peri-

karya are found in the vestibular ganglion, and in part *secondary,* arising from cells in the vestibular nuclei. The former fibers were traced with the Marchi method by Dow (1936), in the cat and rat, to the flocculus, the nodulus, the ventral part of the uvula, and the fastigial nucleus. Following electrical stimulation of the statoacoustic nerve cerebellar action potentials were recorded in the same regions (Dow, 1939). With silver impregnation methods fibers were, in addition, found in the cat to end in the ventral paraflocculus (see Fig. 5-8), while none were found in the fastigial nucleus (Brodal and Høivik, 1964), and it was established that the fibers end as mossy fibers.[7] The *secondary vestibular fibers,* according to Dow (1936), terminate in the same regions of the cerebellum. Probably they end as mossy fibers (Carrea, Reissig, and Mettler, 1947).

It is of interest that the area of origin of secondary vestibulocerebellar fibers (Brodal and Torvik, 1957) is restricted to certain regions of the medial and descending vestibular nucleus as well as to the group x (of Brodal and Pompeiano, 1957) since neither of these nuclear regions appear to receive primary vestibular fibers (Walberg, Bowsher, and Brodal, 1958). The main afferents to the group x come from the spinal cord (see Brodal and Angaut, 1967), indicating that spinal impulses reach the "vestibulocerebellum." The secondary vestibular fibers, therefore, are apparently not substantial in mediating vestibular impulses to the cerebellum.

The primary vestibulocerebellar fibers pass through or close to the superior vestibular nucleus. There are some indications in the literature (see Brodal, Pompeiano, and Walberg, 1962) that the fibers to this nucleus are derived from the cristae of the semicircular ducts, as indeed recently confirmed by Stein and Carpenter (1967). It is likely, therefore, that the vestibular impulses to the cerebellum come mainly from the semicircular ducts (see also Ch. 7).

2. *Spinocerebellar pathways.* One often thinks only of the classical dorsal and ventral spinocerebellar tracts as belonging to this group. However, there are in addition several other routes for impulses from the spinal cord to the cerebellum: the cuneocerebellar tract, a recently discovered rostral spinocerebellar tract, and further pathways which have a synaptic interruption in nuclei of the brain stem and therefore are less direct. Of these the spino-olivo-cerebellar and the spino-reticulo-cerebellar are the most important. The various pathways differ in some respects anatomically and functionally.

The *dorsal spinocerebellar tract and the cuneocerebellar tract.* The former tract has been known for a long time to arise from the cells of Clarke's column or the nucleus dorsalis (see Fig. 2-7), found in the base of the dorsal horn (in Rexed's lamina VII, see Fig. 2-2) at levels from

[7] The termination of primary vestibular fibers outside the flocculonodular lobe makes it clear that the "vestibulocerebellum" exceeds the territory of this lobe (see Brodal and Høivik, 1964; Brodal, 1967a).

Th_1 to L_2 in man (in the cat it extends to L_3-L_4). The rather thick and myelinated axons of the tract turn laterally into the ipsilateral lateral column, where they ascend dorsolaterally to the area of the lateral cortico-spinal tract (Fig. 2-7), arranged in a segmental manner (Yoss, 1952). Via the restiform body, the fibers enter the cerebellum where they terminate in its "spinal regions" (see below).

The *column of Clarke* is slender rostrally and increases in volume caudally. This is related to its supply by afferent fibers, i.e. branches of dorsal root fibers. These branches may ascend ipsilaterally in the dorsal column for many segments before ending in the nucleus (Pass, 1933; Liu, 1956; Grant and Rexed, 1958; and others; Hogg, 1944, in man), and its caudal part is, therefore, charged with receiving the afferents not only from its own segments but also from the segments below (where the column is not present). The contribution of afferents from the upper thoracic levels is modest. The afferent fibers are distributed in a regular segmental somatotopical pattern (Szentágothai, 1961), the fibers from each segment occupying an area which winds spirally along the column. The primary fibers end with large boutons (Szentágothai and Albert, 1955), providing for a potent synaptic action. Cells situated in the gray matter of the cord appear to give off axons to the column as well (Szentágothai, 1961).

It follows from the course of the afferents to the column of Clarke that the dorsal spinocerebellar tract cannot be concerned in the mediation of impulses from the forelimb and only to a lesser extent from the upper part of the trunk. It is now established that *the cervical cord equivalent of the column of Clarke is the external (or accessory) cuneate nucleus* (also called Monakow's nucleus), situated in the medulla lateral and a little rostral to the cuneate nucleus (Fig. 5-11). This nucleus appears to send all its efferents to the cerebellum via the ipsilateral restiform body since practically all its cells disappear following appropriate cerebellar lesions (Ferraro and Barrera, 1935a, in the monkey; Brodal, 1941, in the cat). Its sensory afferents are branches of dorsal root fibers entering in the segments C_1-Th_{4-5}, and they are distributed in a segmental pattern within the nucleus (Ferraro and Barrera, 1935b; Walker and Weaver, 1942; Liu, 1956). The fibers from the nucleus to the cerebellum are usually referred to as the *cuneocerebellar tract*. Anatomically this is for the forelimb, neck, and upper trunk what the dorsal spinocerebellar tract is for the hindlimb and lower trunk. Studies of the terminations within the cerebellum of the two tracts and physiological studies of their functional properties confirm this.

In Marchi studies of the dorsal spinocerebellar tract almost all authors found it to terminate chiefly ipsilaterally in the anterior lobe, covering the vermis and the region which is now referred to as the intermediate zone, and in the posterior vermis, chiefly the pyramis. This has been found also in human material (Brodal and Jansen, 1941;

Marion Smith, 1961). A few authors traced some fibers to the paramedian lobule. Although the presence of a somatotopical mode of termination of spinocerebellar tracts had been suggested on the basis of such material (Vachananda, 1959) it was only by using silver impregnation methods that Grant (1962a) succeeded in demonstrating that in the cat the *dorsal spinocerebellar fibers end only in the cerebellar "hindlimb regions"* (and part of the trunk area, which appears to be small and is difficult to outline) of the anterior lobe and the paramedian lobule as shown in Fig. 5-8. Some fibers end in the caudal part of the pyramis. Likewise, while it has been shown that the external cuneate nucleus projects onto the cerebellar vermis (Brodal, 1941), Grant (1962b) demonstrated that the *termination of the cuneocerebellar tract coincides with the cerebellar "forelimb regions"* as seen in Fig. 5-8. These observations have been substantiated in physiological studies by Lundberg and Oscarsson and their collaborators (for a review see Oscarsson, 1965).

It has been known for some time that the dorsal spinocerebellar tract mediates impulses from proprioceptors (Grundfest and Campbell, 1942; and others). By recordings from single fibers in the dorsal spinocerebellar tract, Lundberg and his associates (see Lundberg and Oscarsson, 1960) have been able to distinguish *several functional components.* The tract conveys information from muscle spindles, tendon organs, pressure receptors in the hairless pads, and from touch and pressure receptors in hairy skin. Many of the fibers of the tract have small receptive fields. Thus some units activated from hairy skin may have receptive fields of only about one square cm, or they may be activated from a single muscle (Lundberg and Oscarsson, 1960). Finally some units convey information from flexor reflex afferents.[8] Corresponding findings have been made concerning the cuneocerebellar tract (Holmqvist, Oscarsson, and Rosén, 1963).

It appears that some neurons of the column of Clarke are modality specific, i.e. they are activated by one kind of receptor only, for example cutaneous, while on other cells information converges from different kinds of receptors (Lundberg and Oscarsson, 1960; Eccles, Oscarsson, and Willis, 1961). Further interesting details of the functioning of some of these cells have been brought forward by Jansen, Nicolaysen, and Rudjord (1966). The activity in the column of Clarke may be influenced from supraspinal levels (Holmqvist, Lundberg, and Oscarsson, 1960). Since descending fibers from supraspinal levels have not been found to end on the

[8] The flexor reflex afferents (often abbreviated to FRA) are defined as those myelinated afferents which, in the spinal animal, evoke the classical flexor reflex, i.e. they give excitation to ipsilateral flexor motoneurons and inhibition to ipsilateral extensor motoneurons (Eccles and Lundberg, 1959). This definition may, however, be too narrow.

272

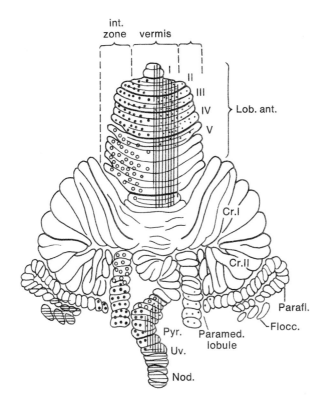

primary vestibulocerebellar fibers

dorsal spinocerebellar tract (hindlimb)

cuneocerebellar tract (forelimb)

ventral spinocerebellar tract (hindlimb)

spino-olivocerebellar fibers

FIG. 5–8 Diagram of the cerebellar surface of the cat showing to the left the sites of termination of dorsal spinocerebellar and cuneocerebellar fibers as determined by Grant (1926a, 1962b). Note somatotopical pattern. The terminal area of primary vestibulocerebellar fibers (Brodal and Hoivik, 1964) is included. On the right are shown the terminal areas of the ventral spinocerebellar fibers according to Grant (1926a) and of the spino-olivo-cerebellar pathway (after Brodal, Walberg, and Blackstad, 1950).

cells (see Nyberg-Hansen, 1966a) this action is presumably indirect, by way of cells in the dorsal horn.

The dorsal spinocerebellar tract in man appears to correspond

273

rather closely to that in the cat and the monkey, as is learned from Marion Smith's (1957, 1961) careful studies of a number of human cases of chordotomies. However, a somatotopical cerebellar termination has not been found (Marion Smith, 1961). Of practical consequence is a shifting of position of the tract as it ascends in the cord.

The *ventral and rostral spinocerebellar tracts* in many ways differ from the two tracts considered above, although like these they are direct pathways from the cord to the cerebellum. The *ventral spinocerebellar tract* (often called Gower's tract) was known to the classical anatomists. It arises from cells in the gray matter of the cord and ascends, segmentally arranged (Yoss, 1953; Marion Smith, 1957, in man), in part ipsilaterally, in part contralaterally, in the lateral funiculus of the cord (see Fig. 2-7), ventral to the dorsal spinocerebellar tract. Unlike this, however, the ventral tract does not enter the cerebellum in the restiform body, but ascends throughout the medulla and most of the pons. It then makes a bend over the trigeminal root fibers and turns dorsolaterally to enter the cerebellum in the superior cerebellar peduncle (Fig. 5-11). According to Marion Smith (1957), in man many fibers join the dorsal spinocerebellar tract.[9] In Marchi studies the fibers of the ventral spinocerebellar tract have been shown by a number of authors to end in the vermis of the anterior lobe, chiefly its anterior portions (for a review, see Jansen and Brodal, 1958). Some students have traced fibers to the posterior vermis and the paramedian lobule. Using silver impregnation methods Grant (1962a) could establish that in the cat the fibers terminate only within the physiologically identified "hindlimb regions" of the anterior lobe and paramedian lobule and in part of the posterior vermis, as shown in Fig. 5-8. On the whole the fibers are distributed somewhat more laterally than those of the dorsal spinocerebellar tract. Some contralateral terminations indicate that some fibers cross the midline in the cerebellum. As one might expect from the site of termination, ventral spinocerebellar fibers have been conclusively demonstrated only from levels of the cord below midthoracic levels. *The tract is thus concerned with transmission of impulses from the hindlimb and lower trunk only,* as confirmed physiologically (see Oscarsson, 1965). The fibers are of different calibers, but on the whole much thinner than those of the dorsal spinocerebellar tract (see Häggqvist, 1936). The cells of origin of the tract have so far escaped anatomical identification, but by recording

[9] In the literature mention is sometimes made of a so-called intermediate spinocerebellar tract. Different opinions have been held about this "tract" which is quantitatively modest (see Marion Smith, 1957; Jansen and Brodal, 1958, for some data).

274

intracellularly in the cord Hubbard and Oscarsson (1962) found cells fulfilling the criteria for cells of origin of the tract in what appears to be Rexed's (1952, 1954) laminae V–VII, chiefly VII, in lumbar segments 3–6 in the cat.

Since the ventral spinocerebellar tract is thus apparently related only to the hindlimb and posterior trunk, it is of great interest that a *forelimb equivalent* has recently been discovered by physiological methods (Oscarsson and Uddenberg, 1964). This tract, which has so far not been anatomically studied, is named the *rostral spinocerebellar tract*. It terminates in the "forelimb" regions of the cerebellum, and appears functionally to correspond in most respects to the ventral spinocerebellar tract (see Oscarsson, 1965). Both tracts have been found to be monosynaptically activated by tendon organ afferents. They are, furthermore, strongly activated polysynaptically by flexor afferent impulses and appear to carry information which is highly integrated at the segmental level. Their cells of origin are acted upon from supraspinal levels, particularly the reticular formation. These tracts differ also from the dorsal spinocerebellar and cuneocerebellar tracts in another respect. While all four tracts appear to end as mossy fibers (see Miskolczy, 1931; Brodal and Grant, 1962; Grant, 1962a; Grant, 1962b), there is physiological evidence that impulses mediated by single fibers in the dorsal spinocerebellar and cuneocerebellar tracts are distributed to much smaller cerebellar areas than are those from the two other tracts, indicating that probably the mossy fibers of the latter branch more amply (see Oscarsson, 1965).

In addition to the spinocerebellar pathways considered above, there are, as already referred to, others which are synaptically interrupted in nuclei of the brain stem. They may collectively be referred to as *indirect spinocerebellar pathways*. One of them has a relay in the inferior olive, the other in the lateral reticular nucleus. Both of these nuclei in addition receive fibers from higher levels, to be considered in the following section of this chapter.

The *inferior olive* is found as a folded gray mass in the medulla, dorsolateral to the pyramid (see Fig. 7-3). It consists of a principal and a dorsal and medial accessory olive, and sends all its axons to the cerebellum. They cross the midline and enter the contralateral restiform body. Henschen, Jr., in 1907, first maintained that the *olivocerebellar projection* in man presents a topical localization, and additional human cases have been described which have verified this. Thus, Holmes and Stewart (1908) were able to collect nine such cases (see further references in Jansen and Brodal, 1958; see also Jakob, 1955). By utilizing the retrograde changes in the inferior olive resulting from circumscribed lesions of the cerebellum in nearly newborn cats and rabbits the olivocerebellar projection has been mapped out in detail (Brodal, 1940b). From the diagram in Fig. 5-9, representing a summary of the findings, it will be seen that the *olivocerebellar localization is astonishingly sharp.* Furthermore, *all parts of the cerebellar cortex and also the intracerebellar nuclei receive olivary fibers.* This has been concluded also from electrophysiological studies (Dow, 1939). As mentioned earlier the olivocerebellar fibers end as climbing fibers. This, as well as the precise topographical pattern in its projection onto the

FIG. 5–9 A diagram of the olivocerebellar connections in the rabbit, based on experimental investigations. Corresponding areas of the inferior olive and the cerebellum are labeled with identical symbols. The inferior olive is imagined unfolded in one plane, as indicated in the section through the inferior olive below. This projection is a good example of the precise topographical relationship which exists between many parts of the nervous system. From Brodal (1940b).

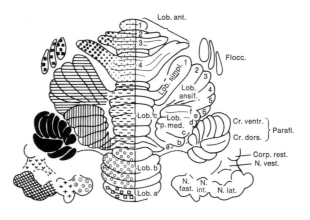

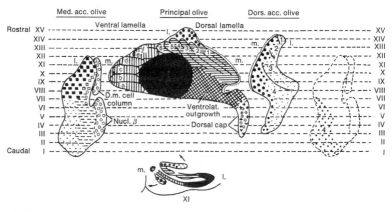

cerebellum, distinguishes the olive from other "precerebellar nuclei." Like recent physiological studies these anatomical features indicate that the inferior olive must play a particular role in cerebellar function. This view is further supported by studies of the *afferents to the olive*. The regions projecting onto particular lobes and lobules of the cerebellum are each supplied from one or more specific sources. Most of the afferents reach the olive from higher levels and will be considered below. As to the *spinal afferents*, precise mapping of their termination shows them to end in those regions of the medial and dorsal accessory olives which send their fibers to the *vermis proper of the anterior lobe and the pyramis and rostral part of the uvula* (Brodal, Walberg, and Blackstad, 1950; Mizuno, 1966), i.e. the *"spinal regions"* (see Fig. 5-8). They supply forelimb as well as hindlimb regions. The fibers arise in the gray matter of the cord and ascend mainly in the contralateral ventral funiculus.

On account of the recent interest in the function of the climbing fibers, the spino-olivary tract has been the subject of several physiological studies. According to Grant and Oscarsson (1966) the tract is activated by cutaneous afferents and high threshold muscle afferents, probably also tendon organ afferents. Oscarsson (1967) has concluded from physiological studies that impulses ascending to the dorsal funiculus reach the "spinal parts" of the olive also via the dorsal column nuclei.[10]

This tract (called the dorsal spino-olivary tract) appears to be activated by the same kind of impulses as the previously known (ventral) spino-olivary tract. According to recent physiological studies (Oscarsson and Uddenberg, 1966; Oscarsson, 1967) both spino-olivo-cerebellar pathways are somatotopically organized. However, it is remarkable that the pattern of localization is longitudinal, thus crossing the somatotopical pattern in the distribution of the direct spinocerebellar paths. The functional significance of this arrangement has been the subject of some speculation, particularly in view of the different types of endings of the fibers, climbing and mossy fibers, respectively (e.g. by Oscarsson, 1967; Eccles, Ito, and Szentágothai, 1967).

The other indirect spinocerebellar pathway involves a synapse in the *lateral reticular nucleus* (nucleus funiculi lateralis) and differs in many respects from the pathways through the inferior olive. The lateral reticular nucleus, situated just lateral to the inferior olive (Fig. 6-2), is composed of cells of different sizes and types. In most mammals a ventrolateral parvicelullar part and a dorsomedial magnocellular part can be distinguished (Walberg, 1952). (Often a subtrigeminal part is

[10] Grant and Boivie are quoted by Oscarsson as having found degeneration in the olive following lesions of the dorsal column nuclei, as has been mentioned in a preliminary report also by Hand and Liu (1966).

also present.) The nucleus appears to send all its efferent fibers via the ipsilateral restiform body to the cerebellum (Blakeslee, Freiman, and Barrera, 1938; Brodal, 1943), where they probably end as mossy fibers (see Miskolczy, 1934). This *reticulocerebellar projection* shows a faint degree of localization, in so far as, for example, the parvicellular part and the adjoining region of the magnocellular part project onto the vermis, the remainder of the latter part to the hemisphere (Brodal, 1943). Like the inferior olive the nucleus receives descending as well as ascending afferents, but in contrast to the olive, the various afferent contingents overlap widely. The *spinal afferents*, which ascend in company with spinothalamic fibers and fibers to other parts of the reticular formation, terminate in a segmental pattern, and chiefly in the region sending fibers to the vermis (Brodal, 1949; and Morin, Kennedy, and Gardner, 1966, in the cat; Mehler, Feferman, and Nauta, 1960, in the monkey; and others). Bohm (1953) and Combs (1956) found that the nucleus is concerned in the transmission of impulses of cutaneous origin. According to Grant, Oscarsson, and Rosén (1966) the spinal afferents to the lateral reticular nucleus carry information concerning flexor reflex patterns. The receptive fields of neurons of the spinoreticular pathway are large and may include all four limbs (Oscarsson and Rosén, 1966b), there is no modality specificity, and the neurons are subject to supraspinal influences from the vestibulospinal as well as the corticospinal pathways. We will return to this and other spinocerebellar pathways in a later section.

In addition to these two indirect spinocerebellar pathways described above mention may be made of some others. In the cat the *paramedian reticular nucleus,* a small but characteristic group of cells in the reticular formation (Brodal, 1953), sends its efferent fibers to the cerebellar vermis (Brodal and Torvik, 1954) and receives some fibers from the cord (Brodal and Gogstad, 1957). The small cell groups surrounding the hypoglossal nucleus, the *perihypoglossal nuclei,* likewise project to the cerebellum (Brodal, 1952) and, at least chiefly, to the vermis (Torvik and Brodal, 1954) and may receive some spinal afferents. Corresponding findings have been made in the monkey (Mehler, Feferman, and Nauta, 1960). Nothing is so far known of the functional role of these nuclei, but it is of some interest that they all receive afferents from the cerebellum.

3. *Pathways mediating impulses to the cerebellum from "higher parts" of the central nervous system.* The expression "higher parts" is here used in a very loose sense, mainly to indicate regions rostral to the spinal cord. There are several connections to be considered under this heading. Among supraspinal regions acting on the cerebellum, the *cerebral cortex* is the most important. It has at its disposal several pathways leading to the cerebellum, all of which ultimately relay cerebral cortical impulses mainly (but not exclusively) to the cerebellar hem-

ispheres. They are all of them interrupted synaptically: in the pontine nuclei, the inferior olive, the lateral reticular nucleus, or in some other cell groups. Direct cerebrocerebellar fibers have never been convincingly demonstrated.

The *most massive cerebrocerebellar route is the cortico-ponto-cere-bellar projection, which has a relay in the pontine nuclei.* In phylogenesis these nuclei increase in size in proportion to the development of the cerebellar hemisphere. The pontine nuclei (see Fig. 7-14) may be sub-divided into several cell groups, although without clear borders, differ-ing with regard to the types and sizes of their cells. It appears from a number of studies, experimental as well as in human material, that all cells of the pontine nuclei send their axons to the cerebellum via the brachium pontis, mainly but not entirely, the contralateral one. The fibers are relatively thin (Szentágothai-Schimert, 1941b) and end as mossy fibers (Snider, 1936; Mettler and Lubin, 1942). Anatomical studies (see Jansen and Brodal, 1958, for a review) indicate that the cerebellar hemispheres are amply supplied with pontine fibers, and that there is a somewhat smaller contribution to the vermis (in these studies the vermis proper and the intermediate zone have not been kept apart). Physiological studies (Dow, 1939; Jansen, Jr., 1957) are in agreement with this. The connection with the hemispheres appears to be contra-lateral, while the projection onto the vermis is bilateral. There is some degree of localization in the pontocerebellar projection, as appears par-ticularly from experimental studies of the changes in the pontine nuclei following lesions of the cerebellum (Brodal and Jansen, 1946). Voogd (1964) made largely corresponding findings following lesions of the pons and in addition advocates the presence of some pontine fibers to the flocculus. Broadly speaking, the lateral and most medial regions of the pontine nuclei project to vermal regions, while the central parts, surrounding the fascicles of the pyramidal tract, send their fibers to the cerebellar hemispheres. In man the situation appears to be similar (for references, see Jansen and Brodal, 1958). It is extremely likely that closer studies may reveal a more detailed pattern in the pontocerebellar projection, an item of considerable interest from the point of view of the cerebrocerebellar functional relationships.

The *corticopontine projection* has been studied by classical anato-mists and is known in broad outlines (for a review, see Jansen and Brodal, 1958). In man and animals these fibers take their origin from all four lobes of the cerebrum and descend with those of the corticospinal tract to the ipsilateral pons. In the cerebral peduncle most of them are situ-ated on either side of the pyramidal tract, as mentioned previously (see Fig. 4-2). The precise termination of the various contingents and their

279

relative quantitative proportions are, however, not yet sufficiently known. Nyby and Jansen (1951), in a Marchi study in the monkey, found that the various contingents have their preferential sites of termination (see also Sunderland, 1940). Thus, the fibers from the occipital and temporal lobes end chiefly in the lateral-most part of the pontine nuclei (which project onto the vermis). There is, however, little doubt that the most massive corticopontine fiber contingent comes from the central region of the cerebral cortex, as appears also from physiological studies (Dow, 1942b; Jansen, Jr., 1957).

As referred to previously (p. 268), physiologically, a somatotopical localization has been demonstrated within the cerebrocerebellar projection onto the "spinal regions" of the cerebellum. It appears from the studies of Jansen, Jr., (1957) that the pathway most likely involves the pontine nuclei. In a recent study of the degeneration in the pontine nuclei (Nauta method) following small lesions of the primary sensory and motor cortices in the cat (P. Brodal, 1968a) it has been shown that the fibers coming from each of these two cortical areas have their particular circumscribed sites of ending within the pontine nuclei and, furthermore, that both contingents betray a clear somatotopical pattern. These anatomical findings leave little doubt that the functionally observed somatotopical relations between the cerebral and cerebellar cortices are indeed chiefly mediated via the pons, the more so since the other cerebrocerebellar routes (see below) are quantitatively very modest.[11]

The fibers from the cerebral cortex are the main afferents to the pontine nuclei. In addition the pons receives some fibers from the tectum, chiefly from the superior colliculus (see Jansen and Brodal, 1958; Pearce, 1960). Finally some fibers have been traced from the spinal cord in the cat (Walberg and Brodal, 1953b; Kerr, 1966).

In connection with the pontocerebellar projection the *pontobulbar body* and the *arcuate nuclei* should be mentioned, both of which appear to be related to the pontine nuclei (Essick, 1912). They are well developed only in man but show individual variations. It appears that they send their efferent fibers to the cerebellum and receive fibers from the cerebral cortex (for references, see Jansen and Brodal, 1958).

The *other cerebrocerebellar pathways* are, as already mentioned, quantitatively far inferior to the corticopontocerebellar. A relatively

[11] It remains to be seen whether the particular pontine regions receiving fibers from various bodily "regions" in the cerebral cortex send their fibers to the corresponding cerebellar regions, but it may almost be predicted that such an arrangement will be found when properly sought for. Not only the primary sensorimotor cortex but the secondary sensory region as well project in a topographically orderly manner onto the pons (P. Brodal, 1968b). This is in agreement with physiological findings.

small number of cortical fibers, chiefly from the primary sensorimotor region, end in the magnocellular part of the *lateral reticular nucleus* (Brodal, Maršala, and Brodal, 1967). Within this *corticoreticular* pathway there is no evidence of localization, and its area of termination in the nucleus overlaps in part with those of fibers from the spinal cord (considered above), from the red nucleus (Courville, 1966a), as well as from the fastigial nucleus (Walberg and Pompeiano, 1960) and the vestibular nuclei (Ladpli and Brodal, 1968). The role of the cortico-reticular fibers in the transmission of information from the cerebrum to the cerebellum has so far not been settled. It should be recalled that the red nucleus, sending fibers to the lateral reticular nucleus, receives a contingent of cortical fibers (see Ch. 4) and thus may also be involved in cerebrocerebellar co-operation via the lateral reticular nucleus.

As referred to above, the *inferior olive* receives some fibers from the cerebral cortex. They end in restricted parts of the olive and will thus be able to influence only certain subdivisions of the cerebellum, among these the intermediate zone of the anterior lobe. This is one of the results of Walberg's (1956, 1960) experimental studies in the cat, which, furthermore has shown that *several nuclei may influence the cerebellum via the olive:* the caudate nucleus, the pallidum, the red nucleus, and the periaqueductal gray. However, the various contingents of olivary afferents end in particular regions of the olivary complex, and thus the various cerebellar lobes differ with regard to the source of information relayed to them via the olive. Such differences must have functional consequences, but almost nothing is known about this so far. It is particularly interesting that the crus I and crus II differ with regard to their olivary afferents. Only the latter is acted upon by the cerebral cortex via the olive.

In a recent anatomical study of the cortico-olivary projection in the cat (Sousa-Pinto and Brodal, 1969) it was shown that the fibers from the "central" region of the cortex, in contrast to the corticopontine fibers, come only from the "motor" region. These fibers are distributed in a somatotopical pattern to restricted parts of the principal olive and the dorsal and medial accessory olives. When this distribution is compared with the map of the olivocerebellar projection (Fig. 5-9) it follows that somatotopically organized impulses may be transmitted from the "motor" cortex via the olive to the intermediate part of the anterior lobe, to the posterior vermis, and to the crus II of the hemisphere. The former two projections agree with the well-known somatotopical pattern in the cerebellum. The somatotopical pattern in the crus II corresponds to that observed by Jansen Jr. (1957) in physiological studies.

The cortico-olivo-cerebellar pathway established anatomically is pre-

2 8 1

sumably involved in the somatotopically organized cerebro-cerebellar impulse transmission even if the cortico-olivary projection is relatively modest. The anatomical differences between the cortico-olivo-cerebellar and the corticopontocerebellar pathways make it appear likely that they differ functionally. A satisfactory correlation of the new anatomical observations with physiological findings is not yet possible, and further research is needed (for some comments see Sousa-Pinto and Brodal, 1969).

The inferior olive and its afferent and efferent connections present several still unsolved problems. As is apparent from the above, particular regions of the olivary complex are related to separate cerebellar lobules or lobes, but each of these olivary regions has its own pattern of afferents. On closer scrutiny it appears that there are at least two types of cells in the olive, which differ with regard to their dendritic patterns (Scheibel and Scheibel, 1955). Furthermore, four kinds of afferent fibers may be distinguished which differ with regard to their terminal patterns and branching within the olive, and presumably, therefore, have different functional properties. However, a study of the distribution of different types of cells and terminations within the olive (Scheibel, Scheibel, Walberg, and Brodal, 1956) did not permit specific correlations between, for example, types of afferent endings and particular sources of afferents. There are, furthermore, differences between certain olivary regions with regard to the degeneration of boutons (Walberg, 1964). Obviously the various parts of the olive differ in anatomical organization, a feature which deserves attention in physiological studies. In order to explain some findings made in recent electrophysiological studies it is postulated that there are interneurons in the olive, and that the axons of the olivary cells (see Eccles, Ito, and Szentágothai, 1967) give off recurrent collaterals. Neither of these features have so far been verified anatomically (see also the physiological study of Crill and Kennedy, 1967). As referred to above, because of their termination as climbing fibers, the olivary afferents are likely to play a special role in the activation of cellular elements in the cerebellar cortex, particularly the Purkinje cells.

In addition to its pathways via the pons, the lateral reticular nucleus, and restricted parts of the inferior olive, the cerebral cortex may act on the cerebellum by way of descending fibers to certain minor cell groups which send their fibers to the cerebellum, such as the paramedian reticular nucleus and the perihypoglossal nuclei. The functional role of these pathways is unknown.

As referred to in the beginning of this section, *action potentials can be recorded in the middle part of the cerebellar vermis following acoustic and optic stimuli, as well as on stimulation of the trigeminal nerve.* As to the other afferent cranial nerves, there is some electrophysiological evidence that vagal and glossopharyngeal impulses reach the cerebellum (see Dow and Moruzzi, 1958), but anatomically little is known of the connections involved. Particularly the acoustic and optic responses have been the subject of extensive physiological studies (see Fadiga and Pupilli, 1964, for a recent exhaustive review). However, our knowledge of the pathways used by the impulses is far from complete.

The Cerebellum

In lower vertebrates fibers from the *trigeminal nerve and nuclei* and some other cranial nerves can easily be traced to the cerebellum (the corpus cerebelli). Such fibers may be assumed to be present also in mammals. In embryos of different mammalian species direct trigeminal fibers can be followed to the corpus cerebelli. According to experimental studies (Whitlock, 1952) there appear to be, in birds, fibers from the principal and spinal trigeminal nucleus, which end in the middle regions of the vermis. Recently Carpenter and Hanna (1961) and Stewart and King (1963) followed fibers to the cerebellum from the spinal trigeminal nucleus in the cat. Since the mesencephalic trigeminal nucleus appears to be concerned in the mediation of proprioceptive impulses from the face (see Ch. 7) it might be assumed that it gives off axons or collaterals to the cerebellum. While such fibers have been described in normal material (Pearson, 1949a, 1949b, in man) attempts to demonstrate their termination experimentally have not given decisive results (see Brodal and Fegersten Saugstad, 1965).

Optic impulses may reach the cerebellum by indirect routes. Fibers of the optic nerve end in the superior colliculus, and it appears (Snider, 1945) that the impulses to the cerebellum are transmitted through this. *Tectocerebellar fibers* may be the link leading to the cerebellum. Such fibers have been described in experimental studies (Ogawa and Mitomo, 1938) as well as in normal material, but their site of ending has not been established, and they appear to be scanty. Another possible and more likely route might be provided by tectopontine fibers (see Pearce, 1960) since these appear to end in regions of the pons which project onto the vermis. For a complete discussion of these problems see Fadiga and Pupilli (1964).

As to the *acoustic impulses,* the routes employed are equally obscure. It appears that destruction of the inferior colliculi prevents acoustic impulses from reaching the cerebellum (Snider and Stowell, 1944).

The action potentials evoked in the middle region of the vermis on stimulation on the acoustic and optic regions of the cerebral cortex most likely reach the cerebellum by way of the cortico-ponto-cerebellar route (see Fadiga and Pupilli, 1964, for particulars).

Efferent cerebellar connections. As described in a preceding section, most Purkinje cell axons end in the intracerebellar nuclei, and this projection is organized in a systematic fashion (see Figs. 5-5, 5-6). When describing the pathways leaving the cerebellum it will be appropriate to consider separately the efferents of the individual nuclei: the fastigial nucleus, acted upon by the vermis proper; the intermediate nucleus, influenced by the intermediate cerebellar cortex; and the lateral nucleus, receiving its afferents from the cerebellar hemispheres. As will be seen, the efferent projections of the three nuclei on the whole have different destinations, a fact further emphasizing the existence of a longitudinal functional subdivision within the cerebellum.

Some of the Purkinje cells, however, do not pass to the intracerebellar nuclei but to the vestibular nuclei. It is appropriate to deal with these *cortical cerebellovestibular projections* first. They *arise in two regions of the cerebellum,* the cortex of the flocculus, nodulus, and the posterior (vestibular) part of the uvula and from the anterior and posterior vermis. The *fibers from the flocculus and nodulus* were investigated in the rat, cat, and monkey by Dow (1936, 1938a) in Marchi preparations. His results have been confirmed and further details revealed by the use of the Nauta method in the cat (Angaut and Brodal, 1967).

The nodulus and the posterior part of the uvula, as well as the flocculus, supply all four nuclei, the floccular projection onto the lateral nucleus being, however, very modest, Furthermore, the flocculus sends fibers to the nucleus of the solitary tract. In keeping with what has been found for other afferents to the vestibular nuclei (see section on the vestibular nerve, Ch. 7), the afferents from the two parts of the vestibulocerebellum concerned in the projection each have their particular sites of termination within the vestibular nuclei, and a correlation of these terminal areas with those of other contingents of afferents is of some interest for functional considerations (see Angaut and Brodal, 1967).

The other contingent of the cortical cerebellovestibular projection, the *pathway from the vermis (proper) to the vestibular nuclei,* is more massive and differently organized. These fibers have been described by several authors, chiefly using the Marchi method, and by some using silver impregnation methods. Walberg and Jansen (1961) in this way could establish two features of considerable interest. In the first place, most of the fibers from the anterior lobe vermis end in the ipsilateral lateral vestibular nucleus, and a few in the adjoining parts of the descending nucleus. Secondly, the projection onto the lateral nucleus is somatotopically organized (Fig. 7-11), fibers from the caudal part of the anterior lobe vermis ending in the "forelimb region" of the nucleus (see also Eager, 1963a; Voogd, 1964). As to the projection from the pyramis and the rostral part of the uvula, the question of a somatotopical arrangement could not be settled. The somatotopical pattern found anatomically is in agreement with the physiological findings of Pompeiano and Cotti (1959). It appears from the above that the two components of the cortical cerebellovestibular projection must obviously be functionally different. Since the lateral vestibular nucleus of Deiters is the source of the massive vestibulospinal tract to the cord (see Ch. 4), the cerebellar vermis by its projection onto this nucleus may act on the spinal cord, while this can be true to a limited extent only for the vestibulocerebellum.

The *cerebellar vermis has, however, other pathways by which it may influence the cord, namely some of the efferent fibers from the fastigial nucleus.* These fibers have been studied by many authors, more recently with silver impregnation methods (Thomas, Kaufman, Sprague, and Chambers, 1956; Carpenter, Brittin, and Pines, 1958; Cohen, Chambers, and Sprague, 1958; Walberg, Pompeiano, Westrum, and Hauglie-Hanssen, 1962; Walberg, Pompeiano, Brodal, and Jansen, 1962). Only some main points will be summarized. The fibers from the rostral part of the nucleus, making up almost half of all fastigiobulbar fibers (Flood and Jansen, 1966), leave the cerebellum in the ipsilateral restiform body. Those coming from the caudal part cross the midline in the cerebellum, in part thereby (unfortunately for experimental studies) passing through the opposite fastigial nucleus. They form the *hook bundle of Russell* (uncinate fasciculus) which bends around the superior cerebellar peduncle. The terminal distributions of the two components differ to some extent, indicating functional differences between the anterior and posterior parts of the fastigial nucleus. Their *main targets are the reticular formation and the vestibular nuclei.*

Many fibers, most of them coming from the caudal part of the fastigial nucleus, are distributed throughout the *medullary and pontine reticular formation,* chiefly contralaterally, without any pattern of localization (Walberg, Pompeiano, Westrum, and Hauglie-Hanssen, 1962). Thus the cerebellar vermis may act on the cord by way of the reticulospinal projections, considered in Chapter 4. Some fibers derived, at least mainly, from the rostral part of the fastigial nucleus, end in the magnocellular part of the lateral reticular nucleus (Walberg and Pompeiano, 1960), which, as we have seen, projects back to the cerebellum. Other components of the fastigiofugal fibers end in all four main *vestibular nuclei.* The projection from the vermis via the fastigial nucleus to the lateral vestibular nucleus is somatotopically organized (see Fig. 7-11).

When this projection is studied in detail (Walberg, Pompeiano, Brodal, and Jansen, 1962) it turns out that the fibers passing ipsilaterally from the rostral part of the fastigial nucleus end in other parts of the vestibular nuclei than do those from the caudal part leaving in the hook bundle (see Fig. 7-11). For example, in the lateral vestibular nucleus the former fibers supply the dorsal half (as do the direct fibers from the anterior lobe vermis), the latter the ventral half. Since the projection from the rostral part of the fastigial nucleus is somatotopically arranged (the same appears to be the case for the posterior part), the anterior lobe vermis (and probably parts of the posterior lobe vermis as well) has at its disposal two somatotopically organized pathways to the lateral vestibular nucleus, one direct and one involving the fastigial nucleus. In addition to efferents to the reticular formation and the vestibular nuclei, the fastigial nucleus also gives off some fibers ascending in the brachium conjunctivum and passing beyond the red nucleus (Jansen and Jansen, Jr., 1955; and others). These appear to end in some of the thalamic nuclei (Thomas et al., 1956; Cohen, Chambers, and Sprague, 1958).

In concordance with the anatomical data, the results of stimulation or destruction of the rostral and caudal parts of the fastigial nucleus are different, as shown in a series of studies by Moruzzi and Pompeiano and collaborators (see Pompeiano, 1967, for a review).

Thus destruction of the caudal part (like ablation of the pyramis and uvula) results in atonia of the contralateral limbs in decerebrate animals (crossed fastigial atonia, Moruzzi and Pompeiano, 1956). Furthermore, the effects from the medial and lateral parts of the rostral half of the nucleus differ, stimulation of the former giving augmentation, of the latter inhibition of postural tonus (Batini and Pompeiano, 1958). In the caudal part there are corresponding differences between medial and lateral regions, but the augmentatory and inhibitory regions are found in the reverse order (Pompeiano, 1962). An anatomical counterpart to these observations of mediolateral differences has not yet been found, but they tally with other findings which indicate that the longitudinal zones of the cerebellum (in this case the vermis proper) can be further subdivided. It is in accord with anatomical data (see above) that the responses following stimulation or localized destructions of the fastigial nucleus are somatotopically organized (see Pompeiano, 1962, 1967).

The literature on the *efferent connections from the nucleus interpositus* is in part difficult to evaluate, since most authors have used rather large lesions which may have interrupted fibers from other nuclei than that said to be damaged. Furthermore, differences in nomenclature and in drawing the border between the nucleus interpositus and the lateral nucleus (see p. 264) have given rise to conflicting statements. It is probably fair to say that information on the precise termination of fibers from each of these nuclei is not yet available. Only some main points will be considered here.

The *nucleus interpositus,* as referred to above, actually consists of an anterior and a posterior nucleus. Like the fastigial, it has turned out to be far more complexly organized than formerly believed. All its efferent fibers appear to leave the cerebellum in the brachium conjunctivum [12] and to course to the *contralateral red nucleus,* where most of them end. Others appear to proceed further as indicated by the presence of retrograde cellular changes in the interpositus following lesions above the red nucleus (Jansen and Jansen, Jr., 1955). Terminations have been described in the ventral lateral thalamic nucleus (VL) as well as in other "specific" and "nonspecific" thalamic nuclei (see Cohen, Chambers, and Sprague, 1958; Jansen and Brodal, 1958). The main influence of the nucleus interpositus (and accordingly the intermediate part of the cerebellar cortex) appears, however, to be on the red nucleus, and via this it may act on the spinal cord.[13] This effect concerns the flexor motoneurons (see Pompeiano, 1967, and Ch. 4 here). In this connection it is of interest that the projection from the nucleus interpositus to the red nucleus (like the rubrospinal tract, see p. 166) is somatotopically arranged as shown anatomically (Courville, 1966c) as well as physio-

[12] The term brachium conjunctivum is here used as a common designation for all ascending fibers in the superior cerebellar peduncle. The latter is a macroscopical anatomical term, and the superior peduncle contains also cerebellar afferents.

[13] Some fibers from the red nucleus pass to the VL and VA of the thalamus (Bowsher and Angaut, 1968), establishing a synaptically interrupted interpositothalamic route in addition to the direct one.

logically (Pompeiano, 1959; Maffei and Pompeiano, 1962a). The red
nucleus cells are monosynaptically excited from the interpositus (see
Tsukahara, Toyama, and Kosaka, 1967), and stimulation of the nucleus interpositus gives responses in flexor muscles in the decerebrate
cat (Pompeiano, 1959). As in the fastigial nucleus, so also in the nucleus interpositus, medial and lateral zones may be distinguished which
differ functionally, and there are functional differences in the pattern in
the anterior and posterior interpositus (see Pompeiano, 1967).

Like the vermis the intermediate part of the cerebellar cortex thus
is able to act on the spinal cord by way of its efferent fibers. This fits in
well with the fact that the main afferents to both these cerebellar zones
transmit information from the spinal cord.

The *lateral (dentate) nucleus,* in contrast to the others, is chiefly
concerned in carrying information from the cerebellum (its hemispheres)
to the cerebral cortex (via the thalamus). The efferent fibers from the
lateral nucleus make up the bulk of the brachium conjunctivum and
cross the midline in the brain stem through the red nucleus. Some authors (Cohen, Chambers, and Sprague, 1958; Voogd, 1964; and others)
have advocated that some of the fibers end here. The majority of fibers
from the dentate proceed rostrally to the thalamus, where their main
terminal station is the nucleus ventralis lateralis (VL, see Fig. 2-12), as
found by the early students (for a review of the literature until 1957,
see Jansen and Brodal, 1958) and confirmed by silver impregnation
studies. However, the terminal area is not restricted to the VL. Some
authors (Cohen et al., 1958) found it to extend into the anteriorly
situated nucleus ventralis anterior (VA). It may also be mentioned
that fibers have been said to end in some of the "nonspecific" thalamic
nuclei. Fibers passing from the rostral part of the red nucleus to the
VA and VL have recently been advocated (Bowsher and Angaut,
1968).

Several authors have traced degeneration to one or more of the "nonspecific"
thalamic nuclei, for example, the centromedian-n. parafascicularis. According to
Mehler's (1966a; 1966b) studies these findings are, however, not valid, a view in
agreement with the conclusions reached by Le Gros Clark (1936) and Walker
(1938a). In man Hassler (1950) advocates terminations in the centromedian and
the mesencephalic tegmentum. In the monkey, fibers from all parts of the dentate
nucleus have been traced to the oculomotor nuclei and the small nuclei in its
vicinity (Carpenter and Strominger, 1964). Finally there is a descending limb of
the brachium conjunctivum which by some has been traced caudally to the level
of the inferior olive, while most authors describe it as ending in the nucleus
reticularis tegmenti pontis (for references, see Jansen and Brodal, 1958).

While the main cerebellar influence on the cerebral cortex occurs via
the lateral (dentate) nucleus, the interpositus and to some extent the

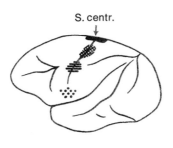
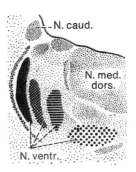

FIG. 5–10 A diagram of the thalamocortical projection to the central region of the cerebral cortex in the monkey, showing the somatotopical pattern in the projection. Corresponding areas of the thalamus and cortex identically labeled. Redrawn from Walker (1934).

fastigial nucleus may also be involved by way of the projections from these nuclei onto the nucleus ventralis lateralis (VL) of the thalamus. This projects onto the precentral gyrus, especially areas 4–6. Within this projection there is a somatotopical pattern (Fig. 5-10), as shown by studies of retrograde cell degeneration (Walker, 1934; see also Chow and Pribram, 1956). It is of particular interest that this pattern has been confirmed in man by recordings of action potentials in the precentral gyrus following stimulation of the VL (Uno et al., 1967). The cortex of the cerebellar hemisphere thus acts primarily on this part of the cerebral cortex. It appears that the cerebellum chiefly facilitates the motor cortex (see Dow and Moruzzi, 1958). From experimental studies in animals (Cooke and Snider, 1953) as well as from studies in man (Snider and Wetzel, 1965) it is learned that stimulation of the cerebellum may influence the electroencephalogram (EEG). However, the cerebral cortex, as we have seen, may act back on the cerebellum by way of the cortico-ponto-cerebellar (and to a lesser extent the cortico-olivo-cerebellar and cortico-reticulo-cerebellar) routes. There is thus a two-way circuit between the cortex of the cerebellar hemisphere and the contralateral "motor" region of the cortex, indicating possibilities for a close cooperation. It has been suggested that the neocerebellum exerts a "stabilizing influence" on the motor cortex. However, while several physiological studies have been devoted to the action of the spinal regions of the cerebellum on the cerebrum, relatively little has so far been done on the influence of the cerebellar hemispheres.

A composite diagram, showing some of the main fiber connections of the cerebellum is reproduced in Fig. 5-11. Before attempting to present, in as integrated a form as possible, the current views on cerebellar func-

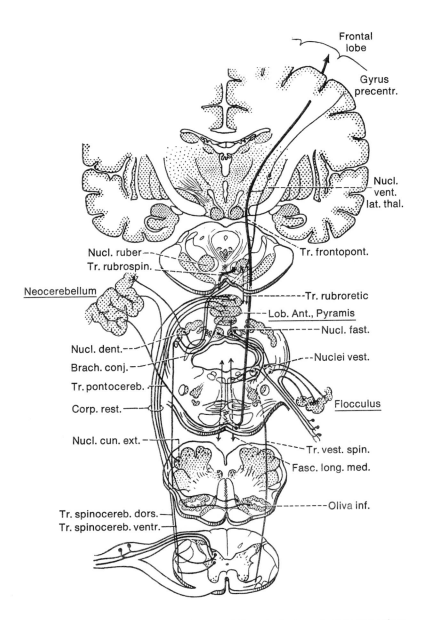

FIG. 5–11 A simplified diagram of some of the principal cerebellar connections. The lateral reticular nucleus and its connections are not included, nor are the spino-olivary and certain other connections shown. Modified and redrawn from Rasmussen (1932).

tion, based largely on experimental evidence, it will be appropriate to describe the symptoms met with in cerebellar affections in man.

Cerebellar symptoms. The classical study of cerebellar symptomatology is still the paper by Gordon Holmes (1939). In recent years relatively few authors have been interested in the subject (see, however, Wyke, 1947; Brown, 1949; Wartenberg, 1954). It has been extensively reviewed by Dow and Moruzzi (1958) and Dow (1969). Leaving for a later section the question whether particular symptoms can be related to specific parts of the cerebellum, the symptoms most commonly observed in cerebellar lesions will be briefly described.

Hypotonia. The tonus of the muscles is reduced; this can usually be ascertained either by palpating the muscles or by examining their resistance to passive movements. When hypotonia is present, the tendon (myotatic) reflexes are usually less brisk than normal, and they may be pendulous. In a unilateral lesion these changes occur on the side of the lesion.

A certain degree of *asthenia* and increased fatigability of the muscles is commonly present together with the hypotonia, and is by some (see Holmes, 1939) regarded as one of the fundamental disturbances in cerebellar lesions.

Other symptoms may be ascribed to a lack of co-operation between the muscles in voluntary contractions, affecting the rate, regularity, and force of the movements. Symptoms of this kind are somewhat difficult to analyze, and have been given different names by various neurologists. However, it appears doubtful that they really are more than different aspects of the same fundamental disturbance. Among such symptoms may be mentioned:

Asynergia. This is defined as a lack of capacity to adjust correctly the impulses of innervation in the various muscles participating in a movement. The different stages of a compound movement are performed as isolated, successive movements, and not as a single synchronous, harmonic performance (*décomposition des mouvements*). The excursions of the movements may be excessive or too small, *dysmetria,* frequently then followed in the next performance by a compensation, leading to an exaggeration in the opposite sense. (Dysmetria is a phenomenon which probably should be included under the more comprehensive heading of asynergia.) The impairment of performing rapid alternate movements, such as pronation and supination of the hand, *dysdiadochokinesis,* is probably also a feature of asynergia.

Tremor. This occurs in voluntary movements, but as a rule not when the extremity is at rest. This "cerebellar tremor" is coarse and

290

arrhythmic and of a different type than the tremor seen, for example, in paralysis agitans.

Spontaneous past pointing. When the patient is told to point in a certain direction with his eyes closed, e.g., to the finger of the examiner, he points to the side, below, or above the right point. Most frequently the deviation is outward.

Deviation of gait may be observed when the patient is made to walk with his eyes closed; usually the deviation occurs in the same direction as the past pointing. When taking some steps alternately forward and backward the phenomenon of compass gait may become evident.

Unsteadiness of gait, staggering (titubatio), may be accompanied by a tendency to fall to one particular side, or it may occur without any definite directional preponderance.

Nystagmus is occasionally observed in cerebellar lesions. (See also section on the vestibular nerves, Ch. 7.)

Speech disturbances are seen particularly with rapidly developing and severe lesions. There may be defects in the proper co-operation of articulation, phonation, and respiration, slowness, explosiveness, and so-called scanning speech (for particulars, see Zentay, 1937).

The function of the cerebellum as inferred from experimental studies. In the course of time a number of studies have been performed to elucidate the function of the cerebellum. The subject is fully and critically considered in the monograph of Dow and Moruzzi (1958). As it gradually became clear that various parts of the cerebellum differ with regard to their connections, experiments were performed to study the function of the various subdivisions specifically, and considerable progress has been made. However, the course of the afferent and efferent cerebellar fibers is such that in experiments with ablations or stimulations of various parts of the cerebellum there is considerable risk of stimulating or destroying connections which are not immediately relevant to the cerebellar subdivision under study. On account of the geography of the cerebellar connections, this is often unavoidable, but the fact should be kept in mind when the functional changes observed are interpreted. Furthermore, it is to be expected that the different development of the cerebellar subdivisions among animal species will be reflected in functional studies.

In the preceding sections of this chapter, mention has been made of a number of findings concerning the origin and terminations of cerebellar connections and of physiological studies of recordings of afferent impulses to the cerebellum and of results of stimulation or destruction of particular structures. This new data bears evidence of the extremely complex organization of the cerebellum and is still difficult to fit into a coherent picture. Much of this data is so far of little immediate relevance to the diagnosis of cerebellar diseases in man, mainly for two reasons: 1) The lesions of the cerebellum met with in patients are usually not restricted to one minor region which appears to have its particular functional role (for example the rostromedial part of the fastigial nucleus). 2) The methods available for the diagnosis of cerebellar disorders in man are rather crude. Therefore, mainly the results of stimulation or ablation of the major principal cerebellar subdivisions will be considered in the following.

As we have seen, it is reasonable to distinguish between three main cerebellar regions, which may be loosely referred to as the "vestibulocerebellum," the "spinocerebellum," and the "pontocerebellum," even if the distinction is not sharp and there are possibilities for co-operation between the main subdivisions.

Thus, on the afferent side, pontocerebellar fibers end in considerable numbers in the cortex of the "spinocerebellum." Spinal afferents may act on the "vestibulocerebellum" by way of endings in certain parts of the vestibular nucleus, such as the group x, which projects onto the flocculus and nodulus-uvula. On the efferent side the overlap is equally evident, as witnessed for example by the fibers from the vermis and fastigial nucleus to the vestibular nuclei, the pathways to the thalamus from the interpositus and fastigial nucleus. Possibilities for direct interactions between the main subdivisions, however, appear to be scanty since the *cerebellar cortical association fibers* are sparse and most of them interconnect neighboring folia (Jansen, 1933; Eager, 1963b). According to Frezik (1963) the association fibers are recurrent collaterals of Purkinje cell axons. In functional analyses it is further important to recall that a number of nuclei which are acted upon by cerebellar efferents send fibers back to the cerebellum (the lateral reticular nucleus, the tegmental pontine nucleus, the red nucleus, the vestibular nuclei, and others).

The *vestibulocerebellum* (consisting of the flocculus, nodulus, caudal part of the uvula, and probably the ventral paraflocculus, see p. 270 and Fig. 5-8) is difficult to approach, particularly the flocculus. If a *lesion* in the monkey is restricted to the *nodulus* (Dow, 1938c), or to the nodulus and the adjoining parts of the uvula (Botterell and Fulton, 1938), disturbances of equilibrium appear, but none of the other cerebellar symptoms are observed. The animal sways when standing and walks unsteadily. However, if the trunk is supported, as when the animal is sitting in a corner of its cage, movements of the extremities are performed without ataxia. There are no signs of asynergia or tremor, and there is no hypotonia of the muscles. If the same operation is performed in animals whose labyrinths have been destroyed bilaterally, no additional symptoms appear following the ablation of the nodulus. These results were confirmed by Carrea and Mettler (1947). In the cat, Fernández and Frederickson (1964), following lesions of the nodulus (and the adjoining part of the uvula), observed disequilibrium without ataxia, as well as positional nystagmus (nystagmus influenced by the position of the animal) and prolonged vestibular reactions to rotatory and caloric tests (see section on the vestibular nerve, Ch. 7). Their findings following attempts to destroy the flocculus were inconclusive, while Carrea and Mettler (1947) in the monkey noted disturbances resembling those following lesions of the nodulus. In *stimulation experiments* with rabbits Aschan, Ekvall, and Grant (1964), using electronystagmography (see p. 392), found that stimulation laterally in the nodulus resulted in positional nystagmus. Correspondingly, Grant, Aschan, and Ekvall (1964), like Fernández and Frederickson in the cat, observed positional nystagmus following unilateral *lesions* of the nodulus and caudal uvula. (In the right lateral position the nystagmus was beating to the left following a lesion on the left side.) From these and other observations it is concluded that the nodulus-uvula exert an inhibitory effect on vestibular responses, at least as concerns their influence on vestibular elicited eye movements.

It is not possible to explain the physiological observations reported above in detail. It seems likely, however, that the influences on nystagmus are mediated by the efferent fibers from the nodulus-uvula to the vestibular nuclei, and their specific distribution within the nuclei (Angaut and Brodal, 1967) may be of relevance. Since the connections from the flocculus differ in their terminations from those from the nodulus-uvula, it appears likely that these two parts of the vestibulocerebellum differ functionally. Some suggestions that it is so are to be found in the literature, but more specific studies are needed. With reference to the disturbances of equilibrium observed following lesions of the nodulus-uvula it is of interest that the projection from the vestibulocerebellum to the lateral vestibular nucleus of Deiters, giving off the vestibulospinal tract, is very modest. This makes it appear unlikely that a disturbance in the function of this nucleus contributes to any large extent to the disequilibrium.

The *"spinocerebellum,"* when defined as the region receiving spinal impulses, covers most of the vermis and intermediate zone of the cerebellum (see Fig. 5-8). These parts of the cerebellum are chiefly concerned in the control of posture. Studies from recent years have shown that the "spinocerebellum" is not an entity, but that several minor regions are to be distinguished as has appeared from data mentioned in previous sections. One of the first important demonstrations of this were the studies of Chambers and Sprague (1955a, 1955b) which showed that the longitudinal subdivision distinguished in the corpus cerebelli on the basis of anatomical findings (see Figs. 5-5 and 5-6) has its functional counterpart. These authors undertook an analysis of the functional disturbances following ablation of the vermis proper, the intermediate zone, and the lateral parts in the cat. They concluded that the vermal zone "controls the posture, tone, locomotion, and equilibrium of the entire body"; the intermediate zone "controls the postural placing and hopping reflexes, tone, and individual movements of the ipsilateral limbs"; the lateral zone in the cat "does not appear to be involved in the regulation of posture or progression," but its function "is limited at most to a regulation of placing and hopping reflexes and volitional movements of the ipsilateral limbs." Further studies have brought additional data which support the presence of a longitudinal functional subdivision, but in addition have demonstrated differences between rostral and caudal parts within the vermis and intermediate zone, as is evident from what has been described in previous sections. It was found relatively early that *the anterior lobe exerts an inhibitory influence on postural tone.* Most of these experiments have been performed on decerebrate cats, in which the presence of an extensor rigidity provides a useful background for testing a reduction in extensor tone. Following ablation (or temporary cooling) of the anterior lobe in a decerebrate cat there is an increase of decerebrate rigidity, while stimulation reduces it. Later studies have shown that this effect is strictly a property of the anterior lobe vermis only, while the intermediate zone has an opposite effect. In total ablations of the anterior lobe the latter effect is, however, not evident, presumably because the vermal action is the strongest. The situation is similar with regard to the posterior part of the spinocerebellum, the pyramis, rostral part of the uvula, and the paramedian lobule, but on the whole these regions appear to be less potent than the corresponding zones in the anterior lobe. For all subdivisions *the effect following localized ablations or stimulations has been shown to be somatotopically localized.*

In the light of many detailed studies it seems possible to explain the main features of these changes as follows (see Pompeiano, 1967): The Purkinje cells of the anterior and posterior cerebellar vermis exert an (at least predominantly) inhibitory action on the cells of Deiters' nucleus, which have a monosynaptically excitatory action on extensor motoneurons (in addition, however, the vermis acts on the nucleus of Deiters via the fastigial nucleus, see p. 285). The loss of this inhibition increases the extensor tone. The intermediate part of the anterior lobe normally inhibits the nucleus interpositus, which has been shown to have a monosynaptic excitatory action on the cells of the red nucleus, which again, via the rubrospinal tract, activate flexor motoneurons. As referred to in Chapter 4, in both instances α as well as γ neurons are acted upon.

This simplified scheme does not take into account the projections from the fastigial nucleus onto facilitatory as well as inhibitory regions of the reticular formation, which act on the motoneurons (cf. Ch. 4 and 6). The actions of these connections are not known in sufficient detail, but among other things the fact that the influences of the vermis proper as well as the intermediate zone are somatotopically organized indicates that the action via the lateral vestibular nucleus and the red nucleus are by far the most important in the cerebellar control of muscle tone. The simplified presentation given above, furthermore, does not take into account the many detailed physiological observations, particularly of Moruzzi and Pompeiano and their collaborators, partially described previously, which show that minor parts of the fastigial nucleus and the nucleus interpositus have different actions. Furthermore, symptoms following lesions of the nuclei do not mirror those seen after lesions of the cortex projecting onto the particular nucleus. It is still not possible to fit all this data into a coherent picture of how the cerebellum controls muscular tone. It should not be overlooked that in this control the cerebellum co-operates with other parts of the brain receiving information from vestibular receptors and cutaneous and proprioceptive receptors from the body. This is evidenced, for example, by the influence of the cerebellum on postural reflexes.

Postural reflexes, some of which have been referred to in Chapter 4, have been found to be influenced by lesions of the anterior lobe. Another of these reflexes may be mentioned here, the so-called positive supporting reflex. This consists of an extension of the extremity in response to a light pressure on the pad. It is in keeping with the anatomy of the spinocerebellar pathways and of its efferent connections that the cerebellum may influence postural reflexes. According to Chambers and Sprague (1955a, 1955b) the intermediate zone is particularly involved in these functions, a point of interest in view of the termination of the dorsal spinocerebellar and cuneocerebellar tracts chiefly in this zone (Fig. 5-8). That the tactile placing reactions are likewise influenced fits in with the demonstration that tactile stimuli give rise to action potentials in the spinocerebellum. In general it appears that lesions of the spinocerebellum, especially the intermediate zone, result in exaggeration of the postural reflexes, particularly the "positive supporting reflexes," while loss or reduction of some other postural reflexes have been described.

Relatively little is known of the functional role of the *middle part of the vermis and intermediate zone,* receiving impulses from the face as well as optic and acoustic impulses. Following lesions of this part, cats show reduced startle responses to loud noises (Chambers and Sprague, 1955b). It may be conjectured (see Dow, 1969) that the role of this part is to exercise "a measure of control on a neural mechanism which in all instances is capable of its own independent activity." Studies on the possible role of the cerebellum on sensory functions are difficult to perform, but the suggestion of Dow does indeed appear to be a likely one.

The *"pontocerebellum"* is the part of the cerebellum which is so far known in least detail. In cats and dogs the symptoms following ablations of the ansoparamedian lobule (making up most of the "pontocerebellum") are not very marked (see Bremer, 1935b; Chambers and Sprague, 1955a, 1955b; Dow and Moruzzi, 1958), but of the same type as seen in monkeys with their far more developed cerebellar hemispheres. Ablations of the hemisphere in monkeys result in disturbances which are different from those following lesions of the spinocerebellum (Botterell and Fulton, 1938; Carrea and Mettler, 1947). Hypotonia and clumsiness develop, as well as atactic movements of the extremities (asynergia). These symptoms are always seen on the the side on which the lesion is performed. In the upper extremity ataxia is particularly evident when the animal uses its hand for grasping or seizing an object; in the lower extremity it is mainly revealed when the animal is walking. If the dentate nucleus is damaged in addition, these symptoms are more enduring and a tremor also occurs. The tremor is not evident unless the animal performs voluntary movements. In monkeys these symptoms disappear in the course of some three weeks, but in apes they persist much longer (Botterell and Fulton, 1938). The tremor following a lesion of the dentate nucleus or a transection of the brachium conjunctivum (Walker and Botterell, 1937) is a coarse, irregular tremor, which is increased at the termination of the movements. It may be designated as a typical intentional tremor.

In this connection some experiments by Aring and Fulton (1936) are of interest. These authors showed that when the contralateral "motor" area is removed immediately following the cerebellar lesion, the tremor is much reduced concomitant with the appearance of paresis of voluntary movements which follows the cerebral extirpation. If then the homolateral "motor" area is also removed, the tremor again becomes more conspicuous, since the animal will now use its first paralyzed arm to a greater extent. If areas 4 and 6 are ablated bilaterally in a monkey its capacity of performing voluntary movements is practically abolished, although reflex movements of different types, e.g. walking movements, can be elicited. However, when the cerebellum is also extirpated in the animal, *no tremor* is present in the reflex movements which can be provoked. These findings tend to stress the relation between cerebellar tremor and voluntary movements.

Many attempts have been made to explain the "mechanism" of cerebellar symptoms following lesions of the cerebellar hemispheres. Most of the hypotheses set forth are based on studies of the effects of cerebellar lesions combined with lesions of other parts of the central nervous system (see for example the recent studies of Growdon, Chambers, and Liu, 1967). The latter authors conclude, for example, that ataxia and tremor "represent a single neurologic disturbance," while others hold a different opinion. These controversial questions will not be considered here.

In spite of several attempts to demonstrate a somatotopical pattern within the cerebellar hemisphere as suspected by Bolk, no convincing evidence in favor of this view has so far been produced. The authors who have made positive findings have probably made lesions which involved the intermediate zone, as pointed out by Chambers and Sprague (1955b).[14] Ablations of the paraflocculus have not given clear results, either in the monkey (Carrea and Mettler, 1947) or in the guinea pig (Manni, 1950).

While the main disturbances following lesions of the cerebellum are thus in the motor sphere, there are indications from some physiological studies that the cerebellum may influence *autonomic functions* as well (see Dow and Moruzzi, 1958), such as cardiovascular regulation (for example the carotid sinus reflex, Moruzzi, 1940), respiration, pupillary size, and not least the urinary bladder. According to Chambers (1947) the points influencing the micturition reflex are in the rostral part of the fastigial nucleus. (Bladder disturbances have been found in human cases as well.) *Eye movements* have been repeatedly reported to follow electrical stimulation of various parts of the cerebellum (see Cohen et al., 1965).

The results of physiological studies lend support to the inference, mentioned in the introduction to this chapter and drawn from a scrutiny of the cerebellar fiber connections, that the cerebellum probably influences almost all functions of the nervous system. Although our present knowledge of how this occurs is scanty some general considerations may be of interest.

On account of the uniformity of the cerebellar cortex it seems a likely assumption that its mode of operation is principally identical all over. Its influence on different functions is a consequence of differences in the efferent projection from the particular parts of the cerebellum.

It is worthy of notice that the number of axons leaving the cerebellar cortex (axons of Purkinje cells) is comparatively modest as compared to the vast number of afferent fibers. Furthermore, other cellular elements by far outnumber the Purkinje cells. As pointed out by Dow and Moruzzi (1958, p. 373) this "suggests that only a comparatively small amount of energy and a limited number of cerebellar neurons are devoted to transmitting information or to sending orders to other portions of the central nervous system." The activity within each part of the

[14] Via the dentate nucleus the cerebellar hemisphere acts mainly on the nucleus ventralis lateralis (VL) of the thalamus. The projection of this onto the cortex presents a somatotopical localization (Fig. 5-10). In view of this it is intriguing that a localization has not been found in the dentatothalamic projection. However, this problem does not appear to have been studied in sufficient detail, and it is not unlikely that after all there may be a detailed dentatothalamic topographic relation. If such is demonstrated it might give clues to the existence of a somatotopical pattern in the cerebellar hemispheres. The reason that this has not been found may well be that the lesions have not been restricted to the proper parts of the dentate nucleus. It should be recalled in this connection that the crus I and crus II differ with regard to sources influencing them via the inferior olive (Walberg, 1956), and that some physiological (Jansen, Jr., 1957) as well as anatomical (Sousa-Pinto and Brodal, 1969) observations strongly suggest the presence of a localization within the crus II.

cerebellar cortex will be determined largely by the afferent information which reaches it. As we have seen, the sources of afferents differ among subdivisions, but each subdivision receives afferents from a number of sources. Obviously, the cortex elaborates and integrates these afferent messages in a very complex manner. (Thus the spinal regions receive information via several routes from tactile receptors, muscle spindles, Golgi tendon organs, and from flexor reflex afferents from the cord, as well as impulses arising in the cerebral cortex and basal ganglia.) The cortex then formulates its outgoing "orders" on the basis of the incoming information. Considering that various parts of the cerebellar cortex differ with regard to their afferent as well as efferent projections it is to be expected that the functional role of the various subdivisions is not identical, even if the intrinsic "circuitry" of the cortex appears to be the same all over.

It will appear from the foregoing account that the consequences of ablations of various subdivisions of the cerebellum are in fairly close agreement with other known data on the anatomy and physiology of the cerebellum. On the basis of experimental studies *three rather characteristic cerebellar syndromes may be distinguished,* each of them representing the changes following a lesion of one of the three main subdivisions of the cerebellum.

1. *The flocculonodular syndrome.* This occurs in lesions of the nodulus (and probably also the flocculus) and the adjoining part of the uvula. It is characterized by difficulties in maintaining equilibrium (sometimes called "trunk ataxia," but in fact not really ataxia). There is no ataxia of the extremities if the body is supported, no tremor, and no hypotonia. Positional nystagmus may occur.

2. *The lobus anterior syndrome.* This is distinguished by an increase of postural reflexes and decerebrate rigidity (when the anterior lobe is ablated). Whether other symptoms may also occur in this case is not yet definitely settled. The changes are somatotopically localized, affecting the hindlimb with anterior lesions, the forelimb with posterior lesions.

3. *The neocerebellar syndrome.* Here homolateral hypotonia and atactic movements, asynergic and clumsy, appear, and when the dentate nucleus is involved tremor also develops. The tremor is an irregular, coarse, intentional tremor. There is no somatotopical pattern.

It should be emphasized that this is a very crude scheme. It is obvious that coordination of voluntary movements requires a precisely organized activity of postural mechanisms, and the latter again are not only dependent on the integrity of the lobus anterior (or more properly the "spinocerebellum") but on the vestibular mechanisms as well. In order to make this evident, it will suffice to recall how practically every voluntary movement will alter the equilibrial status of the whole body and therefore will necessitate several adjustments in the muscular apparatus of the rest of the body. This intimate collaboration, of course, makes it difficult to analyse the disturbances of cerebellar functions, observed clinically as well as experimentally. The fiber connections of the cerebellum bear witness that there are possibilities for such collaboration. Nevertheless, the three syndromes listed above serve a practical purpose since they are found in cases of cerebellar affections in man and, therefore, are also of diagnostic value.

Cerebellar affections in man. There is a vast literature on symptoms of cerebellar diseases in man (see Dow and Moruzzi, 1958, for references). Several authors have attributed certain symptoms to lesions of definite parts of the cerebellum, but opinions are often divergent. In view of the co-operation between various parts of the cerebellum referred to above, this is only what one would expect, the more so since the lesions are often large and not restricted to particular functional regions. There appears, however, to be agreement on certain points. Thus, a picture corresponding to the *flocculonodular syndrome* may often be met with in a special type of glioma, the so-called *medulloblastoma,* which occurs most often in the cerebellum in children between five and ten years of age. With these tumors there is usually an initial period of general symptoms of increased intracranial pressure (headache, vomiting, etc.). When cerebellar symptoms appear, they are at first limited to unsteadiness of gait and standing (Bailey and Cushing, 1925). As a rule, however, there is no incoordination of the extremities when the child is lying in its bed. These tumors practically always arise in the vermis ("midcerebellar tumor"), and in the most posterior part of it, the nodulus, according to Ostertag (1936). They have been assumed to arise from undifferentiated cells at this place, and Raaf and Kernohan (1944) have verified the common occurrence of groups of undifferentiated neuroblasts at the attachment of the posterior medullary velum to the nodulus in human embryos and infants. As will be seen, this origin and symptomatology fit in well with the findings in experimental animals, the clinical picture in the early stages corresponding to the flocculonodular syndrome as described above. When the tumor grows, eventually the cerebellar hemispheres will also be damaged and neocerebellar symptoms appear in addition (apart from symptoms due to increased intracranial pressure, among which should be remembered enlargement of the head in these cases, since the tumors affect children).

In experimental animals positional nystagmus has been seen following unilateral lesions of the nodulus (see p. 293). Positional nystagmus may be observed in cerebellar lesions in man, but it is often impossible to decide whether it is due to the cerebellar lesion or to involvement of vestibular nuclei or pathways (see Nylén, 1950).

A clinical picture which corresponds to the experimentally produced *lobus anterior syndrome* has not yet been clearly defined in man. However, there is reason to believe that in cases in which the postural reflexes are exaggerated this indicates an involvement of the anterior lobe (see Brown, 1949). The type of cerebellar atrophy named after Marie, Foix, and Alajouanine (1922), their *"atrophie cérébelleuse tardive à predominance cortical,"* affects primarily the anterior lobe. These patients usually walk with a wide base and stagger to both sides, while they have little or no symptoms in the upper extremities. The myotatic reflexes in the legs may be increased. The atrophy appears to begin in the anterior part of the anterior lobe. Victor, Adams, and Mancall (1959) have published an exhaustive clinical and pathological analysis of cerebellar cortical degeneration in alcoholic patients. This disease appears to have a similar localization and a corresponding symptomatology to the atrophy of Marie, Foix, and Alajouanine. and the authors consider it likely that the affection which occurs first and is most marked in the legs may be explained by the predominant and early involvement of the anterior parts of the anterior lobe.

In cerebellar diseases in man, symptoms belonging to the *neocerebellar syndrome* as defined in animals are mostly commonly found. In unilateral lesions the symptoms occur on the side of the lesion. If this is restricted to the hemisphere, hypotonia, asynergia, dysdiadochokinesis, and (if the dentate nucleus is involved) intentional tremor usually occur. It appears probable that past pointing and deviation of gait, both to the affected side, belong to the same group of symptoms, since they have been observed in pure hemispheral lesions, e.g. in war injuries (Holmes, 1917). In a lesion restricted to one hemisphere the ensuing ataxia on the homolateral side occurs in the lower as well as in the upper extremity, but the characteristic titubatio, the staggering gait, is not present unless other parts of the cerebellum are also damaged (directly or secondarily by pressure, edema, or circulatory disturbances). Detailed descriptions of the symptomatology and of tests for cerebellar functions have been given by Holmes (1939), Dow and Moruzzi (1958), and Dow (1969). Speech disorders might be expected to occur chiefly in lesions involving the middle part of the vermis, but conclusive data is not available (see Zentay, 1937). It may finally be mentioned that occlusion of the superior cerebellar artery is likely to affect the fibers in the brachium conjunctivum with resultant cerebellar symptoms, especially ipsilateral incoordination of voluntary movements. If the posterior inferior cerebellar artery is occluded cerebellar symptoms are likewise usually present, in combination with signs of involvement of the medulla, e.g. in Wallenberg's syndrome.

The diagnosis of cerebellar diseases.   It appears from the preceding account that an analysis of the cerebellar symptoms in man in some instances will yield information concerning the part of the cerebellum affected. It should be realized, however, that the pure cerebellar syndromes, as they have been defined experimentally in animals, will not very frequently be encountered in man. There are several reasons for this. The pathological processes affecting the cerebellum will frequently have reached a considerable magnitude before they are diagnosed or can be diagnosed, and by that time they are apt to affect more than one of the functionally different subdivisions of the cerebellum. Because of their size the hemispheres will as a rule soon be involved, even if the process starts in one of the other subdivisions. Furthermore, even if the lesion itself is confined to one of the subdivisions, the others may be secondarily affected by pressure, dislocation, or obliteration of vessels with ensuing circulatory disturbances. It is a common experience that pressure effects are particularly apt to occur in diseases in the infratentorial part of the cranial cavity, where the possibilities of unhindered expansion are limited. Such pressure effects may be due to a vascular incident or more frequently to a tumor. For the same reason symptoms due to mechanical pressure may appear from structures outside the cerebellum itself, the medulla or pons, such as signs of pyramidal tract injury without direct involvement of the pyramidal tract, or symptoms of vestibular disturbances or cranial nerve affections. On the other hand, extracerebellar lesions not infrequently give rise to cerebellar symptoms on account of their pressing on the cerebellum. Particularly important in this connection are the tumors of the cerebollopontine angle, most frequently the *acoustic nerve neurinomas* (cf. Ch. 7).

It is to be expected that cerebellar symptoms may also appear when the large afferent and efferent pathways to and from the cerebellum are injured. This has been observed both clinically and experimentally in animals. Thus transection of the superior cerebellar peduncle, as has been mentioned, gives rise to a neocerebellar syndrome on the homolateral side, and following transection of the restiform body, which, *inter alia,* carries the vestibular fibers to the cerebellum, symptoms appear which are reminiscent of the flocculonodular syndrome.

The latter facts raise the question as to whether the symptoms usually designated as cerebellar are specific to lesions of the cerebellum. With several of them this is clearly not the case. Thus hypotonia and weakened tendon reflexes are also met with in lesions of the dorsal roots, and unsteadiness of gait and standing is seen in lesions of the vestibular apparatus. In this case past pointing may also occur (cf. Ch. 7). Disturbances of coordination will be present in lesions of the dorsal columns of the cord or of the dorsal roots, although typical dysmetria and asynergia are as a rule not conspicuous.

No wonder, then, that the diagnosis of a cerebellar disease may be made without any primary affection of the cerebellum being present. As an example may be mentioned *internal hydrocephalus,* in which the dilatation of the ventricles, particularly the 4th, may produce cerebellar symptoms.[15] Not infrequently *tumors of the frontal lobe* may be accompanied by cerebellar symptoms. In this case the cerebellar symptoms occur contralateral to the side of the tumor. The chronological development of the symptoms may give a clue to the correct diagnosis, since frontal lobe tumors commonly start with mental symptoms. When these appear in cerebellar lesions they usually occur late, and are due to the effects of the increased intracranial pressure. As a rule ventriculography and angiography will be able to yield decisive information. The reason for the appearance of cerebellar symptoms in frontal lobe affections is not quite clear, but it appears most reasonable that they are due to an affection of the frontopontine tract.

The few features mentioned will suffice to make clear that the diagnosis of a cerebellar lesion is not always an easy task, particularly not without resorting to special diagnostic measures. The symptoms are sometimes very difficult to evaluate and may be very slight (cf. below), and may be produced by lesions of structures other than the cerebellum. In the etiological diagnosis the case history must be taken into account just as in other cases, and a knowledge of the chronological development of the different symptoms may also give hints concerning the topographical diagnosis. This, for instance, applies to the so-called *heredo-ataxias,* an ill-defined group of slowly progressing degenerative changes, which may affect the cerebellum or its afferent and efferent tracts and also other systems such as the pyramidal tract.

A peculiar feature which contributes to making the diagnosis of cerebellar lesions difficult should finally be emphasized, namely, the *remarkable degree of compensation which occurs in lesions of the cerebellum.* This compensation may be practically complete, with the consequence that some time after the initial lesion only traces are left of the original cerebellar symptoms. As a general rule it can be stated that the more rapidly a pathological process develops in the cerebellum, and the more widespread the damage, the more clear-cut are the symptoms. In slowly progressing affections the symptoms may be very scanty and feeble, be-

---

[15] In cases in which the hydrocephalus develops very early in fetal life it may be accompanied by, and is probably the cause of, a defective development of the cerebellar vermis (see Brodal, 1945). The anomaly is often referred to as the Dandy-Walker syndrome and believed to be due to a congenital atresia of the foramina of Magendie and Luschka. However, these may be found patent in such cases (Brodal and Hauglie-Hanssen, 1959; Portugal and Brock, 1962). This rare developmental anomaly has also been observed as a hereditary condition in mice (Bonnevie, 1943; Bonnevie and Brodal, 1946; see also Portugal and Brock, 1962).

cause they are masked by the compensation which takes place. The compensation is particularly marked in children and young individuals. In cerebellar defects arising in fetal life or early childhood all signs of cerebellar malfunction may be lacking, but nevertheless autopsy may reveal the absence of a cerebellar hemisphere, or other grave defects. It is assumed that the compensation in cerebellar lesions is due to other systems taking over the function of the cerebellum or that intact parts of the cerebellum are able to cope with the functions of the damaged or deficient parts as well. However, nothing definite is known of the mechanism of compensation, in spite of its great importance in clinical neurology.

6

The Reticular Formation

THE RETICULAR formation of the brain stem was recognized as a separate part of the central nervous system by the classical neuroanatomists. By the turn of the century some of its connections were known in broad outline, and speculations upon its functions were ventured. However, neither anatomists and physiologists nor clinicians devoted much attention to it during the first half of htis century. Following the publication of the now classical paper by Moruzzi and Magoun: "Brain stem reticular formation and activation of the E.E.G.," in 1949, this situation was radically altered, chiefly because it appeared that the reticular formation is involved in the maintenance of the enigmatic function which we call consciousness. In the following years further physiological investigations confirmed and extended the original observations of Moruzzi and Magoun (for an extensive review, see Rossi and Zanchetti, 1957). Since we will have to refer to these problems at many places in the following a brief outline is appropriate.

The reticular formation and the "ascending activating system." Following high frequency electrical stimulation of the brain stem in chloralosane-anesthetized cats, the synchronized discharges of high voltage slow waves in the electroencephalogram (EEG) are replaced by low voltage fast activity, closely resembling the corresponding changes observed in the human EEG on transition from a relaxed or drowsy state to attention or alertness. These changes are generally referred to as

304

desynchronization, activation, or *the arousal reaction.* They occur diffusely over the entire cortex, are assumed to be mediated via the "diffuse thalamic system" (mentioned in Ch. 2 and to be considered later in the present chapter). These changes can be obtained by stimulation of the medial bulbar reticular formation, pontile and midbrain tegmentum, and dorsal hypothalamus and subthalamus. The same changes can be produced by natural or electrical stimulation of spinal nerves, the trigeminal, the splanchnic, vagus, acoustic, and some other cranial nerves (for references see Rossi and Zanchetti, 1957). Impulses entering the reticular formation by way of these channels are assumed to produce a state of activity in the reticular formation, where potentials can be recorded on such stimulation. Electrical stimulation or strychninization of the cerebral cortex likewise gives rise to potentials in the reticular formation, and may also produce EEG arousal in sleeping *"encéphale isolé"* cats (cats in which the spinal cord is separated from the rest of the brain). Stimulation of the fastigial nucleus influences the electrocortical activity via the reticular formation. Following transection of the "specific sensory paths" in the brain stem (the medial lemniscus and the spinothalamic tract), activation of the EEG can still be obtained on stimulation of nerves or of the reticular formation. Lesions in the central parts of the brain stem, however, result in behavioral somnolence and electrocortical synchrony, and activation cannot be obtained with stimuli which are effective when the central part of the brain stem is intact. Corresponding results were obtained in monkeys (French, von Amerongen, and Magoun, 1952).

From these and other observations it was concluded that there is an "ascending reticular activating system" in the brain stem. The concept was further elaborated in subsequent studies. The system was found to be tonically active, its level of activity depending on the amount of afferent impulses from a number of sources as well as on humoral agents, such as adrenaline and carbon dioxide. The activity of the system is reflected in the EEG and was assumed to determine the level of consciousness in all its variations from complete alertness and attention to drowsiness and sleep. The system was assumed to be entirely diffusely organized, in contrast to the "specific" sensory "system." The structural basis of the ascending activating system was assumed to be the reticular formation of the brain stem and the "nonspecific" thalamic nuclei, including ascending connections from the former to the latter and further projections from the thalamus to the cortex. Physiological observations on the ascending conduction led to the postulate that the ascending pathways were composed of series of short-axoned cells. Furthermore, it was concluded that activation of the system occurred primarily by "collateral spread" from the specific sensory pathways. The reticular formation was

305

assumed to be diffusely organized, since potentials could be led off from large territories following stimulation of afferents from a particular source, and since impulses from several sources were found to reach the same region. Its capacity for integration was especially stressed.

While the existence of an "activating system" in the brain stem has been definitely established, and its discovery has greatly improved our understanding of important functions of the brain, some of the deductions made by the early workers in the field have had to be modified, especially their assumption concerning the anatomical substrate of the system. Moruzzi and Magoun (1949) clearly stated that on this point their conclusions were tentative, since little information on necessary anatomical details was available. However, in subsequent studies the reservations made by the original workers—as usually happens—have often been disregarded.[1] It is unfortunate that the authors included the word "reticular" in the designation. This is a morphological term and refers to the netlike appearance of the central part of the brain stem (reticular formation). It is clear from the physiological findings that the structures mediating the activation extend rostrally beyond the reticular formation as anatomically defined (see below). Even if there is a nucleus in the thalamus which, on account of its structure, was named the reticular nucleus by the old anatomists, and even if this may be involved in the mechanism of activation, this does not justify the use of the word "reticular" as an epithet to the term "ascending activating system," and even less to speak of parts of the thalamus as belonging to the reticular formation. Much confusion has arisen on account of this lack of clarity in designations. To use the term "reticular system" as synonymous with the "activating system," as is often done, serves only to confuse the issue. *It should be made perfectly clear that the "activating system" is a functional concept, the "reticular formation" a morphological one, and it has been obvious for many years that these do not correspond.* For this reason, when referring to Moruzzi and Magoun's concept in the present text, the word "reticular" will not be used. To retain the term "ascending" might likewise be misleading since it is known that regions related to the ascending activation have a corresponding action on the spinal cord. When speaking of the "activating system," it is further advisable to delete the words "of the brain stem." This designation may be confusing

---

[1] Moruzzi (1963) points to the fact that the hypothesis made possible an understanding and correlation of physiological, pharmacological, and clinical data which had so far appeared to be unrelated, and adds: "It was probably because of this success that the distinction between direct experimental proof and suggestive evidence, a discrimination which should always remain clear in our minds, was frequently forgotten." (Moruzzi, 1963, p. 235.)

since the term *"brain stem"* is defined in different ways. In agreement with common usage it *will here be employed in its gross macroscopical sense, comprising the medulla oblongata, the pons, and the mesencephalon.* Following an account of the structure and fiber connections of the recticular formation we will return to questions of its functions and of the activating system.

Anatomy of the reticular formation.   A reticular formation is found only in the medulla, pons, and mesencephalon and is a phylogenetically old part of the brain. It was named by the old anatomists, and is generally taken to comprise those areas of the brain stem which are characterized structurally by being made up of diffuse aggregations of cells of different types and sizes, separated by a wealth of fibers traveling in all directions. Circumscribed cell groups, such as the red nucleus, the superior olive, or the cranial nerve nuclei are not included. Thus the chief criterion for considering a cellular area of the brain stem as being part of the reticular formation is its structure. From this point of view some fairly well circumscribed nuclei, such as the lateral reticular nucleus (nucleus of the lateral funiculus) and the nucleus reticularis tegmenti pontis of Bechterew, when studied in Nissl-sections, rightly belong to the reticular formation, although they are usually omitted when one speaks of the reticular formation in a general way. This may be justified because these nuclei (as well as the paramedian reticular nucleus), in contrast to the rest of the reticular formation, project onto the cerebellum as described in Chapter 5, and thus differ functionally from the remaining part.[2] On the other hand, there are some minor cell groups, for example those of the raphe, which in spite of having a reticular structure have got their particular names and, therefore, are often not included. Since these nuclei resemble other parts of the reticular formation with regard to their connections, it appears likely that they are functionally closely related to it. Occasionally it may be a matter of taste whether a cell group is considered as belonging to the reticular formation or not.[3] In the following account *the term "reticular formation" will be employed as a general denominator for those areas of the brain stem (as*

[2] In Golgi sections the cerebellar projecting nuclei are found to differ with regard to the dendritic patterns of their cells from the reticular formation proper (Leontovich and Zhukova, 1963).

[3] Because of this, Olszewski (1954) has suggested that the epithet "reticular" should be omitted altogether when speaking of cell groups in the reticular formation, the more so since it can be subdivided into a number of fairly well circumscribed cellular areas which can be referred to as nuclei. A discussion of the criteria for distinguishing the reticular formation as a particular part of the brain is given by Ramón-Moliner and Nauta (1966), who stress the dendritic patterns of the nerve cells as an important feature.

defined above) *which have a reticular structure, with the exception of the three cerebellar projecting nuclei mentioned above.* Nuclei having special traditional names will, however, be referred to under those names. Broadly speaking the region to be considered will cover the central areas of the brain stem. Peripherally, each half of the reticular formation borders on the long ascending and descending fiber bundles traversing the brain stem (medial longitudinal fasciculus, medial lemniscus, spinothalamic tract, etc.) and on particular nuclei, which in certain places intrude somewhat into its territory.

Although some early neuroanatomists had described certain regions of the reticular formation as having their particular structural features, it was generally held that it was a rather diffuse mass of cells. However, in systematic studies of the cytoarchitectonics of the brain stem of the rabbit and man, Meessen and Olszewski (1949) and Olszewski and Baxter (1954), respectively, were able to distinguish a number of cell groups within the reticular formation.[4] The main groups which they recognized can be found in other mammals as well, for example, in the cat (Brodal, 1957; Taber, 1961), the rat (Valverde, 1962), and the guinea-pig (Petrovicky, 1966). There are certain species differences, and the borders between the groups are not equally clear everywhere. Furthermore, the borders between the reticular formation and many nuclei, for example the vestibular and sensory trigeminal nuclei are in places rather indefinite. The main point is, however, *that there are obvious architectonic differences between relatively small areas of the reticular formation.* This makes it appear likely that there are other differences as well between these areas, with regard to fiber connections and function, as has indeed been found to be the case (see below). Fig. 6-1 shows a drawing of a section from the human reticular formation, Fig. 6-2 a series of drawings from the cat's brain stem. The latter gives an impression of the general arrangement. A prominent feature is that the large cells of the reticular formation are restricted to its medial part, approximately the medial two-thirds, where they are intermingled with small and medium-sized cells. In the lateral one-third there are only small cells. Furthermore, large cells are found particularly at certain levels (see Fig. 6-4). One of the large-celled nuclei is the nucleus reticularis gigantocellularis (R. gc.) in the medulla. Rostral to this is another, the nucleus reticularis pontis caudalis (R.p.c.). The latter passes rather gradually into the nucleus reticularis pontis oralis (not seen in Fig. 6-2), which lacks giant cells.

Studies of the reticular formation with the Golgi method give addi-

[4] Some of the findings of Olszewski and Baxter (1954) in man have been criticized by Feremutsch and Simma (1959). See also Koikegami (1957).

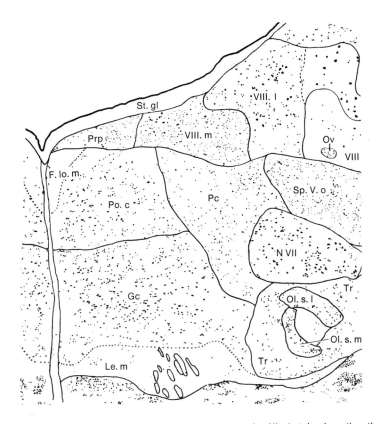

FIG. 6–1 Semischematic representation of part of a Nissl-stained section through the human brain stem at a low pontine level. The facial nucleus (*N. VII*), the rostral part of the spinal trigeminal nucleus (*Sp. V.o*), parts of the vestibular nuclei (*VIII.l* and *VIII.m*), the nucleus praepositus (*Prp*), the medial longitudinal fasciculus (*F.lo.m*), and the medial lemniscus (*Le.m*) surround the reticular formation. Within this three subdivisions can be separated at this level, the nuclei gigantocellularis (*Gc*), pontis caudalis (*Po.c*), and parvicellularis (*Pc*). From Olszewski and Baxter (1954).

tional information about the cells present and their dendritic and axonal patterns. From such studies (Scheibel and Scheibel, 1958; Leontovich and Zhukova, 1963) it has been concluded that there are in the reticular formation no typical Golgi II cells (cells with short axons branching profusely close to the perikarya and considered as prototypes of internuncial or association cells). All axons "appear to project at least some distance rostral and/or caudal" (Scheibel and Scheibel, 1958, p. 37). In the rat Valverde (1961b) found an exceedingly small number of Golgi II cells in the lateral parvicellular region. It is further remarkable that all long

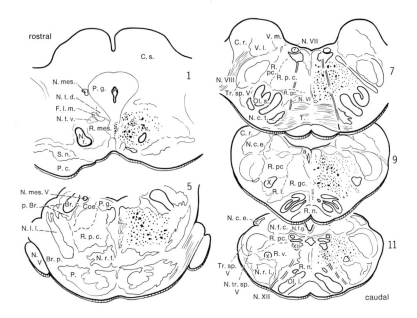

FIG. 6–2 A cytoarchitectonic map of the reticular formation of the cat. In a series
of transverse sections are plotted the various cell groups and their composition of
small, medium-sized, and large cells. Some abbreviations: *Coe.:* nucleus subcoeruleus; *F.l.m.:* medial longitudinal fasciculus; *N.c.e.:* external cuneate nucleus;
N.f.c.: nucleus cuneatus; *N.f.g.:* nucleus gracilis; *N.r.:* red nucleus; *N.r.l.:* lateral
reticular nucleus (nucleus of lateral funiculus); *N.r.t.:* nucleus reticularis tegmenti
pontis; *N.tr.sp.V:* spinal nucleus of trigeminal nerve; *P.:* pontine nuclei; *P.g.:* periaqueductal gray; *R.gc.:* nucleus reticularis gigantocellularis; *R.mes.:* reticular
formation of the mesencephalon; *R.n.:* nuclei of the raphe; *R.p.c.:* nucleus reticularis pontis caudalis; *R.pc.:* nucleus reticularis parvicellularis; *R.v.:* nucleus reticularis ventralis. From Brodal (1957).

axons appear to give off several collaterals along their course and that
collaterals from the same axon may vary with regard to their pattern of
branching. The dendrites are usually long and radiating, characterizing
the cells as being of the so-called isodendritic type (Ramón-Moliner and
Nauta, 1966; and others). It is characteristic that most of the dendrites
of reticular cells are spread out in a plane perpendicular to the long axis
of the brain stem (Fig. 6-3). These and other features of interest for
functional correlations will be considered later.

Along the midline of the brain stem there are collections of nerve
cells, together referred to as the *raphe nuclei.* They may be subdivided
into a number of minor units, which in part are characterized by differences in cytoarchitecture (see Taber, Brodal, and Walberg, 1960).
With regard to cell types and in several other respects these nuclei re-

3 1 0

semble the reticular formation. Some of these cell groups are seen in Fig. 6-2, to the left.

In recent years some authors have studied the *neurochemistry of the reticular formation*. In the medullary and pontine reticular formation some neurons have been found which are excited by acetylcholine while others are inhibited (Salmoiraghi and Steiner, 1963; Bradley, Dhawan, and Wolstencroft, 1964; and others). Other cells are influenced by 1-noradrenaline (Bradley and Wolstencroft, 1962) and most neurons respond to 5-hydroxytryptamine (5-HT). Using fluorescence methods for identifying neurons containing catecholamines and 5-HT, Dahlström and Fuxe (1964) have mapped their distribution in the brain stem. 5-HT cells are numerous in certain of the raphe nuclei. In many papers dealing with neurochemistry, however, the region studied is unfortunately not identified precisely, a fact which makes correlations with observations from other fields difficult. It is to be expected, however, that in the future neurochemical studies will bring much important information, but careful anatomical identification of the cells studied is essential. The scattered data so far available will not be considered in the present text.

Fiber connections of the reticular formation.   These link the reticular formation, directly or indirectly, with many other parts of the central nervous system. The *efferent fibers* pass chiefly to the spinal cord, to the thalamus, and to other nuclei within and above the brain stem. The

FIG. 6–3 A drawing of a Golgi-impregnated parasagittal section through the lower brain stem of a young rat, illustrating the orientation of the dendrites of cells in the reticular formation in planes perpendicular to the long axis of the brain stem. Collaterals of axons descending in the pyramid (*Pyr.*) take off in the same plane as do also the collaterals of a long axon (*a*) of a reticular cell. (Note different organization of the dendrites in the hypoglossal nucleus, XII.) *Ol.i.*: inferior olive; *P*: pons; *R.gc.*: nucleus reticularis gigantocellularis. The inset below to the left shows how the reticular formation may be considered as a series of neuropil segments. (Cf. text) From Scheibel and Scheibel (1958).

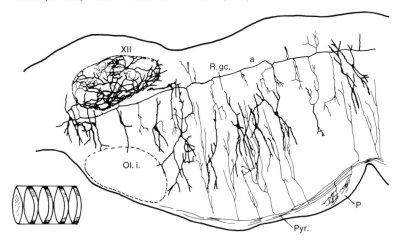

efferent projections may be studied by making lesions in the reticular formation and tracing the ensuing descending or ascending degeneration of fibers. With this approach there is considerable risk of damaging by-passing fibers and thus getting misleading results. Or one may look for retrograde cellular changes in the reticular formation following inter-ruption of its efferent fibers. In this way the sites of origin of the fibers may be established accurately, but the sites of termination can not be determined precisely. If lesions are placed in regions which are known to give off efferents, more unequivocal results can be obtained in studies of anterograde fiber degeneration.

Fibers passing from the reticular formation to the spinal cord were established by the old anatomists with the Marchi method. Present knowl-edge of these tracts, which is fairly complete, was reviewed in Chapter 4 (p. 174 ff). As will be recalled, reticulospinal fibers come from small as well as large cells, chiefly in two regions in the medial two thirds of the reticular formation, one in the pons, the other in the medulla (Fig. 6-4). The latter descend crossed as well as uncrossed, the former chiefly uncrossed. In the cord the fibers do not appear to end in synaptic contact with motoneurons, but end in laminae VII to VIII, the pontine fibers terminating more ventrally than the medullary (see Fig. 4-7). No somato-topical pattern has been found within the areas of origin (Torvik and Brodal, 1957).

Contrary to what has often been assumed, particularly in the early physiological studies of the ascending activating system, *there is an abundant projection of long ascending fibers from the reticular forma-tion.* Many studies have been devoted to these projections. Like the long descending fibers, the ascending ones do not arise in equal numbers from all parts of the reticular formation, but have their preferential sites of origin. Following lesions rostral to the mesencephalon in newborn kit-tens, a mapping of the ensuing retrograde cellular changes (Brodal and Rossi, 1955) shows that although scattered fibers arise from almost all parts of the medial two thirds of the reticular formation, the majority come from two regions, one in the medulla, the other in the lower pons— upper medulla (Fig. 6-4). Both regions give off crossed as well as un-crossed ascending fibers. However, in the caudal region giant cells do not take part in the rostral projection, indicating that the giant cells here act only on the cord. It appears that at least one third of all cells in the regions mentioned have long axons ascending beyond the mesen-cephalon. In addition there are ascending fibers from the mesencephalic reticular formation (Nauta and Kuypers, 1958). The presence of a con-siderable number of long ascending fibers from the medial part of the reticular formation has further been confirmed in studies with the Nauta

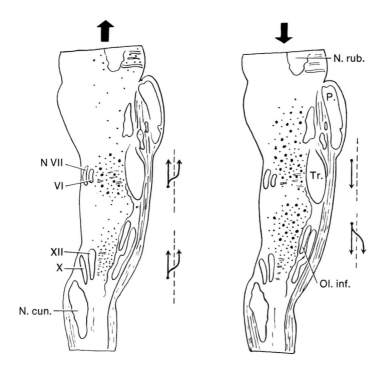

FIG. 6–4 The distribution of cells of the reticular formation sending long axons to the spinal cord (right) and of cells having long axons ascending beyond the mesencephalon (left) is mapped in parasagittal sections of the cat's brain stem. Large dots indicate giant cells. Note that, although both types of fibers take origin from practically the entire longitudinal extent of the reticular formation, they both have their maximal regions of origin. In spite of some overlapping these maximal regions are different. The arrows to the right of each drawing indicate that the pontine reticulospinal fibers descend homolaterally, while all other contingents are crossed as well as uncrossed. From Brodal (1956).

method (Nauta and Kuypers, 1958) as well as in Golgi studies (Scheibel and Scheibel, 1958; Valverde, 1961a). Such studies have further indicated that there are cells also in the lateral small-celled third of the reticular formation which give off ascending axons, but these are relatively short.

As to the *terminations of the long ascending fibers* from the reticular formation, there are still open questions. In general, fibers arising in the mesencephalon pass further than those coming from more caudal regions. There appears to be agreement among authors using the Golgi method (Scheibel and Scheibel, 1958; Valverde, 1961a) and the Nauta method following lesions of the reticular formation (Nauta and Kuypers, 1958) that a fair number of medullary and pontine ascending fibers end in some

313

of the "nonspecific" thalamic nuclei, as will be discussed in a later section (see Fig. 6-9). Fibers from the mesencephalic reticular formation (chiefly its medial parts) have been traced to the hypothalamus, preoptic area, and the medial septal nucleus. Some fibers pass even to the caudate and lentiform nuclei. These mesencephalic fibers do not pass through the thalamus but below it, a point of some interest as will be considered later.

Two features in the anatomy of the long ascending and descending projections deserve particular emphasis. In the first place it is learned from Golgi studies (Scheibel and Scheibel, 1958; Valverde, 1961a) that a considerable number of the cells give off an axon which dichotomizes and has a long ascending, as well as a long descending, branch (see Fig. 6-6). In the mouse and rat one branch of such cells has been traced to the cord, the other to the thalamus (Fig. 6-5). Thus, the same cell will act in a rostral as well as a caudal direction. From a quantitative analysis of the retrograde cellular changes following lesions of the spinal cord or lesions above the mesencephalon in the cat it has been conservatively estimated that in the rostral region of origin (see Fig. 6-4) more than half of the cells must be of this type (Torvik and Brodal,

FIG. 6–5 Drawing of a sagittal Golgi section from the brain stem of a 2-day-old rat, showing a single large cell in the magnocellular nucleus. It emits an axon which bifurcates into an ascending and a descending branch. The latter gives off collaterals to the adjacent reticular formation (*N.gc.,* nucleus reticularis gigantocellularis), to the nucleus gracilis (*N.g.*) and to the ventral horn in the spinal cord. The ascending branch gives off collaterals to the reticular formation, the periaqueductal gray (*P.g.*) and then appears to supply several thalamic nuclei (*Pf. & Pc.;* parafascicularis and paracentralis; *Re.:* reuniens, and others), the hypothalamus (*H*) and the so-called zona incerta (*Z*). *MD:* dorsomedial thalamic nucleus. From Scheibel and Scheibel (1958).

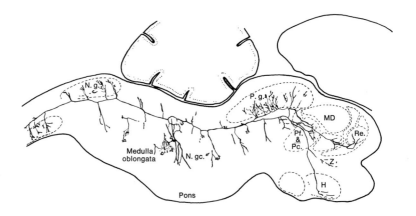

1957). Such cells have been identified also physiologically (Magni and Willis, 1963). The other noteworthy feature is that the rostrally projecting cells are on the whole situated more caudally than those projecting to the cord although there is some overlapping of rostrally and caudally projecting regions. Since the long axons give off collaterals along their course, this must mean that impulses passing to the cord may act on cells projecting rostrally, and vice versa, as shown in Fig. 6-6. The two morphological features mentioned indicate that *there must be a very close integration between the influences exerted by the reticular formation in the rostral and caudal direction.*

In addition to acting on the spinal cord and/or the thalamus and other rostral structures the reticular formation may influence nuclei in the brain stem by collaterals of ascending or descending axons, or by way of the apparently relatively few cells which do not have long ascending or descending axons. Scheibel and Scheibel (1958) traced collaterals to all cranial nerve nuclei in the brain stem.

Afferent connections to the reticular formation come from many sources. Most impressive are the *afferent connections from the spinal cord.* Contrary to what was inferred in early physiological studies, only some of the spinal activation of the reticular formation appears to take place via collaterals of secondary sensory fibers. Thus several anatomical studies have failed to demonstrate collaterals to the reticular formation of the fibers of the medial lemniscus (Matzke, 1951, in the cat; Bowsher, 1958; Nauta and Kuypers, 1958, in the monkey; Valverde, 1961a, in the rat). Supporting evidence comes from physiological studies (see for example, Morillo and Baylor, 1963). Nor do collaterals from the spinothalamic tract appear to be of great importance since this tract is poorly developed (except perhaps in man, see Ch. 2). However, there is *a massive influx of direct spinoreticular fibers* which ascend in the ventrolateral funiculus intermingled with the spinothalamic ones. In the brain stem the fibers take off in a dorsomedial direction, and as stated above, their terminal branches and collaterals run approximately perpendicular to the long axis of the brain stem, in the same plane as most dendrites of the cells (see Fig. 6-3). The termination of many fibers in the reticular formation following transection of the ventrolateral funiculus has been demonstrated by early neuroanatomists using the Marchi method, and more recently with silver impregnation methods in the cat (Rossi and Brodal, 1957; Anderson and Berry, 1959), in the monkey (Mehler, Feferman, and Nauta, 1960) and in man (Bowsher, 1957, 1962; Mehler, 1962). It should be noted that although some spinoreticular fibers appear to reach almost all parts of the reticular formation bilaterally, the majority are distributed to its medial two thirds and, further-

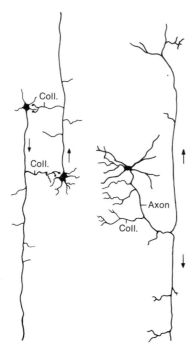

FIG. 6–6 Diagram illustrating two anatomical features which make possible a close correlation of caudally and rostrally directed influences of the reticular formation. To the left a simplified drawing of a typical cell in the medial reticular formation. Its axon gives off a long ascending and a long descending branch provided with collaterals (cf. Fig. 6–3). To the left a diagram showing how cells giving off ascending and descending axons, respectively, may influence each other by way of collaterals. From Brodal (1964b).

more, to particular levels of this. In the cat (Rossi and Brodal, 1957) there is one maximal area of termination in the medulla (corresponding approximately to the nucleus reticularis gigantocellularis) and another in the pons (within the nuclei reticularis pontis caudalis and oralis). These two regions correspond approximately to those giving off long ascending afferents (see Fig. 6-4) indicating that there is a direct route from the spinal cord to the thalamus via the reticular formation. From Bowsher's (1962) study of the brains of seven patients subjected to chordotomy or medullary tractotomy (1 case) it appears that in man there is, in addition, a third maximal terminal region at the transition from the pons to the mesencephalon.[5] In animals as well as in man there appears to be no somatotopical pattern in the distribution of the spinoreticular fibers.

The courses followed by *sensory impulses in the cranial nerves entering the reticular formation* are not completely known. A small number of primary sensory fibers have been traced to it following lesions of the vagal, glossopharyngeal, and trigeminal nerves (see Torvik, 1956b;

[5] In the cat, as well as in the monkey and man, quite heavy degeneration is also found in a particular nucleus dorsal in the upper pons, the nucleus subcoeruleus (*Coe.* in Fig. 6-2).

Clarke and Bowsher, 1962, in the rat; Kerr, 1962, in the cat). This has been confirmed in man for the two former nerves (Kunc and Maršala, 1962). However, such fibers appear to be relatively scanty and to have a restricted distribution. *Secondary sensory fibers,* however, have been shown in Golgi studies to give off collaterals to the reticular formation (see Brodal, 1957; and Rossi and Zanchetti, 1957, for reviews), and some of these connections have been studied experimentally, making it possible to decide their areas of distribution more specifically. This is true for the nucleus of the spinal trigeminal tract (see Carpenter and Hanna, 1961; Stewart and King, 1963), and the vestibular nuclei (see Ladpli and Brodal, 1968). Collaterals of the ascending acoustic pathways have likewise been found to end in the reticular formation (see Ch. 9). Optic impulses presumably reach it via optic nerve fibers to the superior colliculus (see Ch. 7) from which tectoreticular fibers originate. The route followed by olfactory fibers is less clear, but fiber connections have been described which may presumably be utilized (see Guillery, 1956, 1957; Nauta, 1956, 1958).

As described in the preceding chapter, *fibers from the cerebellum,* particularly the fastigial nucleus, are distributed throughout the medial two thirds of especially the medullary reticular formation (see Walberg, Pompeiano, Westrum, and Hauglie-Hanssen, 1962). These fibers supply both rostrally and caudally projecting areas.

Among *fibers to the reticular formation from "higher levels"* there appear to be some from the *lateral hypothalamus* (see Nauta, 1958) and from the *pallidum* (see Johnson and Clemente, 1959), both groups ending chiefly in the mesencephalon. *Tectoreticular fibers* were mentioned above. More impressive are the *corticoreticular fibers,* which presumably mediate the short latency responses recorded in the reticular formation following stimulation of the cerebral cortex (2–6 msec according to Hugeline, Bonvallet, and Dell, 1953; for further data see Brodal, 1957; Rossi and Zanchetti, 1957). The existence of these fibers was established by early neuroanatomical workers. They come chiefly from the "sensorimotor" cortex with contributions from other regions, and descend with the corticospinal fibers, leaving these during their course in the brain stem. (Some of the corticoreticular fibers may be collaterals of corticospinal fibers.) When the terminal distribution of the corticorectircular fibers is studied with silver impregnation methods, it is learned that, like so many other afferent connections, they do not supply the reticular formation in equal density throughout. In the cat (see Fig. 6-7) there are two chief terminal regions (Rossi and Brodal, 1956a), a caudal one which coincides approximately with the nucleus gigantocellularis, and a rostral (covering the nucleus reticularis pontis caudalis and the caudal part of the nucleus reticularis pontis rostralis). In subsequent studies in

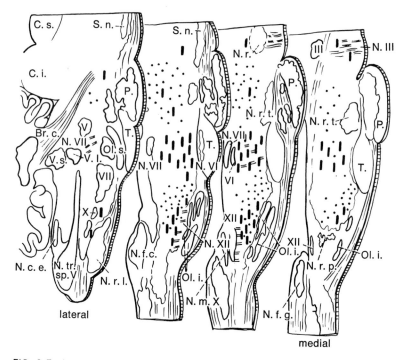

FIG. 6–7 In parasagittal sections through the cat's brain stem are plotted the regions of the medial two thirds of the reticular formation which receive the maximum of fibers from the cerebral cortex (dots) and the regions from which the majority of long ascending fibers take origin (vertical bars). Note overlap in the region dorsal to the middle part of the inferior olive. Some abbreviations: *Br.c:* brachium conjunctivum; *N.f.c.* and *N.f.g.:* nucleus cuneatus and nucleus gracilis; *N. VII:* facial nerve; V, VI, VII, X and XII: motor nuclei of cranial nerves.

the cat, the monkey, and man (Kuypers, 1958a, b, c, 1960) and in the rat (Valverde, 1962, 1966) largely corresponding findings have been made, and evidence has been obtained that the distribution may be even more specific. Thus most fibers to the medial magnocellular reticular formation appear to come from cortical regions situated more frontally than those which supply the lateral parvicellular reticular formation with its more modest projection (Kuypers, 1960, in the monkey; Valverde, 1962, in the rat). There are also direct corticofugal fibers to the mesencephalic reticular formation (Szentágothai and Rajkovits, 1958; Pearce, 1960; Valverde, 1962).[6]

[6] Several physiological studies (see Rossi and Zanchetti, 1957, and later in the present chapter) have demonstrated that following stimulation of various cortical areas potentials can be recorded in the reticular formation. A systematic anatomical mapping of the sites of origin of corticoreticular fibers has so far not been undertaken, and a complete correlation with the physiological data is not yet possible.

318

The Reticular Formation

It is of some interest for functional considerations that although most of the corticoreticular fibers end in regions of the reticular formation which give off reticulospinal fibers, their terminal area in the medulla covers part of the region which gives off long ascending fibers (Fig. 6-7). We will return to this and oher anatomical features of the organization of the reticular formation later.

The raphe nuclei were referred to above. On the whole they receive fibers from and give off fibers to the same parts of the nervous system as does the reticular formation, but the nuclei differ individually in this respect as well as with regard to cytoarchitecture (see Brodal, Taber, and Walberg, 1960; Brodal, Walberg, and Taber, 1960).

Organization of the reticular formation. It is seen from the preceding account that what is known of the fiber connections of the reticular formation supports the notion that it is not diffusely organized. Maximal sites of endings of some main afferents, as well as sites of origin of long efferent fibers, can be indicated fairly precisely, even if these areas of termination or origin do not correspond exactly to particular nuclear groups. Furthermore, there are noteworthy differences between the medial two thirds and the lateral one third of the reticular formation. In the latter part there are only small cells, and their ascending or descending axons are relatively short. The medial two thirds alone, containing many large cells, give rise to long ascending and descending fibers in considerable numbers. It appears, therefore, that what we may call *effector functions of the reticular formation* are mainly mediated by its medial two thirds, while the lateral one third appears to act to a large extent on the former, by medially directed axons of its cells. It seems a likely assumption that the lateral part of the reticular formation functions particularly as what is often referred to loosely as an area of association. Within the medial two thirds there is, furthermore, a segregation, although incomplete, between levels which are equipped to exert their main action on the spinal cord and levels which may act preponderantly on more rostral parts of the brain (see Fig. 6-4). These features in the anatomical organization of the reticular formation argue strongly against the assumption that the reticular formation is functionally a diffusely organized entity.

Studies of cytoarchitectonics and fiber connections, however, give us only part of the picture. Important additional information is derived from studies of Golgi preparations. As mentioned previously, several of the observations made in Golgi studies are in complete accord with those obtained in experimental investigations. However, there are features which can only be studied in Golgi material, such as dendritic patterns and arborizations of axons. As referred to previously the typical cell of the reticular formation has fairly long dendrites, and in Golgi preparations it

319

is striking to see how the "dendritic fields" of cells overlap. Furthermore, it can be seen that collaterals of fibers belonging to different afferent systems overlap extensively. As emphasized by Scheibel and Scheibel (1958) this occurs predominantly in the medial parts of the reticular formation, from which the long ascending and descending projections arise. This overlap of axonal branches "makes it difficult to see how any specificity of input can be maintained" (Scheibel and Scheibel, 1958, p. 34).

There are other features which likewise leave one with the impression that the reticular formation is diffusely organized. On many places dendrites from cells in the reticular formation extend into neighboring nuclei and vice versa (see Ramón-Moliner and Nauta, 1966). It appears that all cranial nerve nuclei give off axons or collaterals to the reticular formation, just as cells in the reticular formation send collaterals or axons to all these nuclei (Scheibel and Scheibel, 1958). The absence of cells of the Golgi II type was mentioned above (most cells have axons which project for some way along the length of the brain stem). Scheibel and Scheibel (1958) have presented an interesting discussion of the intrinsic organization of the reticular formation, and reach the conclusion (loc. cit. p. 42) that "Rather, it can be said that the fine structure of the brain stem core is such that given the proper physiologic conditions an impulse pattern can probably describe any conceivable path within the reticular formation, so extensive is the interconnectivity of the elements." They draw attention, however, to an interesting feature which is of relevance if one attempts to correlate the conclusions made on the basis of Golgi sections with the results of experimental studies. As stated above, the majority of dendrites of reticular cells are oriented in the transverse plane in the brain stem (see Fig. 6-3). The collaterals entering the reticular formation run in the same plane, taking off from the parent fibers at approximately right angles (Fig. 6-3). The reticular formation may thus be described as being composed of a series of segments, as illustrated in the inset of Fig. 6-3. However, even if the fundamental pattern of dendrites and axons is thus fairly uniform throughout the reticular formation, and each segment appears to be principally organized in the same manner, the segments may well differ functionally. In the first place, the cells in different segments do not send their axons to the same destinations (at some levels, for example, most axons are descending, at others ascending, see Fig. 6-4). Secondly, the afferents do not come from the same source at all levels. This is so far best known as concerns the spinal afferents, which supply chiefly certain "segments." It seems a likely assumption that collaterals coming from different afferent fiber systems end predominantly at particular levels, but this problem has so far not been extensively studied.

Physiological studies performed in recent years, have brought forward a great deal of data in good accord with the anatomical findings summarized above. Like the latter they make it clear that the reticular formation is not a functionally homogeneous unit. Some relevant gross functional features will be considered in following sections. Studies of single units have brought further support for the view mentioned above. Even if in many of these studies the sites recorded from have not been precisely indicated some data obtained is of interest.

The afferent input to the reticular formation is often said to be diffuse since sensory information from various sources appears to reach the entire reticular formation. This, however, is not strictly correct. Scheibel, Scheibel, Mollica, and Moruzzi (1955) performed microelectrode recordings of the responses of neurons in the medullary reticular formation to stimulation of the cerebellum, the cerebral cortex, peripheral nerves (proprioceptive and exteroceptive), the vagus nerve, and to acoustic stimuli. While no units were found which responded to acoustic and vagal stimuli, most units could be influenced from several of the other sources, although in different combinations. Units responding to acoustic stimuli are, however, easily found in the mesencephalon (Amassian and de Vito, 1954). Convergence of somatosensory, acoustic, and vestibular impulses on the same units have been observed (Duensing and Schaefer, 1957b). It was concluded by Scheibel, Scheibel, Mollica, and Moruzzi (1955) that even if there is widespread convergence of afferent impulses on units of the reticular formation, this convergence is not unlimited. Patterns of convergence vary markedly among individual units. Further evidence on the minute functional organization of the reticular formation comes from studies in which the neurons recorded from have been identified.

In the medial medullary and pontine reticular formation, neurons projecting to the spinal cord (see Fig. 6-4) have been identified electrophysiologically. About half of them were excited by somatic stimuli from all parts of the body (Wolstencroft, 1964; Magni and Willis, 1964b). For some neurons stimuli applied to different parts of the body were not equally effective (Wolstencroft, 1964). Some neurons were excited from one part of the body and inhibited from others. Magni and Willis (1964a) found that most reticular neurons which project to the spinal cord were excited on cortical stimulation, as were reticular neurons with axons projecting both rostrally and caudally, while neurons with long ascending axons were only occasionally influenced. Even if there was a widespread convergence of excitatory actions from many areas of the cerebral cortex upon individual reticular neurons, the pattern of convergence varied among the neurons. With regard to units responding to stimulation of spinal nerves, Pompeiano and Swett (1962a, 1962b) found that a majority of them are located in the nucleus reticularis gigantocellularis (where many spinoreticular fibers terminate). Not all kinds of spinal impulses are equally effective in influencing the reticular formation. The relatively few single unit studies which have been undertaken (see, for example, Wolstencroft, 1964;

321

Pompeiano and Swett, 1962a, 1962b, 1963; Magni and Willis, 1964b) indicate that cutaneous impulses and group II muscle afferents are effective, while proprioceptive impulses mediated by group I fibers do not influence reticular neurons. Some of the units studied and identified as reticulospinal neurons have been found to respond to nociceptive cutaneous stimuli (Wolstencroft, 1964). Obviously the interplay of impulses entering the reticular formation from various sources is extremely complex, and involves excitatory and inhibitory actions. On stimulation of a particular source of afferents a particular neuron may show excitation, followed by inhibition (see, for example, Magni and Willis, 1964b), or from the same source some neurons may be excited, others inhibited, as found for reticulospinal neurons (Wolstencroft, 1964). It appears that reticular neurons may periodically alter their responsiveness to incoming stimuli (Scheibel and Scheibel, 1965), indicating a flexibility in the impulse passages within the reticular formation.

The above data is compatible with the view of the organization of the reticular formation derived from anatomical studies, but further studies are needed, in which a precise mapping of the distribution of units responding to particular kinds of sensory stimulation is done. A number of microelectrode studies in addition to those mentioned have been performed in recent years, but it is scarcely possible as yet to put the results together into a coherent picture of the modes of operation of the reticular formation. Although a knowledge of the function of the reticular formation at the cellular level is highly desirable, other findings are of more immediate relevance from a neurological point of view.

Functional aspects. A number of functions are known to be influenced from the reticular formation. In fact, it appears that this, like the cerebellum (see Ch. 5), may be of importance for almost all "functions" controlled by the nervous system, as might indeed be expected when one considers its interconnections with other parts of the brain. Only some aspects of the functional role of the reticular formation will be considered in this text. Due to the many problems connected with the studies and concepts of the ascending activating system, this will be dealt with separately in a following section. Here our concern will be mainly with the "descending" actions of the reticular formation, i.e. its influence on spinal cord mechanisms, somatic and visceral.

The beginning of a more systematic approach to this problem was made by Magoun and his collaborators, starting with the papers of Magoun and Rhines (1946) and Rhines and Magoun (1946). It was shown that *electrical stimulation of the reticular formation could alter all kinds of motor activity*. Stimulation of the ventromedial part of the medullary reticular formation (in cats and monkeys) inhibited myotatic reflexes and muscular tone (the rigid limbs in decerebrate animals became flaccid). Likewise, movements evoked by cerebral cortical stimulation were inhibited. Opposite, facilitatory, effects were obtained on stimulation of the reticular formation lateral to the inhibitory region and at more rostral levels, in the pons, mesencephalon, and even from midline structures in the thalamus, the central gray, and the subthalamus and hypothalamus. The effects were assumed to be mediated via a final link of reticulospinal projections. According to Magoun and his collaborators (see Sprague, Schreiner, Lindsley, and Magoun, 1948) the effects involved the entire skeletal musculature, and it was assumed that the two regions of the brain exerted a generalized inhibitory or facilitatory effect, respectively (being thus an exception to Sherrington's principle of reciprocal innervation). Further studies (Sprague and Chambers, 1954; and others, for references see Rossi and Zanchetti, 1957) have, however, shown that most of the responses obtained on stimulation of the lower reticular formation are reciprocally organized. As mentioned in Chapter 4 (p. 177) α as well as γ motoneurons can be influenced, facilitated or inhibited, from the reticular formation. The complexity is well illustrated by findings, such as those of Lindblom and Ottosen (1956), that some reflex activity can be inhibited and some facilitated from the same bulbar point. Recent research tends to support the suggestion of Rossi and Zanchetti (1957), that the reciprocity depends chiefly on properties of the spinal cord and not on the intrinsic organization of the reticular formation. In modifying motor activity the reticular formation collaborates with several other supraspinal structures, such as the vestibular nuclei, the red nucleus, the superior colliculus, the fastigial nucleus, and the cerebral cortex, all of which may act on the spinal cord. Some of these structures act directly on the reticular formation as well.[7] These difficult problems have been touched upon in Chapter 4 (see also Ch. 7).

In spite of a voluminous literature on the spinal actions of the reticular formation (not to be considered here), there are many unsolved questions. From an anatomical point of view it is of interest that the "inhibitory region" coincides fairly well with the medullary region which gives rise to reticulospinal fibers (see Fig. 6-8). The inhibitory effects are therefore presumably mediated directly via reticulospinal fibers. As to the facilitatory effects, the situation is more complex. The area of the brain stem which has been found to yield facilitation extends far outside the regions from which reticulospinal fibers originate, although it includes part of the pontine region. It appears likely, therefore, that stimulation of reticular neurons projecting directly onto the cord can only to

---

[7] By way of ts projections onto the vestibular nuclei, and via connections leading to the cerebral cortex, the reticular formation may act on the spinal motor apparatus indirectly. The role of these mechanisms in the intact animal is not yet clear. However, the fact that the effects described above can be obtained in decerebrate animals shows that, first and foremost, direct reticulospinal pathways are concerned.

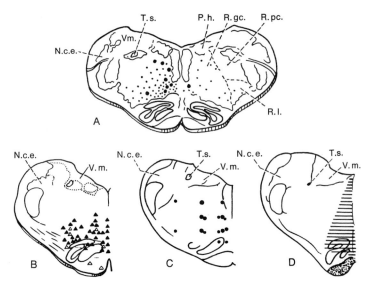

FIG. 6–8 A comparison between the areas in the medulla of the cat shown to give off reticulospinal fibers (*A*, cf. Fig. 6–4) and the maps given in physiological papers of areas which on electrical stimulation yield inspiratory movements (*B*), inhibition of the patellar reflex (*C*) or lowering of blood pressure (*D*). Diagrams *B*, *C* and *D* from Pitts, Magoun, and Ranson (1939), Magoun and Rhines (1946) and Alexander (1946), respectively. Symbols in the original drawings referring to other effects than those mentioned have been omitted. (Cf. text.) From Brodal (1957).

a slight extent be concerned in the facilitatory effects, and that most of these must occur by way of fibers originating in the facilitatory areas and terminating on reticulospinal neurons. Since many of the cortico-reticular fibers end in those regions of the reticular formation which give rise to reticulospinal fibers, it appears likely that the muscular inhibition and facilitation obtained on stimulation of the cerebral cortex are in part mediated via the corticoreticulospinal pathways. Physiological studies, some of which have been mentioned above, are in agreement with this (for further references, see Brodal, 1957; Rossi and Zanchetti, 1957).

Mention was made in Chapter 2 of the *effects exerted by the reticular formation on the central transmission of sensory impulses* entering in the spinal nerves, and in Chapter 7 corresponding observations concerning the cranial nerves will be considered. The pathways involved are presumably reticulospinal projections and reticular fibers entering the cranial nerve nuclei, respectively.

Respiratory movements and cardiovascular functions are influenced from the reticular formation. These mechanisms will not be discussed here, but from the point of view of anatomical correlations it is interesting to consider the regions found to influence respiration and cardiovascular functions. Various *respiratory "centers"* have been claimed to exist in the brain stem. There is an inspiratory area, located in the medulla (see Fig. 6-8), and rostral and lateral to this there is a more extensive region which on electrical stimulation gives rise to expiratory movements. (This region is outlined somewhat differently by various workers). Other respiratory "centers" situated more rostrally in the brain stem have been described: a "pneumotaxic center" which by some has been assumed to be located in the locus caeruleus (see Fig. 6-2), and a more extensive "apneustic center" in the middle and caudal pons. These "centers" are assumed to exert their action on the more elementary inspiratory and expiratory regions. Of these, the inspiratory "center" as mapped physiologically, appears to be almost coextensive with the muscular inhibitory region, and thus covers an area which gives rise to reticulospinal fibers (see Fig. 6-8). The expiratory region, however, is largely situated outside the spinal projecting areas of the reticular formation. In much the same manner, the *cardiovascular depressor region* coincides with the inhibitory region, while the *pressor area* (from which elevation of blood pressure and acceleration of heart rate is obtained on stimulation) extends further laterally and rostrally. It appears from this that the inspiratory and vasodepressor effects which can be obtained on stimulation of the bulbar reticular formation are most likely the result of stimulation of reticulospinal neurons (as are the inhibitory muscular effects), while reticulospinal neurons are only involved as final links in the mediation of expiratory and vasopressor effects.[8] The "centers" in the brain stem considered above appear to be relatively elementary. When changes in respiratory movements, blood pressure and heart rate, and other autonomic functions are elicited on stimulation of certain parts of the cerebral cortex and the hypothalamus (see Ch. 11) these effects appear to be mediated via the lower "centers." The latter are also influenced by afferent impulses entering in spinal and cranial nerves. As far as respiration and cardiovascular control are concerned afferents in the vagus nerve appear to be particularly important, i.e. the solitary tract and its nucleus must be involved (see Ch. 7). Furthermore, alterations in the oxygenation of the blood may influence the "centers" directly in addition to acting on the chemoreceptors, for example in the carotid sinus.

The spatially similar locations of areas giving muscular inhibition, inspiratory movements, and depressor effects (see Fig. 6-8), as well as

[8] According to Wang and Ranson (1939) the pressor impulses descend in the ventrolateral funiculus of the cord, where reticulospinal fibers are present. It must be assumed that in the cord all effects considered above are mediated via interneurons, since reticulospinal fibers do not appear to end on either motoneurons or cells of the intermediolateral cell column (see Ch. 4).

the less striking coincidence of the regions having opposite effects, are indeed remarkable. Simultaneous changes in all three spheres may occur on stimulation of the same point. Whether different reticular neurons are involved when muscle tone, respiratory movements, and blood pressure are influenced, appears so far to be an open question. However, the situation is far more complex than appears from the above brief account (see Bach, 1952).

The ascending activating system and the "nonspecific" thalamic nuclei. The original views on the organization and function of the ascending activating system were summarized in the introduction to this chapter. As alluded to, continued research has necessitated revisions on some points and, in particular, has brought forward a quantity of data demonstrating that matters are far more complex than originally assumed. Since the early 1950's a countless number of papers have appeared on this subject, and there has been a continuous change in views. What was originally conceived of as one particular "system," concerned first and foremost with the maintenance of consciousness, has turned out to be a very differentiated complex, anatomically as well as functionally. It is becoming more and more obvious that it is untenable to consider an ascending activating system as separate from other parts and functions of the brain.

The latter circumstance, as well as the misuse of the designation "reticular formation," may have contributed to the tendency to widen the concept of the reticular formation almost without limits, as exemplified by the contents of the Henry Ford Hospital Symposium "The Reticular Formation of the Brain" (1958). The situation was properly characterized at that symposium by the late Sir Geoffrey Jefferson (1958, p. 729) when he remarked: "I confess that three or four years ago I thought that I understood the concept of the reticular formation, but now I find that it has turned into a system which, like a big flourishing and expanding business, has bought up all its competitors." Alluding to another feature in the development he added: "It would not be too absurd to say that wherever any really interesting fun was going on in brain research, that part was immediately claimed as part of the reticular formation."

Under these circumstances and on account of the complexities of the problems and the overwhelming literature on the subject, it is impossible to give a comprehensive and synthesized presentation of the ascending activating system. In the following, emphasis will be put on some recent data, and an attempt will be made to draw attention to those aspects which are of particular interest from a clinical point of view. A number of specialized physiological and other observations will not be considered at all. It may be practical to start with some of the findings made in the early 1950's and then pass rapidly to the most recent information. Although the "nonspecific" thalamic nuclei are not covered by the heading of the present chapter, it is appropriate to consider them in this connection. They were briefly referred to in the general discussion of the thalamus in Chapter 2 (p. 69).

It was mentioned in the introduction to this chapter that the cortical desynchronization (activation) occurring on high frequency electrical stimulation of the brain stem was assumed to be mediated via the "nonspecific" thalamic nuclei. This assumption was based on several lines of evidence. Thus stimulation of "nonspecific" thalamic nuclei (Dempsey and Morison, 1942; Morison and Dempsey, 1942) gives rise to widespread long-latency recruiting responses in the cerebral cortex, while stimulation of "specific" thalamic nuclei results in localized short-latency responses, the distribution being determined by the cortical projection of the nucleus stimulated. It was well known at that time that there is a parallelism between the EEG (electroencephalographic) records and the state of consciousness. Both in man and animals the alpha-rhythm in the EEG (waves of relatively high voltage and a frequency of 8 to 12 per second) changes to a low voltage fast activity when the animal or man passes from a state of relaxation or drowsiness to an alert, attentive state, for example in response to an external stimulus. As mentioned in the introduction the former pattern, generally referred to as *synchronization* (on the assumption that it represents the synchronous activity of many cortical neurons) was broken and replaced by widespread *desynchronization,* often referred to as EEG *arousal* or *activation*. On the other hand, when an animal passes from wakefulness to sleep, the low voltage fast activity in the cerebral cortex gradually changes to high voltage slow rhythms with so-called spindle bursts. It was further shown that electrical stimulation of the "nonspecific" thalamic nuclei could give rise to both EEG patterns, depending on the frequency of stimulation. Low frequency stimulation of the midline thalamic region produces inattention, drowsiness, and sleep, accompanied by slow waves and spindle bursts; high frequency stimulation will arouse a sleeping animal or alert a waking animal, and there is desynchronization of electrocortical activity.[9]

The essential part of the ascending activating system is located in the brain stem, as appeared from Bremer's (1935a) early observation, that an animal which had its brain stem transected at the mesencephalic level

---

[9] Electrical stimulation with a 3-per-second stimulus was shown to produce a regular wave-and-spike complex as seen in petit mal epilepsy (Jasper and Droogleever-Fortuyn, 1947). The problems of epilepsy and the mechanisms underlying the appearance of different kinds of epileptic seizures will not be considered in this text. For a complete presentation the reader is referred to the monograph of Penfield and Jasper (1954). The generally accepted notion that the "nonspecific" thalamic nuclei are instrumental in the production of seizures has recently been questioned by Williams (1965).

presented a permanently synchronized EEG and behavioral sleep. The fact that lesions in the brain stem result in coma (Lindsley et al., 1950, in the cat; French, von Amerongen, and Magoun, 1952, in the monkey; and others), and that stimulation of the reticular formation may alter the cortical responses following low frequency thalamic stimulation further supported this view (for references, see Rossi and Zanchetti, 1957). There appears to be a tonic activity in the ascending activating system which is upheld by afferent stimuli. However, different kinds of stimuli are not equally effective in influencing it. Acoustic impulses appear to be more potent than optic, for example, and among impulses entering via the trigeminal and spinal nerves, those from pain receptors are particularly effective. Electrical stimulation of certain parts of the cerebral cortex may give electrocortical desynchronization by acting on the reticular formation (see Rossi and Zanchetti, 1957, for a review). Some general anesthetics, such as pentobarbital, have been shown to block the ascending transmission in the activating system while leaving transmission in the "specific" sensory pathways relatively unchanged. Adrenaline as well as CO_2 increase the activity of the system.

In the studies on the ascending activating system, attention was early focused on the "nonspecific" thalamic nuclei. Attempts were made to specify the nuclei involved and their mutual connections and relations by studying the physiological effects of lesions in various regions of the thalamus and neighboring structures. Differing opinions were expressed and hypotheses were set forth to explain the phenomena.[10] This is no wonder, considering the structural complexities of the thalamus, the difficulties involved in producing small and precisely located lesions, the risk of interrupting fibers of passage, and other technical difficulties in the experimental work. These studies will not be reviewed here. Suffice it to mention that until some years ago the most generally accepted view of the mechanism of EEG and behavioral arousal (see, for example, Hanbery, Ajmone-Marsan, and Dilworth, 1954) appeared to be the following: by reticulothalamic connections the reticular formation of the brain stem influences the midline and intralaminar nuclei. These project onto the thalamic reticular nucleus. Projections from this to the cortex are responsible for the widespread cortical distribution of the EEG desynchronization. However, already in the pioneer study of Moruzzi and

[10] A vast number of studies have been undertaken to clarify the neural events occurring in the thalamus and the cortex during synchronized and desynchronized activity. This complex subject is outside the scope of the present text. It appears that there are still many unsolved problems and differences of opinion among authors. For a recent account the reader is referred to the monograph of Andersen and Andersson (1968).

Magoun (1949) it was emphasized that other mechanisms than the diffuse thalamic projection may be involved in the cortical activation following stimulation of the reticular formation. Rather early some authors maintained that the ventral anterior thalamic nucleus (VA) may be concerned.

The problems are still far from being solved, but research from the last few years has clarified some points. Some of the recent findings will be presented below in a rather simplified way. It is appropriate to start with a survey of present anatomical knowledge of the "nonspecific" thalamic nuclei, since lack of information on their anatomy has greatly hampered progress in the field.

According to their location, three groups of *"unspecific" or "nonspecific"* thalamic nuclei (sometimes called reticular, diffuse, or recruiting nuclei) may be distinguished: *the intralaminar nuclei, the midline nuclei,* and *the reticular thalamic nucleus* (see Fig. 2-11). Within the former two groups a parcellation into a number of minor nuclei is possible (see Fig. 6-9). They will not be considered separately here, except for the centromedian nucleus (CM), and the reticular nucleus.[11] The different architecture of the small groups, as well as our, so far fragmentary, knowledge of their connections makes it a likely assumption that they are not functionally identical, but concerning this question information is still very scanty.

As referred to previously (p. 314), *fibers arising in the medullary, pontine, and mesencephalic reticular formation have been traced to several of the "nonspecific" nuclei* (as well as the hypothalamus, the septal area, and the caudate and lentiform nuclei). However, some "specific" thalamic nuclei also receive ascending fibers from the reticular formation (Nauta and Kuypers, 1958; Scheibel and Scheibel, 1958, 1967). In a corresponding manner some spinothalamic fibers have been traced to "nonspecific" thalamic nuclei, although authors are not in complete accord as concerns particulars in the distribution (see Gerebtzoff, 1939; Getz, 1952; Anderson and Berry, 1959; Mehler, Feferman, and Nauta, 1960; Bowsher, 1961; Scheibel and Scheibel, 1967; and others). In addition, efferent cerebellar fibers have been traced to these nuclei (see Ch. 5). Some authors have described terminations of reticulothalamic and spinothalamic fibers in the centromedian nucleus, while others are in-

[11] Some authors include the nucleus ventralis anterior (VA), the nucleus ventralis medialis (VM), and the nucleus suprageniculatus (SG) among the "nonspecific" thalamic nuclei. According to Ajmone Marsan (1965) the following groups have so far not been properly placed in either category: the nuclei limitans, submedius, parafascicularis, paraventricularis anterior, parataenialis· and subparafascicularis. As will be seen from the following, it is scarcely possible to maintain a clear distinction between "specific" and "nonspecific" thalamic nuclei.

329

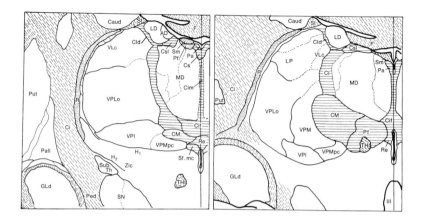

FIG. 6–9 Drawings of transverse sections through the thalamus of the macaque monkey, showing the arrangement and subdivisions of the "nonspecific" thalamic nuclei. The reticular nucleus indicated by dots, the intralaminar and midline nuclei by horizontal hatchings. The section to the left is placed most rostrally. Some abbreviations: *Ci:* internal capsule; *Cif:* nucleus centralis inferior; *Cim:* nucleus centralis intermedialis; *Cl:* nucleus centralis lateralis; *CM:* centromedian nucleus; *Cs:* nucleus centralis superior; *Csl:* nucleus centralis superior lateralis; *GLd:* nucleus geniculatus dorsalis; *LP:* nucleus lateralis posterior; *MD:* dorsomedial nucleus; *Pa:* nucleus paraventricularis; *Pf:* nucleus parafascicularis; *R:* nucleus reticularis; *Re:* nucleus reuniens; *Sf.mc:* nucleus subfascicularis pars magnocellularis; *Sm:* stria medullaris; *SN:* substantia nigra; *St:* stria terminalis; *THl:* tractus habenulointerpeduncularis; *VLc:* nucleus ventralis lateralis, pars caudalis; *VPl:* nucleus ventralis inferior; *VPLo:* nucleus ventralis posterior lateralis, pars oralis; *VPM:* nucleus ventralis posterior medialis; *VPMpc,* nucleus ventralis posterior medialis, pars parvocellularis. From Olszewski (1952).

clined to interpret the degenerating fibers found in this nucleus as fibers of passage. Mehler (1966a) emphatically denies their existence. These divergencies may in part be due to semantic problems.[12] In physiological studies responses (although of relatively long latencies, 10 to 20 msec) have been recorded in the parafascicular-centromedian complex following stimulation of peripheral nerves (see for example, Albe-Fessard and Bowsher, 1965).

The *efferent connections of the intralaminar and midline nuclei* are particularly difficult to clarify with the methods of anterograde degeneration, since the lesions must be small and there is considerable risk of

[12] As recently reviewed by Mehler (1966b) the nucleus centrum medianum of primates consists of a small-celled ventrolateral region and a large-celled dorsomedial region. There is evidence from phylogenetic studies that only the former should be considered as the CM, while the latter corresponds to the parafascicular nucleus, which is relatively better developed in nonprimate species.

interrupting fibers of passage. Nauta and Whitlock (1954) were careful in interpreting their results in a study of this kind. Among the conclusions they felt could safely be made were the following: there are longitudinal interconnections between the various nuclei, predominantly directed rostrally, but there are also transversely running associational connections, and there are interconnections with the adjacent "specific" nuclei. The centromedian nucleus was concluded to send fibers to all other "nonspecific" nuclei, including some contralateral connections and a projection to the rostral part of the reticular nucleus. Furthermore, the centromedian has a fairly massive projection to the ventral nuclear complex of the thalamus, including the ventralis anterior (VA). Fibers could further be traced from the centromedian to the putamen and in lesser numbers to the globus pallidus, caudate nucleus, and claustrum. Some of these connections are described also by Kaelber and Mitchell (1967). Using the method of retrograde cell changes Cowan and Powell (1955) in the rabbit, and Powell and Cowan in the monkey (1956), found evidence for a topically organized projection of the centromedian and parafascicular nuclei to the putamen, while intralaminar nuclei project onto the head of the caudate nucleus. As to projections to the cerebral cortex (a point of particular relevance for physiological interpretations) Nauta and Whitlock (1954) deny a cortical projection from the centromedian nucleus, but conclude that the rostrally situated complex of midline and intralaminar nuclei project to phylogenetically older parts of the cortex, among these the prepiriform cortex, the "limbic" cortex (see Ch. 10), and the entorhinal area. Some of these projections were found also by Powell and Cowan (1956). In a recent study Murray (1966), in the cat, concludes that the paracentral nucleus projects onto the cortex of the cingulate gyrus and the orbitofrontal cortex, while the centralis lateralis projects to the parieto-occipital region. It should be noted that according to Nauta and Whitlock (1954) the afferents to the cortex, described as "nonspecific" afferents according to their mode of termination (see Ch. 12), do not arise only from "nonspecific" but also from "specific" nuclei.

In view of the many sources of error inherent in experimental studies of the fiber connections of the "nonspecific" thalamic nuclei, the recent extensive studies of Scheibel and Scheibel with the Golgi method are highly welcome (Scheibel and Scheibel, 1966c, 1966d, 1966e, 1967). Their observations are based on a large material of preparations, chiefly of brains of mice, rats, kittens, and some other animals, and in the main agree with the conclusions drawn by Nauta and Whitlock (1954). As concerns the midline and intramedullary nuclei (Scheibel and Scheibel, 1967) the following may be noted. The neurons of these nuclei resemble those of the reticular formation of the brain stem (see p. 309) and their richly branching axons enter neighboring "specific" and "nonspecific" nuclei. No Golgi II type cells appear to be present. From the rostral part of the nuclei axons enter the medial portions of the VA and the rostral part of the reticular nucleus, and some axons could be traced to the orbitofrontal cortex. Of particular interest is the observation that there is a considerable contingent of fibers which take off from the rostrally projecting bundle from the "nonspecific" nuclei and turns back toward the mesencephalon (see Fig. 6-10).

The *reticular thalamic nucleus* (see Fig. 6-9) has played an important role in attempts to explain the mechanisms involved in the elicitation of cortical activation or desynchronization from the thalamus. As referred to previously, it was for a long period generally assumed to be the final link in the cortical projections from the "nonspecific" nuclei. (Stimulation of the reticular nucleus gives rise to diffuse recruiting responses in the cortex, see Jasper, 1949; and others.) Following localized cortical lesions topically distributed cell changes (anterior part of the cortex—anterior part of the reticular nucleus, etc.) have been found by Rose and Woolsey (1949a) and others in the reticular nucleus. However, the possibility that the changes found in the nucleus are not retrograde but transneuronal has been emphasized by Rose (1952) and others. The results obtained by Carman, Cowan, and Powell (1964b) strongly support this view, since the reticular nucleus receives a topically arranged projection from the entire cerebral cortex, as shown in experiments in the rabbit with silver impregnation methods. The Golgi studies of Scheibel and Scheibel (1966d) leave *little doubt that the reticular nucleus does not project onto the cerebral cortex.* Only very few axons of the multipolar cells of the nucleus were found to proceed in a rostral direction, and these could not be traced further than to the striatum. More than 90 per cent of the cells have *caudally* directed axons, some of which could be traced to the mesencephalon. The axons give off abundant collaterals which supply both "specific" and "nonspecific" thalamic nuclei. It is characteristic of the reticular nucleus that the dendrites of its cells are largely oriented in the plane of the flattened nucleus. On account of its position the reticular nucleus is traversed by virtually all fibers interconnecting the thalamus and the cerebral cortex. When these fibers penetrate the dendritic neuropil of the reticular nucleus they give off collaterals at right angles which appear to establish synaptic contacts with the dendrites (characterized by having long and filamented spines) of the cells in the nucleus.

It appears from these studies that the *thalamic reticular nucleus cannot be considered as a final relay in the projection of "nonspecific" thalamic nuclei upon the cortex.* From an analysis of their observations,

Scheibel and Scheibel (1966d, 1967) conclude that the reticular thalamic nucleus has presumably another function: to integrate thalamocortical and corticothalamic impulses (entering it by collaterals of the perforating fibers) and to act back on other "nonspecific" and "specific" thalamic nuclei and the mesencephalon and to modify their patterns of activity.

What is then the final link in the "nonspecific" thalamocortical projection? Several physiological studies (for example, Starzl and Whitlock, 1952; Hanbery, Ajmone-Marsan, and Dilworth, 1954; Weinberger, Velasco, and Lindsley, 1965, see also below) indicate that the ventral anterior thalamic nucleus (VA) plays an essential role. This nucleus, as referred to above, receives fibers from many "nonspecific" thalamic nuclei (in addition to fibers from the pallidum) and projects to the cortex, although its projection area is not quite certain (see Ch. 4). Its efferents to the cortex penetrate the anterior part of the reticular nucleus. This might explain the cortical responses obtained on stimulation of the anterior part of the reticular nucleus but, as pointed out by Scheibel and Scheibel and others, there may be additional possibilities for an impulse transmission from "nonspecific" thalamic nuclei to the cortex. The associational connections between "nonspecific" and "specific" thalamic nuclei may be involved.[13]

The diagram of Scheibel and Scheibel shown in Fig. 6-10 summarizes the recent anatomical observations (see legend). It is of interest that there appear to be two routes for rostrally projecting impulses from the reticular formation. One (2 in the figure) goes via midline and intralaminar nuclei from which efferent fibers pass to the VA. From this fibers, penetrating the reticular nucleus (4 in the figure), continue rostrally to the cortex. Another ventral or caudal route of ascending projections from the reticular formation passes outside the thalamus, through the subthalamus and hypothalamus. (The connections of these regions with the cortex are not fully clarified, but the hypothalamus sends fibers to the dorsomedial nucleus (MD) which projects onto the frontal lobe, see Ch. 11).

At present it does not seem possible to reach definite conclusions as to the role played by the various components of the diffuse thalamic system in its action on the cerebral cortex and to correlate physiological and anatomical observations in a fruitful manner. However, some recent ob-

---

[13] Since the caudate nucleus and the putamen both project onto the pallidum (cf. Ch. 4) which again sends its most massive efferents to the thalamus, especially the nucleus ventralis anterior (VA), the impulse passage from the intralaminar and midline nuclei to the cortex may occur along this route. According to Hassler (1964) the cortical projection areas of the relevant thalamic nuclei correspond with the cortical regions from which recruiting responses are most easily obtained.

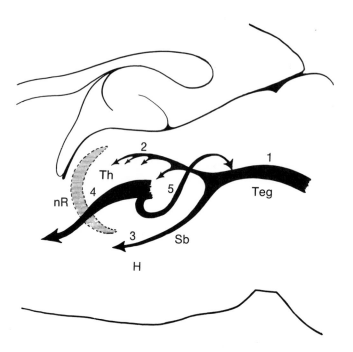

FIG. 6–10 Schematic drawing of some main features in the fiber projections assumed to be related to the ascending activating system. Fibers from the reticular formation of the brain stem (1) ascend through the tegmentum (*Teg*). Caudal to the thalamus they bifurcate into a dorsal leaf (2) which is lost in the intralaminar (*Th*) and dorsomedial thalamic fields and a ventral leaf (3). This runs ventral and lateral through the subthalamus (*Sb*) and hypothalamus (*H*) and thereby swings ventral to the thalamic reticular nucleus (*nR*). Axons of cells in the "nonspecific" thalamic projections have a rostral component (4) which perforates the reticular nucleus and continues rostrally in the inferior thalamic peduncle. Another component (5) turns caudally and runs back to the tegmental level. (Cf. text.) From Scheibel and Scheibel (1967).

servations appear promising. Extending findings made by previous authors, Skinner and Lindsley (1967) found that lesions, or temporary block by local freezing, of the ventral anterior nucleus, the inferior thalamic peduncle (where the rostrally projecting fibers pass), or the orbitofrontal cortex reduce or abolish the recruiting responses. However, such rostrally placed lesions do not affect the desynchronization in the EEG following high frequency thalamic stimulation, as lesions of the mesencephalic reticular formation do (see also Weinberger, Velasco, and Lindsley, 1965). These observations may be correlated with the demonstration of a descending projection from the "nonspecific" nuclei to the mesencephalon (5 in Fig. 6-10). It appears that separate paths are involved in the production of cortical desynchronization (the ventral route) and the recruitment phenomena (the dorsal route). The suggestion that the ventral ascending route (3 in Fig. 6-10) may be concerned with cortical desynchronization may further be correlated with the observation that most of the ascending fibers to the subthalamus, hypothalamus, and septum come from the mesencephalic reticular formation (see p. 314), since this has been shown to be the most potent part in the brain stem in producing cortical desynchronization.

It appears that current thinking on the activating system is rapidly changing. Some anatomical data has been referred to previously, which shows that a clear distinction between "specific" and "nonspecific" thalamic nuclei cannot be made. Physiological findings tend to support this (see Andersen and Andersson, 1968). Other observations demonstrate intimate functional relations between the caudate nucleus and certain parts of the thalamus. Among cortical regions attention has recently been focused on the orbital cortex as an important region in receipt of the diffuse thalamic projection system. The orbital cortex has been shown to have a potent inhibitory effect on motor and autonomic functions (see Kaada, 1951, 1960). According to Sauerland, Nakamura, and Clemente (1967) the inhibition of reflexes which can be obtained on stimulation of the orbital gyrus is mediated via the brain stem regions considered to be inhibitory (see Fig. 6-8).

It appears from the above as well as other data that the ascending activating system may influence the cortical electrical activity by way of the "nonspecific" thalamic nuclei. Since the reticular formation exerts a potent influence on the thalamus it is of great interest that an increasing body of evidence indicates the presence in the reticular formation of regions which do not activate the cortex and are not correlated with behavioral arousal but which have the opposite effect, causing electrocortical synchronization and behavioral sleep.

Sleep and consciousness. Before proceeding a few comments on the subjects of sleep and consciousness are appropriate. Sleep is generally considered as a particular state of consciousness. To give a satisfactory *definition of consciousness* has so far not been possible, in spite of a vast literature in which the problems of consciousness have been approached from philosophical, psychological, and biological points of view.[14] Any discussion of consciousness inevitably leads to another problem, the "mind-body relationship." This probably is—and will forever be—in-

---

[14] An exhaustive and critical account of relevant problems has been given by Kuhlenbeck (1957). Other enlightening papers can be found in "Brain Mechanisms and Consciousness" (1954). See also Kuhlenbeck (1959).

soluble. As Kuhlenbeck (1957, p. 93) phrases it: ". . . any attempt to explain how nervous impulses can be translated into a mental experience is an impossible attempt." Hebb (1954) has expressed a similar opinion. Nevertheless, from a practical point of view a few features of consciousness may be mentioned. In the first place it is important to distinguish between the "level" of consciousness and its "content." As to the latter, we cannot imagine a state of consciousness without "content." Kubie (1954, p. 447) has stressed: ". . . *consciousness of something* exists; but *consciousness* is merely an abstraction." This aspect of the problem of consciousness can only be studied in man, who is able to communicate his perceptions and thoughts to the investigator.[15] The problem of factors which influence the *level* of consciousness, however, may be approached in animal studies. The aim of such studies has been expressed by Kubie (1954, p. 446) as follows: "The psychologist and psychiatrist must challenge the neurophysiologist with the necessity of undertaking to explain not 'Consciousness' but the multiple phenomenology of varied conscious states."

As to the levels of consciousness it is common to undertake a gradation in attention, alertness, relaxed mood, drowsiness, sleep, stupor, and coma, but clear-cut criteria for these various states are difficult to establish since there are fleeting transitions. (An attempt to define characteristics of various degrees of reduced consciousness in human beings has been made by Mollaret and Goulon, 1959, and Jouvet, 1964.) A final aspect of the problem is to define in structural terms those parts of the nervous system which are involved. Anatomical studies cannot by themselves give information of this kind. The task for the morphologist will be restricted to making an attempt to answer the following question: To what extent are anatomical data compatible with conclusions drawn from physiological and clinical studies as to the structural organization of those regions of the brain which are believed to bear some relation to consciousness?

As discussed elsewhere (Brodal, 1964b), this is not an easy question to answer, for several reasons. In the first place, our knowledge of the anatomy as well as the physiology of the brain is still too fragmentary to permit a close correlation between findings made in the two fields of research. Furthermore, the approaches of the anatomist and the physiologist are different. The physiologist of necessity concentrates upon a particular region or function at a time, since it is impossible to record everything that goes on in the brain during an experiment, and he may be tempted to oversimplify the matter. The anatomist, being familiar with the innumerable pathways for impulse transmission which are available, is apt to be skeptical about simple hypotheses of functional organization and parcellations of the brain, and may be inclined to "overcomplicate" the issue.

[15] Some relevant data will be discussed in Ch. 12.

For some time it was generally held that it is the activity in the ascending activating system which determines the level of consciousness. The functional importance of the system would be to act as an "energizer," to exert a facilitatory influence on other parts of the nervous system.[16] It would be concerned mainly with maintaining, in the cortex, an optimal level of activity which could be modulated by the specific sensory impulses. The impulses entering the reticular formation from different sources were assumed to merge and lose their specificity within this. A cessation or reduction of the amount of these impulses would reduce the activity in the system and eventually produce sleep. This, of course, is a rather simple concept.

At the symposium on "Brain Mechanisms and Consciousness" in 1953 (printed 1954) Lord Adrian appropriately raised the question whether one should regard the ascending activating system "as just coming in to wake us up in the morning and to send us to sleep at night, to do non-specific activation," or whether it has "something to do with the direction of attention, with the actual work of the conscious brain." At the same meeting Moruzzi in the final discussion pointed to the fact that research so far had been concerned with the studies of the extremes of the functions of the reticular formation only, and he argued that the intermediate ranges of activity deserve attention as well. Only in this way could one hope to disclose a more detailed and particular functional fractionation.

As has been seen, anatomical data strongly suggests that the reticular formation is not an entity. Physiological data (some of which has been mentioned) has been forthcoming and points in the same direction. It appears that the reticular formation is concerned not only in activation, but also in "deactivation," and that the two opposing functions are related to different regions. Recent observations on sleep mechanisms are particularly illuminating.

The *"mechanism" of sleep* has attracted much interest in recent years, and several symposia have been devoted to the subject.[17] As referred to above, during quiet sleep the EEG shows synchronization (different phases are distinguished, see Kleitman, 1963). From the early 1950's it was realized that during quiet sleep there are intermittent phases of desynchronization in the EEG. Since these are combined with rapid eye movements one often speaks of REM sleep (or paradoxical or desynchronized sleep). These sleep phases are generally accompanied by dreams, and in addition to the rapid eye movements there are other

---

[16] The same factors which produce an activation with desynchronization in the EEG and behavioral arousal will also act on the spinal mechanism, increasing muscular tone and myotatic reflexes, heart rate, and blood pressure. Furthermore, an increased excretion of ACTH from the hypophysis occurs.

[17] See, for example, the Ciba Symposium "The Nature of Sleep," 1961, and "Sleep Mechanisms," 1965.

bodily changes: a reduction or abolition of muscular tone with occasional twitches, weakening of spinal reflexes, and changes in blood pressure and heart rate. These phases of sleep are often referred to also as deep sleep, since the thresholds for sensory stimuli which produce behavioral arousal appear to be increased (see Jouvet, 1962).

According to the concept of the ascending activating system outlined above, sleep would be a passive process, due to a reduced input of afferent impulses to a tonically active excitatory mechanism. This view contrasts with several previous observations which indicated that sleep may be an *active* process, due to an active inhibition originating from regions often referred to as "sleep centers." In clinicopathological studies of lethargic encephalitis, von Economo (1929) found that lesions affecting the posterior hypothalamus and rostral mesencephalon were usually associated with hypersomnia, while lesions in the anterior hypothalamus often resulted in insomnia. The latter region would then be a "sleep center," the former a "waking center." In a review of the literature, Akert (1965) reports further cases in which lesions producing hypersomnia involved the medial thalamus, subthalamus, and even the pons and medulla. In his pioneer studies with implanted electrodes in cats, Hess (1944) could induce "natural" sleep by low frequency stimulation of points in the medial thalamus, the caudate nucleus, and the preoptic and supraoptic parts of the hypothalamus.[18] (High frequency stimulation of the same points gave an awakening reaction.) Lesions of the anterior hypothalamus in rats (Nauta, 1946) result in an almost complete insomnia and hyperactivity which eventually is fatal. Subsequent studies have confirmed that areas in the anterior hypothalamus and neighboring regions are of importance in the induction of sleep (see for example Hernández Peón and Chávez Ibarra, 1963; Clemente and Sterman, 1963), and a general activation and behavioral arousal have been obtained from regions assumed to belong to the "waking center," in agreement with the findings of Moruzzi and Magoun (1949) and others.

The observations referred to above make it clear that *the theory of sleep as being a purely passive process is not satisfactory.* Certain mechanisms in the brain appear to play an active role in inducing sleep. Evidence has been produced in recent years that the reticular formation is involved in these processes. Only some of the relevant observations will be mentioned. (For a recent and lucid account, see Moruzzi, 1963.) In experiments in cats it was found that the effects of transections of the

[18] It should be noted that on stimulation of the sleep inducing regions other inhibitory actions occur, such as inhibition of muscular activity, myotatic reflexes, respiration, and lowering of blood pressure. It appears that the active region comprises also the subcallosal gyrus and some neighboring parts of the cortex (see Kaada, 1951, 1960).

brain stem at the midpontine of rostropontine level differ. In the first case the animal is alert for most of the time and shows an activated desynchronized EEG (Batini et al., 1959). These observations lead to the conclusion that there are synchronizing structures in the lower brain stem, which are tonically active. In the following years these results were confirmed and extended. Following low frequency stimulation of the medulla in the region of the solitary tract (Magnes, Moruzzi, and Pompeiano, 1961), a widespread bilateral cortical synchronization was obtained (in Bremer's *encéphale isolé* preparations, with a transection between the medulla and spinal cord). The responsible cells do not appear to belong to the nucleus of the solitary tract. However, synchronizing responses could be obtained also from other regions of the medullary reticular formation, thus from the nucleus reticularis ventralis (see Fig. 6-2). Signs of behavioral sleep were found to accompany EEG synchronization on low frequency stimulations (in unanesthetized animals) in several regions of the reticular formation (Favale, Loeb, Rossi, and Sacco, 1961). Continued studies by Rossi and his collaborators and others have brought further information of synchronizing structures in the brain stem (see Rossi, 1965, for particulars). Based on evidence of electrical stimulation and of lesions in various parts of the brain stem, the conclusion was reached that there is a region medial in the lower pons which facilitates cortical EEG synchronization. This region seems to coincide with the pontine region which gives off abundant long ascending fibers (see Fig. 6-4, and Fig. 12 in Rossi, 1965) as determined anatomically (Brodal and Rossi, 1955). Further support was derived from studies on injections of small doses of barbiturates in the vertebral artery in *encéphale isolé* cats when the basilar artery was clamped at the midpontine level (Magni, Moruzzi, Rossi, and Zanchetti, 1959). This caused an immediate suppression of EEG synchronization. This is interpreted as being due to a temporary elimination of caudal synchronizing structures while the desynchronizing region in the mesencephalon is unaffected by the anesthetic. Synchronization reappeared when the action of the barbiturate had vanished. These and other findings strongly suggest that there are two regions in the brain stem, both apparently belonging to the reticular formation, which exert a synchronizing effect on the electrocorticogram and, when activated, have a sleep-inducing effect. Certain data supports the assumption (see Rossi, 1965) that the pontine cortically synchronizing region is tonically active, while the medullary regions have a mainly phasic function.[19]

The views outlined above can so far not be considered as being more

---

[19] One may speculate upon whether these functional differences are related to the fact that giant cells contribute to the rostral projection only in the pontine rostrally projecting region of the reticular formation (see Fig. 6-4).

than hypotheses. However, they lead to a less rigid conception of the sleep-waking mechanism. The existence in the reticular formation of a dual system, one having an activating (EEG-desynchronizing), the other a deactivating (EEG-synchronizing) effect, is an attractive hypothesis from several points of view. It is compatible with the observation that other regions of the brain may be concerned in regulating the sleep-waking relations, and will probably make it easier to understand the interrelations between the various sleep and waking "centers." It is, for example, of interest that the long ascending projections from the "synchronizing regions" of the medulla and pons pass chiefly to the intralaminar and midline nuclei, while the mesencephalic projections pass largely outside these. The activating region of the reticular formation appears to be chiefly its mesencephalic part. The problems related to the structural and functional interrelations between cortically "synchronizing" and "desynchronizing" systems are, however, extremely complex, and as yet far from being solved.

The facilitatory action of certain brain stem regions on EEG synchronization has been assumed to occur in two ways. It may be due to a direct excitation of the thalamocortical synchronizing mechanisms or it may occur by inhibition of the ascending activating regions of the brain stem. Final conclusions are as yet not possible, and it may well be that both mechanisms may coexist, as suggested by Magnes, Moruzzi, and Pompeiano (1961) and Favale, Loeb, Rossi, and Sacco (1961). Certain observations seem to indicate that the facilitation of EEG synchronization produced by the pontine region is mainly due to inhibition of the activating part of the reticular formation, while the medullary region close to the nucleus of the solitary tract acts directly on the thalamocortical mechanisms (see Rossi, 1965).

The existence of regions in the reticular formation exerting opposite effects on the electrocorticogram and behavior (arousal-sleep) raises the question of the way in which these opposing regions are brought into play by different kinds of stimuli. From this point of view it is interesting that according to Pompeiano and Swett (1962a, 1962b) EEG synchronization, and often behavioral sleep, may be induced by low rate stimulation of low threshold cutaneous fibers, belonging to group II (while high rate stimulation of these, as well as of group III afferents, gives arousal). The synchronizing impulses were shown to influence especially the nucleus reticularis gigantocellularis, and appear to ascend in the spinoreticular tract (Pompeiano and Swett, 1963). Vagal afferent impulses may induce synchronization (but may also give rise to desynchronization, see Chase et al., 1967). Synchronization of the EEG obtainable by stimulation of the orbitofrontal cortex may be mediated via the medullary reticular formation (see Dell, Bonvallet, and Hugelin, 1961), which, as shown in Fig. 6-7, receives cortical fibers.

340

Further support for the existence of a dual mechanism within the reticular formation comes from pharmacological studies. Extending previous studies of this type, Cordeau, Moreau, Beaulnes, and Laurin (1963) found that small quantities of adrenaline (or related substances) injected directly into the brain stem of sleeping cats usually produces arousal and EEG desynchronization, while injection of acetylcholine is usually followed by synchronization and drowsiness or sleep. It is of particular interest that the points responding to acetylcholine were situated more caudally than the adrenaline-positive points. The authors suggest that the two groups of substances raise the level of activity of two different "systems."

Concerning the *REM phases of deep, desynchronized, sleep* it is so far not clear whether they are due to activity in a particular region. Rossi and his collaborators, as well as Jouvet (1962), have suggested that the caudal part of the nucleus reticularis pontis oralis and immediately caudal, neighboring areas may be responsible. Destruction of this region abolishes both EEG and somatic manifestations of deep sleep.

Jouvet (1965) has further suggested that the raphe nuclei are particularly important "sleep inducing" structures, and that they are involved in regulating the level of serotonin. A reduction of cerebral serotonin leads to a prolonged waking state, as does destruction of the raphe nuclei. Paradoxical sleep is thought to be related to the nucleus coeruleus which has neurons rich in noradrenaline.

There is some evidence that the episodes of deep sleep are caused by sudden outbursts of activity, possibly in the pons (see Jouvet, 1962; Moruzzi, 1963), and it appears that during these phases there is an active inhibition of the thalamocortical synchronizing system. The vestibular nuclei are important in mediating some of the somatic phenomena of deep sleep as shown by Pompeiano and Morrison in a series of studies. Complete destruction of the vestibular nuclei on both sides does not prevent the appearance of the different phases of synchronized or desynchronized sleep. However, the bursts of rapid eye movement and the related phasic inhibition of monosynaptic reflexes are abolished when the medial and descending vestibular nuclei are destroyed bilaterally (see Pompeiano and Morrison, 1966). For some further observations on desynchronized sleep see Gassel and Pompeiano (1967).

The recent studies on sleep are of immediate interest for the problems related to the level of consciousness in general. Rossi (1964, p. 187) has suggested that: "The regulation of the level of consciousness under physiological conditions is achieved by the interplay of two opposite, competing neural mechanisms, a facilitatory activating arousing system and an inhibitory deactivating sleep-producing system with the most important structures involved lying in the brain stem." This means that a decrease in the level of consciousness may depend not only on a reduced activity of the activating structures, but may also occur when the deactivating influences are brought into action (representing a passive and an active reduction of the level of consciousness, respectively). As Rossi (1964, 1965) emphasizes, this is so far only a hypothesis, and it

341

will presumably need modification and elaboration when further studies are made.

It is not yet quite clear whether *conditions in man* are exactly similar to those in the cat. As referred to previously, there are some anatomical differences between the reticular formation in the two species. For example, the spinoreticular fibers appear to extend further rostrally in man and to have three maximal sites of termination. Studies on the behavioral and EEG effects of injecting quickly acting barbiturates into the vertebral artery in human patients are of relevance. The injection produces a temporary "anesthesia" in the areas supplied by the vertebral arteries. Its distribution within the brain stem can be judged approximately from examination of function of the cranial nerves. Following such injections the patient is alert (he is, for example, able to push a button) and his EEG is desynchronized (Alemà, Perria, Rosadini, Rossi, and Zattoni, 1966). If the injection was made with the patient relaxed and with a mild EEG synchronization, as occasionally was possible, there was an immediately clear-cut desynchronization. These findings were interpreted as evidence that the desynchronizing activating part of the reticular formation in man is situated at the mesencephalic level. They are compatible with the assumption that deactivating (EEG synchronizing) structures are present in the lower part of the brain stem (as in the cat) but do not prove this. The consequences of brain-stem lesions in man are in agreement with the above conception, in so far as in man lesions of the brain stem involving the mesencephalon are regularly followed by EEG changes of synchronization and loss of consciousness, indicating involvement of the activating system (see also the following section).

Even if there are still many open questions, it appears that in man as in experimental animals the reticular formation is important in controlling the level of consciousness. That it has a dual influence seems indeed likely. However, it would be *entirely misleading to consider the reticular formation as the "seat of consciousness."* Anatomical studies show that the reticular formation has connections with many other parts of the nervous system, not least the cerebral cortex. Furthermore, as has been pointed out elsewhere (Brodal, 1964b), in the brain stem there are gray masses, especially the raphe nuclei and the periaqueductal gray, which with regard to their connections resemble the reticular formation and have connections with this. It is difficult to imagine that any activity in the reticular formation would not be correlated and integrated with activities going on in some of these gray masses.[20] Integration of impulses

[20] Some physiological observations appear to support this view. For example, Hara, Favale, Rossi, and Sacco (1961) found no substantial differences between the central gray matter and the reticular formation of the mesencephalon as con-

from various sensory sources may occur in many regions of the brain stem apart from the reticular formation, for example in the nucleus of the spinal trigeminal tract (see Rossi and Brodal, 1956b). These functional implications, made on the basis of anatomical data, are supported by physiological observations.

In recent years much attention has been paid to the role of the reticular formation and the ascending activating system in processes such as sensory perception and discrimination, learning, adaptation, habituation, modification of behavior, etc.[21] These functions are all closely related to consciousness, and a number of experimental studies have been made in this field, not least behavioral studies of animals. The use of implanted electrodes permits observations in the unanesthetized state, and radio control may be used for stimulation and recording (telemetry). (For an illuminating study of this kind see Delgado, 1963.) These studies leave no doubt that the reticular formation co-operates with many other parts of the brain in influencing functions such as alertness, attention, perception, discrimination, etc. Changes in many of these functions have, furthermore, been observed following lesions or stimulation of many other parts of the brain, such as the entorhinal area, the nucleus amygdalae, the caudate nucleus, the hypothalamus, and others. (These observations have apparently contributed to the creation of a new foggy concept, "the limbic system," to which reference will be made in Chs. 10 and 11.) The problems are extremely complex, and it is probably right to say that no clear conception can as yet be formulated. The only safe conclusion which can be drawn from all these observations is that *a number of brain regions are of importance for consciousness,* even for its most simple aspect, its level; a conclusion in agreement with clinical observations.

It ought finally to be emphasized, as will have appeared from several data mentioned in this chapter, that *it is no longer possible to maintain a distinction between "specific" and "unspecific" systems.* In an experimental study, Sprague et al. (1963), following bilateral lesions of the rostral midbrain without significant involvement of the reticular formation, found marked effects on functions which are generally thought to be influenced from the reticular formation, such as affective behavior and attention. They conclude (loc. cit. p. 226) that "there is probably a continuous gradient in the functional organization of ascending systems between the most highly localized lemniscal path and the most diffuse of

---

cerns their responsiveness to afferent somatic stimulation. See also the observations of Jouvet (mentioned above) on the role of the raphe in sleep mechanisms.

[21] See, for example: "Neurological Basis of Behaviour," 1958; "The Physiological Basis of Mental Activity," 1963.

the reticular paths. Anatomically there is intermingling of the two. Thus the best placed lesion can achieve no perfect separation of specific and reticular systems."

Clinical aspects.   Even if much remains to be learned before we can say that we "understand" the reticular formation, the many *recent experimental studies have cast light on phenomena which are common in daily life.* The alerting effect of a sudden noise, a light flash, or a painful stimulus is well known, and may be explained by the influence of such stimuli on the ascending activating system. It is likewise a common experience that increased attention and alertness are accompanied by an increased heart rate and often also other autonomic phenomena. This is easily explained by the general, ascending and descending, actions of the activating system (cf. axons with dichotomizing, ascending and descending branches in the reticular formation). On the other hand, monotonous and usually weak stimuli, such as gentle stroking of the skin, slow rhythmic movements (rocking chair!), monotonous sounds and quiet music, are well known to have a relaxing and often sleep-inducing effect. Physiotherapy, especially massage and exercises aiming at muscular relaxation have a beneficial effect in favoring reduction of mental as well as physical tension. It seems a likely assumption that all these procedures owe at least part of their effect to an influence on the synchronizing parts of the reticular formation. The cerebral influence on the reticular formation can, however, scarcely be overrated. Our general alertness is influenced by words we hear, scenes we see, processes which require consciousness and interpretation of perceptions and which certainly are dependent on cortical activity (e.g. the awakening effect on a drowsy audience of a humorous or otherwise engaging remark by the lecturer). More impressive even is the common experience that mental imagery and daydreaming may have a general alerting effect as marked as that following any external stimulus. It appears very likely that the corticoreticular projections are involved in these processes. These connections, presumably in collaboration with others, appear further to be important in the inhibition and facilitation of sensory impulses, which make it possible for us to concentrate upon a particular sensory stimulus and neglect all others. (The most illuminating illustration is perhaps what everybody will have experienced at a lively cocktail party: among a number of loud voices one is able to pick out a single voice and perceive this, without paying attention to all the others.)

Turning to more direct *clinical aspects* it may be noted that there are good reasons to believe that several *anesthetic agents* exert at least part of their action by reducing the activity of the activating (ascending and descending) systems (see Domino, 1958). It appears further that the

344

actions of some *psychopharmaca* are, in part, due to their influence on the reticular formation (see Domino, 1958). These subjects are beyond the scope of the present text. It should be stressed, however, that studies in these fields are complicated by the fact that all these substances, as well as neurohumors, scarcely affect the reticular formation in isolation.

When turning to the symptoms following pathological affections of this part of the brain we meet with a similar complexity and corresponding difficulties in interpreting results. It is certainly true also for the human brain that the reticular formation co-operates with many other parts in influencing functions such as alertness, attention, perception, discrimination, etc. It is no wonder, therefore, that disturbances in such functions may be seen in man with lesions affecting various parts of the brain, not least the cerebral cortex. Clinical observations may serve as a warning against putting too much emphasis on the reticular formation in these complex functions. It appears that in recent years there has been a tendency to overrate the role of the reticular formation, and to underrate the importance of the cerebral cortex as maintained by Sir Geoffrey Jefferson (1958).

A *pathological process affecting the reticular formation* will probably never be restricted to the reticular formation alone. A tumor, a vascular disturbance, or an inflammatory process is extremely likely to involve other structures as well, with resulting signs and symptoms from cranial nerves, long ascending and descending pathways, and various nuclei. These symptoms have been considered in other chapters. Here our concern will be with symptoms which may be related to affections of the reticular formation.

In *poliomyelitis* changes are often found in the reticular formation (Barnhart, Rhines, McCarter, and Magoun, 1948; Bodian, 1949, and others). Pathologic anatomical studies have shown that the changes may extend throughout the brain stem. Whether these changes are responsible for the "spasms" often occurring in the acute stages of poliomyelitis has been debated. In a study of 80 cases, Baker, Matzke, and Brown (1950) point to the frequent affection of the area dorsal to the inferior olive and present evidence that somewhat different regions are involved in the control of respiration and cardiovascular functions. On the basis of predominant injury of various regions they suggest a symptomatological subdivision of bulbar poliomyelitis into four types.

From a clinical point of view the *possible relation of the reticular formation to consciousness* has attracted considerable interest. The role which may be played by a deranged function of the reticular formation in conditions such as diabetic, hepatic, or uremic coma and in disturbances of consciousness in general asphyxia, appears to be little known. It seems likely that the general metabolic and humoral changes in these conditions affect widespread areas of the brain. More information has been obtained from studies of relatively local damage to the brain stem in cases of tumors or vascular affections. It appears to be the general experience of neurosurgeons that tumors involving the mesencephalon and diencephalon are generally followed by loss of consciousness which often may last for months (Cairns, 1952; French, 1952; M. Jefferson, 1952, and others). The EEG may show synchronization. According to Cairns (1952) the most common disturbance in these cases is hypersomnia. This condition may also occur in tumors below the floor of the third ventricle, arising from remnants of the craniopharyngeal pouch, and if the tumor is cystic and is emptied by aspiration, the stupor may promptly disappear (Cairns, 1952). In other instances of tumors in the upper mesencephalon-diencephalon, decerebrate rigidity may be present together with loss of consciousness. This may also occur in occlusion of the basilar artery, which will affect the brain stem (and in which possible pressure effects may be excluded). Disturbances of consciousness, from slight confusion to deep coma, are an early and constant feature in the clinical picture (Kubik and Adams, 1946). Occasionally "akinetic mutism" may be seen in lower brain stem lesions (see Cairns, 1952; Cravioto et al., 1960).

It appears from a relatively large number of observations on patients with tumors of the upper brain stem and diencephalon that these regions are essential for the maintenance of what is sometimes referred to as "crude consciousness." The clinical findings as well as the accompanying EEG changes are compatible with the view that these brain regions are concerned in a general activation of the brain in man, as in experimental animals.

The situation as to the importance of the lower brain stem for consciousness is less clear. On account of the role played by the medulla and lower pons in the regulation of respiration and cardiovascular functions, lesions of the lower brain stem are apt to be rapidly fatal. Unconsciousness in these cases is usually accompanied by disturbances in breathing, lowering of blood pressure, and signs of involvement of other structures in the brain stem. According to Cairns (1952) the loss of consciousness is usually sudden in onset and deep, and it may be that the cerebral anoxia resulting from the deranged cardiovascular and respiratory functions is the cause of the coma. However, some cases have been reported in the literature in which patients with lesions of the pons and medulla have survived for longer periods, and in which the EEG has shown a desynchronized pattern, as in the waking state. Behaviorally, however, in most instances the patients have shown a reduced level of conscious-

346

ness or have been in stupor or coma (see, for example, Loeb and Poggio, 1953; Lundervold, Hauge, and Løken, 1956; Kaada, Harkmark, and Stokke, 1961; Chatrian, White, and Shaw, 1964; Marquardsen and Harvald, 1964; also Aléma et al., 1966). Observations of this kind, as well as the results of intravertebral injection of barbiturates, referred to above, seem at least to indicate that "in man the neurons having a tonic activating function are not located in the whole brain stem, but only in its rostralmost part (i.e. rostral midbrain) and diencephalon" (Rossi, 1965, p. 275). The presence of a synchronizing region in the lower brain stem has so far not been proved, and the relation between loss of consciousness with lesions in this region and the accompanying changes in the EEG is not clear.[22]

From a clinical point of view it is important to recall that *disturbances of consciousness,* as found in lesions of the brain stem and diencephalon, *may be caused by processes outside the brain stem when this is subjected to compression or traction or there are secondary vascular disturbances.* Cairns (1952) in discussing this subject draws attention to the frequent occurrence of compression of the brain stem against the tentorium when a tumor, particularly in the temporal lobe or in the upper cerebellar vermis, produces a displacement of the brain. Release of these brain herniations by operation may often be followed by immediate return of consciousness. The disturbances of consciousness occurring with intense rise of intracranial pressure are probably due to tentorial herniation or tonsillar herniation (downward protrusion of the cerebellar tonsilla into the foramen magnum). In such cases, as well as with local lesions of the brain stem, intermittent attacks of unconsciousness may occur, most likely due to transitory circulatory disturbances (ischemia). The attacks may be accompanied by tonic fits.

There is abundant clinical evidence that *consciousness may be disturbed and reduced in man in affections of the brain which do not involve the brain stem.* In some patients who had shown prolonged altered states of consciousness for months or years, following severe head trauma, no focal lesions were found in the brain stem at autopsy, but there was a diffuse degeneration or often a necrosis of the white matter in the cerebrum, with degeneration of descending tracts (Jouvet and Jouvet, 1963; Kristiansen, 1964; and others). In traumatic head injuries disturbances of consciousness are commonly seen. However, in a great proportion of such cases which take a fatal course no evidence of structural damage of the brain stem is found at autopsy (Tandon and Kristiansen, 1966).

[22] Gastaut (1954, p. 279) early drew attention to the fact that the changes in EEG and in the level of consciousness "are not directly dependent on each other and may evolve independently."

The structural basis of the symptoms in cases of blunt head injury are often difficult to evaluate, since secondary brain changes commonly develop, but obviously disturbances of consciousness are by themselves no reliable criterion of damage to the brain stem in such cases. Some other regions appear to bear a rather close relation to disturbances of consciousness. G. Jefferson (1958, 1960) emphasizes the frequent occurrence of hypersomnia passing into coma in cases of bleeding from aneurysms of the anterior cerebral and anterior communicating arteries. He speaks of the region around the lamina terminalis (in front of the third ventricle) as an "anterior critical point" in contrast to the "posterior critical point" at the level of the tentorium. Reference was made above to the frequent occurrence of hypersomnia in cases of tumors below the floor of the third ventricle. That lesions around the hypothalamus may affect the ascending activating pathways (by pressure or bleeding) can scarcely be denied, but more often it appears that this is not the case and does not explain the changes in consciousness. Disturbances of "crude" consciousness may be seen, although less often, in lesions in many other parts of the brain (see Kristiansen, 1964). In some of these the alterations in the "contents" of consciousness are marked. While it is a general observation by neurosurgeons that quite extensive parts of the cerebral cortex may be ablated without overt signs of a reduced level of consciousness, certain aspects of consciousness, taken in its broader sense (for example those related to perceptual processes), may be affected by cortical lesions. This is particularly well illustrated by lesions of the temporo-parietal cortex (see Ch. 12) and in epileptic seizures in such cases, often appearing as so-called psychical seizures (see Penfield and Jasper, 1954). These may occur as an aura to a larger epileptic attack. Little is known of the mechanisms underlying these and other varieties of disturbances of consciousness, and these subjects will not be discussed here. Suffice it to mention that it is generally held that the petit mal attacks, with their brief loss of consciousness, are produced by a pathological activity in the midline thalamic nuclei. These and other observations in a large number of patients suffering from various types of epileptic seizures form the basis of Penfield's hypothesis of a "centrencephalic system," in which the intimate collaboration of the neuronal networks in the brain stem, thalamus, and cortex is a crucial point (see Penfield and Jasper, 1954; Penfield, 1958).

In closed head injuries unconsciousness is a frequent and important symptom. The depth and duration of unconsciousness may vary. Many attempts have been made to explain the pathogenesis of cerebral concussion. The frequent occurrence of transitory signs of disturbances in cranial nerve functions, in coordination, and in spinal reflexes (Kristian-

348

sen, 1949) suggests that there are reversible changes in the brain stem in many of the patients. The mechanism of these changes has so far not been clarified. The transient disturbances of consciousness which occasionally occur during vertebral angiography (see Hauge, 1954) are presumably due to a temporary ischemia of the brain stem.

As will be apparent from the few data considered in this section, there appears to be good evidence that in man, as in animals, the activity of the reticular formation is important in regulating the *level* of consciousness. However, in this function it certainly collaborates with other parts of the brain, not least the thalamus and the cerebral cortex. Concerning those parts of the brain which are related to the many other, more subtle, aspects of consciousness little can be said except that certain cortical regions are necessary for those aspects of consciousness which are related to acoustic, visual, or other sensory perceptions. It may be wise to be very careful in drawing conclusions about particular anatomical structures related to these complex functions, and Penfield's (1958, p. 232) words: "There is no room or place where consciousness dwells," should be borne in mind.

7

The Cranial Nerves

THE structure of the spinal cord is in general much the same throughout its length, and the plan of organization of its cell groups and fibers can be quite clearly recognized. The brain stem, continuing the spinal cord in the skull, at first glance shows only a slight resemblance to the cord. However, a closer analysis reveals many common principles of organization in these two parts of the central nervous system. Present knowledge of these principles is based mainly on comparative anatomical investigations, for the fundamental pattern of organization is more clearly discernible in animals low in the evolutionary scale. Among the anatomists who have contributed most to this subject, C. Judson Herrick should be especially mentioned.

During evolution the cranial part of the body assumes a steadily increasing importance, due primarily to the development of the special sense organs. This is reflected in the structure of the nervous system. The dominant influence of the cranial parts of the body reaches its peak with the development of a cerebral cortex, which especially in the higher mammals and man, not only in regard to its mass but also to its structural complexity, is an organ of overwhelming importance for the function of the entire nervous system. It follows from this that the primitive pattern of the brain stem is most easily discerned and most completely preserved in its caudal part, the medulla oblongata.

The Cranial Nerves

In the myelencephalon and metencephalon, the *sulcus limitans* is present in man also in the fully developed brain. It is clearly seen in the floor of the 4th ventricle. In accordance with its functional significance in the development of the spinal cord, it indicates also in the brain stem the borderline between the zone of efferent nuclei in the floor plate and the zone of terminal nuclei of the afferent fibers in the alar plate, which is here bent laterally. In embryonic development the cells giving origin to efferent and afferent nuclei are arranged in longitudinal columns, which later become partly broken up into distinct cell groups or nuclei. However, most of them retain approximately their original place, and even in the adult, therefore, nuclei derived from the different primary columns are found arranged in a columnar manner.

Whereas in the spinal cord only four functionally separate categories of fibers are present—somatic efferent, visceral efferent, visceral afferent, and somatic afferent—the development in the cranial part of the body of the special senses and the gill apparatus with the branchial arches is accompanied by a corresponding complexity of fiber categories and nuclei.

However, the composition of the different cranial nerves is not identical, some having only efferent fibers, others only afferent, whereas some are mixed.

The arrangement is presented diagrammatically in Fig. 7-1. The sulcus limitans marks the boundary between efferent and afferent nuclear zones. Within these zones a further differentiation is possible. The medialmost column of efferent nuclei corresponds closely to the groups of ventral horn cells and is embryologically continuous with them. Like them the efferent fibers innervate striated muscle, derived embryologically from the myotomes of the somites. In the head, muscle of myotomic origin, according to most observers, is represented only by the extra-ocular muscles and the intrinsic muscles of the tongue. Accordingly such *somatic efferent nuclei* are the motor nuclei of the IIIrd, IVth, VIth, and XIIth cranial nerves.

The cells of these nuclei are morphologically of the same type as the ventral horn cells, and the nuclei are found immediately ventral to the floor of the 4th ventricle and the aqueduct.

Lateral to the somatic efferent nuclei in the basal plate of the brain stem are found the two categories of *visceral efferent nuclei,* forming two separate columns. The most medial of these, which is displaced somewhat in a ventral direction, is an interrupted column, the fibers of which pass to striated muscles. These muscles are developed from the mesoderm of the branchial arches, and comprise those from the first branchial arch, the masticatory muscles (+ the anterior belly of the digastric and the mylohyoid muscles); those from the second branchial

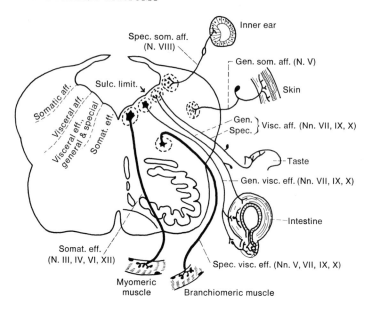

FIG. 7–1 A diagram of the nuclear columns in the brain stem, illustrating the type of structures supplied by the different categories and the nerves containing fibers from the different nuclear columns. The accessory nerve is omitted. Altered from Strong and Elwyn (1943).

arch, the facial, mimetic muscles (+ the posterior belly of the digastric and the stylohyoid muscles); and the striated muscles developed from the third and fourth branchial arches, namely those of the pharynx and larynx. The nuclei are the motor nuclei of the Vth and VIIth cranial nerves, and one of the vagus-glossopharyngeal nuclei, the nucleus ambiguus. Probably the nucleus of the XIth nerve belongs to this group. These nuclei and the fibers they give off are called *special visceral efferent*.

Just as there is a morphological similarity between the striated muscle innervated by these nuclei and the musculature supplied by the nuclei of the somatic efferent group, so their nerve cells also are of the same type. On account of these similarities the name "lateral or special somatic efferent nuclei and fibers" is sometimes applied to them.

Medial to the sulcus limitans are found the nuclei belonging to the *general visceral efferent* category, consisting of the nucleus of Edinger-Westphal of the IIIrd nerve, the superior and inferior salivatory nuclei of the VIIth and IXth nerve, respectively, and the dorsal motor nucleus of the vagus. The cells of these nuclei morphologically resemble those in the sympathetic intermediolateral cell column in the cord and functionally represent the cranial division of the parasympathetic giving rise to preganglionic fibers, which end in autonomic ganglia. The postganglionic neurons supply smooth, unstriped muscle in the organs innervated by the nerves mentioned and glands (e.g. the lacrimal and salivary glands).

Immediately lateral to the sulcus limitans is found a sensory column receiving *visceral afferent* fibers. This consists of only one nucleus, the nucleus of the tractus solitarius, extending throughout the entire length of the medulla oblongata. The afferent fibers ending in it pass through the VIIth (intermedius), IXth, and Xth nerves, have their cells in the ganglia of these nerves, and before entering the nucleus descend as the tractus solitarius. Usually a distinction is made between two types of visceral afferent fibers, and there is some comparative data indicating a corresponding subdivision of the nucleus in certain forms (see Barnard, 1936). Some of the fibers convey impulses of taste and are called *special visceral afferent*. (It may be justifiable to place the olfactory fibers also in this group.) Other fibers convey general impulses from the viscera and are termed *general visceral afferent*.

The *somatic afferent nuclei* are found in the lateralmost part of the alar plate, and here a subdivision can also be made. Fibers conveying impulses of superficial (and probably also deep) sensibility from the face travel through the trigeminal nerve, have their cells in the semilunar ganglion, and end in the principal or superior sensory nucleus of the Vth nerve and in the nucleus of the spinal tract of the trigeminal nerve, after having passed for some distance caudally in the medulla oblongata. The homology of the trigeminal nuclei with the dorsal horns reveals itself morphologically in the continuity of the nucleus of the spinal tract and the gelatinous substance of the dorsal horns. This is the general somatic afferent component. In the vagus, glossopharyngeal, and intermediate nerves some fibers of this type are also present.

The *special somatic afferent* nerves are the vestibular and cochlear, conveying impulses from the sensory apparatus in the inner ear, the former proprioceptive, the latter exteroceptive. Their nuclei are found in the extreme lateral and dorsolateral parts of the medulla oblongata.

It will be seen (cf. also Fig. 7-2) that whereas nearly all of the efferent nuclear columns are broken up into distinct parts, belonging to the different nerves containing fibers of the kind in question, this is not the case with the afferent nuclei. This is particularly evident in the general somatic afferent nuclei of the trigeminal, which forms a continuous cell mass in receipt of fibers from the Vth, VIIth, IXth, and Xth nerves, and in the nucleus of the tractus solitarius, which receives the visceral afferent fibers of the VIIth, IXth, and Xth nerves. This presumably has a func-

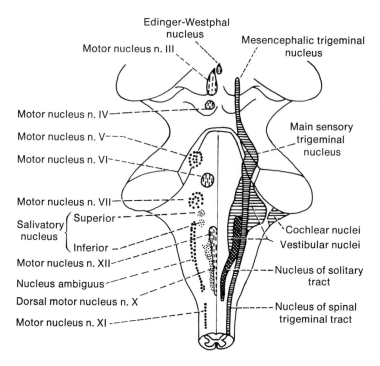

FIG. 7–2 Diagram indicating the columnar arrangement of the cranial nerve nuclei. The nuclei belonging to the same categories are indicated by identical symbols.

tional significance. Kappers has interpreted this as an expression of a general law in morphogenesis: fibers transmitting the same sensory modality and usually stimulated simultaneously tend to take the same course within the central nervous system and end in the same nuclear complex.

The *neurobiotactic* influences (Kappers, 1927) of which the above is an example, are also revealed in other morphological features. Thus the varying position of several of the motor nuclei of the cranial nerves in different vertebrate species has been interpreted by Kappers as being due to the tendency of the perikarya and dendrites of the cells in a center to migrate toward the source of most important impulses, whereas the axons grow out in the opposite direction.[1]

In a general consideration of the cranial nerves it should be remembered that they are not only links in the sensory and effector mechanisms related to the conscious acts subserved by the cerebral cortex. Equally

[1] For some critical comments on the theory of neurobiotaxis, see Harkmark (1954).

354

significant is the role they play in many of the vitally important reflexes, evoked from and partly effected through the mechanisms in the head and its organs. Some of these will be touched upon when dealing with the appropriate cranial nerves.

Regarding the cranial nerves as a whole, it will be apparent that they differ to a considerable degree in their physiological properties, as well as in their anatomical features. From a clinical viewpoint, not all of them are of equal importance. Some of them are highly specific sensory nerves forming links in rather well-defined functional systems. This applies especially to the IInd cranial nerve, the optic (which strictly speaking is not a cranial nerve at all), the cochlear division of the VIIIth nerve, and the olfactory (Ist) nerve. It has on this account been deemed appropriate to treat these cranial nerves in special chapters devoted to the mechanisms of vision, hearing, and smell, respectively. In the following description, therefore, these cranial nerves are omitted. In connection with the description of the other nerves some special problems relating to more than one nerve are more comprehensively treated with only one of them, for example, taste together with the VIIth cranial nerve. The peripheral course of the nerves will be treated only briefly. For a more complete account the reader is referred to the author's book on the cranial nerves (Brodal, 1965b).

The cranial nerve nuclei are acted upon by fibers from many sources. Axons or axonal collaterals of cells in the reticular formation appear to pass to virtually all cranial nerve nuclei (see Scheibel and Scheibel, 1958). Primary afferent fibers, according to Szentágothai (1948), do not pass directly to the efferent nuclei, indicating that at least one neuron must be intercalated in the reflex arcs of the brain stem. Fibers from the nucleus of the spinal trigeminal tract have been described as ending in motor cranial nerve nuclei V to XII (Stewart and King, 1963). Furthermore, fibers from "higher levels," in some cases even from the cerebral cortex, have been traced to the *sensory* nuclei (see later sections). These connections thus indicate possibilities for a central control of the transmission of sensory impulses entering the cranial nerves, just as is the case for afferent impulses entering the spinal cord (see Ch. 2). The *efferent* nuclei likewise are acted upon by fibers from "higher levels." Of particular interest are the connections from the "motor" cortical areas to the somatic and special visceral efferent nuclei. It appears that in man (Kuypers, 1958c), as in the monkey (Kuypers, 1958b) some corticobulbar fibers end in synaptic contact with neurons in the motor cranial nerve nuclei, while in the cat such fibers can be traced only to their vicinity (Walberg, 1957b; Kuypers, 1958a; Szentágothai and Rajkovits, 1958; and others), where they probably end on "internuncial" cells. This, as will be seen, corresponds to the patterns of ending of cortical fibers in the spinal cord.

(a) THE HYPOGLOSSAL NERVE

Anatomy. The fibers of the hypoglossal nerve spring from the hypoglossal nucleus. This belongs to the somatic efferent group of nuclei and is made up of cells of the same type as the motoneurons in the cord. In many animals and embryologically in man the nucleus is continuous with the ventral horn, thus indicating its functional relationship, but after birth in man it becomes separated from this. The nucleus, forming a longitudinal cell column (Fig. 7-2), is found close beneath the floor of the 4th ventricle in the trigonum nervi hypoglossi, and extends rostrally to the striae medullares. Caudally it reaches the caudalmost part of the medulla, where it is found immediately ventral to the central canal (Fig. 7-3). The small nuclei situated in its immediate neighborhood (the nucleus intercalatus of Staderini, the nucleus of Roller, and the nucleus praepositus hypoglossi, collectively referred to as the perihypoglossal nuclei) do not send fibers into the hypoglossal nerve (see Boyd, 1941) but have projections to the cerebellum (see Ch. 5). The hypoglossal nucleus consists of several distinct cell groups. By a study of retrograde changes in the cells after extirpation of various tongue muscles it has been shown that each group supplies certain of the tongue muscles (Barnard, 1940, and earlier authors). Thus a localization pattern is revealed in the structure of the nucleus (cf. similar findings in the ventral horns and other motor nuclei).

The axons from the hypoglossal nucleus emanate as bundles which course in a ventral and slightly lateral direction, traverse the reticular formation of the medulla oblongata, pierce the medial parts of the inferior olive and leave the brain stem in the lateral ventral sulcus, between the pyramid and the olivary eminence (see Figs. 2-9 and 7-6).

The nucleus receives impulses from axons derived from several sources. Fibers of the corticobulbar tract, originating in the central area of the cerebral cortex are presumably involved when voluntary movements of the tongue are performed. In man some fibers appear to end on cells of the nucleus (see Kuypers, 1958c). It appears that most of the corticobulbar fibers acting on the hypoglossal nucleus in man are crossed, since cortical lesions or lesions of the internal capsule give rise only to contralateral changes in the tongue.[2] Furthermore, fibers reach the nu-

[2] According to Mingazzini, uncrossed corticobulbar fibers end predominantly in the medially situated cell groups of the nucleus. This is in harmony with the fact that these groups are concerned with the innervation of the intrinsic lingual muscles, which usually work symmetrically (Barnard, 1940).

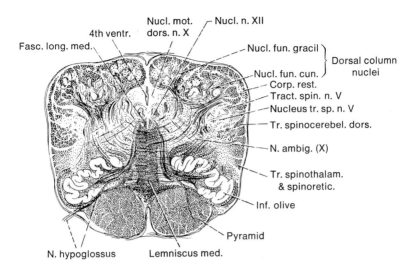

FIG. 7-3 Drawing of a transverse section through the caudal part of the medulla oblongata in man. Weigert's myelin sheath stain. The fibers are clearly visible, the nuclear groups evident as light areas. (Approx. x 4.)

cleus from the reticular formation and possibly also from the sensory trigeminal nuclei (see Stewart and King, 1963) and the nucleus of the tractus solitarius. These fibers are involved in the actions of reflex sucking, swallowing, chewing, etc.

The fibers of the hypoglossal nerve, which are mainly of the larger and medium-sized myelinated type, leave the medulla as 10 to 15 slender rootlets, which soon coalesce and pass through the hypoglossal canal in the occipital bone, surrounded by a plexus of veins.

Turning lateral to the nodose ganglion of the vagus, with which it is usually connected by connective tissue, the nerve descends in a caudally arched course, passes downward and ventrally to reach the tongue near its base, and distributes its fibers to the muscles of the tongue. The hypoglossal fibers supply not only the intrinsic muscles of the tongue, but also the styloglossus, hyoglossus, genioglossus, and geniohyoid muscles (e.g. Pearson, 1939). The fibers terminate with typical motor end plates, *each nerve being limited to the homolateral half of the tongue.* The motor units are small.

From the hypoglossal nerve proper a peculiar closed arch of fiber bundles (the so-called descending hypoglossal ramus) courses downward, and continues in the *ansa hypoglossi.* This, however, is not formed by fibers from the hypoglossal nucleus, but by fibers from the anterior rami of the upper two (or three) cervical nerves. Section of the descending ramus provokes no changes in the hypoglossal nucleus. Some of these fibers join the nerve in the beginning of its extracerebral course but soon leave it again. The fibers of the ansa are distributed to the infrahyoid muscles (sternohyoid, omohyoid, sternothyreoid, and thyreohyoid muscles) which are thus supplied by motor fibers from the upper cervical segments (Fig. 7-4) in the ansa. Clearly a proximal lesion of the hypoglossal trunk will thus not affect the infrahyoid muscles.

From a practical point of view a knowledge of the motor innervation of the tongue as outlined above, is sufficient to interpret disturbances in its function. However, some additional data is of interest for an understanding of the motor function of the tongue.[3] It might be surmised that an organ such as the tongue, employed in chewing and swallowing and in the rather delicate and differentiated movements of speech, should be equipped with a fairly elaborate proprioceptive innervation. A few receptors of a special type ("flower spray") at the origin of the genioglossus muscle have been found in the rabbit by Weddell, Harpman, Lambley, and Young (1940), and Cooper (1953) has demonstrated typical muscle spindles in the human tongue. The possibility exists that there might also be, in the tongue, other types of sensory endings subserving proprioception. The presence of sensory fibers in the hypoglossal nerve has been claimed by several authors, mainly on account of the presence in some animals of a small ganglion on the course of the nerve ("Froriep's ganglion"). Boyd (1941) in a special study of this matter in rabbits found no trace of sensory cells in the hypoglossal nerve. In keeping with this, stretching, deforming, or burning the tongue does not give rise to action potentials in the hypoglossal

[3] The sensory functions, especially the gustatory mechanisms, are treated in connection with the Vth and VIIth cranial nerves.

FIG. 7–4 A diagram of the hypoglossal nerve and its connections with spinal nerve fibers, supplying the infrahyoid muscles via the ansa hypoglossi. (Cf. text.)

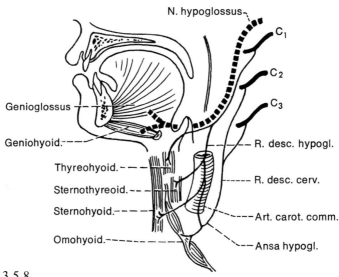

nerve (Barron, 1936). Proprioceptive impulses from the tongue are presumably conveyed by nerves other than the hypoglossal, e.g., the lingual nerves as assumed by Barron. When the lingual nerves are anesthetized in man, proprioceptive impressions from the anterior two thirds of the tongue are abolished (Weddell et al., 1940).

The hypoglossal nerve conveys, however, not only somatic motor fibers to the lingual musculature, but also sympathetic fibers, functionally vasoconstrictors. From anatomical (see Weddell et al.) as well as physiological data it is concluded that these fibers partly join the nerve through an anastomosis with the superior cervical ganglion or the carotid plexus. Unilateral extirpation of the cervical sympathetic chain is followed by degeneration of the fine nerve fibers in the hypoglossal nerve and on the vessels of the tongue on the same side.

Symptomatology. *The trunk of the hypoglossal nerve may be damaged* where it passes through the hypoglossal canal or more distally. The cause may be a tumor, fracture of the occipital bone, or traumatic wounds. As a rule lesions of this type are unilateral. The resulting changes are essentially the same as in lesions of the peripheral motor neurons of the cord. The muscles of half of the tongue on the side of the lesion are paretic or paralytic. This becomes conspicuous when the tongue is protruded. The intact genioglossus muscle (assisted by the geniohyoid) will pull the base of the tongue forward, whereas this will not occur on the paralyzed side. Consequently the *tongue will deviate to the side of the lesion* when it is protruded. When kept in the mouth a deviation will not be apparent. If the paralysis occurs acutely there will at first usually be some difficulty in moving the food within the mouth, and the patient will be unable to press the tip of his tongue against the cheek on the opposite side, but in unilateral lesions swallowing is not severely interfered with and any eventual dysarthria is moderate. *Atrophy* of the paralyzed half of the tongue occurs rapidly, the surface of the tongue becomes wrinkled,[4] and on palpation this side of the tongue is found to be *flaccid*. Fasciculations are usually seen, especially when the tongue is protruded; these appear to be of the same nature as those observed in lesions of the peripheral motor neurons of the cord (cf. Ch. 3).

The symptoms outlined above will also appear in *lesions of the hypoglossal nucleus* on one side. Nuclear lesions, however, because of the close proximity of the right and left nucleus, are most frequently bilateral. They may be caused, for example, by *poliomyelitis,* when the brain stem is involved (bulbar types). Usually in such cases other motor cranial nerves are also affected and the disease often takes a fatal course.

[4] This atrophy of the muscles is not to be confused with the atrophy of the mucous membrane of the tongue, with disappearance of the papillae, seen, for example, in pernicious anemia.

More characteristic is the involvement of the hypoglossal nuclei in *chronic bulbar palsy,* where the motor neurons of the cranial nerves, especially the lower, fall victim to a slowly progressing degeneration. This clinical picture will be more fully discussed in connection with the vagus-glossopharyngeal complex. Not infrequently the first symptom of the disease is fasciculation of the tongue musculature.

Vascular lesions in the medulla oblongata may also affect the hypoglossal nuclei, but more frequently they injure the fibers in their course in the medulla. A peripheral hypoglossal paresis usually occurs in vascular disorders of the anterior spinal artery or the vertebral artery, regularly combined with a complete or incomplete hemiplegia on the other side on account of concomitant damage to long descending fiber tracts.

Because of the crossed path of the corticobulbar fibers to the hypoglossal nuclei, and the usually strictly homolateral peripheral innervation, a *lesion of the corticobulbar fibers above the decussation* will result in a *paralysis of the contralateral half of the tongue.* Thus the common capsular hemiplegias are as a rule combined with a paralysis of the tongue on the hemiplegic side. As this is an "upper motor neuron paralysis," lingual atrophy and fasciculations will be lacking. As a rule there is therefore no difficulty in distinguishing the two types of lingual paralysis. Bilateral affection of the tongue muscles of the "upper motor neuron type" is seen especially in cerebral atherosclerosis where both sides of the brain are usually affected. The clinical picture of this *pseudobulbar palsy* will be referred to later. As always when both sides of the tongue are involved, the disturbances tend to be severe.

(b) THE ACCESSORY NERVE

Anatomy. The XIth cranial nerve, the accessory, is usually regarded as a purely efferent nerve, supplying the sternocleidomastoid and trapezius muscles with motor fibers. It is customary to describe the accessory nerve as having *two parts, a spinal and a cranial.* These fuse in the jugular foramen to form a single nerve trunk which again gives rise to *an internal ramus,* joining the vagus, and *an external ramus,* representing the accessory nerve proper (cf. Fig. 7-5). It is generally agreed that the fibers of the cranial portion which take their origin mainly from the nucleus ambiguus are those leaving the trunk as the internal ramus. Therefore this part may be looked upon as an aberrant vagus fasciculus, and will not be considered more closely.

The efferent fibers of the external ramus arise from the *accessory nucleus,* a column of cells of the somatic efferent type, extending from the 2nd to the 5th–6th cervical segment of the cord. Caudally it is present as a group of cells in the dorsolateral part of the ventral horn, while more cranially it attains a certain degree of independence and approaches the caudal end of the nucleus ambiguus [5] (Pearson, 1938). The fibers pass dorsolaterally and leave the cord as bundles in the lateral funiculus, dorsal to the ligamentum denticulatum, between the dorsal and ventral roots (Fig. 7-5). They bend in a rostral direction and unite to form the spinal part of the nerve which passes through the jugular foramen. Having given off the internal ramus, the remainder descends as the external ramus, bending slightly laterally and dorsally, and reaches the inner aspect of the sternocleidomastoid, pierces it, and then swings from the posterior border of this muscle to the trapezius where it ends.

During its *extracranial course* the accessory nerve is joined by fibers derived from the 3rd and 4th upper cervical ventral rami. On the basis

[5] This fact together with some other findings are taken by some authors to support the view that the accessory nerve belongs to the special visceral efferent group and that the sternocleidomastoid and trapezius muscles are derived from branchial mesoderm.

Fig. 7–5 Drawing of the caudal part of the brain stem with the rootlets of the cranial nerves IV to XII, illustrating particularly the relations of the accessory nerve. (Cf. text.)

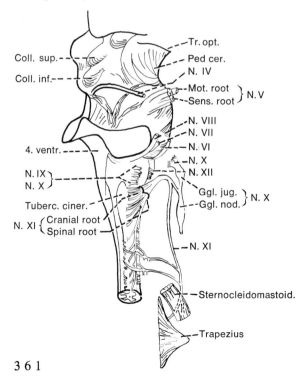

of clinical findings in cases of pure accessory nerve lesions these spinal nerve fibers have been assumed by some neurologists to be concerned chiefly in the innervation of the caudal part of the trapezius, its middle and cranial parts as well as the sternocleidomastoid being supplied predominantly by the accessory nerve.

Besides the motor fibers the accessory nerve also contains some *afferent fibers*. Some of these pass centrally with the accessory nerve, which in its intracranial portion regularly contains some unipolar ganglion cells, in man (Pearson, 1938) as well as in the sheep, cat, and monkey. These ganglion cells undergo retrograde changes after section of the accessory nerve (Windle, 1931). In addition, sensory fibers are found in the spinal nerves joining it. Anatomical and physiological experiments in rabbits by Yee, Harrison, and Corbin (1939) indicate that the fibers are proprioceptive.

Symptomatology. *Lesions of the accessory nerve* are not frequently encountered. The nerve may be damaged by traumatic injury, tumors at the base of the skull, or by fractures. There ensues, in a complete lesion, a loss of motor power in the sternocleidomastoid and the trapezius, less pronounced in its lower part (cf. above). If the lesion is situated distal to the entrance of the nerve into the sternocleidomastoid, as is more common, the trapezius alone will be affected. The paralytic muscles are atrophic and flaccid. The characteristic contour of the sternocleidomastoid in the neck is lost, and likewise the anterior upper border of the trapezius does not reveal itself as distinctly as usual. The atrophy of the sternocleidomastoid is particularly evident when the head is turned to the other side and the chin is elevated. A unilateral paralysis of this muscle as a rule does not inconvenience the patient very much. Bilateral lesions (such as are characteristic of the myotonic type of progressive muscular dystrophy, dystrophia myotonica, which are due, however, to primary muscle changes and not to lesions of the nerve) disable the patient considerably, e.g., when trying to lift his head from the pillow.

Complete paralysis of the *trapezius,* especially if combined with lesions of the upper cervical nerves, is a serious handicap. On account of its widespread origin from the occiput to the 12th dorsal vertebra and the convergence of its fibers to their insertion on the lateral part of the clavicle, the acromion, and the whole of the scapular spine, the muscle is an important assistant to the serratus anterior in elevation of the arm. Elevation of the arm is performed with less power than usual, and frequently cannot be executed to its full extent, mainly because the rotation of the scapula around its antero-posterior axis is reduced. The outward rotation of the arm also suffers, when the scapula cannot be brought as close to the spine as normally. The scapula is frequently displaced a little in a lateral direction and presents some degree of winging ("scapula alata"), as in paralysis of the serratus anterior.

In hemiplegias a contralateral paresis of the muscles supplied by the accessory nerve is a common finding, due to the practically total crossing of the corticobulbar fibers. This paresis, as will be understood, is not accompanied by marked atrophy.

(c) THE VAGUS AND GLOSSOPHARYNGEAL NERVES

Anatomy. On account of the close anatomical and functional relationship of the Xth and IXth cranial nerves they will be treated together. Both contain special and general visceral efferent, general somatic afferent, and special and general visceral afferent fibers. The special visceral efferent fibers of the vagus and glossopharyngeal spring from the nucleus ambiguus, and the general visceral efferent from the dorsal motor nucleus of the vagus and from the so-called inferior salivatory nucleus, respectively. The *nucleus ambiguus,* composed of cells of the same type as the hypoglossal nucleus, forms a longitudinal column in the medulla oblongata (Fig. 7-2). From its original embryonic position it is displaced ventrolaterally and is found in the reticular formation medial to the spinal tract of the Vth nerve and its nucleus (Figs. 7-3 and 7-6). The fibers leaving the nucleus pass backward and then bend sharply forward and laterally to reach the surface of the medulla behind the inferior olive (Fig. 7-6). The nucleus ambiguus is the common special visceral efferent nucleus to nerves IX and X. Most of its fibers pass in the vagus. Some of these make their way through the cranial portion of the accessory nerve to join the vagus again through the internal ramus. A smaller contingent of the fibers runs in the glossopharyngeal nerve. These fibers in the IXth and Xth nerve supply the striated muscles of the pharynx and larynx and the upper part of the esophagus.

The nucleus ambiguus may be subdivided into subgroups with somewhat different cytoarchitecture, in man as well as in animals. Following sections of peripheral branches of the vagus and glossopharyngeal nerves, several authors (Getz and Sirnes, 1949; Szabo and Dussardier, 1964; Lawn, 1966; and others) have studied the ensuing retrograde cellular changes in the nucleus and established a localization within it: the fibers of the glossopharyngeal nerve arise in the rostral regions, the fibers to the laryngeal muscles chiefly caudally. The cricothyroid muscle appears to be innervated from a particular cell group (Lawn, 1966, in the rabbit). According to Szentágothai (1943a) the other laryngeal muscles likewise are innervated from fairly well circumscribed regions of the muscles.

The general visceral efferent *dorsal motor nucleus of the vagus* is found lateral to the hypoglossal nucleus, as a longitudinal column, under the floor of the 4th ventricle (Figs. 7-2, 7-3, and 7-6). Its fibers course

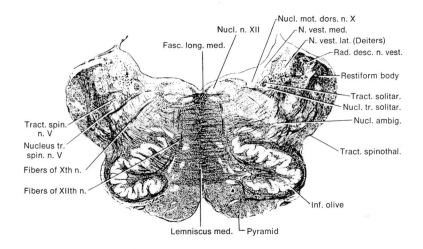

FIG. 7–6 Drawing of a transverse section through the medulla oblongata at the level of the vagus nuclei. Weigert's myelin sheath stain.

ventralward to join those from the nucleus ambiguus. The corresponding nucleus of the glossopharyngeal nerve is the *inferior salivatory nucleus,* which, however, is represented by relatively scattered cells and does not form a proper nucleus. These nuclei give rise to preganglionic fibers in the parasympathetic system, and supply glandular structures and smooth muscle. They will be considered in more detail in Chapter 11 on the autonomic system.

Most of the *afferent fibers in the vagus and glossopharyngeal* are regarded as being of the *visceral type,* conveying impulses of general and special visceral sensations. The latter, the taste fibers, terminate in the same nucleus as do the general visceral afferent fibers, the nucleus of the solitary tract. The fibers have their perikarya in ganglia of the corresponding nerves (the nodose and petrous ganglion, respectively) and having entered the medulla, bend in a caudal direction, thus forming a conspicuous fiber bundle, the *solitary tract,* situated lateral to the dorsal motor nucleus of the vagus nerve and somewhat deeper (Figs. 7-2 and 7-6). This bundle extends throughout the length of the medulla oblongata, and its fibers as well as their collaterals end in a fairly circumscribed cell column, lateral to the tract, forming the *nucleus of the tractus solitarius.* Some visceral afferent fibers of the intermediate nerve join the solitary tract and terminate in the nucleus. The intermediate, glossopharyngeal, and vagal fibers end in particular rostrocaudally arranged, although overlapping, regions of the nucleus of the solitary tract (see Torvik, 1956b; Kerr, 1962). A similar arrangement is found in man

3 6 4

(Schwartz, Roulhac, Lam, and O'Leary, 1951). The nucleus of the solitary tract is made up of small nerve cells, considerably smaller than those in the dorsal motor nucleus of the vagus. Most of their axons ascend in the brain stem, but their destination is difficult to ascertain, since it is almost impossible to destroy the nucleus without damage to neighboring structures, particularly the reticular formation. For several reasons it is, however, likely that some ascending impulses reach the thalamus although efferents from the nucleus have not been traced to it (Morest, 1967). Other fibers, particularly from the caudal parts of the nucleus which contains some larger cells, have been shown, experimentally, to pass to the spinal cord as a *solitariospinal tract* (see Torvik, 1957b). This tract cannot be traced below the thoracic level, and apparently represents an efferent link in the arc of some visceral reflexes, the afferent link of which is formed by visceral afferent fibers.[6]

General somatic afferent fibers are found in the vagus, and are involved in the innervation of the skin in the concha of the ear. These fibers enter the trigeminal nuclei, which represent the terminal station for all general somatic afferent fibers from the face. Some fibers from the glossopharyngeal nerve (as well as some from the intermediate nerve) likewise end in the trigeminal nuclei, in animals as well as in man. This will be considered in more detail in section (f) of this chapter.

The various nuclei treated above are acted upon by fibers from various sources. *Fibers from the corticobulbar tract,* presumably via internuncial cells, act on the nucleus ambiguus. The fibers are partly crossed, partly uncrossed, and are involved in the voluntary movements of the striated muscles supplied by the IXth and Xth nerves (pharynx and larynx, cf. below). In addition, collaterals from afferent visceral and somatic fibers and axons and collaterals from visceral and somatic sensory nuclei (see Stewart and King, 1963; Morest, 1967) mediate the participation of the pharyngeal and laryngeal muscles in reflex acts, such as coughing, swallowing, vomiting, etc. Further, descending fibers from subcortical levels influence the effector nuclei, presumably largely via the reticular formation.

The *roots of the vagus and glossopharyngeal nerves* leave the medulla in a shallow sulcus at the dorsal border of the inferior olive (Figs. 7-5 and 7-6). The upper, fewer, bundles unite to form the glossopharyngeal,

[6] The projection to the spinal cord makes clear that the nucleus of the solitary tract should not be considered as a pure relay station in visceral afferent pathways to higher levels. That a considerable degree of integration can take place in the nucleus appears from the fact that fibers from the cerebral cortex end in it (Brodal, Szabo, and Torvik, 1956; and others) as well as fibers from the spinal cord (Rossi and Brodal, 1956b) and from the vestibular part of the cerebellum (Angaut and Brodal, 1967.)

365

whereas the lower and more numerous bundles fuse to form the vagus nerve. Both leave the skull through the jugular foramen and have two ganglia, each composed of typical (pseudo-) unipolar cells. The IXth nerve ganglia are the superior and petrous, the Xth nerve ganglia the jugular and nodose. Between its ganglia the vagus is joined by the internal ramus of the accessory nerve.

The *peripheral distribution* of the nerves may be briefly outlined as follows: the *glossopharyngeal* descends on the lateral side of the pharynx, bending gradually forward, ultimately penetrating the muscular coat of the pharynx to reach the base of the tongue, the posterior third of which it supplies with sensory fibers; it also supplies the adjacent parts of the mucous membrane, the tonsillar region and posterior palatal arch, and the soft palate. The nerve sends a motor branch to the stylopharyngeus muscle, and partakes with the vagus in the formation of the pharyngeal plexus, in which sympathetic fibers from the cervical sympathetic trunk are also present.

There is some diversity of opinion concerning the relative importance of the vagus and glossopharyngeal in the innervation of the pharynx and the soft palate. In cats, section of the vagus but not of the glossopharyngeal produces a unilateral paralysis of the pharynx (Sjöberg, 1943), and some clinicians have made corresponding findings in human cases of operative sectioning of the IXth and Xth nerves (e.g. Fay, 1927). Sensory loss in the pharynx following intracranial section of the IXth nerve has been described, e.g. by Lewis and Dandy (1930), Reichert (1934) and Bohm and Strang (1962). Foerster maintained that the glossopharyngeal alone is concerned in the innervation of the pharynx, whereas the vagus supplies the soft palate with motor fibers (together with the facial which innervates the levator palati and the trigeminal nerve which innervates the tensor palati).

The glossopharyngeal, besides containing special visceral afferent fibers for taste from the posterior third of the tongue, as already mentioned, also has general visceral efferents to the glands in the region it supplies. In addition, secretory fibers to the parotid gland pass through the small tympanic nerve and the lesser superficial petrosal nerve to the otic ganglion, where the postganglionic fibers have their perikarya. Worthy of mention is a special sensory branch from the glossopharyngeal, the carotid branch, which has constantly been shown to innervate the *carotid sinus* (Boyd, 1937), the dilatation at the beginning of the internal carotid, playing an important role as a receptor mechanism for the regulation of blood pressure.

The peripheral course of the vagus.　　The trunk of the vagus or pneumogastric nerve descends in the sheath common to the internal carotid artery and internal jugular vein in the neck, passes, on the right side anterior to the subclavian artery, on the left anterior to the aortic arch, then on both sides behind the root of the lung, where it is situated posteriorly. Ultimately the left nerve is displaced ventrally onto the anterior surface of the esophagus, the right being found on the posterior surface. Correspondingly the left nerve breaks up into a plexus on the ventral side of the stomach, the right on the posterior. From these plexuses the terminal fibers of the nerve are distributed to the viscera in the upper abdomen (cf. Ch. 11).

The following branches deserve special mention:

The *auricular ramus* leaves the nerve between the two ganglia, frequently anastomoses with the glossopharyngeal, penetrates the mastoid process, and ultimately innervates the skin in the concha of the auricle. This branch is a purely general somatic sensory nerve.

The *pharyngeal rami* join the pharyngeal plexus, referred to above.

The *superior laryngeal nerve,* on the wall of the middle pharyngeal constrictor, gives off a predominantly motor *external ramus* which ends in the cricothyroid muscle, and an *internal ramus.* The latter pierces the thyrohyoid membrane and provides the larynx with sensory fibers.

The inferior laryngeal or recurrent nerve is different on the two sides, the right bending upward posteriorly under the right subclavian artery, the left under the aortic arch. Ascending in the tracheo-esophageal sulcus, it finally divides into an anterior and a posterior ramus which supply all the laryngeal muscles, except the cricothyroid, with motor fibers.

Apart from these more definite branches the vagus gives off the *superior cardiac rami,* usually below the superior laryngeal nerve. They follow the carotids downward to the aorta and partake in the formation of the *cardiac plexus,* which is also supplied by the *inferior cardiac rami* from the recurrent nerve. (The superior, middle, and inferior cardiac *nerves* from the corresponding ganglia of the sympathetic trunk form another component of the cardiac plexus.) From the thoracic part of the vagus emanate the pericardial, bronchial, and esophageal rami, which form nervous plexuses with sympathetic fibers on the organs mentioned and will be discussed in connection with the abdominal branches of the vagus in the chapter on the autonomic system.

It is evident from the above description that the *vagus is preponderantly a visceral nerve,* the somatic afferent constituent being only comprised of the fibers in the auricular ramus. The special visceral efferent component (which functionally at least behaves as a somatic element) is concerned only in the innervation of the pharynx and larynx. This fact is revealed also in the fiber types present in the different parts of the nerve. The auricular branch is composed mainly of thicker myelinated fibers, and at least most, if not all, of them have their cells in the jugular ganglion. After section of this ramus 69 to 77 per cent of these cells show retrograde changes (DuBois and Foley, 1937). Most of the cells of the visceral afferent fibers, representing a far larger number, are thus located in the larger nodose ganglion. Below this the nerve contains predominantly (67–77 per cent) unmyelinated and some small myelinated fibers (Foley and DuBois, 1937). The larger fibers present in this part of the nerve appear to be concerned in the motor innervation of the larynx, and are found in the recurrent nerve, a lesser portion also in the superior laryngeal, supplying the cricothyroid. However, some of the larger fibers do not undergo degeneration after section of the vagus cranial to its ganglia, and are thus afferent and commonly believed to be proprioceptive. Recent studies make it likely that some of the thick afferent fibers are derived from muscle spindles. Paulsen (1958), Lucas Keene (1961), and Grim (1967) have shown that spindles are present in all human laryngeal muscles. In the posterior cricoarytenoid muscle, for example, Grim (1967) in a large material found on an average 5.4 spindles, of the nuclear bag as well as the nuclear chain type (see Ch. 3). Other types of sensory endings have been described (Lucas Keene, 1961). The total number of spindle afferents is, however, relatively modest. In the monkey (Brocklehurst and Edgeworth, 1940) only about 3 per cent of the fibers in the recurrent nerve appear to be afferent against some 30 per cent in the superior laryngeal nerve. In man Ogura and Lam (1953) found the latter nerve to contain some 15,000 fibers, some 30 per cent being thick and myelinated, and from electrical stimulation of the nerve in man they concluded that it mediates sensations of pain and touch. The ample sensory innervation of the larynx by way of the superior laryngeal nerve reflects its importance in the coughing reflex.[7] The co-operation of the laryngeal muscles in phonation is obviously a very complex matter. In an exhaustive electromyographic investigation in normal persons and patients with paralysis of laryngeal muscles, Faaborg-Andersen (1957) has presented much interesting data on this subject.

Symptomatology.   The symptoms due to involvement of the visceral, especially the visceral efferent, components of the IXth and Xth nerves are treated in the chapter on the autonomic system, and will be mentioned here only to complete the descriptions of the clinical pictures. Our concern is here mainly with the somatic functions of these nerves.

A lesion of the supranuclear tracts to the efferent vagus and glossopharyngeal nuclei will, if unilateral, give no clear symptoms. This follows from the bilateral distribution of the corticobulbar and other descending tracts. If bilateral, however, such lesions will be severe (cf. below).

On account of the close spatial relationship between the two nerves

---

[7] It is worthy of notice that sensory impulses from the laryngeal and pharyngeal mucosa are consciously perceived, contrasting with impulses from lower parts of the respiratory and digestive system. Yet the visceral origin of these parts is equally clear. It may be asked whether the usual classification of sensory impulses is appropriate, as it makes no distinction between the consciously and subconsciously perceived stimuli, a functionally important point.

and their nuclei, it follows that symptoms referable to both of them will be more frequently encountered than isolated lesions. However, isolated lesions may occur. The chief *symptoms in lesions of the glossopharyngeal nerve* are those due to interruption of its sensory fibers. They comprise loss of sensibility in the posterior third of the tongue, the palatal arches (especially the posterior), the tonsillar region, the velum, and in most cases at least, the pharynx (cf. above). Taste is lost in the posterior third of the tongue. This has been verified in operative sections of the nerve in man (e.g. Lewis and Dandy, 1930; Reichert, 1934; and others). The motor impairment, according to most authors, will consist of a homo-lateral paresis of the pharynx. When the pharynx is made to contract, e.g. in phonation, the raphe of the pharynx will be drawn over to the intact side (*mouvement de rideau*) due to the effect of the constrictors. The gagging reflex cannot be elicited from the affected side. The causes of glossopharyngeal lesions are the same as those producing affections of the vagus nerve and will be referred to below.

The glossopharyngeal may also be the site of irritative lesions, mani-festing themselves usually as the so-called *glossopharyngeal neuralgia*. As in trigeminal neuralgia this may be caused by local affections of the nerve, for example, tumors, but in most cases the etiology remains obscure. The main feature of the affection is the pain, which usually occurs in paroxysms, starting at the base of the tongue, the tonsil, or in the region of the palatal arches, irradiating eventually to the ear region. "Trigger points" may be present in the areas mentioned, and paroxysms are often elicited on chewing or swallowing. This condition is not frequent, but it is important to distinguish it from trigeminal neuralgia.

In a recent study Bohm and Strang (1962) distinguish two types of glossopharyngeal neuralgia, the otitic and the oropharyngeal, and point to some clinical features of these conditions which differ from those seen in trigeminal neuralgia. (Occasionally pain is felt in the trigeminal area, presumably due to overlapping of glossopharyngeal and trigeminal fibers in the spinal trigeminal nucleus.) Relief may be obtained by intracranial section of the glossopharyngeal nerve (see Bohm and Strang, 1962, for a recent account). However, since the somatic afferent fibers in the nerve join the spinal trigeminal tract, a medullary tractotomy (section of the spinal tract of the trigeminal nerve; see section (*f*) of this chapter) may also be employed. Since the glossopharyngeal fibers occupy a restricted area, dorsalmost within the spinal tract (Torvik, 1956b; Kunc and Maršala, 1962; Kerr, 1962; Rhoton et al., 1966), as shown in Fig. 7-7 it is possible to destroy this part selectively and thus to spare the fibers from the trigeminal nerve, as shown by Kunc (1965).

An isolated *lesion of one vagus nerve* will, according to most ob-

369

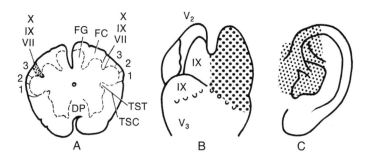

FIG. 7–7 *A:* Diagram showing the position of the fibers from the intermediate, glossopharyngeal, and vagus nerves (VII, IX, X) in the spinal trigeminal tract. *B:* The area of analgesia in the pharynx and palatal arches following a selective tractotomy of the stippled area in *A.* From Kunc (1965). *C:* The analgesic area in the auricle following a medullary tractotomy. From Brodal (1947a).

servers, result in a unilateral paresis or paralysis of the soft palate, which in phonation will not be elevated fully and when at rest will frequently hang somewhat lower on the paralyzed side. In contraction of the velum the uvula will deviate to the unaffected side. In bilateral lesions, particularly, the speech will have a nasal character, and on swallowing, food and especially fluids will enter the nasal cavity as the occlusion of the nasopharynx from the oropharynx, necessary for proper deglutition, will be imperfect. The interruption of the motor fibers to the larynx will produce a unilateral vocal cord palsy. This will also be the case if the damage is restricted to the recurrent laryngeal nerve. Because of its practical significance, recurrent laryngeal nerve palsy will be described more fully.

The *symptoms following unilateral recurrent laryngeal nerve affections are usually transitory.* When the one vocal cord loses its innervation, the intact vocal cord will usually, after some time, adapt itself to the altered conditions, and the initial hoarseness and occasional coughing attacks will disappear. *Therefore, if a unilateral recurrent nerve or vagus nerve affection is suspected, a laryngoscopic examiantion should always be performed, even if there are no symptoms from the larynx.* In paralysis of the recurrent laryngeal nerve due to peripheral injury it is a peculiar feature that the abductor muscles of the larynx are affected first. This circumstance was first described by Semon and consequently is usually referred to as Semon's law. A satisfactory explanation has not been found as yet.[8] Normally, the posterior cricoarytenoid muscles which rotate the

[8] It has been assumed that the fibers to the abductor muscles occupy a particular part of the nerve. However, according to Sunderland and Swaney (1952) the fibers to the various muscles are intermingled in the recurrent nerve.

370

vocal process of the arytenoid cartilages laterally will produce a widening of the rima glottidis and consequently act as abductors. These muscles are supplied by the posterior ramus of the recurrent nerve. The adductors, most important of which is the lateral cricoarytenoid muscle, innervated by the anterior ramus, will act as antagonists and narrow the rima. Consequently the predilection of the posterior ramus to be involved first in affections of the nerve will produce an abductor palsy, and the cord will, by the unopposed action of the antagonists, assume a position in the median line.

Apart from a transitory hoarseness an abductor palsy will usually give rise to no symptoms.[9] If the anterior ramus and the adductor muscles are also affected, the vocal cord will assume the cadaveric position, midway between adduction and abduction. This is usually compensated after some time, as the vocal cord of the intact side can be brought to approach the paralyzed one.

In *bilateral palsies of the recurrent laryngeal nerve,* far more seldom met with, symptoms are always present. A bilateral abductor paralysis will produce an extreme narrowing of the rima, and, especially if it occurs rapidly, it may necessitate immediate tracheotomy, if death resulting from asphyxia is to be prevented. If less pronounced, there will be a marked stridor on inspiration and some degree of asphyxia. In bilateral complete lesions of both nerves, the rima is widened, and as the cords cannot be brought into contact, the voice is lost (aphonia). Whispering, however, is possible.

Partial or total paralysis of the recurrent laryngeal nerve is more frequent on the left side than on the right (the left nerve being longer) and in about two thirds of all cases is due to local processes affecting the nerve. Of such cases may be mentioned *aneurysms of the aortic arch* or the subclavian artery, *enlargement of the tracheobronchial lymph nodes* in tuberculosis, Hodgkin's disease or diseases of the blood (leukemia), and *tumors of the mediastinum.* Recurrent nerve palsy is also a complication encountered in some cases of *thyroidectomy,* where the nerve may be affected by ligature of the inferior thyroid artery, which comes into close contact with the nerve. Isolated paralysis—so-called idiopathic—of the nerve occurs in many cases (one third to one quarter of all) where no definite cause can be ascertained. In some instances it is assumed to be due to a "mononeuritis" of the type far more frequently seen in the facial nerve.[10]

---

[9] On inspiration there normally occurs a moderate widening of the rima glottidis, due to contraction of the abductors. On severe physical exertion a unilateral abductor palsy may therefore cause some dyspnea.

[10] The occurrence of hysterical aphonia should be borne in mind.

By means of electromyography it has been demonstrated that not a few of the unilateral vocal cord palsies, commonly assumed to be due to lesions of the nerve, are virtually not palsies at all but are due to ankylosis of the cricoarytenoid joints. In such cases action potentials are recorded from adductors and abductors, but no movement is seen. The electrodes are inserted through a laryngoscope (see e.g. Weddell, Feinstein, and Pattle, 1944; Faaborg-Andersen, 1957).

It goes without saying that recurrent laryngeal nerve palsies will be a frequent symptom also in lesions of the vagus nerve superior to the origin of the former. In these instances, however, other symptoms usually accompany the vocal cord palsy. Thus the affection of the fibers in the superior laryngeal nerve will produce a partial anesthesia of the larynx and a unilateral paralysis of the velum will be found.

Other symptoms which may be observed are due to the involvement of the parasympathetic fibers, but in unilateral lesions, as a rule, these are negligible. However, it is worthy of notice that isolated paralysis of the laryngeal muscles may also be caused by diseases affecting the medulla oblongata, for example, poliomyelitis. The explanation is found in the arrangement of the motor cells of the nucleus ambiguus, referred to above.

On the whole, unilateral lesions of the extracranial part of the vagus are not common, apart from the recurrent nerve affections already referred to. Tumors, aneurysms of the internal carotid, and enlargement of the deep cervical lymph nodes may be mentioned as causes, as well as traumatic injuries. Unilateral affections of the vagus and glossopharyngeal nuclei may be found, as already mentioned above, in poliomyelitis; furthermore, they are also found in intramedullary vascular disturbances. especially those affecting the posterior inferior cerebellar artery (Wallenberg's syndrome).

It will appear from what has been said that unilateral affections of the vagus and glossopharyngeal nerves give no alarming symptoms. Not so with *bilateral lesions* which, as a rule, prove fatal after some time. It is obvious that such bilateral affections will most frequently be due to diseases of the medulla oblongata. Before turning to these, however, a condition of practical importance should be mentioned, in which the noxious agent probably attacks the peripheral nerve fibers bilaterally, i.e. the common *postdiphtheritic velum palsy*. Diphtheria toxin may damage nerve fibers nearly everywhere in the organism, but, perhaps due to local factors, the fibers to the velum are most frequently involved (see Fisher and Adams, 1956). As a consequence some weeks after the onset of diphtheria the patient's speech will be nasal and difficulties of deglutition will occur (cf. above).

Bilateral lesions of the glossopharyngeal and vagus nerves of central origin as a rule will affect all parts of the nerves, although partial affections of the nuclei may be encountered. Of practical importance are chronic bulbar palsy and *poliomyelitis*. In the latter disease the motor cells of the medulla oblongata may be involved in the same manner as those of the spinal cord.

As the distribution, however, is irregular and fortuitous, all transitions may occur from a selective affection of one small nucleus or part of a nucleus to an involvement of nearly all motor nuclei of the brain stem. In cases of this type death usually ensues rapidly, due frequently to the damage to the vagus and glossopharyngeal nuclei. Briefly mentioned, the symptoms referable to the vagus and glossopharyngeal in these cases will be a paralysis of the velum, with regurgitation into the nose on swallowing. Swallowing itself will also be severely interfered with on account of the paralysis of the pharyngeal muscles. There is aphonia due to a bilateral paralysis of the laryngeal muscles. If the patient does not succumb to a respiratory paralysis, due to concomitant injury to the nucleus of the phrenic nerve, an aspiration pneumonia will regularly result from the lack of coughing reflexes.

In *chronic bulbar palsy* the motor neurons of the brain stem are affected by a slowly progressing degeneration, parallel to that seen in progressive spinal muscular atrophy. The symptoms referable to the vagus and glossopharyngeal nerves are those of most prognostic importance in this disease, but as a rule nearly all motor nuclei in the pons and medulla oblongata are successively affected in a somewhat varying sequence, during the course of three or four years from the beginning of the disease until death. Usually a *dysarthria* is the first symptom, due mainly to lesions of the XIIth and VIIth nuclei. The tongue, the seat of atrophy with fasciculations, cannot be protruded (cf. section (*a*) of this chapter), the mouth cannot be properly closed, and there is frequently dribbling of saliva. The face becomes motionless and acquires an "empty" expression. The dysarthria will be more prominent when the vagus is included, since then the voice grows gradually weaker until complete aphonia occurs, and disturbances in swallowing appear as described above. Finally an aspiration pneumonia ends the sad condition of the patient. It should be remembered that symptoms referable to concomitant degeneration of the motoneurons of the spinal cord are not uncommon.

Somewhat similar clinical manifestations are found in *pseudobulbar palsy*. In this disease, however, the peripheral motor neurons of the bulb are not affected, but the damage responsible for the symptoms is located in the fibers of the corticobulbar tract, usually produced by cerebral atherosclerosis and consequently appearing bilaterally. An important differential diagnostic clue is the lack of muscle atrophy in this disease, most easily ascertained in the tongue. Another peculiarity of pseudo-bulbar palsy is the frequent occurrence of convulsive laughter and weeping (cf. section (e) in this chapter). *Myasthenia gravis,* which also shows a predilection for the muscles of the head, must be borne in mind in the differential diagnosis. Here the morbid alterations are related to the motor end plates, and apart from the frequent diurnal variations in the paresis and the rapid tiring of the muscles, a prostigmine test will aid in the diagnosis.

As a rule *the visceral symptoms* following unilateral lesions of the vagus and glossopharyngeal are negligible. In bilateral lesions, especially if they develop acutely, an acceleration of the heart rate may occur, frequently leading to death. This may be seen in the terminal stages of chronic bulbar palsy. The influence of the vagus on the heart is seen also in some other types of the heredo-degenerative diseases, e.g. Friedreich's ataxia, where electrocardiographic examinations have revealed disturbances, thought to be caused by affection of the vagus nuclei.

(d) The Vestibular Division of the VIIIth Cranial Nerve

The old anatomists called *the VIIIth cranial nerve* the acoustic, since it supplied the internal ear. However, the so-called acoustic nerve is really made up of two functionally different nerves, *the cochlear nerve* and *the vestibular nerve.* The cochlear nerve transmits exteroceptive impulses perceived as hearing, from the organ of Corti. The vestibular nerve transmits proprioceptive impulses from the saccule and utricle of the vestibulum and from the semicircular ducts, which are important for the maintenance of equilibrium and for orientation in space. The impulses conveyed by the vestibular nerve are only to a limited extent consciously perceived, and, therefore, escaped recognition for a far longer period than did the acoustic function of the cochlear division.

The epithelium of the internal ear develops in early embryonic life as a groove of the ectoderm, and later becomes separated from this to form a vesicle. Certain areas of the epithelium later become differentiated into sensory epithelium. The cochlear duct as well as the semicircular ducts and the saccule and utricle are all formed from the original primary otic vesicle. Phylogenetically the vestibular apparatus appeared long before the cochlear. All vertebrates possess some sort of vestibular organ, already fairly well developed in sharks, whereas an organ of hearing makes its appearance first in amphibians.

374

From a comparative anatomical point of view the inner ear of vertebrates can be subdivided into a *pars superior* and a *pars inferior*. Structural features and details in the nervous connections support this conception. Other sensory areas than those usually described in man are present in some vertebrates. The pars superior is assumed to be predominantly concerned in the proprioceptive, "equilibratory" functions of the inner ear, the pars inferior with the exteroceptive function of hearing. To the sensory areas of the pars superior belong the cristae of the three semicircular ducts, the macula of the utricle (and a varying "papilla neglecta"). The pars inferior includes the sensory area of the saccule, the cochlear duct or its forerunner, and another small area. Comparative anatomical studies by Weston (1939) of the relative size of the different sensory areas have given interesting results. The pars superior is rather constant in phylogenesis, but presents variations in the relative development of the macula utriculi and the cristae of the ducts. The pars inferior shows a progressive development, which particularly concerns the cochlear duct. In man the cochlear sensory area constitutes more than half of the sensory area of the pars inferior, and a quarter of the entire sensory areas of the inner ear. There is still some uncertainty concerning the function of the saccule (see Kornhuber, 1966, for references), and it will not be considered in the following description.

The cochlear division of the VIIIth cranial nerve will be discussed in Chapter 9. The impressions mediated by the vestibular part of the nerve are transmitted through various pathways to influence ultimately chiefly the motor apparatus, by means of reflex connections of several kinds. The vestibular apparatus is functionally particularly closely related to the spinal cord and the cerebellum. This has in part been considered in Chapters 4 and 5. In addition, vestibular impulses influence the oculomotor apparatus. In the present section some principal features of the vestibular nerve and its connections will be dealt with, and some anatomical and clinical features not referred to at other places will be described. It should be realized that the vestibular nerve and its connections have widespread influences on other parts of the nervous system.

The vestibular receptors. The vestibular nerve and nuclei. *The vestibular nerve* enters the brain stem (Fig. 7-5) at the lower border of the pons, on the lateral aspect, behind the facial nerve and separated from this only by the tiny intermediate nerve and the cochlear nerve. Together with the nerves mentioned it can be followed in a peripheral direction into the internal acoustic meatus, where it is subdivided into smaller branches, passing to different portions of the labyrinth. Where they pierce the bottom of the internal meatus the vestibular nerve fibers have their perikarya. These, like those of the cochlear nerve, are bipolar ganglion cells of the primitive type and are collectively designated *the vestibular ganglion*. Whereas the central processes of these cells form the vestibular nerve, the distal ones are very short and end in relation to the sensory epithelium of the labyrinth.

It will be appropriate here to recall briefly the *principal features of the structure of the labyrinth* (see Fig. 7-8). The parts of the labyrinth generally assumed to be concerned with *vestibular function* are the two sac-like divisions, the *saccule* and the *utricle,* and the *three semicircular ducts,* which are in open communication with the lumen of the utricle. The whole thin-walled membranous labyrinth, filled with endolymph, is enclosed within the osseous labyrinth, separated from its periosteum by the perilymph. The petrous bone in which these structures are embedded is particularly compact. At five places distinct areas of sensory epithelium are present. In the widened ampulla of each semicircular duct there is a transversely projecting crest, consisting of supporting and sensory cells. The hairs of the latter (the hair cells) are covered by a gelatinous mass, the cupula. The sensory epithelium of the utricle is found in a small area of this only, measuring 3 × 2 mm, and its plane corresponds approximately to that of the base of the skull. The corresponding macula of the saccule has the same size, but its plane is vertical, perpendicular to that of the macula of the utricle. Both these maculae consist of hair cells and supporting cells and are covered by a gelatinous mass, into which the hairs of the sensory cells dip. In this mass small prisms consisting mainly of calcium carbonate are found. These so-called otoliths induce different stimuli to the hairs in various positions of the head, according to the action of gravity on them. The hair cells of the ampullary crests, however, are stimulated by movements of the endolymph in the semicircular canals producing a deflexion of the cupula. Thus the latter will react to movements of the head, the former to alterations in its position. The semicircular ducts (horizontal or lateral, superior, and posterior) are arranged at right angles to each other, and should thus be able to react to movements in all directions. Other relevant data will be mentioned later.

FIG. 7–8   Diagram of the internal ear. The areas containing sensory epithelium are stippled.

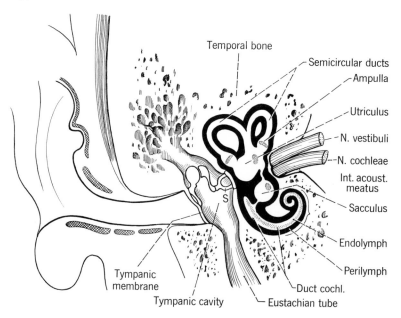

The part of the membranous labyrinth concerned in *hearing* is the *cochlear duct,* which is found as 2½ spiral turns within the bony cochlea. It is in open communication near its blindly ending base with the saccule and its apical coil ends blindly at the apex of the cochlea (Fig. 7-8). The duct is triangular in cross section, attached broadly to the outer walls of the bony cochlear canal, and is separated from the perilymph by the thin vestibular membrane above, and the more solid basilar membrane below. This extends from the bony spiral lamina to the outer wall of the bony duct. On the basilar membrane the sensory apparatus, the organ of Corti, is found. Its sensory hair cells are surrounded by supporting cells. The hair cells are arranged in a single inner row along the duct, and three outer rows. The number of hair cells has been estimated to be about 3,500 and 20,000 in the inner and outer rows respectively. Between the two rows and their adjoining supporting cells the tunnel of Corti is found, traversed by the nerve fibers passing to the outer hair cells. On their free surface the hair cells are in contact with the tectorial membrane.

The majority of the central processes of the cells of the vestibular ganglion, forming together the vestibular nerve, divide into an ascending and a descending branch when they reach the medulla oblongata. Before dividing they pass between the restiform body and the spinal tract of the trigeminal. The branches are distributed to the vestibular nuclei (Figs. 7-2, 7-6, and 7-12).

Within the *vestibular nuclear complex* it is customary to distinguish four large or main nuclei: the *superior* (or nucleus of Bechterew), the *lateral* (or nucleus of Deiters), the *medial* (triangular or nucleus of Schwalbe), and the *descending* (inferior or spinal). The entire vestibular nuclear complex occupies a rather large region just below the floor of the 4th ventricle (see Figs. 7-2, 7-6). On closer analysis it is learned that in addition to the four main nuclei there are several minor cell groups. These have been mapped in detail in the cat (Brodal and Pompeiano, 1957), and most of them can be identified in man as well (Sadjadpour and Brodal, 1968). These groups differ with regard to cytoarchitecture, and there are, furthermore, regional architectonic variations within each of the main nuclei. For example, in the central region of the superior nucleus the cells are on the whole larger and somewhat more densely packed than in the peripheral region. The lateral vestibular nucleus of Deiters is characterized by containing a fair number of large and giant (Deiters') cells; these are (in the cat) more numerous and on the whole larger in the caudodorsal part of the nucleus than in the rostroventral part. The assumption that these and several other architectonic features reflect functional differences is strongly supported by experimental studies of the fiber connections of the vestibular nuclei and by physiological observations, as will appear from the following. The anatomical and functional organization of the vestibular nuclei has been shown to be extremely complex and far more differentiated than was assumed a few decades ago. (For a review, see Brodal, Pompeiano, and Walberg, 1962; for some more recent data, see also Brodal, 1964a, 1967b). Most of the recent information has been obtained from experimental anatomical and physiological studies in the cat. One point of particular interest is the fact, mentioned in Chapter 4, that the nucleus of Deiters presents a somatotopic organization (Pompeiano and Brodal, 1957a) as shown in Figs. 4-6 and 7-9.

As referred to above, the vestibular nerve when entering the vestibular nuclei divides into an ascending and a descending branch due to the fact that most (if not all) primary vestibular fibers divide in a dichotomous fashion. Many of the myelinated parent fibers, most of which are rather coarse, enter the lateral vestibular nucleus, and from here the ascending fibers pass to the superior nucleus (and the cerebellum), the descending ones to the descending and medial vestibular nuclei. Contrary to what has been generally believed, the *primary vestibular fibers do not supply the entire territory of the vestibular nuclear complex*. Within each of the main nuclei there are quite extensive regions which are free from vestibular afferents (Walberg, Bowsher, and Brodal, 1958, in the cat). For example, the rostroventral part only of the nucleus of Deiters (its forelimb region) receives primary vestibular fibers (see Fig. 7-9 and Fig. 1-8A). This has been confirmed physiologically (Wilson et al., 1966). (In the superior nucleus such fibers are restricted to its central regions, and only some of the small groups receive primary fibers.) Obviously the regions which are supplied by primary vestibular fibers

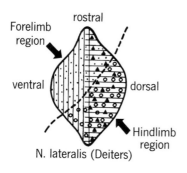

FIG. 7–9 A diagram of the lateral vestibular nucleus of Deiters in the cat in a sagittal view, showing the somatotopic pattern within the nucleus and the approximate distribution within it of some of its main afferents to particular territories. Note restriction of primary vestibular fibers to the "forelimb region." From Brodal (1967b).

must be under a more direct influence of vestibular impulses than the rest of the nuclear complex.[11]

Since the different parts of the vestibular organ are not functionally identical (see also below) it would be of interest to know the central distribution of the fibers from the various receptor regions of the labyrinth. This problem is not yet entirely solved.

From Lorente de Nó's observations, based largely on Golgi material, it appears that, for example, the lateral vestibular nucleus is supplied chiefly from the utricular macula, while the superior nucleus receives fibers only from the semicircular ducts (see Brodal, Pompeiano, and Walberg, 1962, p. 20ff, for particulars). In a recent experimental study in the monkey Stein and Carpenter (1967) have obtained results largely confirming this, except that they favor a termination of utricular fibers chiefly in the descending nucleus. In addition, they present some evidence that fibers from the three semicircular ducts have, in part, separate terminal regions within the superior nucleus. The ducts, furthermore, supply part of the medial nucleus. This is in agreement with physiological studies, since units responding to stimulation of the horizontal semicircular duct appear to be located mainly in the medial and superior nuclei (Shimazu and Precht, 1965). Units responding to tilting have been found in the ventral part of Deiters' nucleus (Peterson, 1967). Thus it appears that the different receptor regions in part have their particular projection areas within the nuclear complex. This is of considerable functional interest, since the various efferent projections from the nuclei arise largely from specific parts of the complex (see below).

In addition to the afferent fibers coming from various subdivisions of the labyrinth an *efferent component* has been demonstrated in the vestibular nerve (Gacek, 1960). The number of efferent fibers is small. According to Rossi and Cortesina (1962) the fibers arise in three small cell groups, one of them in the lateral nucleus. Peripherally the fibers have been traced to the vestibular sensory epithelia (see also below). Presumably these fibers mediate a central control of vestibular receptors (see Sala, 1965; Kornhuber, 1966).

The *vestibular receptors* as mentioned above are the hair cells in the utricular and saccular maculae and in the cristae of the semicircular ducts. Although light microscope studies, particularly by Polyak and Lorente de Nó, had indicated that there are two types of receptor cells in the sensory epithelia and that there are differences in the nerve endings establishing contact with them, electron microscope studies were needed to clarify these problems. These studies in addition have revealed other morphological features which are of functional interest. For particulars the reader is referred to Wersäll (1956), Engström and Wersäll (1958),

---

[11] It may be argued that the term vestibular nuclei should be restricted to those parts of the complex which receive primary vestibular fibers. However, for practical reasons it is advisable to retain the current terminology.

Spoendlin (1964, 1965, 1966), Engström, Lindeman, and Ades (1966) and Wersäll, Gleisner, and Lundquist (1967).

The two types of sensory cells found within the vestibular sensory epithelia and separated by supporting cells, differ in several respects (Fig. 7-10A). The type I cell is bottle-shaped, while the type II cell is slender. The sensory cells do not reach the basal membrane. Both kinds of cells contain several mitochondria and are provided with sensory hairs. On electron microscopic examination it appears that the sensory hairs are stereocilia (40–110 per cell, Spoendlin, 1964), arranged in a regular manner according to their length. In addition, however, each cell is equipped with a peripherally situated kinocilium, having the characteristics of these found in other regions. When the orientation of the hairs is examined it becomes apparent that there is a regular organization (see Flock, 1964; Spoendlin, 1964), a spatial polarization (see Fig. 7-10C), suggesting that the sensibility of the epithelium is not the same to forces acting upon it from all directions. It appears that deviation of the sensory hairs toward the site of the kinocilium (see Fig. 7-10B) increases the firing rate of its afferent nerve fiber, while deviation in the opposite direction reduces the firing rate (see Flock and Duvall, 1965). The cells of type I and II show clear-cut differences with regard to their contacts with the afferent nerve fibers (the distal process of the vestibular ganglion cells). The type I cells are almost surrounded by chalyces of nerve terminals, while the slender type II cells are in contact with smaller bouton-like nerve endings at their bottom (Fig. 7-10A). In addition to these endings there occur small boutons which, in contrast to the two other kinds of endings, are provided with synaptic vesicles. These endings are assumed to belong to the efferent vestibular fibers, an assumption which is supported by the observation that they degenerate following transection of the vestibular nerve.

These morphological observations indicate that the sensory epithelia of the vestibular apparatus are very complexly organized. This is substantiated by neurophysiological studies. Most reliable information is obtained in studies where the receptors are stimulated naturally, by rotatory movements of the animal or tilting of the head. Recordings of action potentials in single fibers in the vestibular nerve have shown that each duct is maximally sensitive to movements in its own plane (Löwenstein and Sand, 1940). Furthermore, such studies have revealed functional differences between the cells in a crista or a macula. Units have been found in the cristae which react with an increase in their impulse frequency at the onset of rotation in one direction, for example to the right, while they are silent at the onset of a rotation to the left. During rest they show a slight resting discharge. A few units respond to rotation in both directions, either by excitation or inhibition (Löwenstein and Sand, 1940; Gernandt, 1949, and others). This data may be related to the polarization of the receptor cells described above. In the case referred to above it is assumed that the potentials recorded arise from stimulation of cells in the cristae. However, strictly speaking, it is not the rotation as such which is the adequate stimulus; it is more correct to speak of *angular acceleration and deceleration* as stimuli. This is exemplified by the following: When a rotation starts a particular unit increases its discharge. In the course of some time, usually about 20 seconds, it gradually reverts to its slow resting discharge frequency, and when the rotation stops its discharge ceases entirely. This can be explained in the following way: a rotation of the head in the plane of a semicircular duct will, on account of the inertia of the endolymph, produce a deviation of the cupula with the sensory

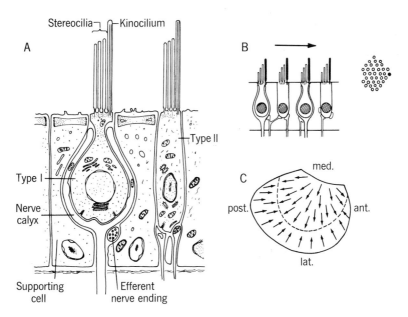

FIG. 7–10 *A:* Schematic drawing of the two types of hair cells in the vestibular epithelia of mammals. Note the different kinds of nerve endings in contact with the cells, the symmetric arrangement of the bundles of sensory hairs, many stereocilia with a single kinocilium in the periphery. From Wersäll, Gleisner, and Lundquist (1967). *B:* A diagram showing the orientation of the sensory hairs, the direction of displacement of the hairs which produces excitation (arrow), and (to the right) a view of the upper surface of a hair cell. *C:* A diagrammatic surface view of the human utricular macula, indicating (arrows) the direction of polarization of the sensory cells in different regions. Figs. *B* and *C:* Courtesy of Dr. H. Lindeman Jr.

hairs. Thus the cell is stimulated. After the rotation has continued for some time the fluid will follow the movement of the head, the cupula resumes its resting position, and there is no stimulus. When the rotation stops the cupula again deviates, but now in the opposite direction. This does not stimulate the particular sensory cell, but silences it. The deviations of the cupula were first observed directly by Steinhausen (1931). The cupula behaves as a highly damped torsion pendulum (see Löwenstein, 1966).

Angular acceleration or deceleration as described above *appears to be the adequate stimuli for the canals. The maculae* appear to be chiefly *position recorders,* which signal the position of the head in space. They are sometimes referred to as the static labyrinth, while the semicircular ducts represent the kinetic labyrinth. (Some data indicates that the maculae may also be vibration receptors.) On tilting the head the otolithic macula of the utricle, on account of its weight, will exert a pull on the sensory hairs, making them respond. These receptors adapt very slowly and most of them continue to fire if the same position of the head is upheld. The spatial polarization within the macula, referred to above (see Fig. 7-10B), gives a rational explanation of the fact that changes of the position of the head in different directions may stimulate hair cells. In one position cells in one area of the macula will be excited, in another position the pull exerted by the otolithic membrane will stimulate cells in another region of the macula. This agrees with results of single unit analyses of afferent fibers, where some units respond to an increase in tilting in one direction, others to tilting in other directions.

The above account is a simplified presentation of a very complicated mechanism which is still not completely understood. The semicircular ducts may be characterized as "bidirectional angular accelerometers," while the utricular macula is more of a "position recorder." However, linear acceleration may influence the semicircular canals to some extent, while it appears doubtful whether angular acceleration affects the macula (see Lowenstein, 1966). The data referred to above makes it appear likely that the central parts of the vestibular pathways are also complexly organized. This, indeed, has turned out to be true. Some main points will be considered in the following.

Fiber connections of the vestibular nuclei. In a general way it may be said that the vestibular nuclei are connected by afferent and efferent fibers with the following regions: *the spinal cord, the cerebellum, certain nuclei in the brain stem, and the reticular formation.* However, the afferent and efferent links in each of these reciprocal pathways with other structures are not quantitatively equal, nor are they related to the same subdivisions of the nuclear complex, a further indication of its intricate organization.

There are two well-known efferent pathways by which the vestibular nuclei may influence the activity of the *spinal cord.* As described previously (p. 170), the *lateral vestibulospinal tract* (see Fig. 4-6) arises only from the ipsilateral nucleus of Deiters and from small as well as large cells; it is somatotopically organized, can be traced to sacral levels of the cord, and terminates chiefly in Rexed's laminae VII to VIII. It exerts a facilitatory action on extensor neurons (α and γ). It appears that the lateral vestibular nucleus in man is likewise somatotopically organized (Løken and Brodal, 1969). The other (*medial*) *vestibulospinal pathway* comes from the medial vestibular nucleus (see Fig. 4-6), descends crossed and uncrossed only to upper thoracic segments and ends in the same laminae of the spinal gray as does the lateral tract. In contrast to these conspicuous vestibulospinal pathways, there is only a modest direct pathway conducting in the opposite direction, from the cord to the

382

vestibular nuclei. The *spinovestibular fibers,* which may to some extent represent collaterals of dorsal spinocerebellar tract fibers, end in a restricted number in the caudalmost part of the descending and lateral vestibular nuclei. Most of them terminate (Pompeiano and Brodal, 1957b; Brodal and Angaut, 1967) in the small group x (of Brodal and Pompeiano, 1957), which does not receive primary vestibular fibers. Physiological studies (Wilson, Kato, Thomas, and Peterson, 1966) have shown, however, that spinal impulses may reach the nucleus of Deiters via other routes, probably chiefly the reticular formation (spinoreticular and reticulovestibular fibers). Wilson et al. found stimulation of mixed and cutaneous nerves to be more effective than stimulation of muscular nerves. According to Frederickson, Schwarz, and Kornhuber (1965) joint movements are particularly effective in eliciting responses.

The relations of the vestibular nuclei with the *cerebellum* have been considered in Chapter 5. Suffice it here to recaptitulate some points. A small number of fibers from the vestibular nuclei pass to the cerebellum and appear to end in its "vestibular part." They are derived from restricted parts of the medial and descending vestibular nuclei (Brodal and Torvik, 1957) which, however, are not supplied with primary vestibular fibers. Nevertheless, vestibular impulses may reach the cerebellum directly via *primary* vestibulocerebellar fibers (see Fig. 5-8) which pass to the nodulus, the ventral part of the uvula, the flocculus (Dow, 1936), and the ventral paraflocculus (Brodal and Høivik, 1964). Thus the cerebellum does not appear to be much influenced from the vestibular apparatus but it exerts a marked influence on the vestibular nuclei. As described in Chapter 5, the "vestibulocerebellum" sends only a relatively modest number of fibers back to certain regions within the complex,[12] but there are two other more massive routes by which the cerebellum may influence the vestibular nuclei. Both these pathways arise in parts of the vermis, one being direct, the other having a synaptic relay in the fastigial nucleus (see Fig. 7-11). Of particular interest is the observation that within the projections onto the lateral vestibular nucleus of Deiters both pathways present a somatotopical localization, as illustrated in Fig. 7-11, from which further details may be seen. By way of these fibers the "spinal parts" of the cerebellum (which do not appear to receive vestibular impulses) may act in a somatotopically localized manner on the motor apparatus of the spinal cord.

The connections of the vestibular nuclei with the *reticular formation*

[12] These cerebellovestibular fibers are distributed in a particular pattern within the nuclei. Thus the flocculus and the nodulus largely project onto different nuclear regions. A comparison of these sites of termination with those of other afferent contingents is of functional interest (see Angaut and Brodal, 1967).

383

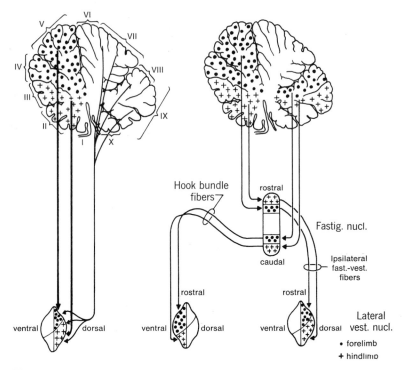

FIG. 7–11 Diagram illustrating major features in the projection from the cerebellar cortex onto the nucleus of Deiters (to the left) and (to the right) in the projections from the cerebellar cortex onto the fastigial nucleus and from this to the lateral vestibular nuclei. Note that the direct cerebellovestibular fibers and the projection from the rostral part of the fastigial nucleus end in the dorsal half of the ipsilateral lateral vestibular nucleus, while the fibers from the caudal part of the fastigial nucleus via the hook bundle supply the ventral half of the contralateral lateral vestibular nucleus. Within each of these projections there is a somatotopic localization. (See text.) Slightly altered from Brodal, Pompeiano, and Walberg (1962).

have largely been studied in Golgi material (see Scheibel and Scheibel, 1958). Axons of cells in the reticular formation appear to reach all nuclei in the vestibular complex, and likewise the latter give off fibers or collaterals to widespread regions of the reticular formation. In experimental studies, where lesions of the individual vestibular nuclei are made (see Ladpli and Brodal, 1968), the projections can be studied in greater detail, and it is also learned that with regard to the projection onto the reticular formation the vestibular nuclei are not identical. For example, only the nucleus of Deiters gives off fibers to the lateral reticular nucleus (which projects back to the cerebellum). By way of the reticular formation the vestibular nuclei may thus influence the activity of the spinal cord as well as certain parts of the thalamus (see Ch. 6) since vestibular efferents pass to regions which give rise to long descending and ascending fibers. The vestibuloreticular connections are presumably involved in vomiting and cardiovascular reactions observed on vestibular irritation (see below).

Connections of the vestibular nuclei with the *higher brain stem,* particularly with the nuclei of the nerves of the ocular muscles, have attracted much interest. Such fibers pass in the *fasciculus longitudinalis medialis.* This is a rather complicated bundle in spite of its course as a distinct fiber tract. It extends from the region of the oculomotor nucleus down the brain stem and continues to the spinal cord. It is phylogenetically very old, and in ontogenesis it stands out very clearly on account of its early myelinization. In the brain stem it is situated close to the median line beneath the aqueduct and 4th ventricle (cf. Figs. 7-3, 7-6, 7-14, 7-18), and is closely related to the nuclei of the eye muscles. In the caudal part of the medulla oblongata it bends ventrally and continues in the ventral funiculus of the spinal cord close to the ventral median fissure. In the cord it is usually called the *sulcomarginal fasciculus* (Fig. 7-12). In addition to fibers from the vestibular nuclei the medial longitudinal fasciculus contains other fibers. Some of these are descending and come from the interstitial nucleus of Cajal in the mesencephalon situated close to the oculomotor nucleus (Fig. 7-12). Some of them end in a restricted part of the medial vestibular nucleus (Pompeiano and Walberg, 1957), while others descend to the cord as the *interstitiospinal tract,* mentioned in Chapter 4 (see Fig. 4-1).

The bulk of fibers in the medial longitudinal fasciculus come from the vestibular nuclei. A smaller proportion passes to the cord as the medial vestibulospinal tract (Figs. 4-6, 7-12), referred to above. While these descending fibers are derived from the medial vestibular nucleus, *all four nuclei give off ascending fibers.* Conflicting opinions have been held concerning these (for a review of the literature, see Brodal and Pompeiano, 1958; Brodal, Pompeiano, and Walberg, 1962). However, there appears now to be unanimity on the main points. Thus the superior nucleus gives rise only to homolaterally ascending fibers (see McMasters, Weiss, and Carpenter, 1966). Other ascending fibers, crossed and uncrossed, come from the medial and, apparently to a lesser extent, from the lateral and descending vestibular nuclei. The majority of ascending fibers pass to the nuclei of cranial nerves III, IV, and VI, innervating the ocular muscles, but a fair number proceed further. Some have been traced to the interstitial nucleus of Cajal (see Fig. 7-12) and to other small nuclei in the same region (nucleus of Darkschewitsch and nucleus of the posterior commissure), perhaps even to the VPM of the thalamus (Carpenter and Hanna, 1962).

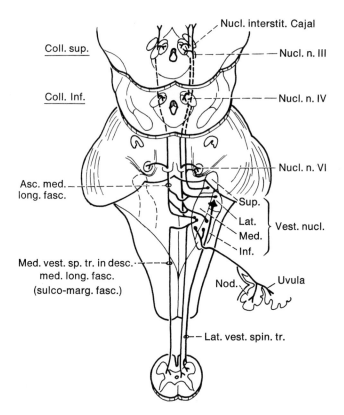

FIG. 7–12 A diagram showing some of the efferent projections of the vestibular nuclei with particular reference to the medial longitudinal fasciculus. The descending fibers in the latter, coming from the interstitial nucleus of Cajal, are not shown.

Natural stimulation of a semicircular duct induces eye movements (nystagmus, see below) in a particular direction, and stimulation of a nerve from a duct results in conjugate deviation of the eyes in the plane of the duct (Fluur, 1959; Cohen, Suzuki, and Bender, 1964; and others). As will be discussed in the section on the oculomotor nerves, conjugate eye movements require a precise co-operation of several muscles of both eyes. Furthermore, the various extrinsic eye muscles appear to be supplied from particular cell groups in the oculomotor nuclei. This strongly suggests that there must be an extremely precise correlation between the sites of ending of primary vestibular fibers from individual receptor organs in the nuclei and the distribution to the oculomotor nuclei of the fibers arising from the particular terminal areas in the vestibular nuclei. Even if it is extremely difficult to clarify the specific pattern in the vestibulo-oculomotor connections there is some evidence to support the above notion. Thus, as referred to above, fibers derived from the cristae end predominantly in the superior nucleus and in the medial, which appear to be the main sources of ascending fibers (see Stein and Carpenter, 1967). Furthermore, the fibers from the various cristae appear to have somewhat different terminal regions within the superior vestibular nucleus. The problem of vestibulo-oculomotor correlations has been reviewed by Szentágothai (1952a, 1964b) on the basis of anatomical as well as physiological studies. It is concluded from such studies that the vestibulo-oculomotor fibers in the medial longitudinal fasciculus are links in elementary three-neuron reflex arcs (primary sensory neuron—ascending vestibular neuron—peripheral motor neuron), but that in addition, vestibuloreticular fibers and fibers ascending from the reticular formation to the oculomotor nuclei are involved when conjugate eye movements occur following vestibular stimulation.

Since vestibular stimulation is well known to give rise to consciously perceived sensations it has been assumed for a long time that there are *pathways from the vestibular nuclei to the cerebral cortex.* Several workers have recorded action potentials from the cerebral cortex in animals following natural or electrical stimulation of the vestibular receptors or the vestibular nerve, but there has been some disagreement concerning the regions of the cortex receiving the vestibular impulses as well as concerning the pathways followed and the laterality of the projections (for some data see Brodal, Pompeiano, and Walberg, 1962). While it was previously assumed that the "cortical vestibular area" is situated in the temporal lobe, recent studies locate it in a small region close to the face subdivision of the first somatosensory area (Fredrickson, Figge, Scheid, and Kornhuber, 1966, in the monkey) in the cytoarchitectonic area 2 of Brodmann. (As described in Chapter 2 this area appears to be concerned chiefly in the reception of sensations from deep tissues, especially joint sensibility.) The cortical projection appears to be almost exclusively contralateral.[13] The pathways followed by the vestibular impulses to the cortex are not known anatomically (for some data see Hassler, 1956; Szentágothai, 1964b), neither are physiological studies of the subject conclusive. It seems a likely assumption (see Fredrickson et al., 1966; Kornhuber, 1966) that the cortical vestibular area is of importance for the conscious appreciation of spatial orientation.

It will appear even from the incomplete account given here that anatomically the vestibular nuclei are organized in a very complex manner. Even within each of the four main nuclei a differentiation is possible, not only with regard to architec-

[13] According to Andersson and Gernandt (1954) stimulation of individual branches of the vestibular nerve gives responses in limited portions of the total "vestibular cortical area," and Massopust and Daigle (1960) found the projections from the medial and descending nuclei to differ spatially in the cortex.

ture but also as concerns the sites of termination of afferent fibers and the sites of origin of efferent projections. This is shown for the nucleus of Deiters in Fig. 7-9, but the patterns within the other nuclei are at least as complex (see Brodal, Pompeiano, and Walberg, 1962; Angaut and Brodal, 1967). Although much data of this kind is now available, there are other features which have not yet been studied in sufficient detail. Some observations which further illustrate the complexity may be mentioned. For example, the afferents from the cerebellar cortex appear to contact preferentially large and giant cells in the nucelus of Deiters (Walberg and Jansen, 1964), while those from the fastigial nucleus first and foremost contact small cells (Walberg, Pompeiano, Brodal, and Jansen, 1962). When studied in the electron microscope it is seen that the speed of degeneration and the appearance of degenerating boutons of the primary vestibular fibers differ from those of the direct cortico-cerebello-vestibular fibers (see Mugnaini, Walberg, and Brodal, 1967, and Mugnaini and Walberg, 1967, respectively). The question of anatomical possibilities for interaction between the various units of the vestibular complex is of great functional interest. In studies with the Golgi method only scattered cells which can be considered as true internuncials have been found (Hauglie-Hanssen, 1968). Physiological studies have demonstrated the existence of a close collaboration between the vestibular nuclei of the two sides. Like the other fiber connections the commissural connections are arranged in a specific manner (Ladpli and Brodal, 1968).

Precise neurophysiological studies with exact identification of the sites recorded from have given much information of the functional organization of the vestibular nuclei, confirming and extending the anatomical findings. These studies likewise bear witness to an extremely complex organization of this nuclear complex. For example, various functional types of neurons may be distinguished (see Duensing and Schaefer, 1958) which have in part different locations in the nuclei. Among those responding to horizontal rotation, the type I neurons increase their discharge on ipsilateral angular acceleration and decrease it on contralateral acceleration, while type II neurons behave in the opposite way (Duensing and Schaefer, 1958). Whether these units are influenced by different kinds of receptor cells in the cristae is unknown. The type I neurons again are of two kinds, tonic and kinetic, according to their response characteristics to horizontal angular acceleration (Shimazu and Precht, 1965). It appears that kinetic neurons are excited monosynaptically, the tonic ones multisynaptically (Precht and Shimazu, 1965). Some of the type II neurons are only excited from the contralateral labyrinth (Shimazu and Precht, 1966). These are located in regions which receive commissural fibers (Ladpli and Brodal, 1968). The picture is further complicated by the fact that the same neurons in the nuclei may be influenced from different vestibular receptors (Duensing and Schaefer, 1959). This is compatible with what is known of the distribution of primary vestibular fibers in the nuclei. Physiological data on some of the other afferent and efferent connections of the vestibular nuclei has been referred to elsewhere in this text (see Chs. 4 and 5).

Functional aspects. Nystagmus. The disturbances resulting from lesions of the vestibular nerve and the labyrinth have particularly attracted the interest of otologists. Increasingly accurate methods of investigation have drawn attention to some special features which are of diagnostic value. However, a satisfactory correlation of the phenomena observed clinically with the new data on the structural and functional organization of the vestibular receptors and their central connections is not yet possible. No attempt will be made here to treat this subject exhaustively, but some main features will be considered.[14]

It is clear from the preceding account that one may with some reservations distinguish between a "static" labyrinth, represented by the utricle (perhaps the saccule), and a "kinetic" labyrinth, consisting of the three semicircular ducts. The former signals the position of the head in space, the latter records angular movements of the head in space. Impulses from the utricle influence chiefly the distribution of muscular tone in various parts of the body, while the semicircular ducts appear to be concerned chiefly in adjusting the position of the eyes so that visual orientation is secured during movements.

Animal experiments which illustrate some features in the function of the *"tonic labyrinth"* have been referred to previously. In Chapter 4 mention was made of decerebrate rigidity (p. 222) as well as of the tonic labyrinthine reflexes, and the role of the cerebellum has been discussed in Chapter 5. The role played by the labyrinth in ocular movements will be considered again in connection with the oculomotor nerves.

It is important to be aware of the fact that under normal circumstances the vestibular impulses interact with impulses from other sources which reach the vestibular nuclei (see Gernandt and Gilman, 1960). The nuclei further collaborate with other parts of the brain. Analysis of this co-operation is, however, difficult. As examples illustrating such collaboration may be mentioned that anesthesia of the upper three cervical dorsal roots in monkeys results in severe disorientation, imbalance, and incoordination, resembling the symptoms appearing in labyrinthectomized animals (Cohen, 1961). This, in addition, demonstrates the great functional role of the tonic neck reflexes considered in Chapter 4. Since the vestibular nuclei have ample projections to the reticular formation (units in the reticular formation responding to vestibular stimulation which produce nystagmus have been recorded; see Duensing and Schaefer, 1957a) it obviously co-operates with the vestibular nuclei when they influence the spinal cord as well as with the oculomotor nuclei.

Some further points of relevance for clinical neurology deserve men-

[14] An extensive review has recently been published by Kornhuber (1966). Here the reader will find a critical evaluation of clinical methods used in the examination of vestibular function, of their anatomico-physiological basis and of their clinical value. Several clinical and theoretical aspects of the vestibular mechanisms have been treated recently in symposia: "Neurological Aspects of Auditory and Vestibular Disorders," 1964; "International Vestibular Symposium," Uppsala 1963, in Memory of Robert Bárány, 1964; "Second Symposium on the Role of the Vestibular Organs in Space Exploration," Ames Research Center, Moffett Field, California, 1966; "Myotatic, Kinesthetic and Vestibular Mechanisms," Ciba Symposium, 1967.

tion. It is obvious from experimental studies that the results of destruction of the labyrinth or transection of the vestibular nerve are not identical to results of destruction of the vestibular nuclei. Nor are the results of stimulation of the nerve and the nuclei the same (see Brodal, Pompeiano, and Walberg, 1962, for some data). It appears that in man the vestibular apparatus is less important than in many animals. Thus, persons with no demonstrable labyrinthine function preserved manage quite well in daily life and may, for example, drive a car. In the absence of information from the labyrinth they rely on visual orientation and on proprioceptive information. It is only when vision is excluded and they have to walk on uneven ground or on a soft mattress that they lose their equilibrium (Martin, 1967).

In view of the complex organization of the vestibular mechanisms it is no wonder that *methods of studying vestibular function in man* are still imperfect, and that diagnostic conclusions often have to be tentative. Attempts have been made to study clinically the influence of the labyrinthine impulses on the spinal motor apparatus. The *stepping test* (see Peitersen, 1965) may give some information in cases of unilateral lesions, but the results must be evaluated with great caution. More objective methods of recording differences in the postural innervation on the two sides of the body have been suggested (Henriksson, Johansson, and Østlund, 1967), but their value is not yet clear. Far better and more precise methods are available for the study of the vestibular influences on the oculomotor apparatus. These are based on the examination of *nystagmus*. On account of its clinical importance it will be appropriate to consider nystagmus and the methods used for its study in some detail. The literature on nystagmus is enormous. While the nystagmus occurring in affections of the labyrinth and occurring in part in affections of the vestibular nuclei is fairly well understood, much less is known of the basis for nystagmus in affections of several other parts of the brain.

The name nystagmus is used for a particular kind of conjugate movement of the eyes, which may be elicited in normal subjects on stimulation of the vestibular apparatus or by a particular kind of optic stimulation (optokinetic nystagmus, see section (*g*)). We are here concerned with *vestibular nystagmus*. This depends essentially on the stimulation of the sensory hairs of the cristae of the semicircular ducts, due to the deflection of the cupula which occurs on angular accelerations and decelerations. As referred to in a preceding section of this chapter, when the head is rotated, at the start the inertia of the endolymph in the semicircular ducts will deflect the cupula in one direction. If the rotation is continued in the same direction the fluid will, after some time, obtain the same velocity of rotation as the canal, and irritation ceases. If then the movement stops short, the inertia of the endolymph will make it continue its flow, with a renewed stimulation of the cupula, but this time in an opposite direction. The correctness of this view, first set forth by Bárány on the basis of clinical studies, has been confirmed, as we have seen, in experimental studies. Since the semicircular canals are situated at right angles to each other, rotation around any axis will induce some change in the endolymph. The stimulation of the vestibular receptors gives rise to potentials transmitted to the vestibular nuclei, and from these impulses are sent to various cell groups of the oculomotor nuclei initiating conjugate movements of the eyes, as discussed above.

The nystagmus elicited from the labyrinth consists essentially in rhythmic conjugate movements of the eyes, the movement being slow in one direction, rapid in the other. In clinical terminology the nystagmus is named according to its fast component, but this is merely for convenience, the slow movement being really the active phase, the rapid being a reflex return to the starting position. In slighter degrees a pathological nystagmus appears only if the patient looks in the direction of the fast component; in the severest forms it is present also when he looks the other way. Among many *variants of pathological nystagmus, positional nystagmus* may be mentioned. This is present only in a certain position of the head, for example, when the patient is lying on his right side. Most commonly a horizontal nystagmus is observed, but it may also be vertical, oblique, or rotatory. The latter type most often occurs in combination with one of the other types.

Nystagmus is always pathological if it occurs spontaneously, but it may be induced by different methods in normal individuals (induced nystagmus). This procedure is much used as a test of the function of the labyrinth. Most employed are the *postrotatory* and the *caloric nystagmus*.[15] When an individual is made to rotate around his axis, the movements set up in the semicircular canals are those described above. (Clinically usually 10 rotations within 20 seconds are used.) During the rotation the impulses try to keep the axis of the eyes fixed at a given point. The eyes will lag behind in the rotatory movement, but when they finally lose sight of the object they perform a quick movement to the original position, another point in the environment is fixed and the process repeats itself. Thus during rotation the quick component will be in the direction of the rotation. When this is stopped, the inertia of the endolymph will produce a stimulation of opposite order to the ampullary crista (of the duct whose plane coincides with that of the rotation).

---

[15] In addition the otogalvanic test may be employed. In this, however, the vestibular nuclei may react to the current, even if the peripheral vestibular apparatus is damaged.

Consequently the postrotatory nystagmus will be one with the quick component opposite to the direction of the rotation. The postrotatory nystagmus normally lasts for a definite time after rotation has stopped.

In the caloric tests movements in the endolymph are produced by irrigation of the external auditory meatus with hot or cold water. To avoid misinterpretations, tests with both hot and cold water should be employed. With the head tilted in different directions the various canals are brought into the most favorable position. For the horizontal canal, which responds most easily to caloric stimulation, this is with the head inclined 60° backward, when the canal is in a vertical position. The nystagmus appears after a short latency and lasts ½ to 2 minutes, depending on conditions such as the temperature of the water and the duration of the stimulus. The effect of cold water is contrary to that of hot. The caloric test has the advantage over the rotatory because it permits the examination of one ear at a time. A reduction in vestibular function will betray itself in abnormal results in these tests. A nystagmus lasting a shorter time than normally, or shorter when elicited from one ear than from the other, thus indicates some reduced function of the corresponding labyrinth. (Examination of nystagmus is usually performed with the patient carrying strong convex lenses to exclude the fixation reflex, see section *g*.)

In recent years a number of methods have been evolved in order to secure a more precise recording of nystagmus movements. Graphic registrations can be made in several ways (see Kornhuber, 1966). Most used of these methods appears to be *electronystagmography,* in which the retinocorneal potential and its changes on movements of the eyes is recorded by electrodes fixed to the skin around the eyes (see Aschan, Bergstedt, and Stahle, 1956; Aschan, 1964). This has the advantage that it may be done with the eyes closed (of interest in some conditions) and in darkness. The graphic registrations permit precise comparison of the results of examinations performed on different occasions. In present-day otoneurology a number of tests for nystagmus are employed, and many variants can be distinguished. To some extent particular patterns of change in the experimentally induced nystagmus may give diagnostic information.

The nystagmus movements elicited in the caloric and postrotatory tests in healthy individuals are, of course, not normal in a restricted sense, since they occur in response to stimuli which are not usually acting on the labyrinth. However, they disclose some principal features of the vestibular control of eye movements. The tests also reveal that the semicircular duct impulses are not only concerned with the adjustment of the gaze in movements of the head, but also influence the muscular status of the body as a whole. Thus the phenomena of *past pointing* which follows both tests mentioned above must be interpreted in this manner. When the individual is asked to touch a certain point with his eyes closed, the arm will be seen to deviate in the opposite direction to the nystagmus. Furthermore, he will have a tendency to fall in this direction.[16] Experimental studies in cats and monkeys (see Suzuki and Cohen, 1964) have shown that following stimulation of single ampullary nerves (by implanted electrodes) there occur ipsilateral forelimb extension and contralateral forelimb flexion as well as some other motor phenomena. This supports the interpretation of past pointing as being a result of stimulation of semicircular ducts.

Nystagmus may be produced in healthy persons in other ways than by employing the tests described above. Thus a *positional nystagmus* may be induced in humans (as well as in rabbits) by alcohol intoxication (see Aschan, 1958; Kornhuber, 1966).[17] Certain drugs have been shown to influence the labyrinth (see, for example, Jongkees and Philipszoon, 1960), a problem of interest in the evaluation of motion sickness drugs. It is well known that experimental as well as spontaneous nystagmus is reduced when the individual is tired, and increases when he is excited. Changes of this kind may occur rather rapidly. During sleep nystagmus ceases. The labyrinths of the two sides must be assumed to collaborate normally, although there is evidence that each labyrinth is concerned primarily in the reactions involving adaptations in one direction. Thus extirpation of the labyrinth in monkeys is followed by nystagmus with the quick component toward the normal side and rotation of head and neck to the same side (see, for example, Dow, 1938b). Following labyrinthectomy in man symptoms of the same kind but of somewhat different order have been observed (Cawthorne, Fitzgerald, and Hallpike, 1942). In man the effects are less, and less enduring, than in monkeys. The chimpanzee appears to hold an intermediate position.

Symptomatology. Disturbances in vestibular function play a more important role in otology than in neurology, even if they are also frequently encountered in patients suffering from diseases of the nervous system. But their diagnostic value in the latter cases is rather limited. In this text the vestibular symptoms provoked by disease of the internal ear

[16] It will be seen that the direction of the past pointing and tendency of falling (e.g. in Romberg's test) are in accord with the fact that the slow component of the nystagmus is the active phase. All phenomena tend to direct the patient to the same side.

[17] It appears that this is due, in part at least, to an action on the labyrinth (Aschan, Bergstedt, and Goldberg, 1964), but in addition there may be a depressing effect on the normally occurring inhibitory action of the nodulus on the vestibular nuclei (Aschan, Ekvall, and Grant, 1964) as discussed in Chapter 5.

will not be considered, nor will the particular differences in symptomatology which in some cases allow the otologist to decide which part of
the labyrinth is affected. It will suffice to point out a few characteristic
features. In *acute vestibular affections* (labyrinthitis, bleedings, etc.) the
vestibular symptoms, such as nystagmus, past pointing, tendency to fall,
and vertigo, are frequently accompanied by symptoms pointing to an involvement of the autonomic system. Nausea and vomiting, lowering of
blood pressure, tachycardia, and excessive perspiration may occur in the
beginning. Following the examination by rotatory or caloric tests the
same symptoms may be provoked, but usually to a more moderate degree. There is good reason to believe that these autonomic effects are
mediated by reflex connections from the vestibular nuclei to the visceral
efferent nuclei of the lower cranial nerves, particularly the vagus.

The most frequently observed symptom of vestibular origin is without doubt *nystagmus.* When this is due to an affection of the labyrinth
or the vestibular nerve it is called "peripheral"; when it is produced by
lesions within the central nervous system it is referred to as "central."
When examining nystagmus, however, some care has to be taken. In
perfectly healthy persons, particularly if they are fatigued, slight *nystag-
moid jerks* may result from gazing markedly in a lateral direction. Irregular movements of the eyes, of an oscillating type and lacking as a rule
the characteristic rhythmic appearance, are common in persons with
severely reduced vision, particularly in congenital amblyopia. This *ocular
nystagmus* is regarded as being due to a defective power of fixation, and
the "miner's nystagmus," which is usually also oscillating, is perhaps of
the same nature. Thus, these types of nystagmus must not be ascribed to
vestibular lesions. The cerebellar nystagmus will be referred to below.

The *peripheral nystagmus* is described as being usually of the combined horizontal-rotary type, with its quick component toward the non-
affected side. It is usually accompanied by vertigo, tendency to falling,
past pointing toward the affected side (cf. above), and autonomic
symptoms. It is transitory, a fact explained by assuming that the vestibular nuclei are able to compensate for the altered distribution of impulses
which results when one labyrinth ceases to function. Apart from appearing in diseases of the labyrinth, these symptoms may occur in *affections
of the vestibular nerve*. The processes affecting this will be the same as
those mentioned as causes of cochlear nerve lesions (cf. Ch. 9). Thus in
an *acoustic nerve tumor,* vertigo may occur, and examination with
vestibular tests may reveal signs of reduced vestibular function. Lesions
of the vestibular and cochlear nerves may give rise to symptoms of
Menière's disease, where attacks of nausea, vertigo, nystagmus, and falling occur and the hearing is reduced following each attack, until the pa-

tient is finally completely deaf on the affected side. Abnormal vessels pressing on the VIIIth nerve may result in tinnitus and vertigo, but this is rare.

Occasionally, most often in the course of a febrile illness, patients complain of episodes of vertigo. These may be associated with objective signs of vestibular dysfunction, such as nystagmus. The condition has been assumed to be due to an affection of the vestibular nerve or the labyrinth and is usually referred to as "vestibular neuronitis," "neuro-labryinthitis," or "epidemic vertigo," since epidemic occurrence has been noted (see Pedersen, 1959). It appears that the pathogenesis is not the same in all cases (see Pedersen, 1959; Harrison, 1962).

"Central" nystagmus differs in certain respects from the peripheral which demonstrates all the symptoms known to be due to disturbed function of the vestibular apparatus. Vertigo is most commonly absent or of slight degree, and the nystagmus is said to be usually to the side of the lesion, but no definite rule can be seen to prevail. The nystagmus in affections of the central nervous system is attributed to lesions involving the vestibular nuclei or the secondary vestibular tracts. It is most commonly observed in *disseminated sclerosis,* in which the nystagmus in combination with a characteristic speech disturbance and intentional tremor forms the classical triad of Charcot. The nystagmus in disseminated sclerosis differs from the peripheral type also in its tendency to persist for years, although remissions may occur as with the other symptoms in this disease. On account of the multiplicity of foci in disseminated sclerosis it has not been possible to decide which structure has to be damaged in order for nystagmus to result. It appears probable that the symptom may follow lesions of several localizations, since nystagmus is a rather constant and frequently an early symptom. On the basis of clinical experience the medial longitudinal fasciculus has frequently been held to be responsible. However, experimental studies by Bender and Weinstein (1944) in monkeys did not give much support to this contention. Following bilateral small lesions to the medial part of the fascicle they observed nystagmus only on lateral gaze. It appears that lesions of the medial longitudinal fasciculus may give rise to so-called *internuclear ophthalmoplegia* (see Carpenter, 1964; Carpenter and Strominger, 1965; Harrington et al., 1966; Ross and deMyer, 1966). Here a paresis of the medial recti muscles of the eye is a prominent feature, associated with particular types of nystagmus. Lesions of the vestibular nuclei may be followed by alterations in induced nystagmus, as shown for example by Shanzer and Bender (1959) in the monkey, and by Carmichael, Dix, and Hallpike (1965) in man. Nystagmus may also appear in *other lesions of the brain stem* (syringobulbia, vascular disorders, tumors) but usually in

combination with symptoms of widespread damage. Finally it may occur in conditions of increased intracranial pressure, presumably on account of affection of the vestibular nuclei.

In cerebral lesions so-called *directional preponderance* of nystagmus is often seen. Attempts have been made to utilize these and other disturbances of nystagmus in the focal diagnosis of brain lesions. Fitzgerald and Hallpike (1942) found a directional preponderance of caloric nystagmus to the side of the lesion only when this was situated in the temporal lobe, but not in any of the other lobes. However, in spite of much work and much speculation, little is yet known of the mechanism of the observed changes. In view of the complex collaboration between certain parts of the cerebral cortex, the brain stem, and the vestibular nuclei in the control of ocular movements this is not astonishing. For some observations and interpretations the reader is referred to Carmichael, Dix, and Hallpike (1954, 1965).

Much discussion has been devoted to the question of the existence of a *cerebellar nystagmus*. It is clear that the "nystagmus" seen in many cases of lesions to the cerebellum is not a true nystagmus movement. It should probably rather be interpreted as ataxia of the eye muscles. In addition, it should be remembered that cerebellar lesions frequently affect the brain stem, directly, by pressure or secondarily by vascular disturbances, and a typical nystagmus might thus be due to damage to the vestibular nuclei. If there is a true cerebellar nystagmus, it appears most likely that it would be seen in lesions involving the flocculonodular lobe or the nucleus fastigii, on account of the intimate connections between these structures and the vestibular nuclei. As described in Chapter 5, positional nystagmus has been found to occur following stimulations and ablations of the nodulus in animals. The nodulus is assumed to exert an inhibitory control on the vestibular nuclei. It is in keeping with this that clinical observers have drawn attention to the occurrence of vestibular hyperirritability in cerebellar lesions (particularly abscesses). They have further emphasized the importance of testing for nystagmus with the patient in different positions.

It may be mentioned that in severe damage to the brain stem sometimes a condition resembling decerebrate rigidity in animals may be seen, presumably when the vestibular nuclei are released from impulses from higher levels. In such cases the tonic labyrinthine reflexes may be demonstrated in man. "Vestibular sensations" have been occasionally reported in man following cortical stimulation close to the primary acoustic area (Penfield and Jasper, 1954).

It will be seen from the account in this chapter that although the vestibular apparatus is of considerable importance in the normal functioning of the organism and is extremely precisely organized, the inferences of diagnostic value for the neurologist which can be drawn from lesions of these structures are limited.

(e) THE INTERMEDIOFACIAL NERVE

Anatomy. The VIIth cranial nerve, the facial, or better, the intermediofacial nerve, is a mixed nerve. Quantitatively the motor (special visceral efferent) fibers supplying the facial mimetic musculature form the most important part, the *facial nerve strictly speaking;* but in addition a minor portion made up of visceral and somatic afferent and general visceral efferent fibers joins it. This minor part is called the *nervus intermedius* and is commonly spoken of as the sensory root of the facial. It will be appropriate to consider the motor root first.

The *fibers of the motor root* spring from the *motor facial nucleus,* which belongs to the special visceral efferent nuclear group (Figs. 7-1 and 7-2). It is found just rostral to the nucleus ambiguus in the caudal part of the pons as a column 4 mm in length, in the lateral part of the reticular formation, dorsal to the superior olive and medial to the nucleus of the spinal tract of the Vth nerve. Its cells are of the usual motor type found in the ventral horns and the somatic efferent cranial nerve nuclei. The axons of these cells do not pass ventrally at once but form a loop (Figs. 7-13 and 7-14). The first part of this is directed dorsomedially, where the fibers approach the floor of the 4th ventricle and then ascend immediately dorsal to the abducens nucleus. In a transverse section at this level of the pons this part of the nerve stands out clearly as a com-

FIG. 7–13   Diagram of the pons illustrating, *inter alia,* the intrapontine course of the facial nerve.

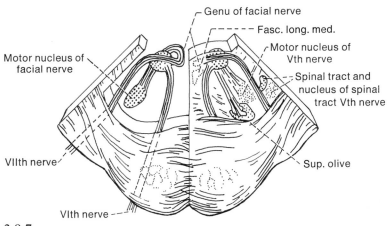

Genu of facial nerve

Fasc. long. med.

Motor nucleus of Vth nerve

Motor nucleus of facial nerve

Spinal tract and nucleus of spinal tract Vth nerve

VIIth nerve

Sup. olive

VIth nerve

pact bundle (Fig. 7-14 to the right). At the rostral part of the abducens nucleus it bends over its dorsal surface (forming the genu of the facial nerve) and then passes directly ventrolaterally and somewhat caudally to its point of exit at the caudal border of the pons on the lateral aspect of the brain stem. Together with the intermedius and the VIIIth cranial nerve it enters the internal auditory meatus, passes through this to its bottom, covered by the meninges in a sheath common to these nerves. The facial and intermediate nerves then enter the facial canal, which in its first part is directed laterally, then at the geniculate ganglion performs a sharp bend in a dorsolateral direction, and after a short course in this direction ultimately proceeds in a caudal direction to leave the skull through the stylomastoid foramen. In the last part of the dorsolateral and the first part of the caudal course the facial canal lies close to the tympanic cavity, separated from it only by a thin bony lamella, a fact of practical importance. The fibers belonging to the intermedius are given off at various places to be considered below.

After leaving the stylomastoid foramen the facial nerve pierces the substance of the parotid gland and is here split into several branches which spread out in a fanlike manner to reach all the superficial, mimetic muscles of the head. These muscles are derived from the second branchial arch, the nerve of which is the facial. Apart from innervating the mimetic (e.g. orbicularis oris and oculi, buccinator, zygomaticus, frontalis, oc-

FIG. 7–14   Drawing of a section through the caudal part of the pons in man. Weigert's myelin sheath stain.

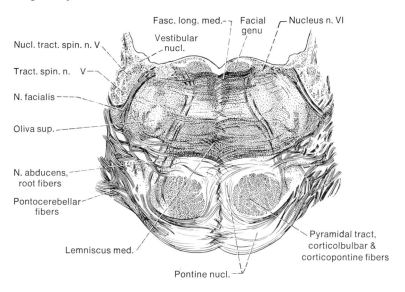

cipitalis, etc.) muscles, the facial nerve also gives off motor fibers to the stapedius muscle in the middle ear and extracranially to the stylohyoid, the posterior belly of the digastric muscle, and the platysma.

In view of the finely differentiated movements performed by the facial musculature, determining the extremely variable expression of the face, it is no wonder that the facial nucleus presents a subdivision into several cellular groups, each of which is concerned in the innervation of certain facial muscles. This question has been studied rather extensively in animals by recording the distribution of retrograde changes in the different parts of the nucleus after section of individual branches of the nerve. The results of various authors using this approach agree fairly well (see Vraa-Jensen, 1942; Courville, 1966b). Some human cases have also been reported.[18] The facial nucleus is more differentiated in man than in other mammals, a fact in harmony with the importance of the facial muscles in speech and emotional facial expression. The oral muscles particularly show a considerable development both in regard to their number and the finer differentiation of the individual muscles. These are supplied by a lateral cell group which is particularly large in man. The frontalis, corrugator supercilii, and orbicularis oculi muscles are innervated by a clearly delimited part of the nucleus, the pars intermedia. The anatomical independence of this part is of interest in view of the clinical findings in supranuclear lesions of the facial nerve (cf. below).

It is in keeping with the almost infinite variations in facial expression in man that the motor units in the mimetic muscles are small, in the platysma 25 muscle fibers per nerve fiber (Feinstein et al., 1954). The total number of fibers in the human facial nerve is some 7,000, and most of them are relatively thick, 7 to 10μ (van Buskirk, 1945). The *afferent innervation of the facial muscles* is relatively little known. One would assume, a priori, that the mimetic muscles are amply provided with proprioceptors. However, the number of muscle spindles in the mimetic muscles appears to be small. Voss (1956) found 6 in the human stylohyoid muscle. The perikarya of the γ fibers to the spindles have not yet been identified (see Courville, 1966b, for a discussion), nor is it known along which route the afferents from the muscle spindles and other possible proprioceptors reach the brain stem. According to Bruesch (1944) in the cat a small number of afferent fibers (140) is found in the branches of the facial nerve to the mimetic muscles. Some clinical studies (for example Huber, 1930; Carmichael and Wollard, 1933) indicate that proprioceptive sensations are preserved even if the trigeminal nerve is anesthetized. It has been suggested that the proprioceptve fibers from the mimetic muscles have their perikarya in the mesencephalic trigeminal nucleus (Kimmel, 1941; Pearson, 1945).

[18] A full review of earlier literature is found in the monograph by Vraa-Jensen (1942) who besides performing experimental studies has pointed out the phylogenetic correspondence between the nuclear and the muscular groups, confirming and extending Huber's (1930) earlier findings.

399

The motor facial nucleus is played upon by impulses from different sources. The facial musculature is involved in several *reflexes,* which are initiated by optic and acoustic stimuli, as well as by sensory impulses from the face and mouth. Fibers entering the nucleus or ending in its vicinity have been traced from the superior colliculi, an optic reflex center, from the superior olive (acoustic impulses) as well as from the sensory trigeminal nuclei and the nucleus of the solitary tract. Reflexes mediated by these fibers are, for example, blinking and eventually closing the eyes in response to strong illumination, closing of the eye on touching the cornea (corneal reflex), contraction or relaxation of the stapedius muscle in response to varying intensity of sounds, and chewing and sucking on introduction of food into the mouth.[19] In addition, the motor facial nucleus is influenced by descending fibers from higher levels, among these some of the "motor" cortex. In man some of these corticobulbar fibers may end on cells of the nucleus (Kuypers, 1958c). The corticobulbar tract presumably mediates the voluntary movements of the face. From clinical findings it appears that these fibers are crossed, except some of those going to the nuclear division supplying the muscles above and around the eye (see above), since lesions of the corticobulbar tracts, e.g. in hemiplegia, result in paralysis only of the lower part of the facial muscles. Some support for this view has been obtained in an anatomical study of human brains by Kuypers (1958c). Among afferents to the facial nucleus from other "higher" regions, the presence of fibers from the red nucleus has been definitely established (Courville, 1966a, in the cat). This projection is crossed and the fibers end only in certain subdivisions (not in those supplying the perioral muscles). In addition there appears to be a bilateral projection from the mesencephalic reticular formation. Other pathways, for example directly, or more likely indirectly, from the globus pallidus, may exist but are so far little known. Such connections have been assumed to be involved in emotional facial movements (see below).

The composition of the *intermediate nerve* is more complex than that of the motor facial. Since it is a small nerve and the contingents belonging to the different fiber types are relatively scanty and the peripheral

---

[19] In electromyographic studies of the corneal reflex in man Magladery and Teasdall (1961) found its reflex latency to be relatively long, 40 to 64 msec on the side ipsilateral to the stimulation. This strongly suggests that the reflex arc is multisynaptic. These authors found only slight increase of reflex latency in patients with cerebral lesions. Other authors (for example Oliver, 1952) report a diminished reflex response in such cases, and have suggested that the corneal reflex has a supranuclear arc. It appears more likely, however, that a delay or a weakening may be due to an affection of descending connections acting on the brain stem nuclei involved.

400

course complicated, it is no wonder that it has been difficult to establish the details of its anatomy, some of which are of some practical
relevance. Most of our present-day knowledge has been obtained from
experimentation with animals. Some of the principal features will be
mentioned below. Concerning the general visceral efferent fibers which
supply the lacrimal, the submaxillary and the sublingual glands and the
glands of the nasal and part of the oral cavity, and which convey preganglionic parasympathetic (secretory) fibers to them, the reader is referred to the chapter on the autonomic system. Here our concern is with
the *sensory components* of the nervus intermedius.

The sensory fibers of the intermediate nerve have their perikarya in
the small *geniculate ganglion,* referred to above. The cells are of the
usual pseudo-unipolar type. A considerable number of the sensory fibers
are special visceral afferent, conveying taste impulses from the anterior
two thirds of the tongue. In addition the nerve also contains other sensory
fibers. The branches from the intermediate nerve are firstly the *greater
superficial petrosal nerve* passing to the sphenopalatine ganglion, then the
chorda tympani leaving the nerve in the tympanic cavity and anastomosing with the lingual nerve to reach the tongue. But not all afferent fibers
are distributed to these two branches. Some, as referred to above, follow
the facial nerve in its further course. In cats, according to Foley and
DuBois (1943), about 33–34 per cent of the sensory fibers, which are
mainly small and myelinated, pass with the great superficial petrosal
nerve; 45 to 55 per cent with the chorda tympani; and 12 to 15 per
cent proceed further with the facial nerve. Whereas at least a considerable
number of the sensory fibers in the two above-mentioned branches are
gustatory (to be treated in more detail below), those passing with the
facial nerve proper cannot be so, but must be general sensory afferents.
From comparative anatomical data (see Kappers, Huber, and Crosby,
1936) as well as from experimental findings (Foley and DuBois, 1943;
Bruesch, 1944) it is apparent that most of these fibers are distributed to
the external ear, partaking in the sensory cutaneous innervation of the
concha of the auricle and sometimes an area behind the ear. (These
regions are also supplied by the auricular ramus of the vagus nerve.) This
cutaneous sensory branch of the facial nerve is present also in man
(Larsell and Fenton, 1928; Pearson, 1945). As early as 1907 Ramsay
Hunt had postulated the existence of such fibers based on a study of
the symptomatology of herpes zoster oticus and a certain type of neuralgia called by him geniculate neuralgia (cf. below). These fibers must
be regarded as somatic sensory and are probably among those which have
been found to end in the trigeminal nuclei (Woodburne, 1936; Kimmel,
1941; Torvik, 1956b; Kunc and Maršala, 1962; Kerr, 1962), as do also

some fibers in the glossopharyngeal and vagus nerves as previously mentioned. All three nerves, contrary to what is often stated, thus contain a *somatic* afferent fiber component. In the case of the vagus these fibers (as well as some glossopharyngeal fibers) are concerned in the innervation of the areas, already mentioned, in the external ear, whereas most of the fibers of the IXth nerve must be those which supply the posterior third of the tongue, the palatal arches, and the pharyngeal wall. This is learned from findings in cases of medullary tractotomy (operative sectioning of the spinal tract of the trigeminal nerve, cf. p. 417), since this is followed by analgesia in the areas mentioned as well as in the trigeminal field proper (Brodal, 1947a; Falconer, 1949, and others). The practical consequences of this distribution of the somatic afferent fibers in the facial intermediate nerve will be mentioned below.

The pathways for taste.   The last sensory quality conveyed through the intermediate nerve is the *sense of taste* from the anterior two thirds of the tongue. On account of the practical importance of taste sensations for the topical diagnosis of a lesion of the facial nerve, the question of the gustatory pathways will be considered in some detail (cf. Fig. 7-15).

It is especially in regard to the part played by the facial nerve that diversity of opinion has prevailed. In considering the cause of these controversies it is worth remembering that the examination of taste, like the examination of other sensory functions, is dependent on the mental power of the patient and his willingness to co-operate, and that several sources of error are involved in the technical side of the examination. Lastly the number of taste buds on the anterior two thirds of the tongue is not very large, and their number decreases progressively with age. Consequently the acuity of taste shows considerable individual variations in normal persons. In man the most important nerve concerned in the mediation of taste is the glossopharyngeal, which supplies the vallate papillae.

Although most investigators agree that operative interruption of the trigeminal nerve does not affect taste (e.g. Lewis and Dandy, 1930; Schwartz and Weddell, 1938), some reports to the contrary are found, but in many of these cases the reduction of gustatory acuity has been found to be slight or transient. The more enduring reduction, or loss in some instances, is reasonably explained as Rowbotham (1939) expressed it, "The taste impulses lack the background of common sensations." A third possibility is that the geniculate ganglion or the greater superficial petrosal nerve may be damaged in the operation. This nerve is mentioned in this connection because in some instances it appears to be concerned in transmitting taste sensations.

4 0 2

In most persons interference with the chorda tympani, for example in mastoid-ectomy, has been observed to lead to loss of taste in the anterior two thirds of the tongue, in accordance with the current conception of the course of the taste fibers. However, Schwartz and Weddell (1938) have reported cases where the chorda tympani was destroyed without ensuing gustatory disturbances. This indicates that in some persons taste fibers from the anterior two thirds of the tongue take another course. This pathway appears to be through the greater superficial petrosal nerve, since the same authors have observed some cases where this nerve was damaged but the chorda remained intact, with resulting loss of taste in the anterior two thirds of the tongue. The fibers are believed to follow the chorda for a short distance and then to leave it through a small anastomotic branch to the otic ganglion. From here they are assumed to pass by another anastomosis to the greater superficial petrosal nerve and then centralward as usual. This variation is apt to cause confusion in diagnostic reasoning in some cases of facial nerve affections. In Fig. 7-15 the usual course of the gustatory fibers of the intermedius is indicated by heavy lines, the alternative by dots.

That the glossopharyngeal nerve is concerned in the transmission of taste impulses from the posterior one third of the tongue is generally agreed upon. Several cases of intracranial section of this nerve have given conclusive evidence of this (e.g. Fay, 1927; Lewis and Dandy, 1930; Reichert, 1934). Likewise taste sensations from the soft palate and palatal arches, where some taste buds are found, presumably pass by the glossopharyngeal, but others may pass via the sphenopalatine ganglion (cf. Fig. 7-15). It is furthermore generally assumed, mainly on an anatomical basis, that the vagus carries some special visceral afferent taste fibers from the extreme dorsal part of the tongue and the superior surface of the epiglottis. These regions are, of course, very difficult to examine with regard to taste, and their taste buds disappear in early infancy.

All taste fibers, those of the intermediate as well as the glossopharyngeal and vagus nerve, are *distributed to the nucleus of the solitary tract* and, as anatomical evidence shows, its rostral part (cf. section (*c*) on glossopharyngeal-vagus). The central course of the secondary gustatory fibers is not well known (see, however, Gerebtzoff, 1939), but it is established that gustatory impulses are transmitted to the thalamus and ultimately reach the cerebral cortex. Some secondary fibers appear to end in the hypothalamus and must be assumed to influence autonomic functions. Previously *the cortical area for taste* was generally assumed to be closely related to the cortical olfactory regions, but recent research has made it clear that the cortical taste area is located in close relation to the focus for somatic sensibility of the tongue.

It is customary to distinguish four elementary taste qualities: salt, sour, bitter, and sweet. Tests of gustatory sensibility are made by applying substances of different kinds to small spots on the tongue. The subjective sensations experienced

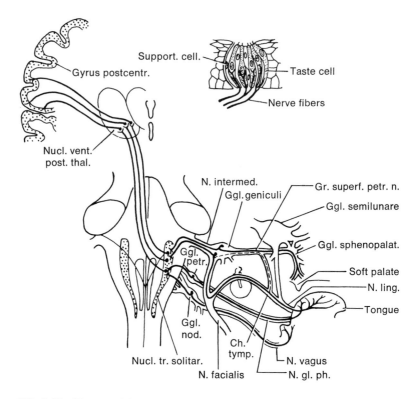

FIG. 7–15 Diagram of the course of the gustatory fibers. Heavy lines indicate the usual paths, stippling the alternative route taken by fibers from the anterior two thirds of the tongue in certain cases. Above to the right a diagram of a taste bud.

bear no clear relation to the chemical composition of the test substance. In experimental animals recordings of action potentials in fibers of the nerves conveying taste impulses can be made. Likewise potentials may be picked up in the central nervous system by the insertion of fine electrodes. From studies of this kind it has been found, in agreement with anatomical data on the central distribution of fibers in the nerves conveying sensations of taste, that the rostral part of the nucleus of the solitary tract is the first relay in the taste pathways (see Makous et al., 1963). Most units found respond to the application of taste stimuli of more than one of the elementary qualities, and often they respond to other kinds of stimulation as well. As referred to previously the course of the secondary gustatory fibers is not definitely settled anatomically. However, following gustatory stimuli action potentials occur in the thalamus, more precisely in the medialmost part of the VPM. According to Blomquist, Benjamin, and Emmers (1962) and Emmers, Benjamin, and Blomquist (1962) in the monkey as well as in the rat the "taste" region is separate from the region which is activated by other stimuli of the tongue. Destruction involving this part of the thalamus is followed by impairment of taste (Patton,

Ruch, and Walker, 1944; and others). From the VPM thalamocortical fibers transmit the impulses to the cerebral cortex, where action potentials can likewise be recorded on gustatory stimulation. Most authors found the "cortical taste region" to be situated below and a little in front of the "face area" of the sensori-motor cortex. In contrast to Cohen et al. (1957) in the cat, Benjamin and his co-workers found that in the rat this area is separate from the nongustatory lingual area (see, however, Emmers, 1964). Furthermore, the taste areas for the inter-mediate and glossopharyngeal nerve are separate in the rat, as they are in the squirrel monkey (see Benjamin, 1962). Ablation of this area in the rat abolishes taste discrimination (Benjamin and Akert, 1959) as does destruction of the ap-propriate thalamic region. (However, in monkeys corresponding cortical ablations did not have this result.) There are obvious but still poorly understood species dif-ferences concerning the central mechanisms of taste.[20]

Experiences in man are in agreement with the results of anatomical studies. Thus cases have been described of contralateral impairment of taste following tumors involving the VPM of the thalamus (Adler, 1934). On stimulation of the anterior portion of the second sensorimotor cortex where it approaches the insula, subjective sensations of taste have been recorded (see Penfield and Jasper, 1954), and occasionally a gustatory aura heralds an epileptic convulsion starting from this part of the cortex (Shenkin and Lewey, 1944; Penfield and Kristiansen, 1951). Finally, lesions of this part of the cortex have been shown to be accompanied by impairment of taste in the contralateral half of the tongue (Börnstein, 1940).

Symptomatology. *Lesions of the central pathways of the somatic and visceral afferent components of the intermediate nerve* are not fre-quently recognized, partly because the ensuing symptoms are usually in-significant and are obscured by more prominent signs. From what has been stated above it is clear, however, that disturbances of taste may be observed when sought for in certain cortical and more deeply situated lesions of the brain, and such cases have been described. Lesions of the central parts of the *efferent* facial mechanism, however, are not uncom-mon, and lesions of the peripheral intermediofacial nerve belong to the most common of the affections which the neurologist encounters. It will be readily understood that according to the site of the lesion the symptoms will be somewhat different and will depend on whether the intermediate nerve is also affected or not. It will be appropriate to treat the pure motor facial paralysis first, and then supplement the account of this with a description of the features which accompany it when the intermediate

[20] In recent years considerable attention has been devoted to this subject. The interested reader will find much information in the monographs *Olfaction and Taste* (1963 and 1967) which carry reports from international symposia. For a recent experimental anatomical and physiological study see Benjamin, Emmers, and Blomquist (1968).

nerve is also involved, and finally discuss some symptoms ascribable to an affection of the intermediate nerve alone.

The most frequent type of *peripheral facial nerve palsy* is that usually spoken of as being "rheumatic," setting in acutely sometimes in the course of an infection of the upper air passages or in connection with exposure to draught or cold. Little is known concerning the true etiology of this condition, the so-called *Bell's palsy*. The assumption that the nerve is compressed due to edema in the facial canal has prompted operative intervention with opening of the canal. This has been reported to give good results in many cases, but the results are difficult to evaluate on account of the frequent occurrence of spontaneous recovery. There appears, however, to be ample room for the nerve in the canal, since about 50 per cent of the space in the canal is occupied by loose connective tissue and vessels (Sunderland and Cossar, 1953). According to Langworth and Taverner (1963) the prognosis of a facial palsy can be reliably established in the first few days by studying the conduction time in the nerve branches. This may thus aid in a decision on whether operative decompression is likely to be of benefit.

If the paralysis, usually unilateral, *is complete,* which is the rule, all movements of the mimetic facial muscles are abolished, and the face is asymmetrical at rest as well as in motion. The patient cannot frown or raise his eyebrow on the affected side, he cannot close his eye on account of the paralysis of the orbicularis oculi, and the palpebral fissure is widened. On attempting to close his eye the eyeball will be seen to deviate upward and slightly outward (Bell's phenomenon), due to a relaxation of the inferior rectus and contraction of the superior rectus. This also occurs normally when the eyes are closed but becomes more distinctly visible when the closure of the eye is impossible. The blinking reflex (corneal reflex) is abolished, and this is of practical relevance since it necessarily leads to a drying of the cornea with resulting ulceration. Therefore one of the most important therapeutic measures of Bell's palsy is the protection of the eye from drying. The most efficient therapy is to perform a tarsorrhaphy. A patient with a peripheral facial palsy cannot properly close his mouth, and the affected oral angle is usually lower than the other, sometimes with dribbling of saliva. On speaking, laughing, weeping, etc., the affected side does not partake in the movements. As the paralysis is of the peripheral type, the flaccidity of the mimetic muscles will betray itself in a more or less complete loss of the habitual wrinkles, which are due to the insertion of several of the facial muscles in the skin, and the affected side of the face will on this account appear smoother than the other. The paralysis and lack of tone of the buccinator muscle will frequently reveal itself on eating as a tendency to accumulation of food within the cheek.

On account of the paralysis of the buccinator it is, for example, difficult for the patient to blow out a candle. After some time the muscles will fall the victim of atrophy. Fasciculation may be seen and can be recorded electromyographically. The diagnosis of a complete peripheral facial palsy is easy. If the palsy is bilateral, difficulties arise in articulation and partly in eating.

In *incomplete lesions* the distribution of the paresis can be variable and the testing of power is important (power of orbicularis oris on closing the mouth, of the frontalis on raising the eyebrow, the power of keeping the eyes closed when the eyelids are forcibly drawn apart, etc.) as in slight affections movements on inspection may appear to be normal, and a slight asymmetry of the face is a normal occurrence. Furthermore, the determination of the location of the paretic muscles is important in order to distinguish a peripheral from a central facial palsy. In the latter the upper part of the face is usually not affected. Electromyography may be of value in diagnosis and prognosis (Weddell, Feinstein, and Pattle, 1944; Taverner, 1955; see also Langworth and Taverner, 1963; Buchthal, 1965).

A feature peculiar to peripheral facial paresis is the frequent occurrence of *contractures of the muscles* when the paralysis is complete and of somewhat longer duration. On inspection the contracted side appears at first to be normal; only when testing for movements is the real state revealed. Electromyographic studies suggest that the contracture is due to abnormal activity of some residual motor units (Taverner, 1955).

Less frequently than these "rheumatic" palsies, a peripheral facial palsy is seen in *affections of the middle ear*. In uncomplicated otitis as well as in mastoiditis, or middle-ear tuberculosis, the nerve may be affected as it passes in the facial canal in the posterior wall of the tympanic cavity. The nerve may be affected with edema and circulatory disturbances, or it may be directly involved in the inflammation when the bone covering it is encroached upon by the disease process in the middle ear. The prognosis will vary according to the pathological alterations of the nerve.

Among other causes of a peripheral facial palsy may be mentioned *traumatic injury* to the nerve at the stylomastoid foramen of the temporal bone, and even *closed head injuries*. The facial palsy in the latter is assumed to be due to an ischemia of the nerve and the prognosis is good (see Weddell, Feinstein, and Pattle, 1944). In *tumors of the parotid gland* an eventual paralysis will usually not be complete, at least not in the beginning. *Operations* aimed at removing or incising submaxillary lymph nodes may cause a partial paralysis affecting the muscles of the lower lip. Another cause of partial facial palsy, although not frequently encountered now, is *leprosy*. In both the maculoanesthetic and the tuberous forms of leprosy, partial affections of the branches of the facial nerve are a common and early symptom (Monrad-Krohn, 1927).

In its *intracranial course* the facial nerve may also be injured, as in diseases of the meninges, e.g. syphilis. Another cause is the affection of the nerve by a *neurinoma of the VIIIth nerve.* Here a facial palsy is one of the symptoms which frequently signal the disease. Usually the paresis progresses slowly, accompanied or preceded by signs of damage to the VIIIth nerve (cf. the latter).

The *motor nucleus of the facial nerve* and its fibers within the pons may be affected by pontile hemorrhages or other *vascular changes,* when there will be motor and frequently also sensory symptoms (resulting in, for example, a "crossed hemiplegia"). The facial nucleus is not infrequently involved in *poliomyelitis.* Cases are not rare in which the facial nucleus alone is affected, or, if other structures are involved in addition, only symptoms due to the damage of this nucleus are manifest as a unilateral peripheral facial palsy (Wallgren, 1929; Schumacher, 1940). In other instances the facial nucleus is affected together with other cranial nerve nuclei (bulbopontile form of poliomyelitis). The frequent affection of the facial nucleus in *chronic bulbar palsy* has already been referred to on p. 373. (Facial palsy is also common in pseudobulbar palsy, but then of the central type.) *Congenital facial palsies,* usually bilateral, are occasionally found, and are due to an aplasia or hypoplasia of the nucleus. When the palsy is only partial the aplasia affects only part of the nucleus (see, for example, Henderson, 1939). Similar aplasias and congenital paralyses may occur concomitantly also in other motor cranial nerves, particularly the abducens.

Before leaving the peripheral motor facial nerve, reference should be made to the frequent occurrence of *involuntary facial movements.* These may appear as a facial hemispasm, consisting of irregularly occurring contractions of the muscles on one side, usually increased by emotional stimuli but absent during sleep. The etiology of this phenomenon is obscure.[21] It may occur following a fascial palsy, but usually no preceding disease can be ascertained. It ought to be remembered, however, that involuntary movements of this type without accompanying paresis may be an early sign of an acoustic nerve tumor (personal observation).

A supranuclear paralysis of the facial nerve is a very frequent feature of *capsular hemiplegia.* The damage at the internal capsule interrupts also the corticobulbar fibers destined for the facial nucleus. As repeatedly mentioned, this central paresis is characterized by being limited to the

---

[21] Ehni and Woltman (1945) conclude from a study of 106 cases that the lesion causing hemifacial spasm may be in the facial nucleus or the proximal portion of the facial nerve.

lower part of the face. Thus a hemiplegic patient can close his eyes and frown, but is somewhat hampered in speech. This central paresis is not followed by marked atrophy of the facial muscles, and is situated on the side opposite the lesion, on the same side as the other paralyses which may be present. This ensues from the crossing of the corticobulbar and corticospinal fibers. A similar paresis or paralysis of the facial muscles may occur in *lesions of the face region of the precentral cortex.* In these instances it is not so frequently accompanied by total hemiplegia, as is easily explained by the larger space occupied by the cortical motor region compared with the narrow zone taken up by the corticobulbar and corticospinal fibers in the internal capsule.

Reference was made above to the *emotional involuntary innervation of the facial muscles.* It is well known that in paralysis agitans and postencephalic Parkinsonism the patient is able to show his teeth, whistle, frown, etc., i.e. there is no facial palsy, but his emotions are not reflected in his mimics, and he usually has a stiff, masklike facial expression (poker face). On the other hand, a hemiplegic patient, suffering from a damage to the corticobulbar fibers and having a complete central paresis of the lower part of the face, may be able to smile a spontaneous smile, for instance when he enjoys a joke. Monrad-Krohn (1939) has drawn attention to the fact that this spontaneous smile on the paralyzed side is frequently exaggerated, occurring earlier and exceeding that which appears on the nonparalyzed side. This *dissociation between the voluntary and emotional facial innervation* can so far not be adequately explained. It appears a likely assumption, however, that the fibers mediating the impulses to the emotional innervation do not descend in the internal capsule. Possibly hypothalamic and pallidal efferents are involved when the patient smiles emotionally, while a "social" smile requires that the corticobulbar projections be intact. Monrad-Krohn is inclined to interpret these phenomena as due to lack of inhibition by the cortical impulses, which in normal individuals suppress some of the involuntary emotional impulses. In the same manner one can explain the exaggerated emotional expressions frequently met with in the form of weeping or laughing following trifling, normally inadequate stimuli, in cases of capsular hemiplegias. The same explanation may be applied to the attacks of spasmodic laughter or weeping so frequent in pseudobulbar palsy. Here on both sides the corticobulbar fibers to the efferent cranial nerve nuclei as a rule are affected, and presumably the lack of cortical control is still more complete than in the hemiplegias.[22]

Turning now to *symptoms referable to the peripheral part of the intermediate nerve,* it will be clear from the anatomical description that they

[22] Some aspects of emotional expression have been discussed by Brown (1967).

may vary. Apart from deficiency symptoms, irritative symptoms also occur, and are discussed below.

A lesion of the facial nerve anywhere from its origin at the lower border of the pons to the tympanic cavity will be apt to affect the intermedius also. The affection of its general visceral efferent, parasympathetic fibers, will usually not be recognized, unless particularly sought for by special methods used to detect some diminution of secretion of saliva and tears. Interference with the gustatory fibers may also escape the patient's attention, but it is more easily ascertained, and is of a certain importance. As a general rule it may be said that a *lesion of the facial nerve anywhere between the pons and the departure of the chorda tympani will be followed by loss of the sense of taste in the anterior two thirds of the homolateral half of the tongue.*[23] A lesion situated distal to the departure of the chorda tympani will not have this consequence. However, this statement requires the qualification, evident from the anatomical data, that in some instances the nerve may be damaged between the geniculate ganglion and the chorda tympani, and yet no gustatory loss is present. This will appear in those cases where the taste fibers pass by way of the greater superficial petrosal nerve. But it is safe to state that, when loss of taste in the anterior two thirds of the tongue accompanies a facial palsy, the lesion must be situated central to the departure of the greater superficial petrosal nerve and probably central to the chorda tympani. Further clues cannot be obtained from an analysis of taste.[24] Another finding may be of some use, namely, the occurrence of *hyperacusis,* when the fibers to the stapedius muscle are involved. This phenomenon then, when present, points to the location of the lesion as being central to the pyramidal eminence in the tympanic cavity. Lesions situated proximal to the tympanic cavity will frequently be accompanied by symptoms due to involvement of the VIIIth nerve (tinnitus, reduced hearing, or vestibular disturbances).

In later stages of a peripheral facial palsy occasionally the *syndrome of crocodile tears* occurs. On eating or following other stimuli which normally produce secretion of saliva, lacrimation appears in the eye on the affected side. This is seen in lesions of the facial nerve central to the geniculate ganglion and is explained as being due to erroneous regeneration of nerve fibers (see Taverner, 1955). Fibers

[23] This ought to be emphasized since several neurological textbooks still contain the statement that only lesions between the geniculate ganglion and the chorda tympani will cause gustatory loss. Since it has been definitely proved by section of the intermediofacial nerve in man (see, for example, Lewis and Dandy, 1930) that the gustatory fibers enter the brain with the facial, this can obviously not be true.

[24] Of course an affection of the taste fibers to the anterior two thirds of the tongue may be due to a lesion of the chorda peripheral to the tympanic cavity, or where it has joined the lingual nerve. In the latter case the concomitant anesthesia of the same regions of the tongue will settle the matter.

of the intermediate nerve which have originally supplied salivatory glands on regeneration enter Schwann sheaths which belong to degenerated fibers having innervated the lacrimal gland.

Deficiency symptoms due to affection of the general sensory fibers, the cutaneous and alleged proprioceptive fibers in the intermediate nerve, will scarcely be detected clinically. However, irritative phenomena referable to this part of the nerve deserve brief mention. The occurrence of the so-called *geniculate neuralgia* of Ramsay Hunt has already been alluded to. This admittedly is not very frequent, although there is reason to believe that it is often not correctly diagnosed. It may appear following a herpes zoster oticus which, as suggested already by Ramsay Hunt (1907, 1937), is due to an inflammation of the geniculate ganglion, the blisters occurring in the cutaneous field of the nerve, the concha, and eventually in a limited area behind the ear.[25] The herpetic eruption may be followed in some days by a facial palsy or this may appear simultaneously. In other instances the neuralgia sets in without any preceding herpetic eruption. Attacks of pain, frequently very severe and localized to the concha and also felt deep in the ear (involvement probably of a tympanic branch of the intermediate), occur in fits. They may be provoked on touching the external ear or sometimes on swallowing or yawning, and frequently irradiate forward deep in the face. This irradiation is explained as being due to the involvement of fibers of the greater superficial petrosal nerve, passing, *inter alia,* to the posterior parts of the nasal and oral cavities. (The irradiating pain marks a transition to the so-called Schluder's neuralgia of the sphenopalatine ganglion.) Neuralgias of the geniculate type have been observed to disappear in certain cases when the intermediate nerve has been cut, and they may also be attacked by tractotomy as referred to above.

Probably due to an affection of the sensory fibers of the intermediate nerve are the pains in the ear region, which not infrequently accompany an ordinary "rheumatic" *peripheral facial palsy,* especially in its beginning. Likewise it may happen that patients affected with a *neurinoma of the VIIIth nerve* tell a story of their sufferings starting with a pain situated deep in the ear. This symptom has been observed to be the initial single symptom in several cases, and the possibility of a tumor is worth remembering when no otitis or other symptoms of disease of the ear can be ascertained in cases of otalgia. It appears probable that the pain is due to affection of the intermediate nerve, lying closer to the acoustic than the facial.

(f) THE TRIGEMINAL NERVE

The nerve and its nuclei. The Vth cranial nerve, the trigeminal, is

[25] In addition some vesicles may appear on the soft palate, explained as due to an affection of sensory intermedius fibers passing via the sphenopalatine ganglion.

a mixed nerve supplying mainly the masticatory muscles with motor fibers and the skin of the face, the conjunctiva, and a large part of the mucous membrane lining the nasal and oral cavities with sensory fibers. Apart from its first division, the ophthalmic nerve, it is the nerve of the 1st branchial arch, as the facial is that of the 2nd, the glossopharyngeal that of the 3rd, and the vagus the nerve of the 4th and following arches.

The *sensory part of the nerve* is far larger than the motor. At the exit of the nerve on the lateral aspect of the pons (Fig. 7-5) the two parts can clearly be distinguished as a larger, lateral, or sensory root, *portio major,* and a smaller, medial, motor root, *portio minor.* The latter joins the third division of the sensory root. The sensory fibers will be considered first.

The pseudo-unipolar perikarya of the fibers of the sensory trigeminal root are found in the large *semilunar or Gasserian ganglion,* situated on the cerebral surface of the petrous bone near its apex in the middle cerebral fossa. Peripherally this gives off three branches, the three principal divisions of the nerve, *ophthalmic, maxillary,* and *mandibular nerves,* leaving the cranial cavity through the superior orbital fissure, the foramen rotundum, and the foramen ovale respectively. The further peripheral course will not be considered in detail. The cutaneous distribution of the different branches will be evident from Fig. 7-16. These sensory trigeminal fibers are *somatic afferent,* and convey impulses of exteroceptive cutaneous sensations. The overlap between the areas supplied by the three divisions of the trigeminal is very slight (in contrast to the overlapping of the dermatomes), and the borders of the cutaneous fields of the trigeminal to those of the spinal nerves are astonishingly sharp.

The cutaneous distribution of the trigeminal nerve has been ascertained by dissections of the nerve and from the findings in clinical cases. With the advance of neurosurgery it has been possible to check these findings where section of the nerve or extirpation of the semilunar ganglion has been performed. These findings correspond well with the anatomical data. It should be noted that the lower border of the mandibular nerve territory is found several centimeters above the lower margin of the mandible, and that whereas the trigeminal as a rule does not supply the concha of the auricle (innervated by the VIIth, the Xth, and possibly the IXth nerves) it is usually concerned in the cutaneous innervation of the anterior wall of the external auditory meatus and the anterior part of the tympanic membrane (Cushing, 1904). It is frequently overlooked that the trigeminal nerve innervates the mucous membranes of the nasal and oral cavities and the maxillary and frontal sinuses. The dura is innervated by meningeal branches from the trigeminal divisions, except the

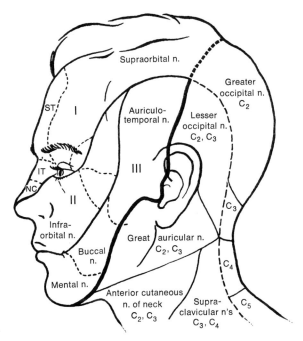

FIG. 7–16 The cutaneous distribution of the trigeminal nerve and its branches, with the adjacent cervical nerves. Modified from Haymaker and Woodhall (1945).

dura in the infratentorial portion of the posterior cranial fossa, which receives its sensory innervation mainly from the vagus.

Just as there are differences in size of the cells in the trigeminal ganglion, so the sensory trigeminal fibers are found to be of widely varying diameter, and partly differ as regards their terminal nuclei. The *sensory nuclei of the trigeminal nerve* consist of three different parts, together extending through the brain stem from the 2nd cervical segment of the cord and upward through the mesencephalon. In a caudorostral direction these nuclei are: the *nucleus of the spinal tract,* the *main, or principal, sensory nucleus,* and the *mesencephalic sensory nucleus* (Fig. 7-2). The fibers of the sensory root, on entering the pons, traverse its basilar portions, coursing dorsomedially, in the direction of the main sensory nucleus. Many of the fibers then dichotomize into ascending and descending branches. Several of the latter are very long and descend as a distinct bundle, the *spinal tract of the trigeminal nerve* (Figs. 7-2, 7-3, 7-6, 7-14, and 7-17), to the caudal end of the medulla oblongata where it fuses with the dorsolateral tract of Lissauer in the spinal cord.[26] As the tract de-

[26] The designation may be confusing, since it is common to use the term

scends, collaterals and terminal fibers are given off to a long small-celled nucleus, lying immediately medial to the tract, the *nucleus of the spinal tract,* which is continuous with the gelatinous substance of the dorsal horn. In the medulla oblongata the tract and its nucleus are situated beneath the surface, its upper part producing the elevation called the tuberculum cinereum (Fig. 7-5). The higher parts of it are covered by the fibers of the brachium pontis (Figs. 7-5 and 7-14). At its rostral end the nucleus of the spinal tract is continuous with the *main sensory nucleus.* The latter nucleus is phylogenetically younger than the nucleus of the spinal tract, and is well developed in most mammals and man. This fact, as well as the knowledge of the central connections of the two nuclei, the distal fusing of the nucleus of the spinal tract with the dorsal horn, and the difference in their afferent fibers and their functions (cf. below) makes it *plausible to regard the main sensory nucleus as being homologous to the nuclei of the dorsal funiculi of the cord, and the nucleus of the spinal tract as being homologous to the dorsalmost laminae of the dorsal horn.*

The details of the distribution of afferent fibers to these two trigeminal nuclei are of practical as well as theoretical interest. From correlated clinical and pathological observations it has, for some forty years, generally been assumed that the main nucleus is concerned primarily in the transmission of tactile sensibility of the face, whereas the spinal tract and its nucleus has to do with pain and thermal sensibility. Experimental findings have on the whole corroborated this, as will be considered below.

The *third sensory trigeminal nucleus,* the so-called *mesencephalic nucleus,* presents several peculiarities. It extends as a slender column of cells from the rostral end of the main sensory nucleus to the superior colliculus, occupying a position somewhat lateral to the upper part of the 4th ventricle and the aqueduct (Figs. 7-2, 7-17, and 7-18). It is made up chiefly of pseudo-unipolar cells resembling those of the semilunar and other ganglia. These cells, for this and other reasons, are generally assumed to be sensory. Their alleged origin in the neural crest is, however, disputed. The cell column is accompanied by a fine tract of fibers, the *mesencephalic root* of the trigeminal nerve. Most of these fibers are derived from the cells of the mesencephalic nucleus and descend. These descending fibers, many of which are of the large myelinated type, have been traced in degeneration experiments to the portio minor and to the branches of the mandibular nerve supplying the masseter, temporalis,

---

"tract" (tractus) for fiber bundles connecting nuclei within the central nervous system, while the spinal trigeminal tract (as well as the solitary tract) is composed of the central processes of cells having their perikarya outside the central nervous system.

and pterygoid muscles, i.e. the muscles of mastication, and have therefore been assumed to mediate proprioceptive impulses. This assumption has gained support from recent studies to be considered below.

The *motor nucleus of the trigeminal nerve* is the uppermost of the special visceral efferent column nuclei (see Fig. 7-2). It is composed of cells of the usual "motor" type, and is situated in the middle of the pons, closely medial to the main sensory nucleus (see Fig. 7-17B). Its fibers, as already mentioned, all leave the pons as the portio minor, join the mandibular nerve and supply the masticatory muscles proper: the masseter, temporalis, and external and internal pterygoid muscles. In addition motor fibers are given off to the tensor tympani, the tensor palati, the mylohyoid, and the anterior belly of the digastric muscle. Like the other motor nuclei in the brain stem, the masticatory nucleus consists of several cell groups, and the particular muscles receive their motor innervation from fairly well circumscribed regions of the nucleus (see Szentágothai, 1949).

The motor trigeminal nucleus is acted upon by fibers from higher levels, among them corticobulbar fibers. Sensory fibers from various cranial nerves, chiefly it appears, by way of intercalated cells, may activate the nucleus in different reflex actions. (Fibers of the trigeminal nerve do not appear to end in the motor nucleus, Kerr 1961). Fibers from the mesencephalic trigeminal nucleus, however, end in direct synaptic contact with the cells of the motor nucleus (see below).

From a clinical point of view the trigeminal nerve and its central connections are of great importance. Research from recent years has greatly increased our knowledge of these subjects. Since many of the observations made, particularly on the sensory trigeminal nuclei, are of relevance to clinical problems, some main points in their anatomical and functional organization will be considered. The complexity is far greater than was previously assumed.

Organization and connections of the sensory trigeminal nuclei. As shown by Olszewski (1950) the nucleus of the spinal tract may be subdivided into three architectonically different portions, called the nucleus caudalis, interpolaris, and oralis, respectively (Fig. 7-17A). These subdivisions can be identified in a number of animal species and in man (Olszewski and Baxter, 1954). Structurally the nucleus caudalis closely resembles the dorsal horn (being made up of a peripheral marginal zone, an intermediate gelatinous part, and a more massive deep part, the subnucleus magnocellularis), and the distribution of afferents appears to be similar. Within the other nuclei, likewise, different subgroups may be distinguished. These features indicate the presence of functional differences between minor parts of the nucleus of the spinal tract.

On entering the brain stem almost half of the root fibers of the trigeminal nerve divide into an ascending and a descending branch (Windle, 1926), the former ending in the main sensory nucleus, the latter in the nucleus of the spinal tract. These fibers are of different calibers, and a considerable proportion are thin. In the spinal trigeminal tract in man approximately 90 per cent have a diameter of less than 4μ (Sjöqvist, 1938). At caudal levels thin fibers appear to be relatively more numerous than more rostrally. It is of some practical interest that the fibers belonging to the three main branches of the nerve are arranged in a definite order within the tract, the ophthalmic being found most ventrally, the mandibular most dorsally (see Figs. 7-7A and 7-17B). This has been repeatedly demonstrated anatomically, in the rat (Torvik, 1956b), in the cat and in the monkey (Kerr, 1963a; and others). It has further been held, chiefly on the basis of studies of clinical cases of vascular disturbances of the posterior inferior cerebellar artery (Smyth, 1939) and electrophysiological studies (Harrison and Corbin, 1942; McKinley and Magoun, 1942), that the ophthalmic fibers extend most caudally, while the maxillary and mandibular fibers end successively more rostrally. Thus the ophthalmic division, in the nucleus as well as in its cutaneous distribu-

FIG. 7–17 *A:* Diagram showing the subdivision of the trigeminal sensory nuclei. The upper region (*N.V.sn.pr.*) is the main sensory nucleus. Below this follow the three subdivisions of the spinal nucleus: the oralis (*N.V.sp.o.*), the interpolaris (*N.V.sp.ip.*), and the caudalis (*N.V.sp.c.*). The latter continues caudally into the dorsal horn. From Olszewski (1950). *B:* A diagram showing the topical arrangement within the spinal trigeminal tract of the fibers belonging to the main divisions of the trigeminal nerve. The fibers terminate in the nuclei according to the same pattern. The successive rostrocaudal terminations of the three groups shown in the diagram is disputed. (Cf. text.)

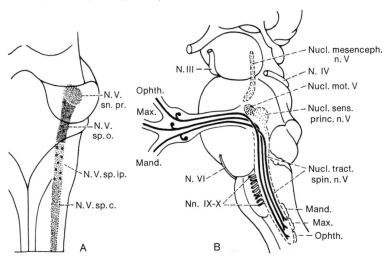

tion, would be in series with the sensory 2nd cervical nerve. However, Torvik (1956b) and Kerr (1963a) found no clear evidence of a successive pattern in the distribution. It is of interest that a fair number of trigeminal fibers descend as far as the upper part of the C_2 segment of the cord and even to C_4 in the rat (Torvik, 1956b). Furthermore, the termination in the main nucleus as well as in the divisions of the spinal nucleus shows the same dorsoventral somatotopical order as found in the spinal tract (Torvik, 1956b; Kerr, 1963a). This agrees with physiological observations (Kruger and Michel, 1962a; Eisenman et al., 1963; see also Darian-Smith, 1966). There appears to be little overlap between the terminal territories of the three branches in the nuclei.

In addition to the primary sensory fibers the main and spinal trigeminal nuclei have other connections. In the first place, as referred to in previous sections, some fibers in the intermediate, glossopharyngeal and vagus nerves join the spinal tract, where they occupy the dorsalmost part (see Fig. 7-7A). These fibers can be traced caudally to the level of C_2 in the cat (Kerr, 1962) or even C_3 in the monkey (Rhoton, O'Leary, and Ferguson, 1966). Furthermore, there are fibers in the spinal tract which pass from the caudal nucleus to the more rostrally situated subdivisions including the main nucleus (Carpenter and Hanna, 1961; Stewart and King, 1963) as well as fibers from the spinal cord (Torvik, 1956b; Rossi and Brodal, 1956b; Mehler, Feferman, and Nauta, 1960; Bowsher, 1962). Dorsal root fibers of the upper cervical nerves end in the nucleus of the spinal trigeminal tract (see Kerr, 1961). Finally, the main nucleus as well as all subdivisions of the spinal nucleus receive fibers from the cerebral cortex, mainly its central region (Brodal, Szabo, and Torvik, 1956, in the cat). It appears that most of these fibers come from the primary sensory cortex (Kuypers, 1960). Reference should also be made to afferent fibers from the reticular formation. Fibers from many different sources thus converge on the main and spinal trigeminal nuclei, suggesting that they are more than pure relay stations. The convergence of trigeminal, intermediate, glossopharyngeal, vagal, and spinal afferents in the spinal nucleus is of some clinical relevance (see below).

As referred to above it has been generally held that the caudal part of the spinal trigeminal nucleus is concerned chiefly in the mediation of impulses arising on stimulation of pain and temperature receptors, while the main nucleus has been related to tactile sensation. (For an account of the receptors involved, see Ch. 2.) This view is based on several lines of evidence, not least on observations of clinical material. It received strong support when Sjöqvist (1938) introduced his method of *medullary trigeminal tractotomy*. Since the majority of the fibers in the caudal part of the spinal trigeminal tract are thin, and pain sensations were assumed to be mediated by thin and in part unmyelinated fibers, Sjöqvist under-took to transect the spinal tract at the level of the obex in patients suf-fering from major trigeminal neuralgia. Following this operation the patients were usually relieved of their pain attacks, and there was a loss of pain and temperature sensibility in the skin and mucous membranes of the face. The great advantage of this operative procedure, compared with those performed on the nerve or the ganglion, is that corneal sensibility is not abolished. Thus the corneal reflex is not lost following the opera-tion, and the complication of corneal ulceration is avoided. Further experiences (see, for example, Grant and Weinberger, 1941; Olivecrona, 1942; and others) indicated that the section of the spinal tract may be performed at a more caudal level than originally proposed by Sjöqvist, thereby minimizing the risk of complications, such as ataxia (on account of lesions of the restiform body), or unilateral vocal cord palsy (damage to the vagus). This indicated that the very caudal part of the nucleus and its continuation in the dorsal horn at the levels of C_1 and C_2 were the regions receiving the fibers mediating sensations of pain. It soon became clear, however, that following the operation there was usually also some loss of tactile sensation (see, for example, Olivecrona, 1942; Weinberger and Grant, 1942; Falconer, 1949). In view of the large number of primary afferent trigeminal fibers which give off one branch to the main nucleus, another to the spinal nucleus, it would indeed not be strange if the separation of sensory modalities within the nucleus is not as distinct as was formerly believed. This has been confirmed in neuro-physiological studies, where a number of students have found units responding to tactile stimuli (for example bending of hairs or light touch) to be present in the main nucleus as well as in all subdivisions of the spinal nucleus (see Darian-Smith, 1966, for references). Most cells have a restricted receptive field and adapt rapidly, and most of them appear to be modality specific. Less is known of the distribution within the nuclei of impulses arising on painful stimulation, more difficult to study than responses to tactile stimulation. Eisenman, Landgren, and Novin (1963) recorded cells responding to noxious stimuli in the main nucleus and in the rostral part of the spinal nucleus (nucleus oralis). These authors found cells of this type to be more common than did Kruger and Michel (1962b) who stress the many sources of error in studies of this kind. It would appear from these and other investigations that there is no clear segregation within the sensory trigeminal nucleus with regard to areas concerned in the transmission of tactile and pain impulses.[27] However, it seems equally clear from clinical experiences that the caudal part of

[27] It is of interest that in trigeminal neuralgia pain paroxysms are often easily triggered by weak cutaneous stimulation while painful stimuli are far less effective.

the spinal nucleus and the upper cervical segments of the dorsal horn are especially important in the conduction of pain from the face. How this is to be explained is not yet clear, but some findings from various fields of research demonstrate that the functional organization of the trigeminal nuclei is extremely complex, and suggest that the mechanism of pain transmission from the face is not a simple process.

The structural differentiation of the main and spinal trigeminal nuclei cannot yet be finally correlated with physiological observations. It is of interest, however, that the nucleus oralis and interpolaris of the spinal nucleus differ in some respect from the main as well as the caudal nucleus. This is the case for example for the neurons responding to tactile stimuli located in the interpolaris (see Darian-Smith, 1966). Afferent "surround" inhibition has been observed in the trigeminal nuclei following peripheral stimulation. Presynaptic inhibition (see p. 13) appears to play an important role in this and to be quantitatively more important in the rostral part of the nuclear complex than in the nucleus caudalis (Darian-Smith, 1965). Following trigeminal tractotomy some students have observed that temperature sensibility may be less affected than pain perception (Weinberger and Grant, 1942; and others), supporting the classical view that temperature sensibility is related to more rostral levels of the spinal nucleus than pain sensibility (see also Smyth, 1939). Other data, for example with regard to the connections of the various parts of the spinal nucleus (see below), are further indications of a certain functional segregation within the nucleus.

It is evident from the afferent connections of the trigeminal nuclei that their activity may be subject to alterations from several sources. Hernández-Peón and Hagbarth (1955) first demonstrated that stimulation of the sensorimotor cortical regions and the reticular formation may inhibit the central transmission of trigeminal impulses through the nucleus, the former phenomenon being presumably mediated via the corticotrigeminal fibers (see above). Subsequent studies by various authors have brought more information. Both the first and second somatosensory areas are concerned, chiefly their "face regions" (see Darian-Smith, 1966; Dubner, 1967), and inhibitory effects appear to be predominant. At least some of this effect is due to presynaptic inhibition (Darian-Smith, 1965; Stewart, Scibetta, and King, 1967). The situation is thus similar to that in other somatosensory pathways (see Ch. 2), where the transmission of sensory impulses is subject to central control. Since the corticotrigeminal fibers end in all subdivisions of the nuclei, this effect presumably concerns all sensory modalities. Furthermore, units in the main sensory nucleus have been found to respond to acoustic and visual stimuli (see Dubner, 1967). Presumably the latter impulses are mediated via the reticular formation. These polysensory units appear to be present only in the medial parts of the nuclei.

The *mesencephalic trigeminal nucleus* differs in many respects from the two other sensory trigeminal nuclei. Some trigeminal afferents from

419

the mandibular division appear to end in its caudal part (Torvik, 1956b), but their functional role is not clear. There appears to be reliable evidence for concluding that the mesencephalic nucleus is concerned in the mediation of proprioceptive impulses. Thus short latency action potentials have been recorded from it on stretching of the extrinsic ocular muscles (see section *g* of the present chapter) as well as on stretching of the muscles of mastication (Corbin and Harrison, 1940; Cooper, Daniel, and Whitteridge, 1953a). In agreement with these physiological observations the peripheral, largely myelinated (sensory) fibers from the cells of the nucleus can, when degenerating, be followed into the muscular branches of the mandibular nerve (Szentágothai, 1948; and others) and appear to supply the muscle spindles which have been identified in the muscles of mastication (see Cooper, 1960). Since the fibers of the mesencephalic root give off collaterals to the motor trigeminal nucleus (Szentágothai, 1948) a two-neuron reflex arch is formed for proprioceptive impulses from the masticatory muscles, analogous to the condition existing in the spinal cord (afferent fibers from the muscle spindles establishing monosynaptic contact with motoneurons). This appears to be the basis for the *jaw reflex* tested in clinical examinations.

Some of the peripheral mesencephalic fibers, however, appear to run in sensory branches of the trigeminal nerve such as the alveolar nerves (Corbin, 1940) and are assumed to mediate sensations of pressure from the teeth and the peridontium. Action potentials can be led off from these nerves when pressure is applied to the teeth (Pfaffmann, 1939) and also from the mesencephalic nucleus (Jerge, 1963a). It therefore appears likely that these fibers may be concerned in a mechanism which controls the force of the bite. Since the structure of the mesencephalic nucleus is in principle identical along its longitudinal extent, it appears likely that it is an entity also in a functional respect. The termination of some mesencephalic fibers in the cerebellum (see Ch. 5) fits in with the view of its function outlined above.[28]

The ascending connections from the main and spinal trigeminal nuclei have been the subject of much controversy. In studies of human cases the lesions have not been circumscribed, and in experimental studies stereotactic placing of lesions has been done only in recent years. However, the main features appear now to be clarified in animals, and it is reasonable to assume that conditions are, in principle, similar in man.

---

[28] It should be recalled that the mesencephalic trigeminal nucleus is not a nucleus in the proper sense, but rather is to be compared with the sensory ganglia. It is possible, but has not so far been proved, that the impulses which are mediated via the mesencephalic nucleus and reach consciousness, have a relay in the principal sensory trigeminal nucleus.

Using the modified Gudden method (see Ch. 1), Torvik (1957a) could establish in the cat that practically all cells of *the main sensory nucleus* give off ascending fibers passing to the thalamus. A smaller uncrossed component comes from the dorsomedial part of the nucleus; a larger crossed component arises in the ventral part. (The former appears to correspond to the dorsal trigeminal tract described by several authors, see Carpenter, 1957.) This explains much of the difference of opinion among students who earlier studied the ascending degeneration following lesions of the main nucleus.[29] At least some of the fibers, apparently those from the ventral part of the nucleus, after having crossed appear to ascend with the medial lemniscus (Walker, 1939) where they (in the medulla) are located dorsomedially (see Fig. 2-9). The ascending fibers from *the spinal nucleus* have been studied by several authors following lesions in the nucleus, most recently with silver impregnation methods by Carpenter and Hanna (1961) and Stewart and King (1963). While the former authors, who made lesions in the interpolaris and oralis parts of the spinal nucleus, found only contralateral ascending fibers, Stewart and King advocate the presence of bilateral ascending projections following lesions restricted to the nucleus caudalis. Fibers from all subdivisions of the spinal nucleus appear to ascend in close association to those of the medial lemniscus, while some of the crossed and uncrossed fibers of the caudal nucleus ascend in the reticular formation (Stewart and King, 1963). With regard to its ascending projections the nucleus caudalis thus differs from the two other divisions of the spinal nucleus, an observation which like others mentioned above indicates that it represents a functionally distinct part. This is further evident from observations of *the thalamic terminations of the ascending fibers*. Those from the nucleus caudalis (Stewart and King, 1963) appear to end in certain intralaminar nuclei, in the magnocellular part of the medial geniculate body and to a lesser extent in the VPM of the thalamus (see Fig. 2-11), while the fibers from the other parts of the spinal nucleus appear to end in the latter nucleus only (Carpenter and Hanna, 1961). This, according to several studies, is also the main site of termiantion of the ascending fibers from the main sensory nucleus (Walker, 1939; and others). As mentioned in Chapter 2, the terminal region is found medial to the sites of ending of spinothalamic and medial lemniscus fibers in the VPL (see Fig. 2-13). Thus the VPM is the face subdivision of the nucleus ventralis posterior of the thalamus.

Physiological studies largely agree with the anatomical data. The

---

[29] A small cell group, situated dorsomedial to the main nucleus and named the supratrigeminal nucleus has attracted some attention. According to Jerge (1963b) it receives proprioceptive impulses from the jaws.

responses following tactile stimulation of the face are restricted to the VPM (Mountcastle and Henneman, 1952; and others). Axons of cells in the main nucleus, mediating tactile stimuli and having restricted receptive fields have been identified as ending in the VPM (see Darian-Smith, 1966, for particulars and references). There is even a somatotopical pattern within the terminal area, the lower jaw being "represented" most ventrally. In agreement with other data mentioned above it has been concluded that some tactile units in the spinal nucleus project onto the VPM. In more posterior parts of the thalamus (the PO region of Poggio and Mountcastle, 1960) some units responding to tactile stimuli applied to the face have also been found, but these units have quite extensive receptive fields and are less specific, some of them responding to acoustic stimuli. Physiological information on the thalamic sites of ending of fibers concerned in the transmission of nociceptive stimuli from the face appears to be scanty and so far undecisive.

The final links in the ascending pathways for facial sensation are parts of the thalamocortical projections. Units responding to tactile stimuli of the face have been found by several authors in the "face region" of somatosensory areas I and II (see Fig. 2-17) and recently even in a third region, S III (Darian-Smith, Isbister, Mok, and Yokota, 1966). In all three areas most of the units were specific as to mode and place. It thus appears that tactile facial sensation has three cortical regions of representation. The functional relationships of the three regions are not yet clear. However, it appears from physiological studies that they all receive projections from the VPM (see Darian-Smith, 1966), and they all show a somatotopical pattern. Anatomically the projection of VPM onto a subdivision of S I appears to be well established, but concerning the thalamic projections to S II and S III little is known. It appears that the nuclei and fiber systems concerned in the transmission of tactile stimuli to the face are organized in a similar manner as are those mediating corresponding stimuli from the body (see Ch. 2). Thus inhibition, in part presynaptic, can be produced in the VPM on cortical stimulation.

It will appear from the preceding incomplete account of present-day knowledge of the sensory trigeminal nuclei that there are still many open questions. It is obvious, however, that the various subdivisions are functionally dissimilar, even if information on their function is incomplete, particularly as concerns the nuclei interpolaris and oralis. While recent anatomical and physiological data support the notion that the nucleus caudalis is homologous to the dorsalmost laminae of the dorsal horn in the cord, the main nucleus to the dorsal column nuclei, spinal cord homologues of the nucleus oralis and interpolaris have so far not been found. It has been suggested (Torvik, 1956b) that the latter divi-

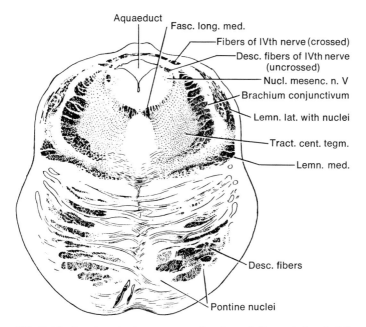

Aquaeduct
Fasc. long. med.
Fibers of IVth nerve (crossed)
Desc. fibers of IVth nerve (uncrossed)
Nucl. mesenc. n. V
Brachium conjunctivum
Lemn. lat. with nuclei
Tract. cent. tegm.
Lemn. med.
Desc. fibers
Pontine nuclei

FIG. 7–18 Drawing of a transverse section through the rostral part of the pons in a 20-day-old infant. Weigert's myelin sheath stain. A large proportion of the fibers from the cerebral peduncle and the pontocerebellar fibers are still unmyelinated and therefore not clearly visible.

sions are concerned particularly in reflex functions mediated via the pons and medulla, in which trigeminal afferents are involved.

Symptomatology. Lesions of the *peripheral branches* of the trigeminal nerve are not very frequently encountered. They may be caused by traumatic injury to the face, by tumors, or by fractures of bones of the face or skull. The infraorbital nerve is frequently damaged in maxillary fractures. Pain is usually absent in such cases, but the ensuing sensory loss in the face and oral and nasal cavities, as a rule, easily permits the determination of the branches affected, the more so as the extent of overlapping between the areas of the three divisions and their separate branches is small. The peripheral distribution is seen in Fig. 7-16, and a detailed description is superfluous.

If the *mandibular nerve* is damaged, e.g. by a skull fracture passing through the foramen ovale, the *motor fibers will usually also be affected,* and there results a homolateral *paresis or paralysis of the masticatory muscles.* The paralysis of the anterior belly of the digastric and the mylohyoid which usually accompany it are of little practical importance, although they may easily be ascertained when looked for. Likewise the eventually concomitant paralysis of the tensor tympani and tensor palati muscles are of little importance. The paralysis of the masticatory muscles is easily recognized. The masseter and temporalis muscles are flaccid, as the paralysis is one affecting the peripheral motor neuron, and their lack of contraction and flaccidity are felt and seen when the patient is asked to bite. After some time the atrophy of these muscles can be seen. If only a partial lesion of the nerve is present, the reduced power on biting can be felt clearly when the closing of the opened mouth is resisted by the examiner. The paralysis of the external pterygoid reveals itself when the patient opens his mouth. This muscle normally pulls the mandible forward on opening the mouth as it is attached to the neck of the mandible and reaches it from the anterior aspect. On this account a *deviation of the jaw to the paralyzed side* will appear, because the paralyzed external pterygoid will not partake in the protrusion of the mandible. The patient will chew on the normal side only. In rare cases the masticatory muscles will be affected on both sides. The lower jaw then droops, but the mouth can be closed with reduced power by means of the facial muscles. Chewing is impossible, and swallowing is difficult.

The lesions of the trigeminal nerve referred to above, affecting peripheral branches of one or more divisions, are usually not accompanied by pain. However, such lesions are far less frequently observed than those where *facial pain* is the outstanding or only complaint of the patient. The facial pain may occur in several forms and may be due to a variety of causes. Some of the more important will be mentioned.

First, on account of its frequency, the typical or *major trigeminal neuralgia* should be remembered. It manifests itself in a characteristic clinical picture. Paroxysms of pain, localized to the peripheral area of one or more of the three divisions of the nerve, and lasting for some seconds only, occur with varying frequency. The pain is severe, even excruciating, commonly described as stabbing, cutting, grinding, or tearing. Between the paroxysms there are no pains. As a rule "trigger zones" are present, most commonly near the eye, the nose, or on the alveolar margins. The slightest stimulus at these points induces a paroxysm. Frequently chewing, swallowing, washing the face, or even the slightest tactile stimulus provokes a paroxysm. Signs of autonomic irritation frequently accompany the paroxysms of pain. Thus lacrimation, conjunctival injection, salivation, or flushing on the painful side of the face is not uncommon. In the typical cases, which occur predominantly in the latter half of life, apart from the pain *no neurological disturbances are present.* There are, for example, no trigeminal areas with altered sensibility.

The etiology of this peculiar and distressing disease is not clear. There appears to be no neuritis of the nerve or the semilunar ganglion. Some authors assume that the symptoms are due to a central process, others believe that changes in the nerve or at its entry into the brain stem are responsible.

On the basis of neurophysiological considerations of observations of 50 patients with trigeminal neuralgia Kugelberg and Lindblom (1959) reached the conclusion that the mechanism responsible for the paroxysmal pain is situated centrally. probably in the brain stem in structures related to the spinal trigeminal nucleus, in support of the view of List and Williams (1957) that the paroxysms are due to a "pathological multineuronal reflex in the trigeminal systems of the brain stem." These views are, however, challenged by Kerr (1963b) who points to certain features in the disease which are difficult to reconcile with the assumption of a central origin, such as the rare occurrence of concomitant neuralgia of the glossopharyngeal or intermediate nerve, the predominant involvement of the third or second divisions, and the age and sex distribution. Kerr draws attention to certain features in the anatomical relation between the semilunar ganglion and the internal carotid artery (Fig. 7-20) and certain changes occurring in this region with age, which he has found in autopsy studies. Carney (1967) reports favorable results of correcting asymmetric protrusion of the jaw, and assumes that traction on the third division in such instances is responsible for trigeminal neuralgia.

In spite of insufficient knowledge of the etiology of trigeminal neuralgia, treatment on an empirical basis has given valuable results. Modern neurosurgery is able to cope with practically all severe cases where medical treatment fails.

The different measures at the surgeon's disposal consist of interruption of the trigeminal pathways, for example, by alcohol injections [30] in the maxillary or mandibular nerves at the foramen rotundum or ovale or into the semilunar ganglion, or by section of the trigeminal nerve between the pons and the ganglion in various technical procedures. The most common method is still the retrogasserian root section introduced by Spiller and Frazier (1901). In most of these cases an ensuing anesthesia of the cornea is a serious danger to the eye of the patient, since keratitis is apt to develop unless special care is taken. In the medullary or trigeminal tractotomy of Sjöqvist this is avoided. Taarnhøj (1952) introduced a method of "decompression" of the ganglion by splitting the dural envelope of the semilunar ganglion, while Shelden et al. (1955) attempted compression of the nerve. It seems a likely assumption that the effect of the latter two procedures depends on destruction of ganglion cells. Experimental support for this view has been produced by Baker and Kerr (1963), who studied the degeneration resulting from compression of the semilunar ganglion in the cat. The trigeminal secondary neurons have been attacked by so-called mesencephalic tractotomy (Walker, 1942b). The latter operation and medullary tractotomy may to a certain extent be regarded as an indirect outcome of anatomical knowledge, as practical applications of theoretical achievements. For an account of trigeminal neuralgia and its treatment see Stookey and Ransohoff (1955).

Pains referred by the patient to one or more of the trigeminal divi-

---

[30] In recent years phenol injections have been recommended (see Jefferson, 1963).

sions may be caused by a variety of diseases in the face. These facial pains are frequently termed *symptomatic trigeminal neuralgia*. This name is misleading since true neuralgic paroxysmal pain is rare in these conditions. Usually there is a more continuous aching that is sometimes intensified as paroxysms. Facial pain of this type may be caused by any process which is apt to irritate the nerve directly. The distribution will commonly, at least in the beginning, be limited to the division or branch involved, but has a tendency to irradiate in the course of time to other divisions.

The mechanism of this phenomenon is not entirely clear. Since fibers from all divisions of the nerve extend to the caudalmost part of the nucleus caudalis and the dorsal horn at C_1 and C_2, irradiation of pain may perhaps be explained in the same way as suggested by Kerr for so-called *atypical facial neuralgia*. Here pain may be felt outside the trigeminal area, including the neck, on the same side. Kerr (1962) points to the convergence of afferents of the trigeminal, intermediate, glossopharyngeal-vagal and spinal nerves in the nucelus caudalis and C_1–C_2 (see Kerr, 1961), and cites clinical evidence in favor of this explanation. Units responding to volleys in both the trigeminal and the first and second dorsal roots have, furthermore, been found in the dorsal horn at C_1 and C_2 in the cat (Kerr and Olafson, 1961). The authors suggest that a similar situation in man may account for a diffuse spread of hemicranial pain.

Of morbid conditions which may be the causal factor of pains in the trigeminal area, *infections of the nasal sinuses* are perhaps the most common. The infra-orbital nerve, and the superior alveolar branches especially, will easily be affected by edema and hyperemia or may even be the seat of real inflammation in sinusitis of the maxillary sinus, as only tiny bone lamellae or even only the mucous membrane cover the nerves.

Other conditions capable of producing trigeminal pain are tumors of the mouth, tongue, nasal sinuses, or in the neck. Dental infections are responsible less frequently than usually assumed. Facial pain of a trigeminal distribution may also be caused by impacted wisdom teeth or diseases of the temporomandibular joint, and likewise diseases of the eye, especially iritis and glaucoma, are sometimes accompanied by pain irradiating in one of the major divisions. These pains are usually assumed to be of the type called "referred pain" (cf. Ch. 11).

Before leaving the topic of trigeminal neuralgia, the occurrence of glossopharyngeal and intermediate nerve neuralgia, referred to previously, should be remembered, as they may be confused with true trigeminal neuralgia. Finally, the so-called *atypical trigeminal neuralgia* should be mentioned. This designation is usually applied to conditions in which facial pain is the outstanding symptom, frequently the only symptom, and where no local affections of the face and skull can be held responsible for the symptom. The etiology is unknown. The main difference from the typical forms is that the pain is more continuous, lasting for hours or even days, but frequently acute exacerbations occur in addition. These paroxysmal pains, as well as the more persistent ones, are usually less clearly confined to one or more divisions of the nerve.

Let us now consider the *intracranial division* of the trigeminal nerve (Fig. 7-19). Apart from its occasional involvement in *diseases of the meninges,* such as arachnoiditis and syphilitic infection, some special instances may be particularly mentioned. *Herpes zoster,* a virus infection, occurs also in the trigeminal ganglion. It manifests itself pathologically as an inflammation of the ganglion with concomitant necrosis of ganglion cells, localized leptomeningitis, and less severe changes within the root and in the gray matter where the root enters. This will result in typical herpetic eruptions, localized to the entire trigeminal area or the area innervated by one of its divisions or an even smaller area. Facial herpes is most commonly seen in the region of the ophthalmic nerve (herpes zoster ophthalmicus) in which case the cornea is also frequently involved. The inflammatory changes, obviously representing a highly abnormal irritation of the ganglion cells and fibers, must be assumed to be the cause of the facial pain which is usually premonitory to the eruption of the vesicles. The appearance of the latter is explained by some as being due to antidromic impulses in the sensory fibers (cf. Ch. 11). Occasionally the inflammation of the motor root or the motor nucleus may cause an accompanying paresis of the masticatory muscles, or in ophthalmic herpes a paralysis or paresis of one of the motor ocular nerves may occur, an indication of the spread of the infection within the gray matter of the cord. When the inflammation recedes, several ganglion cells are as a rule

FIG. 7–19 Diagram of dissection of the cavernous sinus region, displaying the course of the IInd to Vth cranial nerves. In the right half of the diagram the dura is retained, in the left it is removed. (Cf. text.)

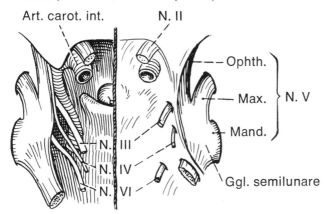

4 2 7

lost and the ensuing scar formation in the ganglion will represent an abnormal irritant to the remaining cells. This explains the occurrence of pains which often last for years after a herpes zoster, frequently of neuralgic type (postherpetic neuralgia) and also the anesthesia of the scars which usually persist in the patches where the eruption has been located. The fibers of the corresponding twigs and branches must be assumed to have been destroyed.

Involvement of the trigeminal nerve may occur in cases of *aneurysms of the internal carotid,* particularly in the so-called infraclinoid carotid aneurysms (Jefferson, 1938). Owing to the intimate relationships of the carotid to the oculomotor, trochlear, and abducens nerves, symptoms from these will usually also be present. The more posteriorly the aneurysm is seated, the greater is the tendency to affect all three divisions of the trigeminal nerve (cf. Fig. 7-20). Apart from the ocular palsies which occur especially in the IIIrd and IVth nerves, trigeminal pain may be an early symptom, usually starting in the first division and hence being located to the forehead and orbit. The first sign of an affection of the first division is often a weakening of the corneal reflex. When the conductive capacity of the fibers is lost, a hypoesthesia or anesthesia will appear.

With increasing growth of the aneurysm, pressure may be exerted on several other structures, e.g. the optic nerve with resulting visual impairment, or the hypothalamic region with autonomic symptoms (see, for example, Nyquist, Refsum, and Torkildsen, 1939). The symptoms referred to above will in some instances develop gradually, while in other cases they become manifest only after rupture of the aneurysm, when this is not immediately fatal. It is a peculiar feature that the facial pains as well as the ocular palsies not infrequently appear intermittently. Probably this must be attributed to changes taking place in the aneurysm. The ensuing symptoms in this case may present themselves as an intermittent painful ocular palsy or "migraine ophthalmoplègique." Following each attack a certain residual paresis is frequent. Ophthalmoplegic migraine may, however, occur in the absence of an obvious structural abnormality (Friedman, Harter, and Merritt, 1962).

FIG. 7–20 *A:* Lateral view of the right internal carotid artery and related nerves in the cavernous sinus. *B:* The alterations seen in cases of aneurysm of the carotid artery (posterior aneurysm of the infraclinoid type). (Cf. text.) From Jefferson (1938).

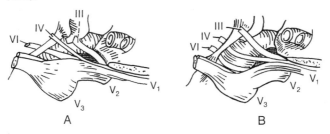

Another condition apt to affect the trigeminal nerve is *inflammation of the pneumatic cells in the apex of the petrous temporal bone,* a not uncommon complication to suppurative otitis. This so-called Gradenigo's syndrome reveals itself as pain in the trigeminal area, usually in the first division, accompanied by a paralysis of the external rectus muscle, due to affection of the abducent nerve. The fact that especially these nerves are apt to suffer will be evident from their close relationship with the apex (cf. Fig. 7-19). Among other possibilities of injury to the intracranial part of the trigeminal may be mentioned *acoustic nerve tumors.* As a rule, however, the trigeminal pain in this instance will first appear late in the course of the disease when the tumor has reached a considerable size.

Lesions of the trigeminal nuclei are met with particularly in two morbid conditions: *syringobulbia* and *vascular disturbances* of the medulla oblongata and pons, particularly of the posterior inferior cerebellar artery. In both instances the lesion will also comprise other structures. The main symptoms due to lesions of the trigeminal nuclei and their secondary tracts will be evident from a knowledge of the anatomical data and have been mentioned in connection with the account of the sensory system. It should, however, be pointed out that on account of imperfect knowledge and the varying distribution and size of the lesions, an exact anatomical diagnosis cannot always be reached in these cases. Lesions of the sensory trigeminal pathways in the thalamus and the cortical area of the face are discussed in Chapter 2.

(g) The Abducent, Trochlear, and Oculomotor Nerves

The three cranial nerves concerned in the innervation of the ocular muscles are conveniently treated collectively on account of their close anatomical and functional relationship.

The nerves and their nuclei.   Morphologically, as well as functionally, there are common features between these three nerves, the VIth, IVth, and IIIrd, usually regarded to be purely efferent. Apart from the parasympathetic division of the oculomotor nucleus, supplying the intrinsic muscles of the eye, the other nuclei belong to the somatic efferent nuclear column (Fig. 7-2) and are composed of rather large polygonal cells like the motoneurons in the cord. Concerning particulars of the three nuclei and the peripheral distribution of their fibers the following data may be noted.

The nucleus of the abducent nerve has already been referred to in connection with the description of the facial. It is situated beneath the floor of the 4th ventricle, covered by the facial fibers, and separated from the median plane by the medial longitudinal fasciculus (Figs. 7-13 and 7-14).

429

The emerging fibers course forward through the pons, pass immediately lateral to the pyramid, and leave the brain stem at the lower border of the pons (Fig. 7-5). The nerve then pierces the dura, traverses the cavernous sinus in its lateral part (Fig. 7-19), enters the orbit through the superior orbital fissure, and ends in the *lateral rectus muscle* of the eyeball, supplying it with motor fibers. In the sinus it is joined by some sympathetic fibers from the carotid plexus.

The nucleus of the trochlear nerve is found in the mesencephalon at the level of the inferior colliculus, a little ventral to the aqueduct (Fig. 7-2) near the midline. Immediately ventral to it is the medial longitudinal fasciculus. The trochlear nerve is the only cranial nerve emerging on the dorsal aspect of the brain stem. Leaving the cells of the nucleus the axons descend somewhat and then cross the median line dorsal to the aqueduct (Fig. 7-18). The nerve emerges slightly above and lateral to the anterior medullary velum, then swings along the upper border of the pons around the cerebral peduncle (Fig. 7-5), and pierces the dura in the anterior attaching fold of the tentorium (Fig. 7-19). After having traversed the cavernous sinus, where it is placed near the lateral wall, it enters the orbit through the superior orbital fissure and innervates the *superior oblique muscle*. It will be seen that the right trochlear nucleus innervates the left superior oblique muscle and vice versa.

The nucleus of the oculomotor nerve, situated at the level of the superior colliculus, is more complex. Like the trochlear nucleus it is situated near the midline, ventral to the aqueduct, and has on its lateral and ventral side the medial longitudinal fasciculus (Fig. 4-4). The axons course ventralward in the mesencephalon in several bundles, which leave the brain stem in the interpeduncular fossa, medial to the cerebral peduncle. The bundles partly penetrate the red nucleus (Fig. 4-4), the most lateral of them even the medial part of the cerebral peduncle. The several bundles then unite to form the oculomotor nerve, which courses forward for a distance before piercing the dura and entering the cavernous sinus. Its superior position here can be seen from Figs. 7-19 and 7-20. Bending then somewhat laterally and downward the nerve enters the orbit in the medial part of the superior orbital fissure. In the orbit a superior ramus supplies the *superior rectus muscle* and the *levator palpebrae superioris,* and an inferior ramus splits into branches to the *inferior rectus,* the *inferior oblique,* and the *medial rectus muscles.* Furthermore branches are given off to the *ciliary ganglion,* where the preganglionic parasympathetic fibers to the pupillary sphincter and the ciliary muscle (cf. below) terminate. In the cavernous sinus the oculomotor and the trochlear nerves are joined by some sympathetic fibers.

4 3 0

Contrary to the abducent and trochlear nerves, the oculomotor is concerned in the innervation of more than one of the extrinsic eye muscles, and furthermore has a contingent of parasympathetic, visceral efferent fibers. Several groups and subgroups have been distinguished (for references see, for example, Pearson, 1944; Warwick, 1953). Broadly speaking the nucleus is made up of a larger *lateral nucleus* situated a little distance from the midline, a *median nucleus,* which is unpaired and extends in front of the lateral, and the *visceral efferent nucleus of Edinger-Westphal* (Fig. 7-2), paired and interposed between the other parts. The latter is composed of small, pyriform cells of the preganglionic autonomic type, whereas the lateral and part of the median nucleus are composed of cells of the somatic motor type as are the nuclei of the abducent and trochlear nerves. In the immediate vicinity of the oculomotor nuclear groups there are several small nuclei, the function of which is incompletely known. One of these is *the interstitial nucleus of Cajal* to which reference was made in the account of the vestibular nerve. It might be expected that definite regions of the somatic efferent part of the oculomotor nucleus should be related to the different extrinsic eye muscles in analogy with the situation, for example, in the facial nucleus.

Several investigators have attacked this problem, but there has been no unanimity of opinion. Two factors may explain this, at least to a certain extent. Firstly, in experimental investigations in animals the different degree of binocular vision in different species may be reflected in the nuclear structure and make comparisons with man difficult. Since one muscle may be active in different movements (cf. below), it might furthermore be surmised that localization in the ocular nuclei will be in terms of movements rather than of muscles as pointed out by Le Gros Clark (1926). The recent studies on the subject, by Szentágothai (1942a) in the cat and Warwick (1953) in the monkey, agree, however, on most points. The former author studied the effects of localized stimulations of small parts of the nucleus, the latter analyzed the retrograde cellular changes which occur after extirpation of the individual extrinsic eye muscles. The cells in the nucleus appear to be arranged in groups according to the muscles they supply. The groups are arranged as columns of cells. When passing from rostrodorsal to ventrocaudal the muscles are represented in the following order: the inferior rectus, the inferior oblique, the medial rectus. The area of the superior rectus is found medial to those of the two former muscles. The levator palpebrae has its representation most dorsocaudally. Human cases showing paresis or paralysis of one extrinsic eye muscle only are rare, and even more rarely have histological studies been made in such cases. Little is known, therefore, concerning a possible localization within the oculomotor nucleus in man (for references see Warwick, 1953). However, it is fair to assume that conditions are in principle as in the monkey, even if some older observations seem to contradict this.

Warwick (1954) has confirmed the general assumption that the small-celled Edinger-Westphal nucleus furnishes the parasympathetic innervation of the eye (pupillary sphincter and ciliary muscle, see also Chapter 11). Part of the median nucleus is often regarded as being concerned in convergence. The justification for this is, however, doubtful (Warwick, 1955).

The efferent fibers from the oculomotor nucleus are partly crossed, partly uncrossed, but exact knowledge of the proportions of crossed and uncrossed fibers from the different parts of the nucleus in man is lacking. In the monkey, according to Warwick (1953), the internal and inferior recti and the inferior oblique are supplied with uncrossed fibers only; the superior rectus receives only crossed fibers, while the levator palpebrae superioris has a bilateral innervation, a point of interest since as a rule both eyelids are lifted simultaneously.

Eye movements. The ocular muscles are brought into play both reflexly and voluntarily. The voluntary innervation takes place through cortical fibers, originating from the cortical eye field (cf. below), passing through the internal capsule and cerebral peduncle. However, most of the movements performed by the eyes are not strictly voluntary. Thus those concerned in fixation, i.e. orientating the ocular axes to a given point, occur reflexly, although the reflex involves the visual cortex. Some of the ocular reflexes will be discussed in some detail below, but before turning to this, the action of the different extrinsic muscles should be mentioned and the question of possible afferent fibers in the ocular nerves should be considered.

It is important to remember that *the action of the particular different extrinsic muscles of the eye is not only mechanically determined by their origin and attachment but that nervous factors are also important. The mechanical features* of the action of the individual eye muscles can be understood in principle when their position relative to the optical axis of the eye is visualized.

The origin of the lateral and medial rectus at the sides of the optic nerve and their insertion onto the lateral and medial aspect of the eyeball, anterior to its equator, make them act practically as a pure abductor and adductor respectively. With the superior and inferior rectus the situation is more complicated, since their longitudinal axes diverge from the optical axis of the eye at rest. Only when the eye is abducted some 25° are these two axes parallel, and consequently the muscles in question will pull the eye purely upward or downward only in this position. With the eye axis directed straight forward, the superior and inferior recti will have an additional effect of adduction. The superior and inferior oblique muscles, with their insertion tendons reaching the eyeball from a medial and anterior direction, will move the eye around its transverse axis when it is adducted, the maximal effect being reached in an adduction of some 50°. In this position the superior oblique has only the effect of lowering the visual axis, whereas the inferior oblique will be a pure elevator. In intermediate positions the superior oblique collaborates with the inferior rectus, the inferior oblique with the superior rectus, the oblique muscles compensating by a component of abduction [31] the adductor tendency of the recti. Thus it is safe to state that in most of the movements of the eye (except in pure lateral and medial movements) an oblique and a rectus muscle collaborate. The components in the action of the individual muscles are represented diagrammatically in Fig. 7-21.

The nervous factors implied in the ocular movements are many, and for details reference must be made to special textbooks. Some principal points only will be mentioned. First, a contraction of one of the eye-muscles is always followed by a relaxation of its antagonist (Sherrington's law of reciprocal innervation). This is clearly seen also in ocular palsies. For example, in a complete pure abducens paralysis, where the paralyzed eye cannot be abducted actively, a slight abduction is nevertheless observed when the gaze is directed to the paralyzed side, due partly to a relaxation of the medial rectus (cf. also later). Secondly, there is always some degree of differential tone of the eye muscles, which tends to keep the axes of the two eyes directed to the same point in space. This compulsory tendency of fusion is temporarily abolished when vision is excluded from one of the eyes. In nearly all normal persons a slight squint then occurs (heterophoria). This is clear evidence that as a rule mechanical factors alone are not sufficient to secure a correct position of the eyeballs. For the same reason a squint is prone to develop when the vision of one eye is so reduced that corresponding visual impressions from both eyes cannot be fused to one image. Heterophoria should be borne in mind as a factor which may make the diagnosis of ocular palsies uncertain in some cases.

Another point which is of a certain practical interest in evaluating changes in ocular movements should also be mentioned. Normally there is a tendency for convergence of the eyeballs with the gaze directed downward, and inversely a tendency of divergence when the gaze is directed upward. There are, however,

[31] The abductor component of the oblique muscles is due to their being inserted behind the equator of the eye.

FIG. 7–21 Starling's diagram of the action of the extrinsic eye muscles.

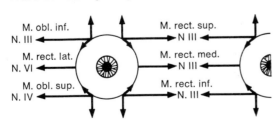

433

other phenomena of a similar nature which occur normally, and which frequently make the exact diagnosis of an ocular muscle palsy a more difficult matter than should perhaps be expected from their rather schematic mechanical arrangement. This will not be discussed further in this text, but it is important not to overlook functional factors when anomalies of ocular movements are to be analyzed.

The extrinsic eye muscles and their innervation present a number of interesting problems related to the capacity of these muscles to produce extremely finely coordinated conjugate movements of the eyes. Several anatomical features are known which cast some light on the basis of this phenomenon. Thus the muscles are amply innervated. In man close to the brain stem the oculomotor nerve has some 24,000 fibers, the trochlear and the abducent nerves about 3,400 and 6,600, respectively (Björkman and Wohlfart, 1936). Furthermore, the muscle fibers are thin and the motor units are small; that is, each nerve cell supplies only a few muscle fibers, probably about 6 (see Whitteridge, 1960). Electromyographic investigations of the human extrinsic eye muscles (Björk and Kugelberg, 1953a, 1953b; see also Teasdall and Sears, 1960) illuminate the finely co-ordinated activity of the extrinsic eye muscles referred to above. They show that there is activity, revealed as motor unit potentials, in the eye muscles in all positions of the eyes, except on maximal contraction of antagonists (for example, in the lateral rectus when the eye bulb is turned maximally inward). On looking straight ahead, all four recti muscles are active, but the activity in the individual muscles varies according to the position of the bulb. Electromyography may be of value in the diagnosis of ocular muscle palsies.

Proprioceptive impulses from the extrinsic ocular muscles. It would appear extremely likely that the eye muscles are endowed with proprioceptors; very elaborate proprioceptive mechanisms appear to be necessary for the performance of the rapid and extremely finely graded eye movements. However, only fairly recently have we got some information on this subject. Daniel (1946), by using very thick sections of silver-stained material, found in human ocular muscles an abundance of spiral nerve endings, which in several turns encircle single muscle fibers. These were assumed to be sensory. In further studies in which the muscles were cut serially, Cooper and Daniel (1949) and Merrillees, Sunderland, and Hayhow (1950) could demonstrate typical muscle spindles in all human extraocular muscles. Impulses from the muscle spindles have further been traced to the mesencephalic trigeminal nucleus.

From 22 to 71 spindles were found in one muscle. The spindles are located only in certain regions, mainly near the proximal ends of the muscles, and have more delicate capsules and thinner intrafusal fibers than those in skeletal muscles. (It is pecular that muscle spindles are not found in the eye muscles of all mammals.) Small motor end plates can be seen at the poles of the spindles (Cooper, Daniel, and Whitteridge, 1955) representing an innervation by γ fibers. In addition to muscle spindles the extraocular muscles of man contain other kinds of nerve endings which are apparently sensory, for example, some which resemble the Golgi tendon organs. Stretch reflexes (see Ch. 3) do not appear to be elicitable in the extraocular muscles, but on stretching the muscles action potentials with short latencies have been recorded from the mesencephalic trigeminal nucleus along its entire length in the goat (Cooper, Daniel and Whitteridge, 1953a; 1953b) and in the cat (Fillenz, 1955; Jerge, 1963a). These potentials apparently are derived from the spindles like those recorded in this nucleus following stretching of the muscles of mastication. (Potentials with longer latencies, having presumably passed one or more synapses, can be recorded from the superior colliculus, the superior cerebellar peduncle and the medial longitudinal fasciculus.) It is not yet definitely settled along which routes the proprioceptive impulses from the ocular muscles reach the brain stem. According to the physiological studies of Cooper, Daniel, and Whitteridge (1951) it appears that some of them may pass in the oculomotor nerve, in agreement with anatomical observations of some efferent fibers from the mesencephalic nucleus in these nerves (Tarkhan, 1934). However, most of the impulses pass from the oculomotor nerve to branches of the trigeminal nerve by way of anastomoses in the orbit or in the cavernous sinus (see Cooper, Daniel, and Whitteridge, 1955). Some fibers from the mesencephalic nucleus can be traced to the nuclei of the extrinsic eye muscles (Pearson, 1949a; and others). It is possible, therefore, that there may exist a two-neuron reflex arc for a stretch reflex in these muscles (neuron of the mesencephalic nucleus—peripheral motor neuron) as for the muscles of mastication. As commented upon by Cooper, Daniel, and Whitteridge (1955), the fact that it has not been possible to demonstrate a stretch reflex experimentally does not exclude the possibility that it may be active under normal conditions and contribute to the control of the eye movements. The γ neurons supplying the extrinsic ocular nucleus remain to be identified, but the efferent innervation of the spindles bears evidence that they are under central control. It appears that proprioceptive impulses from the extrinsic ocular muscles are not, as often assumed, of importance for the "position sense" of the human eye. If the conjunctiva is anesthetized the subject is unable to detect passive movements of the eye if visual clues are excluded (Brindley and Merton, 1960).

There are still many unsolved problems concerning the proprioceptive innervation of the extrinsic ocular muscles.[32] Even if it in many respects resembles that of other striated muscles, certain anatomical and physiological features indicate that there may be important differences, presumably related to particular features in the function of these muscles. The extreme precision occurring in the performance of conjugate movements (simultaneous and differently graded activation of up to 12 muscles) will require an elaborate central control. Several regions of the central nervous system co-operate in this function, but our understanding of how this takes place is far from complete. A large literature and

[32] For a recent study of the stretch receptors in the extrinsic ocular muscles, see Bach-y-Rita and Ito (1966).

much speculation have been devoted to this subject. Some main points will be considered in the following.

The voluntary eye movements and the cortical eye fields.　It has already been mentioned that most of our eye movements are not voluntarily initiated. But some of the reflex ocular movements involve reflex arcs reaching the cerebral cortex, and it is appropriate to consider these reflexes in connection with the cortical eye fields. Reference was made in Chapter 4 to the so-called *frontal eye field,* situated anterior to the precentral face region. It appears to correspond approximately to Brodmann's area 8 (see Fig. 12-2) and appears to play a similar role in the voluntary innervation of the extrinsic eye muscles as does the precentral cortex in the innervation of the other striated muscles of the body. From this region ocular movements have been elicited experimentally in monkeys, apes, and man by a number of investigators. On the whole their findings are in good accord, but in regard to the exact relation of cytoarchitectonic areas to the fields responding with ocular movements on stimulation there has been some difference of opinion. Smith (1944a) reached the conclusion that, in man, eye movements may probably be elicited not only from area 8 but also from portions of areas 6 and 9 (in front of area 8). Studies in monkeys (see Wagman, 1964) are in agreement with this. The threshold to stimulation is lowest in area 8.

The most constantly observed response on electrical stimulation of the frontal eye field is a conjugate deviation of the eyes to the contralateral side. This may be accompanied by a turning of the head in the same direction. However, movements in other directions may be elicited from the frontal eye field as well, for example vertical conjugate movements of the eyes, and occasionally dilatation of the pupils occurs (for a review see Crosby, 1953). The dominant response in all instances, however, is the lateral conjugate deviation of the eyes, a finding which may probably be related to the fact that under normal circumstances lateral movements are functionally most important.

The pathways of the impulses from the frontal eye field to the nuclei of the ocular nerves are not fully known. In Marchi preparations (Levin, 1936) degenerated fibers have been followed in the monkey from this cortical region through the internal capsule and the pes pedunculi. In the former they are found posteriorly in the anterior crus near the genu, in the latter place in the medial part of the peduncle (cf. Figs. 4-2 and 4-8). The frontal corticofugal fibers have so far not been conclusively traced to the motor nuclei of the ocular nerves themselves. It appears that the fibers from the eye fields act on the peripheral motor neurons through an intermediate link. Some authors (see Szentágothai, 1943b) maintain that this is represented by "centers" in the brain stem, to be considered below. Presumably the interstitial nucleus of Cajal in the mesencephalon (see Fig. 7-12) is involved.

Even if the ultimate pathways of the voluntary impulses initiating movements of the eyes are not finally settled there seems to be no doubt that the cerebral cortex, especially the frontal eye field, is essential in initiating voluntary movements of the eyes, as appears indeed from clinical findings, to be considered below.[33] It should, however, be realized that these eye movements, like all other voluntary movements, are influenced by reflex impulses. In the case of the eyes particularly optic and probably also proprioceptive impulses from the eye muscles are important. Furthermore, impulses from the labyrinth, from the neck muscles, and from the occipital cortex play a role.

In man the most important of these reflex connections appear to be the optic reflex arcs involving the occipital lobe. *Movements of the eyes can be elicited on stimulation of the occipital cortex,* from the striate area 17, as well as from areas 18 and 19 (see Fig. 12-2). The resulting movement is essentially a conjugate deviation of both eyes to the contralateral side. (On stimulation of area 17 in man the patient usually has a visual sensation, see Penfield and Jasper, 1954.) However, according to Crosby and Henderson (1948) stimulation of the upper part of the striate area evokes downward movements of the eyes, of the lower part upward movements. This pattern agrees with the "representation" of the retina in the striate area (see Ch. 8). The basis of production of conjugate movements of the eyes must be sought in corticofugal fibers from these areas. At least most of them pass to the superior colliculus and pretectal region (see below).

The occipital motor eye fields are not concerned in the strictly voluntary movements of the eyes. If they are destroyed, the patient is still able to look, for example, to the right when asked to do so, whereas when the frontal eye field (in this case the left one) is damaged this is not possible. On the other hand, reflex movements are not affected in lesions of the frontal eye field. This becomes evident when the patient follows a slowly moving object with his eyes. Then the eyes may deviate to a normal extent to the side to which the patient is unable to direct the gaze on voluntary effort. Before considering these visual reflexes which depend on the integrity of the occipital cortex some more elementary reflexes will be dealt with.

[33] It is of some interest that the thalamic afferents to the frontal eye field are not derived from the VL, which projects, at least mainly, onto the precentral gyrus. They come, at least chiefly, from the so-called paralamellar portion of the MD (see Fig. 2-11), according to Walker (1940b) and Scollo-Lavizzari and Akert (1963). Correspondingly it appears that area 8 projects in part back to the dorsomedial nucleus (Rinvik, 1968c).

Subcortical optic reflexes and reflex arcs.   Vision is the most important of the senses in man. It is therefore not surprising that the ocular reflexes are numerous and functionally important. In order to understand them, and still more the diagnostic value of disturbances of these reflexes, a knowledge of the anatomical substratum, i.e. the reflex arcs, is indispensable. However, on many points there are still gaps in our knowledge.

Reflex ocular movements, as has been mentioned, are initiated from different sources; by visual, vestibular, and acoustic impulses and from the muscles of the neck. The efferent link in the various reflex paths is made up of the efferent neurons from the nuclei of the eye muscles (somatic and visceral), and the *afferent* by fibers in the pathways of the optic, vestibular, acoustic, and ascending spinal fiber tracts. The reflexes may be somewhat arbitrarily subdivided into two groups. One group is concerned in the regulation of the position of the eyes and ensures their appropriate movements, when the position of the object being looked at or of the head are altered. The other is concerned in the finer adjustment of the optic apparatus necessary for visual perception (accommodation and pupillary changes). In many cases, however, reflexes of both types occur simultaneously.

Some of the optic nerve fibers do not follow the course of the majority through the optic tract to the lateral geniculate body, but leave the tract as it enters the latter. These fibers, situated on the medial aspect of the optic tract (and which, probably, mostly have crossed in the chiasma), pass through the superior quadrigeminal brachium to *the superior colliculus* on the same side, but some also cross and reach the contralateral superior colliculus. This is commonly regarded as an important optic reflex center. It has a laminar structure, with alternating cell and fiber layers. The optic fibers are found superficially but bend into deeper layers before ending (see Altman, 1962).

From experimental anatomical studies it is known that a strict localizatory arrangement exists in the projection of the retina on the superior colliculus in several lower vertebrates, as well as in rats (Lashley, 1934), rabbits (Brouwer, Zeeman, and Houwer, 1923; Putnam and Putnam, 1926), and the opossum (Bodian, 1937). In higher mammals the number of optic fibers passing to the superior colliculus becomes progressively reduced and a clear-cut localization has not been established in monkeys (Brouwer and Zeeman, 1926). In the cat the findings in anatomical studies by the Marchi method have not given conclusive results, but Apter (1945) succeeded in demonstrating a localizatory pattern in the retinocollicular projection in this animal by physiological methods. In principle her procedure consisted in recording the action potentials from the superior colliculus when small parts of the retina only were stimulated by flashes of light. The localization mapped out by this method corresponds well with the results of anatomical findings in other animals, and shows that the crossed fibers from the nasal parts of the retina go to the contralateral colliculus, the uncrossed to the homolateral. Thus there is a representation of homonymous visual fields in the contralateral colliculus, similar in principle to the projection on the lateral geniculate body (cf. Chapter 8, where other references to details of the retinocollicular projections may be found). Furthermore, the upper visual field (i.e. the lower retina) is represented nearer to the midline than the lower visual field. The anterior pole of the colliculus is related to the central area of the retina which has a larger projection in the colliculus than the rest of the retina. Largely corresponding results have been obtained by Hoessly (1947) in the cat (see also Laties and Sprague, 1966). Studies of single units have demonstrated similarities in the organization of the superior colliculus and the lateral geniculate body (see Ch. 8), for example the presence of "direction specific" units (see McIlwain and Buser, 1968). The findings mentioned above are of interest in the interpretation of the fixation reflex (see below).

Corticofugal fibers ending in the superior colliculus have been demonstrated by numerous authors (Polyak, 1932; Barris, Ingram, and Ranson, 1935; Mettler, 1935; Szentágothai, 1943b; Crosby and Henderson, 1948; Nauta and Bucher, 1954; Altman, 1962; and others). There is some diversity of opinion among authors concerning details. According to Crosby and Henderson (1948, Marchi studies in the monkey) there is a topical relationship between parts of the cortical visual areas and certain regions of the superior colliculus. In Nauta studies in the cat Altman (1962) could establish the sites of termination more precisely. It appears that corticollicular fibers come from area 17 as well as from the surrounding areas 18 and 19. Other corticofugal fibers end in the reticular formation ventral to the superior colliculus, the so-called *pretectal area*.[34] This is an indistinctly outlined area ventral and slightly rostral to the superior colliculus at the transition between mesencephalon and diencephalon. (In man this area is probably less clearly separated from the colliculus proper, and Kappers, Huber, and Crosby (1936) are inclined to homologize it with the deepest part of the superior colliculus.) In addition to fibers from the cerebral cortex the superior colliculus receives fibers ascending from the spinal cord as well as fibers from stations in the ascending acoustic pathways (see Ch. 9) and other minor contingents of afferents (for references, see Bürgi, 1957; Meikle and Sprague, 1964).

In the reflex functions of the superior colliculus its efferent fiber con-

---

[34] Minor contingents pass to other nuclei in the brain stem, for example the lateral geniculate body, and to the pulvinar (see Altman, 1962).

nections are important. They have different destinations. *The tectospinal tract,* as described previously (Ch. 4) may act on motoneurons in the cervical cord, particularly its upper segments (see Nyberg-Hansen, 1964b) and may be involved in turning of the head in response to visual stimuli. Fibers leaving the tectospinal tract terminate in *the pontine nuclei* (tectopontine fibers), particularly in its dorsolateral part (Bürgi, 1957; Altman and Carpenter, 1961) which projects onto the cerebellum (Brodal and Jansen, 1946). As referred to in Chapter 5 these connections may be involved in the transmission of visual impulses to the cerebellum. Still other descending fibers have been traced to *the reticular formation* (tectorecticular fibers), particularly to the mesencephalic part (see Altman and Carpenter, 1961), including *the pretectal area.* Fibers passing from the superior colliculus directly to the nuclei of the eye muscles have not been convincingly demonstrated, but some have been traced to the vicinity of the interstitial nucleus of Cajal and the nucleus of Darkschewitsch, lying close to the oculomotor nucleus (see Fig. 7-12), most recently by Altman and Carpenter (1961). It has been suggested that these nuclei or the pretectal area are interposed in the reflex arcs via the superior colliculus to the motoneurons of the eye muscles.

It will appear from this incomplete review of the main fiber connections of the superior colliculus that it should be able to mediate a number of reflexes evoked by visual as well as other stimuli. Several experimental studies, performed chiefly in the cat, support this notion. In applying the results of such studies to man some caution is, however, necessary, since the relative development of the various contingents shows considerable changes in phylogenesis. In man the corticocollicular fibers appear to be far better developed than in the cat, while the situation for the retinocollicular projection is the reverse.

In lower vertebrates the superior colliculus, which in these animals receives all fibers from the optic tract, has a highly differentiated structure with several discrete layers. When the cerebral cortex develops in the phylogenetic ascent of animals, the striate area of the cortex eventually becomes the main end station for the visual impulses (via a relay station in the lateral geniculate body). The fibers which terminate in the superior colliculus become gradually reduced in number, coincidentally with a considerable simplification of the structure of the colliculus. Functionally this is reflected in the fact that the superior colliculus in mammals, and particularly in anthropoids, is reduced to a pure reflex center for visual reflexes. The perception of vision previously located to this structure now takes place in the cerebral cortex. A removal of the striate area in higher mammals leads to complete blindness, whereas there is no clear-cut reduction of visual capacity, for example, in the frog after extirpation of the cortex. This is one of many examples of the "migration" of functions to higher levels in the central nervous system, usually referred to as *"corticalization"* or *"encephalization."* It is

440

important to be aware of this fact when experimental physiological results are to be compared with clinical findings in human beings, and it is necessary to be cautious with conclusions concerning analogies.

The mechanism which enables an animal or man to perform precisely co-ordinated conjugate eye movements has been the subject of much experimental and clinical research and has fostered much speculation. The notion that there exist particular *gaze centers* has many proponents. It is commonly held that there is a center for conjugate movements in the horizontal plane in the pontine region in the immediate vicinity of the abducens nucleus, another for vertical movements in the mesencephalon. This view is mainly based on the observation that lesions in these regions result in a *paralysis of gaze:* there is no affection of the peripheral motor neuron, no paralysis of the muscles, but the eyes cannot be directed in a conjugate fashion in a particular direction. Considering that a lesion involving these "centers" will inevitably damage fibers passing to the abducent and oculomotor nuclei, the evidence for such "centers" is far from convincing. Whitteridge concludes in a review (1960, p. 1102): "There are others who consider the suggestion of a pontine center for gaze an unprofitable hypothesis, and it is doubtful if any center for vertical movements need be postulated other than the layers of the superior colliculus."

Following lesions of a superior colliculus in cats, compulsive turning of eyes, head, and body and a neglect of stimuli in the contralateral visual fields have been observed, for example, by Sprague and Meikle (1965). Such findings indicate that the superior colliculus is more than a pure reflex center, but they give little information about its reflex function. However, several authors have recorded conjugate movements of the eyes in different directions following electrical stimulation of various parts of the superior colliculus (see, for example, Hyde and Eliasson, 1957). The presence of a localization within the retinocollicular projection makes it reasonable to presume that this arrangement is concerned in the fixation reflexes, which make it possible to keep the image of the object looked at at the place of best vision in the retina, i.e. the macula in man. The functional significance of this structural organization, which could be inferred from theoretical reasoning, has been demonstrated by Julia Apter in the cat (1946) by applying strychnine to circumscribed small parts of the colliculus.

The strychnine makes the point to which it is applied more sensitive to its incoming retinal impulses than the other regions. When light was flashed into the eye after allowing the strychnine an appropriate time for its effect to appear, it was observed that both eyes moved conjugately to bring the center of the gaze to a definite point in the visual field. By varying the site of the strychninized area

441

the resultant position achieved by the eyes was different. Thus it appears that each small focus of the superior colliculus of the cat is concerned in directing the gaze at a definite point in the visual field and, as the experiments showed, the point which corresponds to the retinal focus projected on the particular part of the colliculus. The map of the superior colliculus worked out on the basis of these experiments is in agreement with the anatomical and physiological findings referred to above.

Whether a similar localization exists in the superior colliculus of man remains unsettled, but even if the reflex function of the colliculus in man is less than in animals, it might well be possible that a similar organization exists in the retinocollicular projection. An observation which conforms with this conception is the fact that in certain cases of lesions of the superior colliculus in man, particularly in pineal tumors, paralysis of gaze in an upward direction is commonly observed, followed frequently in later stages by a paralysis of downward gaze in addition, and eventually also of horizontal gaze.[35] Now the spatial projection of the retina on the superior colliculus and the map of conjugate movements worked out by Apter is such that the foci for upward movements of the eyes are found medially and anteriorly. In the case of a pineal tumor, therefore, these will be apt to be affected first, while later on the lateral anterior part of the colliculus is affected (with the foci for downward gaze). As Julia Apter points out, these conclusions must be regarded as tentative as yet, and it should also be remembered, in addition, that cortifugal fibers are damaged as a rule. Even if in man fixation usually is a cortical reflex, as will be more fully described below, it appears probable for several reasons that the superior colliculus (probably including the pretectal region) is concerned in these reflexes, providing a basic, rather rigidly fixed mechanism, on which the cortical impulses play. For example, the sudden turning of the eyes toward a flash of light is apparently a subcortical reflex, which may well be mediated by the collicular reflex apparatus alone.

Even if there is good evidence that the superior colliculus is a center in reflex arcs mediating conjugate movements in response to visual stimuli (at least in the cat), it is involved in other reflex responses as well, as briefly mentioned above. To what extent the "center" involves the colliculus only or in addition includes other adjacent regions is in part a question of definition of a "center," and is difficult to decide on the basis of available data. As concerns one of the subcortical optic reflexes, the

---

[35] A relevant case has been described by Alpers (1942). Different explanations of the phenomenon are discussed in this paper. In a study of 47 cases of pineal tumor Müller and Wohlfart (1947) found paralysis of upward conjugate movements in 17 cases, in two there was paralysis of upward and downward gaze.

light reflex, there is fairly good evidence that the pretectal area is the important region.

The light reflex, as is well known, consists in constriction of the pupil on illumination of the eye. The efferent link in the reflex arc is represented by visceral efferent fibers in the oculomotor nerve coming from the Edinger-Westphal nuclei. These preganglionic parasympathetic fibers pass to the ciliary ganglion, and from this the postganglionic fibers reach the sphincter of the pupil via the short ciliary nerves (Fig. 11-2). *The afferent link* in the reflex arc is represented by optic nerve fibers which pass via the superior quadrigeminal brachium and the superior colliculus to the pretectal area. The central connections in the reflex arc are not known exactly, but since pupillary constriction occurs on both eyes if light is thrown into one eye (consensual reaction), afferent optic impulses must reach the Edinger-Westphal nucleus of both sides. The afferent fibers cross, in part at least, in the posterior commissure (Magoun and Ranson, 1935; Szentágothai, 1942b). According to Ranson and Magoun (1933) destruction of the superior colliculus does not abolish the light reflex, whereas the reflex disappears when the pretectal area is damaged, and it is probable that axons of cells in this area transmit the impulses to the Edinger-Westphal nucleus (see, for example, Hare, Magoun, and Ranson, 1935). *The reflex center for the light reflex* is, therefore, generally held to be in the pretectal area.

It will be seen that a lesion of the oculomotor nerve or the ciliary ganglion will prevent the impulses from reaching the homolateral pupillary sphincter, i.e. the light reflex will be abolished on the side of the lesion.[36] On the other hand, illumination of the eye on the affected side will elicit pupillary constriction in the other eye (consensual reaction). This is due to the fact that the afferent impulses traveling via the optic nerve are distributed to both sides of the brain stem. On this account a unilaterally absent light reflex due to an optic nerve lesion can be distinguished from one due to lesion of the oculomotor. In the case of an optic nerve lesion illumination of the nonaffected eye causes pupillary constriction in both eyes (direct and consensual reaction to light) but illumination of the affected eye is not followed by pupillary changes in

---

[36] According to Sunderland and Hughes (1946) the majority of the constrictor fibers for the pupil in the proximal part of the oculomotor nerve are found in its upper segment. This has recently been confirmed by Kerr and Hollowell (1964). Based on findings in experimental studies in the dog and the monkey, these authors stress that the oculomotor nerve is the only supratentorial structure which on compression gives rise to pupillary dilatation (mydriasis). Compression of the brain stem results in miosis. These observations may be of diagnostic value. The authors further found that the fibers mediating accommodation run together with the pupillomotor fibers in the third nerve.

443

either eye. If the lesion of the optic nerve is incomplete the reaction may be present, but is reduced in magnitude and rapidity (cf. also Ch. 8, on the diagnostic value of pupillary changes in lesions of the optic tract). Since the efferent fibers from the Edinger-Westphal nucleus appear to be crossed and uncrossed a lesion of only one of these nuclei, which, however, rarely occurs, should not give clear-cut alterations in the light reflex.

The light reflex described above appears to be purely subcortical. However, this does not mean that the size of the pupil is independent of impulses from other sources than the eye. This fact should always be borne in mind when pupillary changes, so frequently met with in neurological patients, are to be evaluated, and it may be appropriate to review briefly some of the main data concerning the factors which influence the size of the pupil.

Everyone is familiar with the current statement in most textbooks, that the size of the pupil is determined by a balance between the sympathetic and parasympathetic system.[37] The pupillary sphincter is innervated by the parasympathetic fibers in the oculomotor nerve, having a relay in the ciliary ganglion, the dilator by sympathetic fibers having their preganglionic perikarya in the upper two thoracic segments of the cord and their postganglionic cells in the superior cervical ganglion, from which the fibers follow the internal carotid (cf. Fig. 11-4). Stimulation of the parasympathetic yields constriction of the pupil, stimulation of the sympathetic results in dilatation. Recent research has brought forward data which tends to complicate this simple scheme to a certain extent, although the anatomical principles of innervation appear to be as assumed. Thus the existence of a true dilator muscle has been questioned. The investigations by Langworthy and Ortega (1943) have shown that the pupillary dilatation following stimulation of the sympathetic is due mainly, and perhaps exclusively, to the constriction of the vessels of the iris which are provided with sympathetic vasoconstrictor nerves. This assumption has also been made by some earlier authors.

Several findings have been made which tend to show that the varying size of the pupil under different circumstances is first and foremost an expression of a varying tonic influence by the parasympathetic fibers of the oculomotor nerve, and that the sympathetic plays a subordinate role in this respect. Thus Kuntz and Richins (1946) as well as other authors have shown that the reflex dilatation of the pupil which follows painful stimuli is not abolished in cats and dogs if the sympathetic impulses to the eye are eliminated, e.g. after section of the cervical sympathetic trunk. This reflex previously was commonly regarded as mediated through the

[37] Although this subject should logically be treated in the chapter on the autonomic system it is considered here for practical reasons. Further reference to the sympathetic-parasympathetic "balance" is made in Chapter 11.

sympathetic fibers to the dilator of the pupil. In view of the recent findings it appears to result from an inhibition of the parasympathetic tone of the sphincter. The same is the case with the pupillary dilatation occurring on stimulation of the frontal eyefields. Pupillary dilatation can still be elicited from the frontal cortex if the cervical sympathetic is removed. The pupillary dilatation on peripheral stimulation appears to be mediated through reflex areas which do not reach above the mesencephalon, since the reaction is not abolished when parts rostral to the oculomotor region are ablated, as shown by Harris, Hodes, and Magoun (1944).

There seems to be agreement that the pupillary dilatation following peripheral, particularly painful, stimulation is first and foremost due to inhibition of the parasympathetic innervation by the oculomotor nerve. The same applies to the dilatation occurring in psychical excitement. However, there is no doubt that active stimulation of the sympathetic is also able to produce a pupillary dilatation, and that, conversely, damage to the sympathetic supply to the eye is followed by reduction of the size of the pupil (cf. also Ch. 11). It is probable that maximal dilatation of the pupil requires both parasympathetic inhibition and sympathetic stimulation, and some findings seem to indicate that conditions are not wholly identical in different animal species. Thus Weinstein and Bender (1941) found that the sympathetic is also concerned in the reflex dilatation following peripheral stimulation in monkeys, but that this is of little importance in the cat. This species difference is of some interest from a clinical point of view, since it has a bearing on the diagnostic value of this reflex in man.

Apart from impulses from the frontal eye fields and the peripheral impulses, both of which may elicit pupillary dilatation, other cortical impulses may produce *pupillary constriction*. This effect is obtained on electrical stimulation of the occipital cortex, and, it appears, most constantly and most easily from area 19 both in man and in animals (Barris, 1936). This area appears to be that sending most corticofugal fibers to the midbrain, and the occurrence of pupillary constriction from stimulation of it is in complete harmony with what is known of the function of the occipital eye fields (areas 17, 18, and 19) known to be concerned in the cortically integrated optic reflexes, among which are those of fixation and accommodation. On account of their practical importance these reflexes will be dealt with in some detail.

Cortical optic reflexes. Fixation. Accommodation. The cortical optic reflexes in man are far more important and elaborate than in any animal and on this account inferences from animal experiments in this field can only be drawn with the utmost care. Mention was made above of the process of encephalization of function in the optic system. This applies not only to the processes of visual perception, but to the optic reflexes as well. Thus the reflex direction of the eye toward an object at-

445

tracting the attention of the animal or man appears in man to be at least predominantly subserved by reflex arcs involving the cerebral cortex, whereas, for example, in cats it appears to be mainly subserved by reflexes having their center in the superior colliculus or tectum of the mesencephalon. In the following we will consider chiefly the *fixation reflex in man*. Most of our information concerning this subject has been obtained from studies of patients suffering from lesions of the central nervous system, and it will be reasonable to postpone the detailed description until the symptomatology is considered. At this place it will be sufficient to draw attention to some of the data revealed by clinical studies. This rather complicated subject may well be approached by making reference to a phenomenon familiar to everyone, namely, the so-called *railway nystagmus*. As is well known, when a person is sitting in a moving train, looking out of the window, his eyes will fix some object in the landscape and keep the image of it in the center of the visual field until it disappears at the border of the window. Then the eyes make a quick movement in the direction in which the train is going and fix another object. It requires a considerable effort to avoid this fixation under these circumstances, a fact which clearly betrays the fact that a tendency to involuntary fixation is present. The same nystagmus may be observed when a person is looking at a series of moving objects. When experimentally induced by making a patient look, for example, at a horizontal revolving screen with alternate light and dark vertical stripes, the phenomenon is referred to as *optokinetic nystagmus*. This may be *subcortical,* mediated, it appears, via the superior colliculi, or *cortical*. The former may be elicited even if the cerebral cortex is destroyed, while the latter is dependent on the integrity of the occipital cortex. It seems to be generally accepted that in man the optokinetic nystagmus is probably purely cortical (see for example, Kornhuber, 1966). This optokinetic nystagmus requires the attention of the individual. It appears that it may be present even if the striate area is destroyed, and there is a hemianopsia (see Ch. 8). The testing of optokinetic nystagmus can often give information of diagnostic value. For particulars the reader is referred to special otological and ophthalmological texts.

The reason for mentioning optokinetic nystagmus at this point is that it so clearly betrays *the strong tendency to fixation* which obtains in normal persons and, furthermore, that this is *reflex in nature*. The fixation aims essentially at maintaining the position of the eyes so that the image of the object looked at is kept on the fovea of both eyes. The fixation reflex displayed in normal persons requires far weaker stimuli than those necessary for eliciting optokinetic nystagmus. The reflex arc involved has its afferent link in the visual pathways, which ultimately reach the striate area. The efferent link must be presumed to be the corticofugal connections to the superior colliculus, pretectal region, and ultimately to the eye muscle nuclei. As concerns the "reflex center" nothing definite can be said except that it must be sought in the occipital lobe and presumably is not limited to the striate area. Under normal circumstances, it is necessary that the optic impulses are consciously perceived if they are to elicit the fixation reflex, and attention and interest for particular objects in the visual field, as is well known, determines which objects will elicit the reflex. It is, for example, brought into action when a person is reading. The importance of the occipital cortex in the fixation reflex is clearly brought out in cases of lesions of this part (cf. below).

In the monkey, conjugate movements elicited on stimulation of the striate area occur in different directions according to the place of the electrode within the area (Walker and Weaver, Jr., 1940; Crosby and Henderson, 1948; and others), and the resulting change in position of the eyes in general conforms with what might be expected if they should serve the purpose of fixation. On the basis of these findings and other data it is tempting to assume that there exists an organization of the occipital cortex as concerns its role in the fixation reflex similar to that present in the superior colliculus. However, the activity of the occipital reflex center apparently is subject to alterations by impulses from the rest of the cortex, presumably the most important being derived from the adjoining areas and being concerned in the role played by the subject's attention and interest.

Evidently the cortical fixation reflex is an extremely precisely working mechanism, which ultimately influences the differential tone and contraction of the external muscles of both eyes. It is a prerequisite for the appropriate perception of the retinal images that the fixation reflex functions satisfactorily since it ensures that the image of the object looked at falls on corresponding parts of the retinae and particularly on the fovea in both eyes. The fixation reflex should, however, not be conceived of as a rigidly organized mechanism, as some of the facts mentioned might suggest. On the contrary, it acts in an extremely finely graded, functionally plastic manner. This is evidenced, *inter alia,* by the fact that normal persons are capable of fusing to a single impression images which are artificially made to fall on noncorresponding parts of the two retinae by placing prisms in front of the eyes. The fixation reflex in this instance will bring the eye axes to the position required to obtain a single image (if the prisms are not too strong), although this means that an entirely unusual innervation of the extrinsic muscles must occur.

The extreme delicacy displayed in the process of fixation is still more astonishing when we consider that fixation is usually maintained even if the head or the head and body are moving. Also in these instances, as is well known, we are able to keep the eyes fixed on an object of interest. To secure this, the cortical fixation reflex is supported by *vestibular reflexes.* These have been discussed in section (d) of this chapter. Impulses from the labyrinth are able to act on the different ocular muscles in an extremely precise manner. The details of these reflex arcs are as yet obscure, but their delicacy will be realized when it is remembered, for example, that the slightest tilting of the head is accompanied by a rotation of the eyeballs around their longitudinal axes (performed by an appropriate interaction between the two oblique and the superior and inferior recti muscles of both eyes). In a similar way *proprioceptive impulses* from the muscles of the neck are concerned in the fixation reflex. These impulses are probably transmitted through the medial lemniscus.

After this account of the fixation reflex, some words must be devoted to another optic reflex which is also dependent on the occipital cortex, namely, the *accommodation reflex*. Accommodation, as will be known, consists in an adaptation of the visual apparatus of the eye for near vision, and is accomplished by an increased curvature of the lens.[38] The smooth muscles of the ciliary body are supplied by the oculomotor nerve by parasympathetic fibers having a relay in the ciliary ganglion. Stimulation of the oculomotor nerve leads to accommodation, i.e. increased curvature of the lens.

Normally accommodation occurs only when a near object is looked at, and thus, if both eyes are utilized, is accompanied by fixation, consisting essentially of converging movements of the eyeballs. Exactly how the accommodation reflex is integrated is not known, but it appears to be established that the reflex involves the occipital cortex. It is a familiar experience that the act of accommodation requires the attention of the individual and the desire to get a clear image of a near object. Although this process in states of fatigue may require some volitional effort, the frontal eye fields appear not to be directly concerned in it. Most probably the efferent link in the reflex path is made up of corticofugal fibers to the pretectal region, from which the appropriate part of the oculomotor nucleus is innervated. The afferent link in the reflex path obviously must be represented by fibers in the optic nerve and geniculocalcarine projection.

It should be remembered that, *under normal circumstances, accommodation is always accompanied by pupillary constriction*.[39] It is reasonable to regard this as a feature favorable to acute visual perception, since the narrowing of the pupil will counteract the chromatic and spherical aberrations of the lens. The assumption that the accommodation and accompanying pupillary constriction are initiated from the occipital cortex

[38] The mechanism appears to be as follows: When the ciliary muscle is made to contract, the pull exerted on the lens by its suspensory ligament (the zonula) will decrease. On account of its elastic properties the lens will then increase its curvature. With advancing age the elasticity of the lens decreases and the power of accommodation is gradually reduced and finally completely lost, usually at an age of about 60.

[39] Although the phenomena of accommodation, pupillary constriction, and convergence normally are closely linked and occur in combination, it has been shown by testing these functions with prisms or lenses in front of the eyes that each of them may occur separately.

is in harmony with the fact mentioned previously, that pupillary constriction may be elicited from the occipital cortex.

Some other reflexes acting upon the eyes have already been mentioned, such as the *vestibular reflexes* and the *proprioceptive reflexes from the neck muscles.* The reflex pupillary dilatation observed on *peripheral stimuli,* particularly of painful nature, has also been described. Other reflexes are of less importance. The turning of the eyes and the head in the direction of a sudden noise clearly is an *acoustic reflex,* mediated probably through the acoustic impulses which reach the superior colliculus (cf. also Ch. 9). The closing of the eyes in response to strong illumination has already been mentioned.

Symptoms following lesions of the abducent, trochlear, and oculomotor nerves.   Among all lesions affecting the oculomotor apparatus including its reflex arcs, those affecting the nerves themselves are by far the most common and practically important. The causes may be of various kinds, a fact which is easily understood in view of the long and partly intracranial course of the nerves.

A lesion occurring acutely and abolishing the conductive capacity of the fibers (with or without anatomical interruption of their continuity) is regularly followed by symptoms which are of the same type regardless of whether the oculomotor, trochlear, or abducent nerve is affected. There occurs *strabismus, diplopia, vertigo,* and an *altered posture of the head.* Diplopia and vertigo usually disappear after some time, even if the paralysis is enduring, because the patient learns to suppress the image of the paralyzed eye. Thus he will no longer be disturbed by dissimilar retinal images, and since probably these are responsible for the vertigo, this will disappear. Diplopia and vertigo occur mainly when the patient is looking in the direction of the action of the paralyzed muscle or muscles. In order to avoid diplopia the patient soon learns to hold the head habitually in a position which does not require the cooperation of the paralyzed muscle for binocular vision. In these paralytic forms of strabismus, the secondary deviation of the eyes is greater than the primary (i.e. the squint is more pronounced when the paralyzed eye is used for fixation than when the sound eye is utilized). This is a differential diagnostic feature which distinguishes these paralyses from cases of concomitant strabismus (developed, for example, on the basis of amblyopia of one eye) where the primary and secondary squint angles are identical.

Some reference should be made to the paralyses of the individual nerves. Since the abducent and trochlear nerves each supply one muscle only, the resultant symptoms are simpler than those following lesions of the oculomotor nerve.

In a pure *abducent nerve palsy* the affected eye cannot be abducted actively. However, when the patient is asked to look to the affected side, some abduction movement of the eye on this side is nevertheless observed, but this is due mainly to relaxation of the internal rectus, which would normally occur under this circumstance, and in addition the two intact oblique muscles have a slight abductor effect (cf. Fig. 7-21). The head is usually turned to the paralyzed side and is kept so habitually in the beginning, as diplopia will be avoided with the head in this position. Abducens paralysis is the ocular palsy most frequently observed and in about 25 per cent of all cases occurs without concomitant signs of injury to the trochlear or oculomotor nerves.

An isolated *paralysis of the trochlear nerve* is not infrequently encountered. The abnormal position of the affected eye will be most conspicuous when the patient is looking downwards and medially with the affected eye, since the superior oblique muscle then should exert its maximal effect as a pure depressor of the visual axis (cf. Fig. 7-21). However, on looking downward in other directions, as well as in abduction and inward rotation, some deviation will occur, since the muscle partakes in these movements (cf. Fig. 7-21). The head is usually kept tilted a little forward and sometimes also rotated to the other side in an attempt to compensate for the lacking action of the superior oblique and thus avoid diplopia.

The symptoms following lesions of the oculomotor nerve are more complex, since it innervates several extrinsic muscles with different actions and in addition supplies the sphincter of the iris and the ciliary muscle with motor fibers. In a *complete IIIrd cranial nerve palsy* there will be a marked ptosis (due to the paralysis of the levator palpebrae). However, the patient usually tries to compensate for this by a contraction of the frontalis muscle (innervated by the facial nerve), visible as wrinkles on his forehead on the affected side. If the lid is elevated passively the eye is found to be in an abducted and somewhat depressed position, due to the combined action of the intact external rectus and superior oblique muscles. The pupil will be found to be larger than on the normal side due to the absence of innervation of the sphincter, and accommodation is abolished. The direct and consensual light reflexes are lost in the affected eye. Usually it appears that the eyeball is protruding somewhat (exophthalmos). This is explained as being due to the lack of retraction by the paralyzed muscles.

Incomplete oculomotor nerve lesions are, however, not infrequently found. They may mark the beginning of a later complete paralysis or remain as incomplete, when the lesion responsible is not of a progressive nature. Their distribution will depend on the parts of the nerve affected, and if due to pathological processes in the orbit may be limited to the superior or inferior branch of the nerve with resulting paralyses of the muscles supplied by them only (cf. above). Such cases are, however, not common. Partial oculomotor palsies are more often observed in cases where the whole nerve has been the subject of damage, but in which, for some cause or other not always clearly understood, some of the fibers only are injured. Most commonly such partial affections reveal themselves as a ptosis, due to paralysis of the levator palpebrae superioris. The ptosis may even be incomplete, or if complete, unaccompanied by other signs of damage to the oculomotor nerve. Two particular types of incomplete oculomotor palsies are the so-called *external* and *internal oculomotor palsies*. In the former the extrinsic muscles to the eye only are paralyzed, while in the latter these are not affected, but there is paralysis of the pupillary sphincter and paralysis of accommodation. These types are, however, more frequently observed in cases where the lesion is nuclear and does not involve the nerve fibers but their nuclei of origin.

By careful examination of the ocular movements, of the pupillary changes, and of accommodation, it will usually be possible to decide which muscles and nerves or parts of nerves are suffering in a particular case. However, this is by no means an easy task in many instances, as has already been pointed out in the description of ocular movements.[40] Apart from the factors mentioned which also come into play normally, the secondary contracture which usually occurs after some time in the antagonists of the paralyzed muscles should be remembered. For details textbooks of ophthalmology should be consulted. Here only some points of particular interest to the neurologist will be mentioned. One of these concerns the *ptosis*. When evaluating the degree of a ptosis the compensatory frontalis contraction should be taken into account. Furthermore, the possibility that the ptosis may be due to a lesion of the sympathetic (cf. Ch. 11) should be remembered. If paralyses of extrinsic eye muscles are not concomitantly present, the condition of the pupil will frequently settle the question. If the ptosis is due to an oculomotor nerve lesion, the pupil will be larger than that of the normal side. In this case the light reflex of the affected eye will also be abolished or weaker than the other (when elicited from both eyes). A ptosis due to a lesion of the sympathetic innervation of the eye leading to a paralysis of the smooth tarsal muscle will be accompanied by a smaller pupil than that in the other eye, and the light reflex will be preserved. This miosis, however, is most clearly seen in the early stages (cf. Ch. 11) and the reduced size of the pupil will make the light reflex less conspicuous than in the intact eye.

Lesions of the abducent, trochlear, and oculomotor nerves in their peripheral course, as is clear from their anatomical features, may be produced by processes of various sites and types. *Orbital disease,* most commonly *tumors* (although these are not very frequent), may damage one or more of the nerves within the orbit. Protrusion of the eyeball is usually present in these cases. More important from the neurologist's point of view are *intracranial disturbances.* The course of the three nerves in the cavernous sinus makes them liable to be damaged in *aneurysms of the internal carotid artery* as described in the section on the trigeminal nerve. The common affection of the abducent nerve in *inflammation of the cells in the apex of the petrous bone* has also been pointed to. It may be added that a *thrombosis of the cavernous sinus* will affect these nerves. The intimate and extensive relations of the nerves to the meninges make them liable to be affected in diseases of these, and ocular palsies are among the most common signs of involvement of cranial nerves in meningeal diseases. In *epidemic meningitis,* as well as in other types of *acute (purulent) meningitis,* ocular palsies are, therefore, com-

---

[40] As referred to previously electromyography may be of diagnostic value in some cases.

mon symptoms. Chronic meningeal diseases are also frequently accompanied by ocular palsies. Particularly common are they in *syphilitic meningitis.* In *tabes dorsalis* a partial oculomotor paresis, betraying itself first and foremost by ptosis and an internal ophthalmoplegia, is one of the most constant symptoms. The pupillary changes, usually present in the form of the so-called Argyll Robertson pupil, will be referred to below.

Apart from these processes and *tuberculous meningitis,* other diseases of the meninges will commonly give symptoms from the ocular nerves. Without going into details as concerns their mode of action, which in most instances is probably by pressure, the following diseases may be mentioned: *subarachnoid hemorrhage, subdural hematoma* (in the latter the changes may give a valuable clue to which side is affected), and *sarcomatosis and other tumor metastases of the meninges.* In this connection should also be mentioned *meningeomas,* which when arising from the tuberculum sellae, the alae parvae of the sphenoid bone, or the olfactory grove, may cause ocular palsies, although usually only late, when other more conspicuous symptoms have been apparent for some time (visual defects, olfactory loss). Other *intracranial tumors* may occasionally also give rise to ocular palsies. Thus tumors of the temporal lobe, if they are situated medially, may affect the nerves, and also neoplasms of the semilunar ganglion will usually soon damage particularly the abducens nerve. In all cases in which extracerebral but intracranial lesions are responsible the ocular palsies are frequently accompanied by other cranial nerve palsies.

The ocular palsies are, however, not always produced by a direct action on the nerves. Thus tumors, particularly in the temporal lobe, or an epidural or an acute subdural or intracerebral hematoma, may press the medial part of the temporal lobe with the uncus through the tentorial notch ("tentorial herniation"). The cerebral peduncle is displaced to the opposite side and caudally and the *oculomotor nerve* is stretched (Sunderland and Bradley, 1953). The oculomotor nerve of the other side may also be affected in this way, but as a rule later. The posterior cerebral artery may also be dislocated and compressed with a resultant infarction of the medial aspect of the occipital lobe.

The diagnostic value of ocular palsies, occurring in intra-cranial tumors, should, however, not be overestimated. This applies particularly to abducens palsy. An abducens palsy is often seen in cases in which the intracranial pressure is increased when the pathological process, particularly a tumor, does not affect the nerve directly. It is often assumed that the paralysis is due to the stretching of the long slender nerve that occurs when the brain is dislocated somewhat. Anatomical studies (Sunderland,

1948) make it probable that it may be due to traction on the nerve exerted by the anterior inferior cerebellar artery which as a rule runs just above it. (Possibly a similar mechanism is responsible for the abducent nerve palsy which occasionally occurs following spinal anesthesia.) Van Allen (1967) presents evidence indicating that the paralysis, which is often transient and recurring, is due in part to ischemia of the brain stem. Of causes of *local damage* to the ocular nerves *cranial fractures* should be mentioned; even *closed head injuries* are not uncommonly accompanied by ocular nerve palsies. These may be due to lesions of the nerves or in other cases to intracerebral lesions of the nuclei and are frequently transitory.

In most of the instances mentioned above a clear-cut local cause is responsible for the paralyses of the ocular nerves. However, it happens that an ocular palsy develops in the course of a few days, and in some days or weeks usually disappears again completely or leaves only traces of the original symptoms. This may occur several times, with intervals of months or years. Even the most thorough examination may fail to reveal any obvious cause of the paralysis which may affect one, or more, rarely several, of the oculomotor nerves. Such cases of *recurring ocular palsies* are usually designated as being "rheumatic" in lack of precise knowledge of their etiology. That the ocular palsies in aneurysms of the internal carotid artery may occur intermittently, under the picture of a *migraine ophthalmoplégique,* has been mentioned in discussing the trigeminal nerve.

Although not dependent on lesions of the peripheral nerves, the pareses of the ocular muscles observed in *myasthenia gravis* should be mentioned, since they are not infrequently misinterpreted. Particularly common is a ptosis, usually one of the initial symptoms in this disease. The diurnal variations, the fatigability of the muscles, the occurrence of other pareses of the same type, and finally the result of the prostigmine test should give the correct diagnosis, if the possibility of this disease is borne in mind. That the abnormal fatigability of the muscles is first revealed in the ocular muscles appears to be due to their being almost constantly innervated when the person is awake, as demonstrated electromyographically (Björk and Kugelberg, 1953b).

Chronic progressive ophthalmoplegia was formerly often assumed to be due to a progressive degeneration of nerve cells in the nuclei of the ocular nerves. However, in recent years several studies have shown that the primary pathological process usually occurs in the muscles and resembles that seen in muscular dystrophies. This appears from anatomical (Kiloh and Nevin, 1951; Nicolaissen and Brodal, 1959; and others) as well as from electromyographic studies (Teasdall and Sears, 1960; Lees and Liversedge, 1962). The intrinsic (smooth) muscles of the eye are not affected, but dystrophic changes have often been found in skeletal muscles.

Symptoms in intracerebral lesions of the oculomotor mechanisms. Apart from lesions of the nuclei of the IIIrd, IVth, and VIth cranial nerves, lesions at other places of the central nervous system may interfere with the proper innervation of the ocular muscles, as will be realized when the widespread connections of these nuclei are recalled. In these instances the symptoms frequently occur bilaterally.

Starting with the *nuclei,* these may be quite selectively affected in rare instances. *Congenital aplasias* or hypoplasias of the nuclei in question may occur and will appear as a congenital paralysis of the respective muscles. Most commonly a *congenital ptosis* is observed. The pupillary reactions are usually not affected.

Inflammatory diseases of the central nervous system may affect also the oculomotor nuclei. Of practical relevance are, in particular, acute poliomyelitis and epidemic (lethargic) encephalitis. The occasional occurrence of isolated cranial nerve palsies in *poliomyelitis* has been referred to previously. The process may be limited to the nuclei of one or more eye muscles. The author has observed a case where only the one abducent nerve was paralyzed. If the general symptoms of the disease are vague or are overlooked, such cases are apt to be misinterpreted. The same may be the case in *epidemic encephalitis,* in which ocular palsies, revealing themselves as ptosis, strabismus, convergence palsies, paralysis of accommodation, or pupillary disturbances, are among the most common symptoms in the acute stages. This is explained by the predilection of the pathological process to attack the gray matter around the aqueduct, and the nature of the process explains that the ocular palsies as a rule are transitory and changing in intensity. Other signs of interference with the oculomotor mechanisms may also be found in this disease, such as involuntary, usually conjugate, movements of the eyes, so-called oculogyric crises. These, however, are scarcely due to lesions of the nuclei themselves, but more probably to interference with supranuclear connections (cf. below).

If the nuclei of the eye muscles are involved in *vascular disturbances* (embolism, thrombosis, or hemorrhage) or *tumors* of the brain stem paralyses or pareses of the appropriate muscles will, of course, occur. Since these lesions as a rule are of a larger extent, there will be other symptoms as well. Thus in a unilateral mesencephalic vascular accident the oculomotor palsy on the side of the lesion will frequently be accompanied by a hemiplegia of the other half of the body including the face, since the pyramidal tract is situated not far from oculomotor nucleus (so-called Weber's syndrome). Other structures in the vicinity (see Fig. 4-4) may also be involved, e.g. the medial lemniscus and the spino-thalamic tract, with a resultant contralateral hemi-anesthesia. Or the red nucleus and the fibers of the brachium conjunctivum may be damaged, producing in addition to the oculomotor palsy, ataxia and other cerebellar symptoms. The different syndromes observed in these and other instances have been designated by the names of those first to describe them, but there is no need to burden the mind with these designations. Occasionally cases have been observed in which partial loss of oculomotor function has been noted, such as isolated loss of convergence and accommodation. Present knowledge in this field is, however, still too scanty to be utilized practically, and in addition such cases are very rare. If the *abducent nucleus* is affected by vascular accidents or tumors there will regularly appear a homolateral facial palsy, since the facial fibers bend around the nucleus (cf. Figs. 7-13 and 7-14).

Lesions of the nuclei of the abducent, trochlear, and oculomotor nerves, or of the nerves themselves, may thus be the cause of ocular palsies. However, ocular movements can be interfered with also by lesions sparing these structures, and it is on this account important not to limit the diagnostic considerations to them, when ocular disturbances are observed. On the whole the symptoms in lesions of the nerves or the nuclei are fairly simple, consisting of more or less widespread and more or less severe paralyses. The *symptoms observed in lesions of other parts of the nervous oculomotor structures* are more complex, more difficult to analyze clinically, and far less fully understood as concerns their mechanism. This is no wonder, since the neuronal connections subserving ocular reflexes, as has been seen, are imperfectly known. *These disturbances are never limited to a single muscle only and practically always affect muscles of both eyes.*[41]

The *nystagmus,* observed in lesions of the vestibular nuclei and tracts, has been considered in section (*d*) of this chapter. It remains to deal particularly with the disturbances of conjugate ocular movements and some pupillary changes which cannot be explained as being due to a pure nerve or nuclear lesion.

It has been mentioned that conjugate movements can be elicited from the frontal eye field and the occipital lobe in man, and when discussing the superior colliculi, it was pointed out that probably this, in man as well as in animals, is concerned in the performance of conjugate movements. *Disturbances of conjugate movements are found, therefore, in lesions of the cerebral cortex (frontal and occipital), in lesions inter-*

[41] Electromyography of ocular muscles may be of some value in these cases (see Reuben and Gonzalez, 1964, for references).

rupting the corticofugal pathways, and in lesions in or near the superior colliculus.

As referred to previously it has been customary to localize "centers" for conjugate vertical and horizontal eye movements in the mesencephalon and pons, respectively. Even if the existence of these "centers" is disputed, it is clinically well known that lesions in the mesencephalon and pons in man regularly are accompanied by disturbance in conjugate ocular movements. The occurrence of paralyses of upward and downward gaze in pineal tumors has been referred to above. Similar phenomena may occur in other lesions in the mesencephalon, for example the *oculogyric crises* seen in some cases of *epidemic encephalitis,* and assumed to be caused by an abnormal irritation of the mesencephalic "centers." These "crises" most frequently reveal themselves in a forcible involuntary upward movement of both eyes, lasting for seconds or minutes. Several hypotheses have been set forth to explain the anatomical connections, the lesion of which will result in such symptoms, but definite evidence in favor of one or another is still lacking.

The pontine gaze "center," assumed to be situated in the vicinity of the abducent nucleus, is assumed to be concerned in conjugate movements to the same side. This assumption rests chiefly on observations of conjugate lateral paralysis of gaze found in pontine lesions. In these cases the eyes cannot be moved conjugately to the side of the lesion. Reflex lateral movements of the eyes are also abolished (when tested, for example, with visual stimuli as in optokinetic nystagmus). As a rule there is a paralysis of the abducent nerve on the same side, but the internal rectus of the other side, which is also concerned in the lateral conjugate deviation, is not paralyzed, as shown, for example, by the preserved capacity of convergence. In addition, a homolateral facial palsy and also a contralateral hemiplegia are frequently present. Some diagnostic value in differentiating between pontine and cortical paralyses of conjugate lateral gaze can be attributed to these accompanying symptoms, as will be described below. In rare cases bilateral paralyses of conjugate gaze occur. These are usually due to midline pontine lesions.

Even if it is unknown which structures have to be injured in the pons in order to elicit the paralysis of lateral gaze, the occurrence of paralysis of lateral conjugate gaze with certain accompanying features (cf. below) points definitely to a lesion in the region of the pons.[42]

[42] Fisher (1967) has recently pointed out that episodic deviation of one or both eyes may occur in transient ischemic attacks associated with cerebrovascular disease in the territory of the basal and vertebral arteries. In the same paper Fisher reports a number of neuro-ophthalmological observations that may be of diagnostic value.

Since conjugate movements, as has been mentioned, can be elicited in man as well as in animals from the frontal eye field and the occipital eye fields, it is to be expected that damage to these cortical regions or to their efferent fiber tracts will be followed by ocular symptoms. This, indeed, is the case. The lateral conjugate deviation of the eyes to the contralateral side which occurs in epileptic seizures originating in these regions is commonly explained as being due to an abnormal *irritation.*

Considering first the *frontal eye field,* a *destructive* lesion of this will be followed by a paralysis of conjugate ocular movements to the contra-lateral side. This has also been observed in animals. In man it is most frequently found in the ordinary vascular accidents which damage the corticofugal fibers in the internal capsule and thus will interrupt the pathway for the voluntary impulses to the eye muscle nuclei. If asked to look to the side opposite the lesion, the patient is unable to do so. The paralysis, however, is not enduring, and if the lesion is a slowly developing one, the symptom may not occur at all. Some sort of com-pensation, presumably from the eye field of the other side, seems to occur. With regard to lateral movements each side of the brain appears usually to be concerned predominantely in the innervations necessary for the eyes to be directed to the opposite side, and when one eye field is destroyed the normal balance is for some time disturbed. At the very onset of a lesion of the type mentioned, it may be seen that the patient's eyes are forcibly directed toward the other side ("the patient looks away from his focus"). This presumably is due to an abnormal stimulation of the damaged fibers, and thus to a certain extent is comparable to the phenomena of ocular deviation seen in epileptic seizures.

Even if voluntary eye movements, particularly in the lateral direc-tion, are completely paralyzed, this does not mean that the eyes cannot be moved in this direction. This is evident from the following fact, which also shows that the eye muscles themselves are not paralyzed. If the pa-tient is asked to look at an object which is placed in front of him, and the object is then slowly moved toward the side to which voluntary move-ments are not possible, the eyes can be seen to follow the object as in a normal person. As maintained, for example, by Holmes (1938) the *fixation reflex* is responsible for this. When the object is moved rapidly or irregularly, the patient is no longer capable of following it, since then the image will be removed from the fovea from which the strongest fixation reflex is elicited. That extrafoveal impulses, however, are also able to elicit the fixation reflex, and to bring the image perceived extra-foveally in the focus, is revealed by the fact that such patients are able to read slowly. It may occasionally also be observed that the fixation re-flex is exaggerated when normal volitional control is lacking, making it difficult for the patient to divert his gaze from the object which he has fixed, and patients may be observed to use several kinds of tricks in order to break the "spasmodic fixation," such as blinking, suddenly turning the head, etc. (Holmes). This phenomenon is a parallel to other conditions in which the loss of voluntary control allows the usually subordinate reflex mechanisms to become exaggerated (cf., for example, pseudobulbar paralysis, p. 409).

The occurrence of paralysis of lateral gaze or loss of conjugate lateral movements of the eyes in pontine lesions was mentioned above. Certain features usually enable a differential diagnosis to be made. In a case in which the paralysis of lateral gaze is due to a lesion in the cortex or the subcortical matter, usually fibers from the "motor" area will also be involved. Thus there will be a hemiplegia on the side opposite the lesion, i.e. on the side to which the patient is unable to look voluntarily, since the corticofugal fibers are damaged before they cross. Particularly common will be a facial palsy contralateral to the side of the lesion, since the facial fibers are found anterior to the fibers to the body in the internal capsule. This facial palsy, then, will be of the central type, with sparing of the supra-orbital facial muscles. In pontine lesions, on the other hand, the facial palsy will be of the peripheral type, involving as a rule all facial muscles, since the peripheral fibers or the nucleus itself is damaged in the pons, and, furthermore, it will be present on the side of the lesion (but also in this case on the side to which the patient is unable to look). An accompanying hemiplegia will be contralateral to the lesion. Finally, the fixation reflex will be preserved in lesions of the frontal eye field, as described above, whereas in pontine lesions the eyes cannot be moved to the contralateral side even when a slowly moving object is fixed. Optokinetic nystagmus is lost in the latter case in the direction of the paralysis but preserved in lesions of the frontal eyefield.

In *pseudobulbar palsy* an impairment of voluntary eye movements may be observed, with well preserved reflex movements. The mechanism of the symptom is the same as that just described, i.e., damage to the corticofugal frontal fibers.

Lesions of the occipital cortex or of the underlying white matter may interrupt the corticofugal pathways concerned in the optic reflexes which are dependent on the occipital cortex (fixation, accommodation, and fusion of the two retinal images). However, in such instances very frequently the optic pathways or the striate, peristriate, or parastriate areas (as concerns symptoms see Ch. 8) will be injured in addition, and since these reflexes are dependent on visual impulses reaching the cortex, they will be lost when the visual pathways or cortical areas are damaged. In rare cases, however, the cortico-mesencephalic fibers may be injured without damage to the afferent link in the reflex arc. Then the lesion is most frequently found in the posterior part of the thalamus or the pulvinar, sparing the lateral geniculate body and the optic radiation (cf. Ch. 8). In the rare cases of this type which have been analyzed, it has been found that the eyes can be voluntarily directed in all directions, but it is not possible for the patient to keep the eyes fixed on any particular object. This is most prominent when the patient is to fix an object on the side opposite the lesion. He also has difficulties in obtaining clear vision if he is moving, e.g. in walking or driving a car. As Holmes (1938) has pointed out, this is not due only to diplopia or failure of fusion of the two images, since the difficulty is still present if one eye is closed. In the extremely rare cases of bilateral lesions of this type the disturbances are still more prominent.

The power of accommodation will also suffer in the latter cases. Even if there are no visual defects, and visual acuity is good, the patient experiences difficulties in obtaining a clear image when accommodation is required. That the capacity of fusing the images of the two retinae may also be reduced is evidenced by the fact that the patients may prefer using one eye only, e.g. in reading.

A comparison between the defects following lesions of the frontal and occipital cortical eye fields and their efferent connections gives clear evidence that neither functions appropriately without the aid of the other. Normally an intimate collaboration exists, and it is reasonable to assume that in those activities of the cortical optic reflex apparatus in which mental factors, such as attention, play a role, other cortical areas are also involved.

Some aspects of pupillary function. Argyll Robertson's sign. The size of the pupil under normal conditions, as has been seen, is dependent on several factors. Ultimately it is influenced by parasympathetic impulses to the pupillary sphincter and to a lesser extent by sympathetic impulses, acting certainly on the vessels of the iris and possibly also on a functionally less important dilator muscle. The pupillary size may be varied by factors which act through these nervous pathways, such as changes in illumination, peripheral sensations, particularly painful ones, emotional factors, and lastly impulses reaching it in the act of accommodation.[43] It has already been mentioned that in accommodation there occurs normally a concomitant pupillary constriction and a convergence of the eye axes. These three phenomena appear to be functionally intimately linked together, a fact of which it is important to be aware, e.g. in the ordinary testing for pupillary reactions. As is well known, a light reflex may be falsely assumed to be present when the patient is tested for this with a small lamp close to his eyes, since he then will be inclined to fix the lamp, i.e. accommodate.

[43] The normal variations in pupillary size according to age should be borne in mind, particularly the normally small pupils in old age and the commonly wide pupils in young adults and children.

4 5 9

In pathological cases of damage to the oculomotor nerve, pupillary reflex constriction to light and accommodation and convergence are usually affected in a corresponding degree. Occasionally, however, a dissociation between these phenomena may be observed. Thus the *post-diphtheritic paralysis of accommodation* is not as a rule followed by a corresponding diminution of the light reflex. The most important of these instances, however, is the symptom complex called *Argyll Robertson's sign,* described in 1869. This is found first and foremost in syphilis of the central nervous system, and particularly in tabes dorsalis, where it is stated to be present in some 90 per cent of the patients or even more, according to the duration of the disease. Its presence is, therefore, rightly taken to indicate the probability of a syphilitic infection of the nervous system, even if the symptom may occur occasionally also in other diseases, such as encephalitis, disseminated sclerosis, syringobulbia, tumors of the pineal body (see Müller and Wohlfart, 1947), the superior colliculus, or the 3rd ventricle, and some other rare conditions. The Argyll Robertson pupil is a small pupil, which does not react to light but reacts well on accommodation. In the nonsyphilitic diseases mentioned the pupil is not always small, and thus is not a true Argyll Robertson pupil. It should also be made clear that a necessary prerequisite for designating the pupillary anomalies mentioned as an Argyll Robertson pupil is that vision in the eye in question must not be too much reduced, since this clearly will impair the light reflex. Sometimes, in otherwise normal persons, a pupil is found which reacts to light only very slowly, but the pupil is usually larger than the other and on accommodation it also contracts slowly. This pseudo-Argyll Robertson pupil may be misinterpreted, particularly if the knee-jerks are absent. The combination of such "myotonic" pupils and absent patellar reflexes is usually designated Adie's syndrome, but is a harmless condition which bears no relation to syphilis (see Adie, 1932).

On account of its considerable clinical importance, the Argyll Robertson pupil has attracted a lively interest among neurologists, but in spite of numerous attempts at explaining the underlying mechanism, this is not yet clearly understood. Some authors have interpreted the pupillary changes as being due to basilar meningeal changes, while others have looked for changes in the central gray matter which might be responsible for the symptom, but none of their hypotheses overcome the difficulty of explaining the unilateral Argyll Robertson pupil. Langworthy and Ortega (1943) emphasize particularly the common occurrence of local changes in the iris in syphilis, consisting, *inter alia,* of an atrophy of the stroma and of the vessels. The Argyll Robertson pupil is frequently irregular in outline, a fact which may be due to the local changes, or to partial damage of the fibers, those supplying one or more sectors of the iris only being affected. The probability of local changes as the cause of the irregularity is brought out by the fact that the pupils remain irregular after death. Langworthy and Ortega regard it as probable that a peripheral injury, perhaps changes in the iris itself, may produce the characteristics of the true Argyll Robertson pupil. This hypothesis contains much valuable data, but it does not satisfactorily explain the preserved reaction on accommodation.

8

The Optic System

THE EXAMINATION of the optic system is of great importance in clinical neurology since the findings allow the neurologist to draw conclusions of value with regard to the localization of a lesion and frequently with regard to its nature. The fact that the optic pathways extend from the eyeball to the posterior pole of the hemisphere explains that lesions in various parts of the brain may be followed by symptoms due to injury of the optic system, and that symptoms of this type are relatively frequent. In order to evaluate the symptoms correctly, a knowledge of the anatomical structures is indispensable.

The pathways of the visual impulses in general and the partial crossing of the optic nerve fibers. The receptor organ for visual impressions, *the retina,* is really an evaginated part of the hemisphere. It develops very early in fetal life as the optic vesicle in open communication with the first cerebral vesicle. This origin is reflected in the structure of the retina, which mainly consists of nerve cells. One layer of these, the *bipolar cells,* send their dendrites outward in the direction of the pigmented layer of the retina (formed by the outer wall of the optic vesicle). The dendrites enter into synaptic connection with the *visual receptors, the rod and cone cells* (cf. Fig. 8-1, below to the left). The axons of the bipolar cells, conducting in a central direction, end in synaptic contact with the *ganglion cells,* and the long axons from these transmit the visual impulses as far as the lateral geniculate body (Fig. 8-1). They pass first in the inner,

462

fibrillar, layer of the retina, then pierce the wall of the eyeball at the papilla (optic disk) and collect to form the optic nerve.[1] After a partial crossing in the optic chiasma the fibers continue in the optic tracts to end ultimately in the *lateral geniculate body,* some also in the superior colliculus and adjacent parts of the brain stem. The latter fibers form the basis of optic reflex tracts and are treated in Chapter 7. The further course of the optic impulses from the lateral geniculate body is by means of the axons of its cells, which collect to form the *optic radiation,* passing through the white matter of the hemisphere to reach the cerebral cortex of the occipital lobe, more precisely the *striate area,* a cytoarchitecturally characteristic region on both sides of the calcarine fissure.

There can be little doubt that vision is the most important of the special senses in man. A morphological expression of this may be seen in the fact that the total amount of fibers in the optic nerve of man (about one million) constitutes as much as 38 per cent of the total number of afferent and efferent nerve fibers of all cranial nerves together (Bruesch and Arey, 1942).

From the point of view of practical neurology it is fortunate that the optic fibers are not intermingled irregularly in their course. On the contrary, a detailed orderly arrangement of the fibers and their cells of origin is characteristic of the optic system. The partial decussation of the optic nerve fibers in the optic chiasma has been known for a long time. The fibers originating from ganglion cells in the nasal half of the retina cross in the chiasma to the tract of the other side, whereas the temporal fibers continue in the homolateral optic tract. As a result, *all visual stimuli which impinge upon homonymous halves of the retinae* (e.g. both right halves) *are ultimately transmitted to the lateral geniculate body on the same side and finally to the homolateral striate area.* All light waves coming, for example, from the left will fall on the right halves of both retinae, namely, the temporal half of the right retina, the nasal of the left (cf. diagram in Fig. 8-1). The fibers from the right eye pass without crossing to the right optic tract, those from the nasal half of the left eye cross to continue in the right optic tract. During their further course the two groups of fibers will both reach the right lateral geniculate body and from this the efferent fibers pass to the right striate area. Consequently, *the right striate area is concerned in the perception of objects situated to the left of the vertical median line in the visual fields.* This condition corresponds to the fact that the right cerebral hemisphere is concerned in the motor and sensory

[1] According to the investigations of Arey and Gore (1942) in the dog, all ganglion cells of the retina appear to send their axons into the optic nerve. The existence of internuncial ganglion cells could not be substantiated.

463

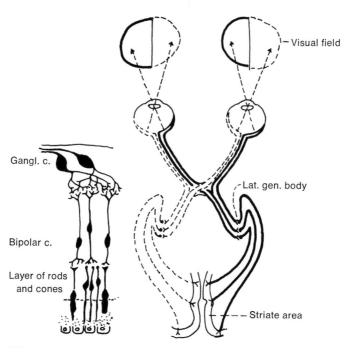

FIG. 8–1 Diagram of the optic pathways, illustrating the partial decussation of the optic fibers in the chiasma. Below to the left, a figure indicating the arrangement of the cells of the retina.

activities of the left half of the body. The significance of this arrangement for symptomatology will be considered below.

Before proceeding it will be appropriate to quote Hubel and Wiesel (1965, p. 229): "To understand vision in physiological terms represents a formidable problem for the biologist. It amounts to learning how the nervous system handles incoming messages so that form, color, movement, and depth can be perceived and interpreted." In recent years considerable advances have been made toward this goal. These studies have revealed an overwhelming complexity in the structural and functional organization of the receptor organ, the retina, as well as of the parts of the central nervous system related to vision. Electron microscopy has clarified a number of structural details in the retina of importance for functional interpretations (see Sjöstrand, 1961, for a review), and physiological studies have given much information on the function of the receptors and the other elements in the retina (for a review see Granit, 1950). However, even if the retina is the starting point for all visual impulses, and its organization, therefore, is fundamental in determining the processes occurring in the central parts of the visual system, the subject is of relatively remote interest for clinical neurology. For this reason it will only be referred to very briefly in the following account, which will deal primarily with the anatomical organization of the visual pathways. Physiological data will be considered chiefly where it can be correlated with anatomical and clinical observations.[2]

Localization within the optic system. The localized arrangement within the optic system goes much farther than to the semidecussation of the fibers in the chiasma. It has been established that *there is a very definite point to point localization of each small part of the retina throughout the entire optic system.* The light impulses which reach the various minute parts of the retina are transmitted through clearly localized paths to the striate area. With a certain simplification it is permissible to say that in the striate area is formed an "image" which is a true copy of the image formed in the retina. On this account Henschen designated the striate area as "the cortical retina."

Henschen (about 1890) was the first to claim the existence of a detailed localization within the optic system. He drew his conclusions from an extensive study of human cases. Since his first papers appeared in a period when most of the leading nuerologists were strongly opposed to the idea of cerebral localization, his views were vigorously championed. Gradually, and particularly since 1920, after experimental investigations of the optic system had been made, his opinion has proved to be correct.

Since the fibers of the optic nerve have their cell bodies in the retina, a destruction of the retina will be followed by a degeneration of the optic nerve fibers from the injured parts of the retina. These degenerating fibers can be traced by the Marchi method, since they are myelinated. By a comparison between the situation of the degenerated fibers when different parts of the retina are destroyed, the pattern of localization can be mapped out. It has been demonstrated that the fibers originating from the different retinal quadrants occupy different parts of the optic nerve and optic tract. In the nerve the situation of the fibers from the four quadrants corresponds approximately to their mutual relations in the retina. Fibers from the upper quadrants are found superiorly, from the lower quadrants inferiorly, whereas the central fibers from the macular region occupy a central position (Brouwer and Zeeman in monkeys, 1926). In the optic chiasma the upper retinal fibers cross dorsally, the lower ventrally. When the partial decussation occurs in the chiasma, crossed and uncrossed fibers are intermingled and there is a certain rearrangement, the fibers

---

[2] Various aspects of the physiology of vision are considered in a report of a symposium in Freiburg, 1960,: "Neurophysiologie und Psychophysik des visuellen Systems," 1961.

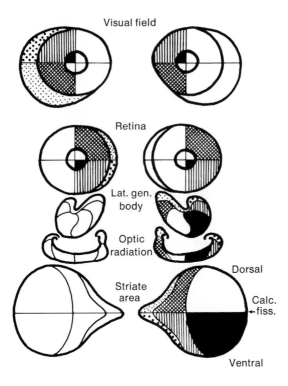

Visual field

Retina

Lat. gen. body

Optic radiation

Dorsal

Striate area

Calc. fiss.

Ventral

FIG. 8–2 Diagram of the projection of the different parts of the retina in the lateral geniculate body, the optic radiation, and the striate area. Redrawn from Polyak (1932).

assuming an arrangement corresponding to their relative end stations in the lateral geniculate body. Therefore in the optic tract the crossed and uncrossed fibers from the homonymous halves of the central, macular regions of the retinae are found to occupy a large area of the cross section dorsolaterally, those from the lower retinal quadrants are found laterally, and those from the upper retinal quadrants are found medially. The same pattern is present in the lateral geniculate body, as will be seen from Fig. 8-2. *The macular fibers end in an extensive area, centrally and posteriorly, in the lateral geniculate body; the fibers from the peripheral parts of the retina terminate more anteriorly,* and, furthermore, the fibers from the upper quadrants end medially, while those from the lower quadrants end laterally.[3] Within the macular area the same distinction between fibers from lower and upper parts of the macula can be found.

[3] For a study of the macular projection in the lateral geniculate body of man, see Kupfer (1962).

466

A more detailed mapping out of the retinogeniculate projection has not been possible by the Marchi method. Experiments by other methods have shown that the localization is virtually very distinct. Thus Le Gros Clark and Penman (1934) succeeded in demonstrating this very clearly in monkeys by means of the transneuronal degeneration method described in Chapter 1. When the ganglion cells of the retina are damaged, the cells of the lateral geniculate body to which their axons are distributed degenerate. Fig. 1-15 demonstrates the circumscribed changes in the lateral geniculate body of a monkey following a lesion of a restricted part of the retina. The sharp boundaries of the changes give evidence that the localization must be very accurate. Another feature, which is seen in the photograph and should also be drawn attention to, is the fact that the cellular degeneration affects only three of the six layers which compose the lateral geniculate body (in monkeys and man). The explanation of this peculiar fact is that the intact areas of the layers between the changed ones are the terminal areas for fibers from corresponding parts of the intact retina, i.e. from the region of the retina which corresponds to the damaged area in the operated eye. If one eye is extirpated, the cells will disappear in one set (three out of the six present) of cellular layers in the homolateral lateral geniculate body, but in the other set in the contralateral body, namely, the layers which are intact on the side of the lesion. In other words, *the crossed and uncrossed retinal fibers end in alternating layers of the lateral geniculate body, but in such a manner that fibers from corresponding parts of the two retinae end in neighboring parts of the different layers* (see Fig. 8-3). The very precise retinotopical projection onto the lateral geniculate nucleus and the distribution of the crossed and uncrossed optic fibers to alternating layers of the lateral geniculate body have also been verified by studies with silver impregnation methods after section of the optic nerve in monkeys (Glees and Le Gros Clark, 1941) and after lesions of the retina in the cat (Hayhow, 1958; Laties and Sprague, 1966; Stone and Hansen, 1966; Garey and Powell, 1968). When the fibers enter the lateral geniculate body, crossed and uncrossed fibers are, however, not yet segregated.

A localization of the same sharpness as in the retinogeniculate projection is also present in the next link of the system, the projection of the lateral geniculate body on the striate area. This projection has been mapped out in detail in animal experiments. If a small lesion is made in the striate area of a monkey and the animal is killed some weeks later, the cells in the homolateral lateral geniculate body which send their fibers to the damaged part will be affected by retrograde degeneration. Figure 8-4 is a photograph from the lateral geniculate body of a monkey in which three small lesions had previously been made in the striate area (Polyak,

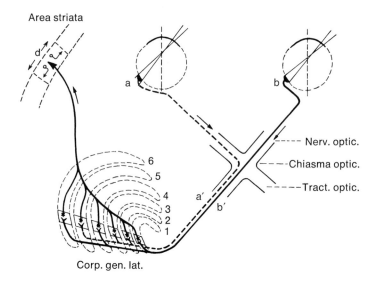

Area striata

Corp. gen. lat.

FIG. 8–3 Diagram to explain the anatomical basis for the impulse propagation from corresponding parts of the two retinae to the same region in the striate area. (See text.) Redrawn from Le Gros Clark (1941a).

1933). Corresponding to the lesions, three small patches of cell loss are found in the lateral geniculate body. On the basis of investigations of this kind the organization of the geniculocortical projection has been determined as it is represented diagrammatically in Fig. 8-2.

In the diagram the projection of the retina on the lateral geniculate body is seen as described above. In the further course the localization is maintained, and it will be seen that *the upper retinal quadrants are represented in the striate area superior or dorsal to the calcarine fissure, the lower quadrants below or ventral to the fissure.* This principle applies to the peripheral parts of the retina as well as to the central, macular region. It will also be seen that *the macular representation comprises a large posterior part of the striate area,* and this area is relatively much larger in proportion to the entire striate area than is the macular region in proportion to the whole retina. Thus *the macula must be more amply represented in the striate area than the peripheral parts of the retina,* a finding in complete harmony with the fact that the macula is the part of the retina in which the visual acuity is highest and in which the sensory cells are most densely packed. Anterior to the macular area the homonymous peripheral retinal quadrants are represented, the upper above, the lower below the calcarine fissure. The extreme anterior part of the striate area is occupied by the representation of the most peripheral nasal parts of the retina, which correspond to the extreme temporal crescent of the visual field where vision is monocular. In man conditions appear to be principally identical with those studied so closely in monkeys. A knowledge of this pattern of localization is of practical value when the visual field defects in lesions of the striate area are to be interpreted, as will be described below.

If the minute localization described above is to have any functional meaning, it must be presupposed that a similar clear-cut localization must be present in the first link of the optic pathways, the conduction within the retina itself from the rod and cone cells via the bipolar to the ganglion cells. This has indeed been demonstrated to be the case. In painstaking investigations of normal preparations from the retina of monkey and man, Polyak (1936 and 1941) has found that each bipolar cell of the retina is in synaptic connection with only a few rods and cones, in the macular region even to some extent only with a single cone cell. The axons of the bipolar cells are similarly not distributed to large numbers of ganglion cells, but only a few; in the macular region partly to only one or two ganglion cells. Owing to this arrangement, the possibility exists that impulses can be conveyed in a central direction by separate paths from a very small number of sensory cells (cones).[4]

The lateral geniculate body. In the simplified presentation given above, the lateral geniculate body has been treated as if it were a pure relay station in the transmission of impulses from the retina to the striate area. Its main task would be to make possible a fusion of the impulses from corresponding parts of the two retinae (see Fig. 8-3). Fibers from

---

[4] However, the cone cells in the fovea which exhibit a one to one relationship to bipolar and ganglion cells are also in synaptic relation to other types of bipolars. The studies of Polyak, collected and commented upon in his monographs (1941 and 1957), have elucidated the immensely complex structure of the primate retina. Concerning details his monographs should be consulted.

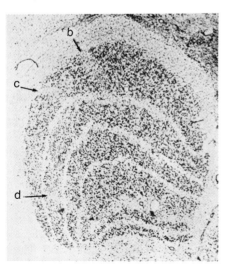

FIG. 8–4 Photograph from a section through the lateral geniculate body of a monkey. In the three small areas, labeled *b*, *c*, and *d*, the cells have disappeared because of three small lesions which were placed in the striate area some weeks before death. From Polyak (1933).

corresponding points (*a* and *b* in Fig. 8-3) of each of the two retinae end in small areas within three of the six laminae of the lateral geniculate body. The patches supplied from corresponding points of both retinae are arranged in a regular manner, representing together approximately a column extending through all layers of the lateral geniculate body. Cells in all six laminae within this column project onto the same small area (*d*) of the striate area, as recently confirmed in the rabbit, by Rose and Malis (1965b). Impulses from corresponding points of the two retinae will therefore meet only when they reach the striate area. This has been confirmed in physiological studies, since in the striate area a majority of the cells respond to stimuli of both eyes (see below), while such cells are only very rarely found in the lateral geniculate body (Erulkar and Fillenz, 1960; Hubel and Wiesel, 1961; and others).

However, it appears from recent research that the lateral geniculate body is more than a pure relay station, and its projection onto the cortex is not as simple as presented above. Although some of the new data concerning this subject is as yet scarcely of practical diagnostic value, some of it deserves mentioning.

As referred to above, in man and monkeys six layers of cells, separated by fibers, can be distinguished in the main dorsal part of the lateral geniculate body (Figs. 8-3 and 8-4). They are usually numbered 1 to 6, beginning ventrally. Layers 1 and 2 are composed of large cells, the others of smaller ones. In the peripheral part (corresponding to the termination of fibers from the periphery of the retina, where rods only are present) some of the layers (3 and 5, 4 and 6) fuse (not shown in Fig. 8-3) so that there are only four laminae, and here the proportion of large to small cells is much greater than in the central regions. It has been suggested that this is related to the absence of color vision in the periphery of the retina (Chacko, 1948), and single unit responses have shown that the large cells of the lateral geniculate body react to a wide spectrum of light stimuli.

The total number of cells in the human lateral geniculate body has been estimated to be about 1 million (Sullivan et al., 1958; Kupfer, Chumbley, and Downer, 1967), a figure whilch corresponds approximately to the number of fibers in the human optic nerve. This gives a 1:1 ratio of afferent optic fibers and cells in the lateral geniculate body, but does not mean that one fiber establishes contact with one cell only. Glees and Le Gros Clark (1941) concluded from an experimental study in the monkey that a single optic nerve fiber establishes contact with only five or six geniculate cells and that the boutons end on the somata. Authors working with the Golgi method (O'Leary, 1940; Bishop, 1953) have likewise found the terminal arborizations of single optic nerve fibers (in the cat) to be very restricted.[5] The dendrites of the geniculate neurons are largely distributed only within their particular lamina (see, however, Guillery, 1966). However, it is obvious from Golgi preparations that not all cells of the lateral geniculate nucleus give off axons to the optic radiation. A fair number are short-axoned cells of the Golgi II type and distribute their axon within their own lamina (O'Leary, 1940; Bishop, 1953; and others).

The *synaptic organization* of the lateral geniculate body appears to be rather complex. Optic nerve fibers end on Golgi II cells as well as on the projecting neurons. Furthermore, there are glomerular synaptic formations, centered around the terminals of optic nerve fibers and resembling the cerebellar glomeruli (cf. Fig. 1-5 G). Other axonal endings in these glomeruli appear to belong to the Golgi II cells, referred to above, and still others to afferents from the occipital cortex (while others of the latter type end on dendrites). Axo-axonic synapses have been observed. The above data is among that reported by authors who have studied the subject with Golgi and electron microscopic methods (in normal and experimental material) (Colonnier and Guillery, 1964, monkey; Peters and Palay, 1966, cat; Szentágothai, Hámori, and Tömböl, 1966, cat; McMahan, 1967, rat). In the main points the results are concordant.

Physiological studies likewise bear witness to the complex organization of the lateral geniculate body. Thus its activity can be influenced from the occipital cortex which presumably may exert a central control of the transmission of optic impulses.[6] Interaction of corticofugal and retinal impulses has been demonstrated in the lateral geniculate body (Hubel and Wiesel, 1961; Widén and Ajmone Marsan, 1961; and others), and stimulation of the reticular formation has been claimed to influence it. Presynaptic cortical inhibition has been reported to occur. It is still not possible to obtain a completely satisfactory correlation between the detailed neurophysiological and neuroanatomical data concerning the organization of the lateral geniculate body. (For a discussion of some points see Szentágothai, Hámori, and Tömböl, 1966). Both kinds of research demonstrate, however, that the lateral geniculate body is far

[5] The lateral geniculate body of the monkey is rather similar to the human. However, the cat's lateral geniculate body differs in several respects from these. It has only three distinct layers. Nevertheless, the main principles of organization appear to be as in monkey and man (see Meikle and Sprague,1964, for an account of the visual pathways in cats).

[6] A central influence on the transmission of impulses from the retina to the brain has been physiologically demonstrated (Granit, 1955b; Dodt, 1956) and is assumed to occur via efferent fibers in the optic nerve. Such fibers and their origin have been conclusively demonstrated in birds (Cowan and Powell, 1963). In electron microscopic studies degeneration of terminal boutons has been found in the retina of the cat and monkey following lesions of the optic tract or nerve (Brooke, Downer, and Powell, 1965).

4 7 1

from being a simple relay station in the visual pathways. Some other recent data on the lateral geniculate body will be considered in the account of the striate area.

The optic radiation. The optic radiation, consisting of the axons of the cells of the lateral geniculate body and ending in the striate area, takes a peculiar course in man, important to the neurologist. After leaving the lateral geniculate body, the fibers pass for a short distance laterally, and to some extent anteriorly, in the most posterior part of the internal capsule, the so-called pars retrolenticularis. In this way the fibers come to occupy a position anterior to the lateral ventricle. Some of them are found anterior to the transition between the temporal horn and the central part (cella media) of the ventricle, while others, the lower fibers of the bundle, are situated anterior to the anterior and upper limit of the temporal horn (see Fig. 8-5). In their further course the fibers are found on the lateral surface of the temporal and occipital horns of the lateral ventricle to finally reach the striate area. In this part of their course they are found immediately beneath the lateral wall of the ventricle, in the so-called external sagittal stratum (Pfeifer, 1925, myelogenetic studies). The original view, that the optic radiation fibers took a straight course to the striate area, has been disproved, by anatomical as well as by clinico-pathological findings. The clinical importance of the complicated course of the optic radiation will be discussed below. It is of interest for the interpretation of the symptoms in lesions of the occipital and temporal lobes.

FIG. 8–5 Diagrammatic representation of the course of the fibers of the optic radiation. The geniculocalcarine fibers are seen to swing from the geniculate body (not visible) around the lateral ventricle to reach the striate area. From Sanford and Bair (1939) after Cushing (1922).

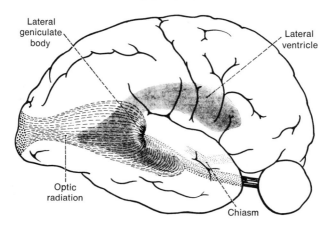

The fibers in the optic radiation are arranged in a localized manner.
The fibers ending in the upper part of the striate area, for example, are
found in the upper part of the optic radiation; the macular fibers from the
central part of the lateral geniculate body occupy the largest central part
of the radiation. Even if there appears to be some degree of intermingling
of fibers from different parts of the geniculate body in the radiation, the
principle of localization appears to be valid. This is learned from anatomical studies (see Polyak, 1957) and confirmed in clinical observations (see especially Spalding, 1952a). Localized lesions of the optic
radiation may result in well-delimited homonymous visual field defects
(scotomas) as will be discussed below.

The striate area. The striate area, receiving the fibers of the optic
radiation, is in man found almost entirely on the medial surface of the
occipital lobe (see Figs. 10-3, and 12-2). In lower mammals it is located
more or less exclusively on the convexity of the cortex, and in monkeys
a certain part, mainly the macular area, is still on the lateral surface. The
area striata has got its name on account of a light strip visible even in
fresh preparations of this part of the cortex. This line of Gennari or Vicq
d'Azyr consists of a layer of myelinated fibers, which appear whitish
within the gray cortex. In myelin sheath preparations it can easily be
recognized as a dark line in the cortex (Fig. 8-6). It is limited to the
striate area. In regard to cytoarchitecture the striate area is also characteristic (Fig. 8-7c). The inner and outer granular layers (cf. Ch. 12) are
well developed. The inner granular layer, IV, is particularly thick, and
can be subdivided into sublayers, IV*a, b,* and *c.* Layer IV*b* corresponds
to the line of Gennari and in Nissl preparations appears poor in cells. The
third cortical layer, the pyramidal layer, also contains predominantly
granular cells. A Vth layer cannot be clearly identified. The ample occurrence of granule cells and the high degree of development of the granular
cortex so characteristic of the striate area is found to a lesser extent also
in other cortical areas mainly subserving receptory functions (cf. Ch. 12).

The fibers of the optic radiation terminate predominantly in relation
to the cells of the granular layers. As described above (see also Fig. 8-3),
it is only in the striate area that the impulses originating from corresponding parts of the two retinae meet.

Surrounding the striate area (area 17 after Brodmann) two other
cortical areas are found which bear some relation to the visual functions
of the brain. Brodmann's area 18 (area parastriata) immediately surrounds the striate area (cf. Fig. 12-2) and is sharply delimited from it.
It contains abundant granular cells, but in addition some pyramidal cells
are present, mainly in the IIIrd and Vth layers. Area 19 (area peristriata)
has a structure somewhat similar to that of area 18, and surrounds it just

473

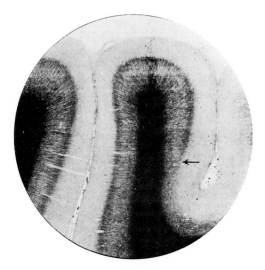

FIG. 8–6 A photograph of a myelin-stained section through the striate area of man. The abrupt transition from the striate area (area 17) with the line of Gennari to the surrounding area 18 is clearly seen (arrow).

as area 18 surrounds area 17. The peristriate area, however, has a larger size than the parastriate, and occupies a considerable portion of the convexity of the occipital lobe.

When the cortex of the occipital lobe is electrically stimulated in conscious human beings, subjective optic sensations are usually elicited. They differ somewhat according to the area stimulated. When the striate area is stimulated simple optic "hallucinations" are usually produced; the patient says that he sees sparks and flashes of light, sometimes in the form of the flicker scotomas occurring in migraine. These visual impressions are commonly observed to arise from different parts of the visual field, according to which part of the striate area is stimulated, and the localization corresponds with the known projection of the visual fields on the striate area. Stimulation of the anterior parts of the area, on which the peripheral parts of the retina are projected, gives rise to "hallucinations" which start in the periphery of the visual field and usually move toward the center, imitating thus a common type of visual prodromata in migraine. They start from the left side when the right striate area is stimulated and vice versa, and from the lower part of the visual field if the superior (supracalcarine) portion of the striate area is the site of stimulation. When the macular region, the posterior part of the striate area, is stimulated, the visual sensations are referred to the center of the visual field (Foerster, 1929).

4 7 4

The Optic System

The visual sensations following stimulation of the area 18, and particularly area 19, were by Foerster (1929) reported to be more complex, although simple visual sensations are not uncommon. The patient may inform the investigator that he sees animals, men, figures, or objects of various kinds. According to Penfield and Jasper (1954) simple visual sensations are the rule. (The designation of these optic sensations as hallucinations is unfortunate, since the patient as a rule is fully aware that the things he sees are not really existing.) From the visual areas movements of the eyes are elicited on electrical stimulation, as has been discussed in the preceding chapter.

From the available anatomical and physiological data, as well as from the findings in clinical cases, to be treated later, it must be concluded that

FIG. 8–7 Photomicrographs from three different cortical areas of the human brain (Nissl stain). The various layers are indicated, the figures in parentheses indicating that the corresponding layer cannot be clearly identified. (x 134). (a) From the area 4. A Betz cell is visible in layer V, and layers II and IV are indistinct. (b) Area 3. The granular layers (II and IV) are well developed. (c) Striate area, 17. Typical granular cortex. Layer IV subdivided by the line of Gennari at the level of IVb. Since the sections are not quite pependicular to the surface, the relative thickness of the cortex of the three areas cannot be judged from the photographs. Note columnar arrangement of cells.

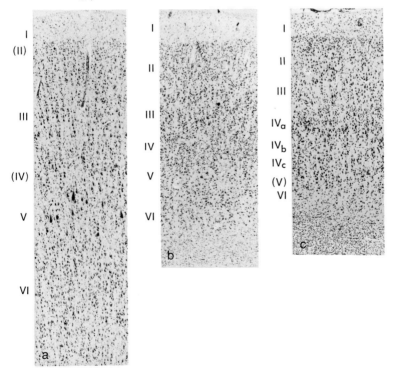

the striate area 17 is the primary visual cortex, to which the visual impressions are relayed (cf. the "cortical retina" of Henschen). The two other areas, particularly area 19, appear to be essential for the interpretation of the visual impressions and their integration with other sensory impressions. Furthermore, the visual areas are concerned in cortical optic reflexes, which are of supreme importance for normal visual function in securing the fixation of the object to which interest is attached. The symptoms following lesions of the occipital cortex have given evidence in accord with the views mentioned, as will be seen below. Information obtained in meticulous studies in animals in recent years is on the whole compatible with clinical observations and has considerably enhanced our understanding of the visual functions of the brain. Particularly illuminating have been the studies of Hubel and Wiesel. Most of this experimental work has been done in the cat. Even if the striate area and the lateral geniculate body in the cat differ in some respects from those of monkey and man it appears that the results are valid also for these species.

In studies with the Golgi method, Sholl (1955, 1956) has brought forward some quantitative data of interest. The fibers from the lateral geniculate body, which make up the majority of afferents to the striate area, branch extensively (see also O'Leary, 1941), and each fiber may directly influence about 5,000 neurons. These fibers end chiefly in the middle layers of the cortex, rich in granular (stellate) cells. It is further of interest that a considerable number of axons of cells in the deeper layers give off recurrent collaterals which may act on more superficially situated cells. It appears from this and other data that the organization of cells in columns in the cortex may be of functional relevance. Support for this view has been provided by Rose and Malis (1965a), since only following cortical lesions involving all layers of the striate area is there a complete cellular degeneration in the corresponding area of the lateral geniculate body (cf. Fig. 8-4).

In a series of extensive and carefully controlled experiments Hubel and Wiesel have studied the responses of neurons in the cat's visual cortex following the application of light stimuli to the retina. A unit in the visual cortex is characterized on the basis of its *receptive field,* defined as the region of the retina (or visual field) over which one can influence the firing of the cell. It turned out that in contrast to the lateral geniculate body, where there are two types of cells, the visual cortex contains a large number of functionally different cell types. One type is called "simple," the others are "complex."

The responses of the cortical units were recorded with microelectrodes in anesthetized cats following exposure of the retina to white light stimuli of different shapes, such as stripes of light, edges between dark and light fields etc., stationary or moving. In the lateral geniculate body the receptive fields are approximately circular, having a center which excites the cell (on-response) and a periphery which inhibits it (off-response), or vice versa. The simple cortical receptive fields likewise have excitatory and inhibitory subdivisions, but in contrast to those in the lateral geniculate they are linear with a parallel arrangement of excitatory and inhibitory areas. These cells thus respond to a stripe of light, and for each cell a particular orientation of the stripe in the visual field is the most effective (Hubel and Wiesel, 1962). In fact, often a slight change in the orientation of the illuminating line will make the stimulus ineffective for the particular cell. Cells have been registered which respond specifically to a vertical, a horizontal, or any intermediate orientation of the illuminating line. The difference in the shape of the receptive fields of the geniculate and striate area neurons can be explained (Hubel and Wiesel, 1962) by assuming that there are a number of cells in the lateral geniculate body which have receptive fields with their circular "on-centers" arranged along a straight line in the retina, and that the axons of all these cells converge on a particular cortical cell and excite it. The cells with simple receptive fields react only to stimuli applied to a particular region of the retina, in agreement with the topical projection onto the striate area.

The "complex" cells respond to an appropriately oriented stimulus regardless of where in the visual field it is positioned. Some of these units respond well to contrasting edges between dark and light but poorly or not at all to stripes of light. Many other variants have been encountered. It is assumed that these "complex" units receive axons from several "simple" cells in the visual cortex. Thus it appears that the latter cells represent an early stage in cortical integration, the "complex" cells a later stage. These findings are illuminating when attempts are made to explain certain features in visual perception. For example, a hierarchy of "complex" cells will make it possible to explain how a form can be recognized regardless of its position in the visual field. For further interesting considerations the original paper should be consulted.

The explanations given by Hubel and Wiesel (1962), receive further support from data obtained by the authors on the location of the units. Cells with common orientation of the axis of their receptive field are not scattered at random through the cortex but tend to be grouped together, arranged in vertical columns which extend throughout the cortex, just as is the case for the modality specific units in the first somatosensory cortex (see Ch. 2). However, within a single column both "simple" and "complex" units occur. It is interesting that the former are particularly abundant in layers III and IV, where so many of the fibers from the lateral geniculate terminate, while "complex" units are scarce in layer IV. These and other findings fit in well with what is known of the anatomical organization of the striate area and its afferent projections. For example, convergence of influences from the two retinae has been demonstrated in 84 per cent of the cells, and the convergent receptive fields for a particular unit are similarly organized with the same longitudinal orientation and occupy corresponding areas in the two retinae, a point of relevance for binocular vision. In continued studies interesting data concerning the results of visual deprivation and other features in the organization of the visual areas have been brought forward (see, for example, Wiesel and Hubel, 1965, Hubel and Wiesel, 1968).

It appears from the studies of Hubel and Wiesel that in the striate area each small part of the retina is "represented" by cell columns, containing "simple" cells responding to linear illumination of a particular orientation. Impulses from these cells converge on "complex" cells within the columns, which integrate the information supplied by the "simple" cells. As the authors point out, this explains the great increase in the number of cells as one goes from the lateral geniculate body to the striate cortex.

As referred to above, there is clinical (and experimental) evidence that areas outside the striate, especially areas 18 and 19, are important for visual perceptions of a more complex order. Recent experimental studies have given interesting information confirming this. It has been known for some time that on stimulation of the retina with light, action potentials can be recorded outside the striate cortex in an area which is often referred to as visual area II. This has been confirmed repeatedly, and recently Hubel and Wiesel (1965) have in addition demonstrated a visual area III. It appears that the visual areas II and III in the cat correspond to the areas which Otsuka and Hassler (1962) on a cyto-architectonic basis have homologized with areas 18 and 19 in primates. The pathways followed by visual impulses to these cortical areas have been disputed but recent anatomical studies have given results which are compatible with the physiological observations.

Some optic nerve fibers have been traced to the so-called pregeniculate nucleus or ventral part of the lateral geniculate body (O'Leary, 1940; Hayhow, 1958; Singleton and Peele, 1965; and others), to the superior colliculus and the pretectal region (see Singleton and Peele, 1965, Laties and Sprague, 1966, and Garey and Powell, 1968, for recent studies and references). Most authors deny the presence of optic fibers to the pulvinar. Projections from some of the nuclear regions mentioned have been claimed to pass to the occipital cortex, but apart from a projection of parts of the pulvinar (to the cortex including probably areas 18 and 19; see also footnote p. 67) these connections are still a matter of dispute. It appears at present unlikely that visual impulses reach areas 18 and 19 via the pulvinar. However, these areas may be activated by optic impulses via the striate area 17, since areas 17, 18, and 19 are mutually interconnected by associa-tion fibers. The association fibers of the striate area appear to be short and to pass only for a little distance outside the area itself (Le Gros Clark, 1941a), according to physiological studies only for a few millimeters (Dusser de Barenne and McCulloch, 1938). Area 18 appears to send ample association fibers to areas 17 and 19 as well as to area 6 and the lateral suprasylvian cortex (Garey, Jones, and Powell, 1968). The associational projections of area 17 appear to be rather spe-cifically arranged, since following small lesions of the striate area degenerating fibers can be traced to restricted parts of areas 18 and 19 (Hubel and Wiesel, Garey, Jones, and Powell, 1968). Physiological evidence supports the assumption that areas 18 and 19 may be activated via area 17 (see Cowey, 1964; Hubel and Wiesel, 1965).

It appears from some recent studies that, in contrast to what has been generally assumed, direct geniculocortical projections pass not only to

478

area 17, but to 18 and 19 as well. Following lesions of the lateral geniculate body in the cat and monkey, Wilson and Cragg (1967) and Glickstein, King, Miller, and Berkley (1967, in the cat) traced degenerating fibers to all three areas, and confirming evidence comes from studies of retrograde cellular changes in the lateral geniculate nucleus after lesions of the visual areas by Rose and Malis (1965a) in the rabbit, and Garey and Powell (1967) in the cat. The latter authors found evidence that small cells project only to the area 17, while large cells have axons which dichotomize and supply areas 17 and 18, and a particular part (the medial intralaminar nucleus) projects to area 19. This may be related to recent demonstrations that there is a representation of each retinal point in three subdivisions of the lateral geniculate nucleus in the cat—the main laminae and in the central and medial intralaminar nuclei (Laties and Sprague, 1966; Stone and Hansen, 1966). It appears further from the recent studies that there is a retinotopical projection onto not only area 17 but areas 18 and 19 as well (see Garey and Powell, 1967; Wilson and Cragg, 1967). This is inferred also from physiological studies in the monkey (Hubel and Wiesel, 1965), which further indicate that the latter areas serve visual integrations of a higher order.

Hubel and Wiesel (1965), using the approach described above, have studied units in these areas and found that most of the cells in area II and half of those in area III are of the "complex" type, discussed above. Cells of even more complex types than those encountered in the striate area were found in addition, named "hypercomplex" cells of lower and higher order. In both areas II and III (18 and 19) the cells are arranged in columns, and the majority of cells are influenced from both eyes. The cells with increasing complexly organized receptive fields are presumably utilized in higher order integration of visual impulses. In this integration both excitatory and inhibitory processes are involved. (For particulars see Hubel and Wiesel, 1965, 1968).

The recent findings give valuable hints concerning important features in visual perception, but as stated by Hubel and Wiesel (1965, p. 286): "How far such analysis can be carried is anyone's guess, but it is clear that the transformations occurring in these three cortical areas go only a short way toward accounting for the perception of shapes encountered in everyday life."

Above, chiefly one aspect of the function of the visual areas has been considered, that related to the neural basis of pattern recognition. Several neurophysiological studies devoted to the striate area have dealt with characteristics of the responses of the cells, with the reception of impulses arising in response to light of different colors, etc. This data is as yet of restricted interest from a clinical point of view and will not be considered. It should be emphasized, however, that the visual areas, like all other cortical areas, cooperate with other regions of the central nervous system. Thus, in the striate area units have been found showing convergence of visual impulses with impulses from the reticular formation and some "unspecific thalamic nuclei" (Creutzfeldt and Akimoto, 1958; Jung, 1958; and others). The visual areas give off efferent fibers to the lateral geniculate body, as well as to the superior colliculus, the pretectum and other nuclei (see Garey, Jones, and Powell, 1968). The fibers to the lateral geniculate, as referred to previously, may be involved in a central control of visual impulses (see, for example, Widén and Ajmone Marsan, 1961). Commissural connections are certainly of importance for the co-operation between the visual areas of both hemispheres. It appears, however, that this function is taken care of by areas 18 and 19, since commissural fibers between the two striate areas have not been convincingly demonstrated. The two areas 18 appear to be particularly amply interconnected by commissural connections (Myers, 1962, in the monkey; Ebner and Myers, 1965, in the cat and raccoon; see also Garey, Jones, and Powell, 1968). It is interesting to note the parallelism with the situation in the first somatosensory area, described in Chapter 2.

Symptoms following lesions of the optic system. Lesions of the optic chiasma. From a knowledge of the anatomical features of the optic system it is easy to understand the symptoms following lesions of its different parts. Most important for the focal diagnosis are the defects of the visual fields which will appear.[7]

Defects in the visual fields occur in diseases affecting the retina and the optic nerve. However, these will not be considered extensively. From a neurological point of view the so-called "axial neuritis" is of interest, revealing itself in a *central scotoma,* frequently at first only for colors, since it is a rather frequent symptom in *disseminated sclerosis* (retrobulbar neuritis). The visual field defects in *glaucoma* should also be recalled. They are due to a compression of the nerve fibers at the margin of the papilla when this becomes excavated. A complete lesion of the optic nerve will, of course, produce complete blindness of the corresponding eye. In incomplete lesions the visual field defects will be partial, their localization being determined by the arrangement of the fibers as described previously.[8]

In *lesions of the optic chiasma* the typical visual field defect will be a *bitemporal hemianopsia.* The crossing fibers will be damaged, whereas the laterally situated uncrossed fibers escape destruction (Fig. 8-8B). The light impinging upon the nasal halves of the two retinae will not be perceived, i.e. the *temporal halves of both visual fields are blind.* This type of lesion of the chiasma is met with most typically in *hypophyseal* or

[7] The occurrence of papilledema or choked disks in cases of increased intracranial pressure will not be considered in this connection. Although it may in some cases aid in the topographical diagnosis (being, for example, usually pronounced and appearing early in tumors of the infratentorial type), its main importance is as a general symptom of increased intracranial pressure.

[8] For an exhaustive account of the symptomatology in lesions of the optic system, see Cogan (1966).

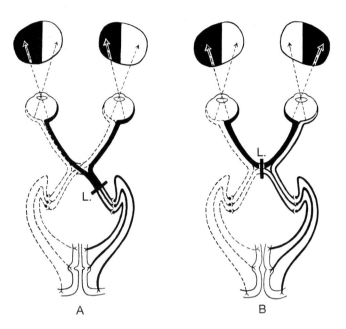

FIG. 8–8 A diagram of the defects in the visual field (black) following: *A*, a lesion of the optic tract (homonymous hemianopsia); and *B*, a lesion of the optic chiasma (bitemporal hemianopsia). *L*, lesion.

pituitary tumors. When the tumor expands it will exert a pressure on the chiasma from below, and consequently the lowermost fibers of the chiasma, namely those derived from the lower regions of both nasal halves of the retinae, will be damaged first. On this account the visual defect usually starts as an *upper bitemporal quadrantanopsia*. As a rule this starts from the periphery, but sometimes the first defect appears somewhat nearer to the center. (On this account it is important to test for visual defects in a radial direction from the periphery to the center, and not to content oneself with making sure that the outer limits of the visual fields are intact.) In the very beginning the defect is only for colors, a finding quite commonly made also in other types of visual defects. Visual acuity commonly remains good for a long time, an expression of the anatomical fact that the macular fibers are not attacked until later, and since these tumors are followed by increased intracranial pressure only late in the course of the disease, the fundi of the eyes will remain normal for a long time, the more so since the atrophy of the fibers occurs slowly. It is not uncommon for the bitemporal defects in the visual field to be the first symptom to make the patient seek medical advice.

Since the pituitary is separated from the cranial cavity proper by the firm diaphragma sellae the tumor must have reached some size before it is able to dislocate the diaphragm and exert a pressure on the optic chiasma. Two other factors, which explain that the bitemporal hemianopsia does not occur as early as might be expected, should also be borne in mind. First, the chiasma is not rigidly fixed, but is capable of a considerable amount of dislocation. Second, the position of the chiasma varies somewhat. It may be found resting on the sulcus chiasmatis, but usually lies more posteriorly, and in some cases extremely so. According to this varying position of the chiasma the length of the intracranial part of the optic nerve will vary from a very short distance to a very long one. Apart from irregularities in the symptomatology due to these conditions, it is obvious that it is possible for the tumor to expand not exactly in the median plane. The visual defects of the two eyes, therefore, are frequently not exactly similar, and additional abberations may be caused by concomitant pressure on one of the optic nerves or optic tracts.

Although bitemporal defects of the visual fields are common in tumors of the hypophysis they may also be observed in other instances. Thus similar defects are seen in cases of *craniopharyngeomas* ("adamantinomas," hypophyseal duct tumors) which arise from remnants of the embryonal Rathke's pouch. Since this tumor, as well as those mentioned below, arises supratentorially, it is apt to exert pressure also on the third ventricle and the hypothalamus, resulting in corresponding symptoms (cf. Ch. 11). The more uncommon *gliomas* arising from the chiasma may give bitemporal hemianopsia, usually of a more irregular type, and combined with signs of lesions of the optic nerve or tracts as well, since the tumors are apt to infiltrate these structures. The so-called *suprasellar meningeomas,* most frequently arising from the sulcus chiasmatis or the dorsum of the sella, should also be mentioned. They will as a rule dislocate the chiasma in an upward, posterior direction, and the visual defect is commonly not purely bitemporal. This is even more the case with the visual defects produced by other tumors in this region, such as *meningeomas from the olfactory groove, gliomas of the frontal lobe,* or tumors in relation to the interpeduncular fossa. However, the examination of the visual fields will usually give valuable diagnostic information.

Far less common than bitemporal hemianopsias are the *binasal hemianopsias,* occurring when pressure is exerted against the lateral sides of the optic chiasma. In this case the uncrossed retinal fibers, arising from the temporal halves of the retinae, will be damaged, and, consequently, visual impulses set up by objects in the nasal halves of both visual fields will not be perceived. The most frequent cause of a binasal hemianopsia is an *aneurysm of the internal carotid artery.* If a binasal hemianopsia is to develop, there must be aneurysms on both sides. Aneurysms may also occur in other arteries of the circulus arteriosus and may give various types of defects of the visual fields.

Of other pathological conditions which less frequently give rise to visual field defects of the chiasmatic type may be mentioned *syphilitic and tuberculous basal meningitis* (direct pressure or impairment of vascular supply) and *localized arachnoiditis* in the cisterna chiasmatis. *Skull fractures* involving the base of the skull may occasionally affect the optic chiasma. In all these instances, however, the defects of the visual fields are rarely purely bitemporal.

Symptoms in lesions of the optic tract. The bitemporal and binasal hemianopsias seen in lesions of the optic chiasma are *heteronymous*. In contrast to this, lesions affecting the optic pathways posterior to the chiasma will always be *homonymous,* i.e. they will affect the same half of the visual fields of both eyes, the right or the left according to whether the lesion is in the left or the right side of the brain. This is a consequence of the partial crossing of the fibers in the chiasma and the intermingling of crossed and uncrossed fibers in the optic tract. The differences observed in the visual defects in lesions of the various parts of the pathways posterior to the chiasma are not always sufficiently marked to allow a detailed diagnosis of the site of the lesion. Generally, a complete hemianopsia is more likely to develop when the lesion affects a part where the fibers are tightly packed, as for instance the optic tract; whereas, when the lesion affects a structure in which the fibers are more widely spread, such as the optic radiation or the striate area, partial defects are more likely to develop in the form of partial homonymous field defects, quadrant scotomas, or smaller scotomas. However, the definite localization throughout the optic system explains that even small, circumscribed lesions may produce rather sharply delimited scotomas, which will be present in corresponding places in the visual fields of both eyes.

A *lesion of the optic tract,* by a tumor or a traumatic injury, as a rule will result in a *complete homonymous hemianopsia.* An interruption of the right optic tract will cut off impulses originating in the right halves of both retinae, and consequently the left halves of the visual fields are blind (Fig. 8-8A). The limit between the intact and the blind halves of the visual fields goes through the point of fixation, and as a rule is completely vertical.

However, a lesion situated more posteriorly may also produce a complete homonymous hemianopsia. A distinguishing feature of some value is the difference observed when testing for the so-called *hemianopic pupillary reflex.* When this is present the pupils react only when light is thrown onto the intact halves of the retinae, but not when the blind halves are illuminated. This indicates a lesion of the optic tract. The explanation of this is to be found in the course of the retinal fibers concerned in the light reflex (cf. Ch. 7). These leave the optic tract to reach the superior colliculus and pretectal region. A lesion of the optic tract will also interrupt these fibers, but they will not be affected when the optic radiation or the striate area is injured. However, unless special precautions are taken it is difficult to make sure that the light will fall only on one half of the retina. Special apparatuses have been designed for this purpose, but on the whole the practical value of the hemianopic pupillary reflex is moderate. More important as a distinguishing feature between optic tract lesions and lesions of the radiation or visual cortex is the fact that an optic tract lesion most commonly will be accompanied by evidence of damage to neighboring structures in addition, such as the cerebral peduncle, since the tract is rather small.

Apart from tumors which may produce a lesion of the optic tract, basal meningitis should be recalled.

Lesions of the lateral geniculate body will result in a complete, or nearly complete, homonymous hemianopsia, if they affect the entire nucleus, or most of it. As a rule other symptoms from neighboring structures will be present.

Symptoms in lesions of the optic radiation and the striate area. A *complete homonymous hemianopsia* will occur in lesions of the *optic radiation* or the *striate area* if all fibers of the radiation are interrupted or the entire area is destroyed. However, owing to the larger extent of these structures, incomplete lesions and *incomplete hemianopsias are far more common than in lesions of the optic tract.* Many authors have stressed that in lesions of the optic radiation and of the striate area, the macular region is frequently spared, in contrast to the condition with lesions of the optic tract. However, this is not an entirely reliable criterion; central vision may occasionally be preserved also in lesions of the tract, and in posteriorly situated lesions the hemianopsia may be complete, without sparing of the macula.

There has been much discussion concerning this "macular sparing" frequently observed in these lesions. Some authors have maintained that the macula is represented bilaterally in the striate area, in contrast to the rest of the retina. Most of the adherents to this view assume that some fibers join the optic radiation on the other side, reaching this through the posterior part of the corpus callosum. There would thus be a second crossing of some of the fibers in the optic system. This of course would explain the macular sparing. This view is, however, based on anatomical investigations of cases of lesions in the temporal and occipital lobes, and it is practically impossible to be sure in such cases that *all* fibers have been interrupted or that the *entire* striate area has been functionless. In monkeys in which the entire striate area has been destroyed, all cells of the lateral geniculate body disintegrate, as was mentioned previously, a fact which demonstrates that crossing fibers of the type assumed to be present in man cannot exist in these animals (monkeys and apes). It appears reasonable that conditions should be essentially similar in man. In investigations aiming especially at tracing the fibers of the optic radiation in man, crossing fibers have not been ascertained (Putnam, 1926). Human cases have also been described in which a total ablation of the occipital lobe was not followed by any macular sparing (e.g. Halstead, Walker, and Bucy, 1940). Following unilateral occipital lobectomy no cellular degeneration has been observed in the contralateral lateral geniculate body (German and Brody, 1940). It should be remembered that it is extremely difficult to ascertain a moderate sparing of macular vision, and that some investigators are inclined to assume that a certain degree of shifting of the fixation point occurs normally. A factor of some importance in this connection is that the macular representation in man occupies a very large proportion of the striate area, and probably even extends anteriorly in the depth of the calcarine fissure. The macular sparing might therefore be explained on this basis as being due to preservation of these regions in some cases. As Putnam and Liebman (1942) emphasized in a review of this problem, what is most urgently needed is a minute anatomical control of relevant cases which have been examined with exact methods during life. Even if such studies have not yet been made, Spalding's (1952b) analysis of 72 cases of traumatic injuries of the striate cortex leave little doubt that in man there is no bilateral representation of the macula, and that when "macular sparing" occurs in lesions of the striate area this is due to incomplete involvement of the macular representation. (See also Kupfer, 1962.)

However, irrespective of the theoretical explanations which may be given, the frequent occurrence of macular sparing in lesions of the striate area has some diagnostic value in distinguishing hemisphere hemianopsias from optic tract hemianopsias. Still greater diagnostic importance may be attributed to the less complete types of homonymous hemianopsias. If, for instance, part of the upper or lower homonymous quadrants are spared, this is a more or less definite indication that a lesion of the tract is not responsible, but that the lesion has to be looked for in more posterior parts of the brain. Purely quadrantic homonymous anopsias point even more to a lesion of the hemisphere, and they are most commonly encountered in lesions of the striate area. The arrangement of the anatomical projection explains that a partial lesion of the striate area will result in partial defects of the homonymous visual fields, varying according to the situation of the lesion. For example, a destruction of the striate area below the calcarine fissure will reveal itself in an upper homonymous quadrantic anopsia contralateral to the side of the lesion. Circumscribed central (homonymous) scotomas will result from lesions of the posterior part of the striate area. Purely peripheral scotomas, homonymous and as a rule congruent in the two eyes, will develop in lesions of the anterior part of the striate area. The different types of such small homonymous scotomas have been observed mainly in traumatic lesions of the occipital lobe, particularly in war time (Holmes and Lister, 1916), but they may occasionally be due to vascular lesions. Details concerning the visual defects in lesions of the striate area and the optic radiation can be found in the papers of Spalding (1952a, 1952b), van Buren and Baldwin (1958), and Falconer and Wilson (1958).

From the anatomical features described previously it will be clear that *diseases affecting the temporal lobe can produce visual field defects of the same type as lesions of the occipital lobe.* This is due to the peculiar course of the optic radiation, and is a fact worth remembering for the clinical neurologist. A tumor of the temporal lobe, even if it is situated only some centimeters behind the temporal pole, will be likely to destroy parts of the optic radiation, particularly the lower fibers (cf. Fig. 8-5). Consequently the visual defect in these cases usually starts as an upper homonymous quadrantic anopsia (see, for example, Falconer and Wilson, 1958). It might be expected that the optical irritative phenomena which may occur should give a clue to the differential diagnosis between temporal and occipital lobe lesions, since electrical stimulation of the striate area gives rise to simple visual sensations only, whereas more complex "hallucinations" are elicited from areas 18 and 19. However, such phenomena of irritation are not very common, and furthermore it should be remembered that the striate area is not a very large region. A tumor involving the striate area will therefore frequently also affect the surrounding areas and the subjective sensations which may occur will be of a mixed type. Other symptoms may give more information (cf. Ch. 9), and ventriculography usually settles the question.

When the defects in the visual fields are due to a tumor, they will gradually increase, and if edema or circulatory disturbances develop, a sudden deterioration may occur. If the cause is a vascular accident or a traumatic lesion, however, a gradual improvment usually takes place. This is due to the fact that fibers which are at first only damaged by edema or pressure due to hemorrhage, so abolishing their conducting capacity but not destroying them, eventually regain their function. In this restitution it is a regular feature that the perception of white is first regained, and only later does the perception of colors reappear. Usually also the definitive scotomas for colors are more extensive than is that for white. As mentioned above, the opposite development is common when the scotomas start. In these cases color vision is affected first and may be severely impaired before any defect can be ascertained by testing the visual field with white objects. The examination of the visual field for colors on this account may give valuable information in cases in which there is reason to suspect a visual field defect.[9]

As mentioned above, it is commonly assumed that the interpretation and the comprehension of visual impressions take place mainly in the areas surrounding the striate area, collaborating in this function with other areas, mainly in the parietal and probably also the temporal lobe.

---

[9] The facts mentioned most probably can be explained by the assumption that the perception of colors is a very complex process, which requires intact pathways, whereas the perception of white may be possible also when a slight damage to the optic pathways is present.

This conception is founded mainly on the phenomena which have been observed in more extensive lesions of the occipital lobe where it borders on the other lobes. In such cases various types of defective visual functions occur, even if the striate area is intact and there is no visual field defect. For example, such patients may be unable to recognize persons whom they know very well, or they may have lost the capacity of reading, although vision is good, or other types of disturbances may occur. These symptoms usually occur only with lesions in the left hemisphere in right-handed persons. They are grouped among the so-called psychosomatic disturbances, which are to be considered in Chapter 12. It should be emphasized that disturbances of the type mentioned very frequently occur in association with other signs of impaired psychosomatic functions.

In focal epilepsy originating in the occipital lobe, especially the striate area, the patient may have a *visual aura,* seeing light, often moving, white or colored, or there may be dimming of vision. The phenomena occur in the opposite visual fields. If the discharge is localized to areas 18 or 19, similar sensations may occur, but the movement is more apt to be twinkling or pulsating (Penfield and Jasper, 1954). These auras resemble the *flicker scotomas* occurring in some patients suffering from migraine, usually at the start of an attack. Most often a semicircular flickering light sensation, sometimes in color, moves from the periphery of the visual field toward the center, indicating a spread of cortical irritation progressing from the anterior part of the striate cortex toward its macular part.

Finally, mention should be made of transient *visual disturbances following vertebral angiography.* There may be blindness lasting for some days with complete or incomplete recovery. Visual "hallucinations," visual agnosia, and other varieties of changes in visual function may also occur as well as mental changes (see, for example, Hauge, 1954; Silverman et al., 1961). Obviously the visual symptoms are due to transitory circulatory disturbances in the territory of the posterior cerebral artery which supplies the striate area.

In evaluating visual disturbances it should be borne in mind that psychological factors are of importance. Recent research has brought forward interesting data concerning these subjects. Since they have, as yet, a moderate practical importance for the neurologist they will not be considered here. The interested reader may be referred to Gassel and Williams (1963) and preceding papers by the same authors.

9

The Acoustic System

ALTHOUGH objections may be raised to the title given above it is used for practical purposes. The main subject to be treated will be the pathways followed by acoustic impulses. Though of great theoretical interest, the anatomical and functional organization of these pathways will be treated rather briefly since they are of limited practical importance to the clinical neurologist.[1]

The cochlear nerve and the acoustic receptors. *The cochlear nerve* enters the brain stem in company with the vestibular nerve at the lower border of the pons immediately behind the facial nerve, separated from this only by the tiny intermediate nerve (Fig. 7-5). The facial, acoustic, and intermediate nerves all pass through the internal auditory meatus. When followed in a peripheral direction the nerves separate at the bottom of the internal meatus. The fibers belonging to the cochlear nerve pierce the bony medial end of the meatus anteriorly and superiorly (Fig. 7-8) where small bundles of fibers produce a spiral of small channels in the bone. These channels can be followed into the modiolus of the cochlea. From the center of the modiolus the fibers bend outward to the osseous

---

[1] For reviews covering various aspects of the auditory mechanisms the reader is referred to Whitfield (1967) and the following symposia: "Neural Mechanisms of the Auditory and Vestibular Systems," 1960; "Neurological Aspects of Auditory and Vestibular Disorders," 1964; "Sensorineural Hearing Processes and Disorders," 1967; "Hearing Mechanisms in Vertebrates," 1968.

The Acoustic System

spiral lamina, and after having pierced this they end on the sensory hair cells of the cochlear duct. The perikarya of the cochlear nerve fibers are bipolar ganglion cells situated in the base of the osseous spiral lamina along its entire course. Collectively all these small groups of ganglion cells represent *the cochlear or spiral ganglion*. The distal arborizations of the ganglion cells lose their myelin sheaths when leaving the bone and are dendrites, while the fibers passing through the modiolus and internal meatus to the rostral part of the medulla oblongata are axons. The fibers of the cochlear nerve, like those of the vestibular, belong to the *special somatic afferent* category (Fig. 7-1).

The main features of the structure of the cochlear duct with the organ of Corti, the receptor organ for acoustic impulses, were described in Chapter 7. A few additional remarks are appropriate. The basilar membrane, on which the organ of Corti rests, increases in width when it is followed from the base of the cochlea to its apex. Since there are connective tissue fibers in the membrane, running across its length, Helmholtz (1863) postulated that the lowest turn and the apical turn were concerned in the reception of high and low frequency sounds, respectively, on the assumption that the connective tissue fibers were set in motion by sounds, like the strings of a piano. Although Helmholtz's "resonance theory" has not stood the test of time it has been definitely proved that his idea of a *tonotopical localization in the organ of Corti* is, in principle, correct. Even though the mechanisms are far more complex than imagined by Helmholtz, there occurs along the cochlear duct from the base to the apex, a regular sequence of responses to tones of progressively lower frequency (from some 20,000 to 16 cycles per second in man).

The receptors are activated by vibrations set up by traveling waves of pressure changes in the fluids (transmitted to these by vibrations of the stapes, which again is set in motion via the other inner ear ossicles from the tympanic membrane). The point of maximum amplitude of the excursions of the basilar membrane moves progressively toward the apex as the frequency of the stimulus decreases. Even with a pure tone stimulus a wide stretch of the basilar membrane will, however, oscillate (and a number of hair cells will be excited). This and other fundamental knowledge we owe largely to von Békésy. Other observations support the idea of a tonotopical localization within the cochlear duct: for example, studies of hearing loss following localized damage to the hair cells by needle punctures of the cochlear duct or by excessive sound stimulation in animals (Held and Kleinknecht, 1927; Schuknecht, 1960). Guild, Crowe, Bunch, and Polvogt (1931) studied the cochlea, post mortem, in a series of patients who had suffered from partial loss of hearing, in some instances as limited defects in the tonal scale only. The sensory epithelium was degenerated or completely lacking exclusively in certain regions of the cochlear duct. The localization of the changes shows that also in man the basal coil of the cochlea is concerned in the perception of sounds of highest frequency, the apical coil mediating those of the lowest frequency (see also Crowe, Guild, and Polvogt, 1931). More precise information has been obtained in neurophysiological studies (see Whitfield, 1967). As will be mentioned in a later section (p. 503 ff) central nervous factors appear to be involved in the capacity to perceive a sound of a particular frequency even though the sound activates a long stretch of the basilar membrane.

The distribution of the terminal nerve fibers to the hair cells of the cochlear duct shows an orderly arrangement. Most of the dendritic fibers from cells of the spiral ganglion are distributed only to small groups of hair cells, and take a direct course toward them (radial fibers). Each ganglion cell, therefore, appears to be related to a small number of sensory cells. Other fibers take a longitudinal course along the cochlear duct (spiral fibers) and end on several cells. These fibers also show an orderly arrangement (Polyak, 1927a; Lorente de Nó, 1933b; Fernandez, 1951). As concerns the anatomical arrangement of the peripheral nerve fibers, the organ of hearing thus appears to be well fitted for differential responses, even if the smallest unit is a small group of cells rather than a single hair cell. In man there are about 25,000 hair cells (Guild, 1932). The number of ganglion cells and nerve fibers is about 32,000 (Rasmussen, 1940a). This gives an average of 1.25 nerve fibers per hair cell. (However, the ratio is not uniform for all kinds of fibers.)

The mechanisms by which the hair cells of the organ of Corti are influenced by the vibrations of the basilar membrane and mediate very precise information to the central nervous system have been the subject of extensive physiological studies, and there are still unsolved problems (for a recent review, see Whitfield, 1967, and "Sensorineural Hearing Processes and Disorders," 1967). These extremely complex processes will not be considered here. Recent anatomical studies, chiefly electron microscopic observations, have clarified a number of details in the structural organization of the organ of Corti which are of relevance for functional interpretations. Among such findings may be mentioned the demonstration of *efferent fibers in the cochlear nerve.* Rasmussen (1946, 1953) traced fibers from the region of the superior olive (see below and Fig. 9-2) which cross the midline of the medulla under the floor of the 4th ventricle, pass ventrally to the cochlear nuclei (where they give off collaterals), and enter the vestibular nerve, from which they finally reach the cochlear nerve via an anastomosis. These efferent fibers can be followed to the sensory hair cells in the organ of Corti (Rasmussen, 1960; Smith and Rasmussen, 1963). In addition there is a smaller uncrossed component of this *olivocochlear bundle* (Rasmussen, 1960). These efferent fibers appear to have an inhibitory action on the sensory outflow from the cochlea (Galambos, 1956; Desmedt, 1962), but their exact

490

functional role is not clear (see Fex, 1967). The bundle is present in man (Gacek, 1961).

Electron microscopic studies, in addition to bringing to light important details concerning the structure of the inner and outer hair cells and supporting cells (see Engström, 1958, 1967), have shown the presence of two types of endings on the hair cells. Apart from relatively large clear synaptic endings there are smaller ones, containing synaptic vesicles and resembling those found in the central nervous system (Engström, 1958; Smith and Sjöstrand, 1961). The assumption that the latter kind of bouton belongs to the efferent fibers is supported by the observation that they degenerate following transection of the cochlear nerve as shown by the electron microscope (Kimura and Wersäll, 1962; Smith and Rasmussen, 1963). An account of the structure of the organ of Corti and the implications of structural features in regard to physiological and pathological problems can be found in the monographs of Engström, Ades, and Andersson (1966) and Spoendlin (1966), and in the symposium "Hearing Mechanisms in Vertebrates," 1968.

The cochlear nuclei and the fiber connections of the acoustic system. The cochlear nerve enters the ventral cochlear nucleus which is situated on the lateral side of the restiform body at the caudal border of the pons (Fig. 9-2). Within this nucleus the fibers bifurcate in a regular manner, sending one branch to the *anterior part of the ventral cochlear nucleus* (the anteroventral nucleus) and one through its *posterior part* (the posteroventral nucleus) to the *dorsal cochlear nucleus*. In man the latter nucleus is situated dorsal to the ventral cochlear nucleus on the dorsolateral aspect of the restiform body. The axons of the second order neurons in the cochlear nuclei transmit the acoustic impulses along different routes (see below).

On closer examination *the cochlear nuclei* are seen to *consist of several subdivisions which differ architectonically.* Harrison and Irving (1965, 1966b) have described a rather detailed parcellation in the rat. Figure 9-1A shows the main features of the nuclei in the cat as described by Osen (1969a). The dorsal nucleus is laminated, having two layers, surrounding a central part which contains some large and many small cells. Within the anteroventral (AVC) and posteroventral (PVC) nuclei several subdivisions can be distinguished by their contents of cells of many different types (see key to Fig. 9-1A).

The assumption that *the various subdivisions differ with regard to their connections* receives support from recent experimental studies. This is especially the case for the efferent connections (see below), but the distribution of the afferent cochlear nerve fibers reflects this as well. It has been known since the early studies of Cajal (1909) and has been particularly clearly shown by Lorente de Nó (1933b) that the bifurcating cochlear nerve fibers are arranged in a very regular fashion within the

4 9 1

nuclei.[2] In all divisions the fibers from the basal turn of the cochlea are distributed dorsomedially, those from the apical coil ventrolaterally (Fig. 9-1A). Lewy and Kobrak (1936) brought forward the first experimental proof of this pattern of termination which has recently been worked out in greater detail by Sando (1965), who like Lewy and Kobrak traced the central fiber degeneration following lesions restricted to small parts of the cochlea. Accordingly, small regions of the organ of Corti supply particular areas in the ventral as well as the dorsal cochlear nuclei. This makes it clear that there must be a tonotopical localization within the cochlear nuclei. The anatomical pattern of the cochlear projection onto the nuclei appears to be in complete agreement with the physiological studies of Rose, Galambos, and Hughes (1959), who mapped the spots giving rise to potentials in the cochlear nucleus following stimulation of the ear by sounds of different frequencies (Fig. 9-1B). For each frequency there are thus at least three separate receptive regions within the nuclei. Even if all details have not yet been worked out the principal pattern appears to be clear.

The *efferent connections from the cochlear nuclei* are at present fairly well known. Most of the axons of the cells of the cochlear nuclei constitute the first link in an *ascending auditory pathway*. Via the superior olive, nuclei of the lateral lemniscus, the inferior colliculus, and the medial geniculate body, this pathway ultimately reaches the cerebral cortex in the superior temporal gyrus. The nuclear stations in which the pathway is synaptically interrupted give off fibers to other destinations. Mention was made above of the olivocochlear bundle. Other fibers pass to the reticular formation. Finally there are descending connections running largely parallel to the ascending fibers. The organization of the various links in

[2] G. L. Rasmussen at a Symposium in Bethesda, 1959, presented a model of his experimental studies of the same subject, but his findings have so far not been published. See, however, Rasmussen, Gacek, McCrane, and Baker (1960).

FIG. 9-1 *A:* A diagram of the cochlear nuclei in the cat in the sagittal plane, showing the distribution within the nuclei of cells of different kinds and the subdivision of the nuclei. *AVC* and *PVC:* anteroventral and posteroventral cochlear nucleus, respectively; *DC:* dorsal cochlear nucleus. The various regions of the nucleus have different connections (cf. text). Note the regular tonotopically organized distribution of cochlear nerve fibers, bifurcating into an ascending (*a.f.*) and a descending (*d.f.*) branch. *g.l.* and *m.l.:* granular and molecular layer in the dorsal cochlear nucleus. Courtesy of Dr. K.K. Osen.

B: Photograph of a saggital section through the cochlear nuclei in the cat showing an example of the tonotopical localization in the nuclei as determined in single unit recordings following stimulation by sounds of different frequencies. Note correspondence with Fig. 9-1A. *Av, Pv* and *Dc:* anteroventral, posteroventral and dorsal cochlear nucleus, respectively. From Rose, Galambos, and Hughes (1959).

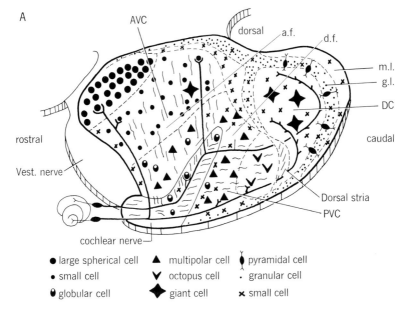

A

AVC
dorsal
a.f.
d.f.
m.l.
g.l.
DC
rostral
caudal
Vest. nerve
Dorsal stria
PVC
cochlear nerve

● large spherical cell   ▲ multipolar cell   pyramidal cell
• small cell   ∨ octopus cell   · granular cell
globular cell   ◆ giant cell   ✕ small cell

B

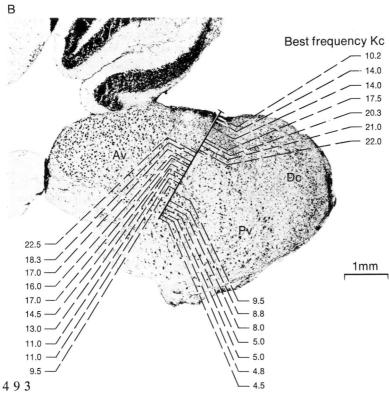

Best frequency Kc
— 10.2
— 14.0
— 14.0
— 17.5
— 20.3
— 21.0
— 22.0

Av

Dc

Pv

1mm

22.5
18.3
17.0
16.0
17.0
14.5
13.0
11.0
11.0
9.5

9.5
8.8
8.0
5.0
5.0
4.8
4.5

4 9 3

the pathway leading from the cochlear nuclei to the cortex is not yet completely known. As might be expected in view of the differentiated structure of the cochlear nuclei, the auditory pathway is organized in a complex manner. It will be possible here to give only a short outline of the subject. The course of the ascending fibers may be depicted as follows.

The efferent fibers leave the cochlear nuclei by three main routes. Some fibers make up the bundle called the *trapezoid body* (Figs. 7-14, 9-2). These fibers come from the main part of the ventral cochlear nucleus and run almost transversely across the pons, closely dorsal to the pontine gray matter. (In man the fibers ascend somewhat during their course and cannot be followed continuously in transverse sections.) When the fibers reach the contralateral border of the pons they make a sharp turn and continue rostrally in the *lateral lemniscus,* which can be followed superficially beneath the lateral surface of the brain stem (Figs. 7-18 and 9-2) until it disappears into the inferior colliculus. The fibers from the *dorsal cochlear nucleus* pass dorsal to the restiform body in the *dorsal acoustic striae* and continue through the reticular formation to join the contralateral lateral lemniscus (Fig. 9-2). Finally some fibers, derived from a specific part of the ventral nucleus, form what is called the *intermediate acoustic striae.*

However, not all of the fibers from the cochlear nuclei ascend to the inferior colliculus. Some end in the superior olivary nucleus, others in the nuclei of the lateral lemniscus (Stotler, 1949; Harrison and Irving, 1966a; Warr, 1966; Osen, 1969b). From these nuclei tertiary neurons then continue rostrally, and some may end in the inferior colliculus. Some features of these structures and their connections will be considered below.

The superior olive consists of several cell groups (see Stotler, 1953) and is therefore commonly referred to as the *superior olivary complex.* It is situated in the caudal part of the pons, ventral to the facial nucleus (Figs. 7-14 and 9-2). The various subdivisions of the olivary complex differ with regard to their connections. These features can in part be related to functional differences.[3] The *lateral* (or main) *superior olive* is conspicuous by its S-shape (in the cat). It receives its afferents from the ipsilateral anterior ventral cochlear nucleus, but only from certain parts. In the rat, Harrison and Irving (1966a) traced them from region III of Harrison and Irving (1964). In the cat, Osen (1969b) correspondingly

[3] The relative development of the various subdivisions of the superior olivary complex differs among mammals (Irving and Harrison, 1967). In monkey and man the lateral division is relatively small, the medial division large, while in the cat (in which most physiological studies have been made) both divisions are relatively large. This data is of interest when correlated with the fiber connections of the superior olive and observations on its function.

494

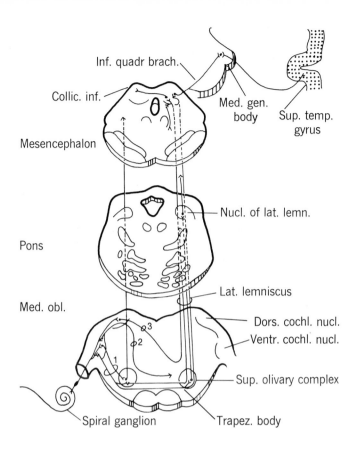

Inf. quadr brach.

Collic. inf.

Med. gen. body

Sup. temp. gyrus

Mesencephalon

Nucl. of lat. lemn.

Pons

Lat. lemniscus

Med. obl.

Dors. cochl. nucl.

Ventr. cochl. nucl.

3

2

1

Sup. olivary complex

Spiral ganglion

Trapez. body

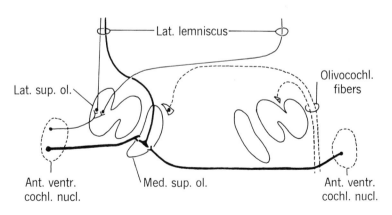

Lat. lemniscus

Olivocochl. fibers

Lat. sup. ol.

Ant. ventr. cochl. nucl.

Med. sup. ol.

Ant. ventr. cochl. nucl.

FIG. 9–2 Above a diagram summarizing the main ascending links in the acoustic pathways. Below a diagram illustrating some details in the connections of the superior olive. (Cf. text.) *1:* trapezoid body; *2:* intermediate acoustic stria; *3:* dorsal acoustic stria.

495

found these fibers to come from a band of small round cells in the ante-roventral nucleus (see Fig. 9-1A) which receives topically arranged primary afferents from the entire cochlea. By comparing the distribution of degeneration following differently placed small lesions in the anteroventral nucleus in the cat, and taking into account the termination within this of the afferents from the cochlea, Warr (1966) concluded that the projection onto the lateral superior olive is arranged according to a tonotopical pattern. This has been more amply shown in a corresponding study by Osen (1969b). Thus an anatomical basis has been established for a tonotopical localization in this part of the superior olive. The pattern agrees with that found in single unit studies following application of tonal stimuli (Tsuchitani and Boudreau, 1966). Units are arranged along the S-shaped band according to the tonal frequencies which excite them. According to Stotler (1953) and other authors the lateral superior olive gives off contralateral ascending fibers (Fig. 9-2, below).

The *medial* (or accessory) *superior olive* is quite differently organized. It receives afferents from the cochlear nuclei of both sides (see Fig. 9-2). Its cells are arranged across the band-shaped nucleus, and usually have two long dendrites, one of which receives afferents from the contralateral, the other from the ipsilateral, cochlear nucleus (Cajal, 1909–11; Stotler, 1953). This arrangement naturally suggests that the medial superior olive might be concerned in the capacity to localize sounds in the environment, a suggestion which has been confirmed in later research (see following section). The special role of the medial superior olive in auditory function is further illustrated by the fact that it receives its cochlear nuclei afferents from a particular group of large spherical cells in the anteroventral cochlear nucleus, as shown by Osen (1969b) (see Fig. 9-1A). This region appears to receive afferents only from the apical parts of the cochlea. The medial superior olive gives off ascending fibers to the ipsilateral lateral lemniscus (Stotler, 1953).[4]

The *nuclei of the lateral lemniscus* (Figs. 7-18 and 9-2) consist of small cell groups along the course of the lateral lemniscus. The fibers from the cochlear nuclei terminating in the nuclei of the lateral lemniscus (and in the so-called nuclei of the trapezoid body) appear to be organized in a specific manner, not yet clarified in all details, and to originate in particular subdivisions of the cochlear nuclei (for some data see Harrison and Irving, 1966a; Warr, 1966). Ascending fibers from these small nuclear groups appear to form further links in the ascending acoustic pathways, in addition to those from the superior olive, mentioned above.

---

[4] The olivocochlear bundles originate in particular small cell groups (see Rasmussen, 1960, 1964). These are further indications of the complexity of the organization of the superior olive.

Presumably fibers from both main divisions of the superior olive reach the inferior colliculus, but there is little positive evidence of this. Some authors have found fibers from the cochlear nuclei ascending only in the contralateral lateral lemniscus to the inferior colliculus (Barnes, Magoun, and Ranson, 1943, in the monkey; Osen, 1969c, in the cat), while others maintain that this projection is bilateral (Woollard and Harpman, 1940; Warr, 1966). In a detailed study of the central projections from the various subdivisions of the cochlear nuclei (Osen, 1969c) a contralateral projection has been shown to come from the pyramidal cells of the dorsal cochlear nucleus (see Fig. 9-1A) and pass in the dorsal acoustic stria, while a projection from the anteroventral nucleus appears to be doubtful.

The *inferior colliculus* has been considered as an important station in the ascending acoustic pathways. Architectonically the inferior colliculus is generally subdivided into a central or main nucleus and an external nucleus. It appears that the fibers of the lateral lemniscus end only (or at least chiefly) in its central or main nucleus (Woollard and Harpman, 1940; Goldberg and Moore, 1967). Single unit recordings following application of tonal stimuli have demonstrated a tonotopical localization within the central nucleus and, less convincingly, in the external nucleus (Rose, Greenwood, Goldberg, and Hind, 1963). Presumably this is made possible by a corresponding organization within the projection from the lateral superior olive or from parts of the cochlear nuclei (both of which show a tonotopical pattern, see above) or by both systems. The studies of Osen (1969c) show that there is indeed a topical arrangement in the projection from the dorsal cochlear nucleus onto the contralateral inferior colliculus. The intrinsic organization of this nuclear region is not known completely (see, however, Goldberg and Moore, 1967), but some information is available of its functional role (see the following section). It gives off fibers which are presumably involved in reflex actions. However, it has long been recognized that its main efferents go to the ipsilateral medial geniculate body. In addition there are commissural connections between the two colliculi.

The massive projection bundle from the inferior colliculus to the medial geniculate body is visible macroscopically as the *inferior quadrigeminal brachium*. Most authors maintain that the bulk of its fibers come from the inferior colliculus (Woollard and Harpman, 1940; Barnes, Magoun, and Ranson, 1943). (According to some authors a few fibers of the lateral lemniscus ascend to the medial geniculate body.) The *medial geniculate body* has generally been considered to consist of a small-celled principal division and a large-celled division, the pars magnocellularis (MGm), situated medioventrally. Morest (1964) has undertaken a more detailed parcellation, on the basis of Golgi studies, of the cells and the plexuses of afferent fibers. In one of these divisions, the ventral, a laminar structure is present in the part of it which is called the ventral nucleus (Morest, 1965a). Morest's analyses, as well as other anatomical and physiological observations, make it clear that the medial geniculate body is rather complexly organized and is not related only to the acoustic system.

The fibers from the inferior colliculus appear to end chiefly in the laminated ventral nucleus of Morest's (1964) ventral division (Rasmussen, 1961; Moore and Goldberg, 1963). The medial, but not the ventral, division appears to receive fibers from the spinal cord (Nauta and Kuypers, 1958; Bowsher, 1961). According to Goldberg and Moore (1967) the fibers of the lateral lemniscus which have been claimed by some to end in the medial geniculate body are actually spinal afferents. It was mentioned in Chapter 2 that the magnocellular part of the medial geniculate body appears to be related to the central transmission of somatosensory impulses. The region in question may perhaps be Morest's medial division. The same division appears to receive afferents from the fastigial nucleus (Carpenter, 1960) and from the superior colliculus (Altman and Carpenter, 1961). In a detailed Golgi and experimental study, Morest (1965b) has mapped the distribution of some afferent systems to the medial geniculate body in the cat, especially the dorsal division. It is clear that various afferent contingents have in part different terminal distributions within the medial geniculate body, and correlations with the Golgi patterns and physiological data lend strong support to the assumption of a functional differentiation within the medial geniculate body (see Morest, 1965b).

Since the ventral nucleus has a laminar arrangement and it projects onto the primary acoustic cortex (see below), Morest (1964, 1965a) has suggested that the ventral nucleus may be concerned in frequency discrimination. This question will be considered below.

Even if the medial geniculate body is not a homogeneous structure, parts of it appear to be the last subcortical relay in the acoustic system, just as the lateral geniculate body holds this position in the optic system. The medial geniculate body gives off fibers to the temporal lobe. These pass laterally in the most posterior part of the internal capsule to end in a circumscribed small area of koniocortex (the type of cortex present where direct sensory projection systems terminate, cf. Ch. 12). From experimental studies, partly in monkeys (Polyak, 1932; Le Gros Clark, 1936b; Walker, 1938b) and chimpanzees (Walker and Fulton, 1938), and electrophysiological investigations (Bremer and Dow, 1939; Ades and Felder, 1942; and others) this area of koniocortex was conluded to coincide closely with the terminal area for the fibers from the medial geniculate body. In man and monkey the terminal area is found in a small region in the superior temporal gyrus, buried in the Sylvian fissure. (In man it would correspond to area 41 of Brodmann, but decisive evidence on this point is lacking.) The cortical region discussed so far is now generally considered to be only one of several *cortical acoustic or auditory areas,* and is generally referred to as the *first acoustic area* or AI. Follow-

498

ing acoustic stimuli potentials occur not only in AI but also in a *second acoustic area,* AII, and in an area referred to as Ep (ectosylvian posterior), on account of its position in the cat, in which most of these studies have been made (see Fig. 9-3). A further area Ea (ectosylvian anterior) has also been described.[5] The various regions differ to some extent cytoarchitectonically (Rose, 1949) and are not functionally identical (for a recent account see Whitfield, 1967). While it was originally assumed that only AI was activated directly by geniculocortical fibers, there is some evidence that AII as well as Ep are influenced by fibers directly from the medial geniculate body. (Compare the rather similar situation as concerns the cortical visual areas discussed in Ch. 8).

Following ablation of AI, clear-cut retrograde cellular changes are found only in certain regions of the principal small-celled division of the medial geniculate body, while they are absent when lesions are restricted to the other cortical acoustic areas (Rose and Woolsey, 1949b; see also Butler, Diamond, and Neff, 1957; Locke, 1961). It has been assumed that some cells in the medial geniculate body give off axons which branch and supply more than one acoustic area, and that these cells do not degenerate unless both branches are destroyed. It appears that the region of the medial geniculate body projecting onto AI covers the terminal region of the fibers from the inferior colliculus, but the pattern of the medial geniculocortical projection is not yet clear.

From an analysis of available data Morest (1964) concluded that his ventral division of the medial geniculate body projects to AI, the dorsal nucleus to the

[5] Responses to acoustic stimuli have been recorded from other cortical regions as well, for example the second somatosensory area, S II (see for example, Woolsey, 1964). It is, however, scarcely justifiable to consider all these regions as acoustic. The situation is similar for other sensory systems. In man responses to clicks have been recorded from the exposed cortex in the superior temporal gyrus and frontal and parietal operculum (see Celesia et al., 1968). This indicates that the acoustic areas in man extend far beyond the area 41.

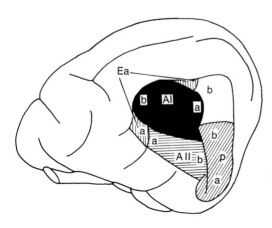

FIG. 9–3 Drawing of the cerebral cortex of the cat, showing the four acoustic areas, *AI, AII, Ep,* and *Ea.* (Some authors use other designations.) The tonotopical pattern is indicated by letters a and b, referring to sites responding to stimulation of the apical (*a*) and basal (*b*) turn of the cochlea, respectively. Slightly altered from Woolsey (1964).

temporoinsular cortex, and a particular cell group to the areas surrounding the ectosylvian gyrus. These projections can only be studied by determining the destination of the fibers which degenerate following lesions restricted to the various small subdivisions of the medial geniculate body, obviously a very difficult task. The clarification of these projections as well as a precise correlation of their areas of origin with the sites of endings of afferents to the medial geniculate body is essential for a complete analysis of many observations on the function of the medial geniculate body and the auditory cortical areas.

Within the first acoustic area AI a *tonotopical localization* was demonstrated by Woolsey and Walzl (1942) by recordings of the potentials in AI following stimulation of groups of fibers of the cochlear nerve in the cat. The basal turn of the cochlea (high frequencies) was "represented" most anteriorly, the apical turn (low frequencies) posteriorly. In AII the representation is found to be reversed. The tonotopical projection onto the cortex was mapped more precisely by Tunturi (1950). Following application of strychnine to the acoustic cortex (in order to raise its excitability) in anesthetized dogs, tones of different frequencies (with low intensities) produce action potentials in narrow strips of the cortex only. The pattern of tonal representation agrees with that established by previous workers, but the discreteness of the responses in Tunturi's experiments shows that the tonal localization in the first acoustic cortex is extremely sharp. Some authors have obtained somewhat different results, and it has been suggested that the methods used "tend to bring out the organization of the underlying fibre pathways rather than of the cortex itself" (Whitfield, 1967, p. 117). There is some anatomical evidence that the geniculocortical projection is topically organized. Polyak (1932), in Marchi preparations from monkeys, described an orderly fanlike distribution of the geniculotemporal fibers; similar observations have been made in man by Pfeifer (1920), utilizing the myelogenetic method (cf. Ch. 1). In a study of retrograde changes in the medial geniculate body following lesions of the first acoustic area Walker and Fulton (1938) constructed a map of the geniculocortical projection.

In *man* auditory sensations can be produced by electrical stimulation of the first temporal gyrus, in a region which appears to correspond to Brodmann's areas 41 and 42 and to cover the transverse gyrus of Heschl (Penfield and Jasper, 1954). The sensations are usually described as ringing, humming, clicking, buzzing, etc. and most often are referred to the opposite ear. A tonotopical localization has not been demonstrated in this way in man. (More complex auditory sensations may occur on stimulation of other parts of the temporal lobe; see Ch. 12.) Pfeifer (1936), from a study of human cases with temporal lobe lesions, was led to conclude that if there exists any tonotopical localization in the primary acoustic cortex of man the highest frequencies must be "represented" medially, those of lowest frequency laterally. This appears to be in agreement with findings in the monkey and chimpanzee by Bailey, von Bonin, Garol, and McCulloch (1943), who studied the action potentials in the acoustic area following auditory stimulation. On the whole the available evidence suggests that there is a tonotopical pattern in the geniculocortical projection, but detailed information is lacking. It is obvious, however, that the organization of the various acoustic areas is far from simple (some functional aspects will be considered below).

Before leaving the ascending acoustic pathways it should be emphasized that even if most of these connections ascend contralaterally, there are also pathways making possible a transmission of impulses from one ear to the ipsilateral cerebral cortex (see Fig. 9-2). This is of some practical importance.

In recent years much attention has been devoted to *descending* (*"efferent"*) *connections within the acoustic system*. Mention was made above of the final link of these connections, the olivocochlear bundles. However, there are continuous chains of connections from the acoustic cortex down to the superior olive and the cochlear nuclei. In general they run parallel to the ascending fibers. For example, fibers from the cortex, coming largely from the acoustic areas, terminate in the medial geniculate body, some also in the inferior colliculus. Fibers from the latter and from the nuclei of the lateral lemniscus pass to the dorsal cochlear nucleus (Rasmussen, 1964) and the superior olive. From the lateral division of this there are fibers to the cochlear nuclei. These connections are not yet known in all details, but those which are better known, the olivocochlear projections, show a very specific pattern (see Rasmussen, 1967, for particulars), just as do the ascending projections. Physiological studies have chiefly been made of the olivocochlear projections, some of which have been mentioned previously. The results obtained so far leave no doubt that the "descending" or "centrifugal" connections are of great functional importance. As expressed by Whitfield (1967, p. 140) when concluding an account of this subject: ". . . it will no longer be worth while to treat the auditory system as if it were a one-way system proceeding to higher and higher degrees of elaboration."

Apart from the connections of the acoustic system described above, most of which form pathways for auditory impulses which ultimately reach consciousness, other connections subserve *acoustic reflexes*. Some reflex fibers are able to influence, presumably via neurons in the reticular formation (see, for example, Rasmussen, 1946), the facial and motor trigeminal nuclei. These connections are concerned in reflex changes in the tone of the stapedius and tensor tympani muscles, respectively. By means of these muscles the position and tension of the ossicles in the middle ear are influenced. Experimental studies have demonstrated that there occurs a reflex contraction of the muscles on stimulation of the ear with sounds of high intensity. The same occurs in man (for some data see Perlman, 1960; Terkildsen, 1960). This is obviously a reflex mechanism which protects the organ of Corti against excessive stimulation, which is known to have a deleterious effect on the sensory epithelia. However, these reflexes are subject to central control, as revealed by several observations. For example, the muscles contract in advance of the sounds in vocalization, and the reflexes may be influenced by previous experience with loud noise (Carmel and Starr, 1963).

The principal center for acoustic reflexes is generally said to be the inferior colliculus. Whether fibers from this descend in the tectospinal tract (see Ch. 4) with fibers from the superior colliculus, some ending in the pons (tectopontine tract), others in the medulla oblongata (tectobulbar tract), has been disputed. According to Woollard and Harpman (1940) and Moore and Goldberg (1966) the contribution of the inferior colliculus to the tectal descending systems is modest (see also Nyberg-Hansen, 1964b). Other fibers from the inferior colliculus go to the superior colliculus and the central gray matter of the mesencephalon (see Moore and Goldberg, 1966). The importance of the inferior colliculus as an acoustic reflex center may in the past have been overestimated.

Functional aspects. In man acoustic reflexes are not of the same importance as in many animals. On the other hand, it is clear that the *analytical aspect of hearing has achieved a higher differentiation in man.* The analytical powers of the acoustic apparatus, as is well known, are considerable, allowing us to discriminate between tones of only slightly different pitch, and in addition, probably by means of an analysis of the simultaneous overtones which determine the timbre of the sound, to discriminate between the sounds of different musical instruments and different voices. Furthermore, we are able to select from a multitude of simultaneous acoustic stimuli precisely those in which we are interested at the moment (cf. Ch. 6), and to determine from where in our surroundings a sound comes.

Little is known of how the brain handles the more complex kinds of auditory information, for example, in perceiving speech. However, experimental studies in animals have given valuable clues to our understanding of the more elementary features of acoustic perception, even though much is still disputed. Three elementary functions have been fairly extensively studied: the ability to recognize frequency of sound, intensity of sound, and the source of sound (its localization in space). In the following some data on these subjects will be briefly considered.

The capacity to discriminate between frequencies of sounds has been touched upon repeatedly in the preceding account, and reference has been

502

made to the existence of a tonotopical localization within the acoustic system. At all levels portions of the ascending pathways and related nuclei are organized according to this principle. However, even if each afferent fiber from the spiral ganglion supplies only a few hair cells, this does not mean that a pure tone excites only a small number of hair cells. On the contrary, at any frequency a considerable length of the basilar membrane is made to oscillate and accordingly a large number of hair cells must be assumed to be stimulated. Two barely distinguishable tones have most of the stimulated cells in common. Accordingly, in recordings from the cochlear nuclei and from higher levels, such as the inferior colliculus, a single unit responds to a wide band of frequencies. Only by applying the "best frequency" (i.e. the frequency of sound which will excite the cell with the least intensity of the sound stimulus) it is possible to demonstrate the tonotopical pattern (as in Fig. 9-1B). The capacity to distinguish closely related frequencies is not a consequence of a topical arrangement within afferent connections only. It requires additional mechanisms of suppression of a number of impulses set up by neighboring receptors. This appears to occur by inhibition, in which presumably the efferent, centrifugal connections at various levels play an important role. (For a discussion see Whitfield, 1967.) These refining mechanisms act upon an elementary and relatively coarse pattern of anatomically tonotopical organized connections.

The problem of which parts and levels of the acoustic system are necessary for frequency discrimination has been approached experimentally. Animals are trained to respond differently to sounds of different frequencies. In studies of this kind Butler, Diamond, and Neff (1957) found that simple frequency discrimination is preserved even if all cortical auditory areas are removed bilaterally. Even if there is a temporary amnesia of the learned habit, the animals are able to relearn auditory frequency discrimination (Goldberg and Neff, 1961). Since cortical ablations are followed by degeneration of cells in the medial geniculate body, it appears that simple frequency discrimination may be related to the inferior colliculus. However, in more elaborate aspects of frequency discrimination the auditory cortex is involved. In the first auditory area Whitfield and Evans (1965) found numerous units which were responsive to *changes* in frequency, and furthermore, *frequency oriented,* i.e. they respond to a rising tone but not to a falling tone, or vice versa, in the same frequency range. (This resembles the situation in the visual cortex, where units responding to lines of light in different orientation have been found; see Ch. 8.) It seems a likely assumption that units of this kind, responding to temporal patterns of sound, may play a role in speech recognition in man.

The view that the auditory cortex has a function in frequency dis-

503

crimination is compatible with anatomical and physiological data which indicate that there is a tonoptopical pattern throughout all levels of the ascending acoustic system. In fact, certain parts of the system are particularly related to frequency discrimination; for example, the lateral superior olive. From this point of view it is of interest that according to Osen (1969b) cochlear fibers to the lateral superior olive come from the small spherical cells in the anteroventral cochlear nucleus (see Fig. 9-1A). This projection is tonotopically organized, and the small spherical cells are contacted in a regular sequence by primary afferents from the entire cochlea.

The discrimination of intensities of sound appears to depend primarily on the number of hair cells stimulated. Experimental studies indicate that the cortex is not necessary for simple intensity discrimination, and it may be that some discrimination of this kind may be mediated even by structures below the collicular level (see Whitfield, 1967, for an account of this subject).

Localization of sound in space is functionally important in man as in animals. As everyone knows, our capacity to localize the source of sound in our surroundings is remarkably precise. Much work has been devoted to the mechanisms underlying this capacity. Several factors appear to be involved. When a sound reaches the ears from one side of the body it will hit the ipsilateral ear with a greater intensity than the contralateral ear and also a little earlier. Both factors appear to be of importance, according to physiological studies (see Whitfield, 1967). Among structures involved in this function, the medial (or accessory) superior olive has been shown to be essential and to provide the initial analysis. As described in a previous section (see also Fig. 9-2), the cells of the medial superior olive receive afferents from the cochlear nuclei of both sides, establishing contact with dendrites extending either medially or laterally. These neurons are therefore influenced from both ears, and the impulses from both sides will interact. In view of this specific function of the medial olive it is of interest that its afferents from the cochlear nuclei, as shown by Osen (1969b), come from the group of large spherical cells in the anteroventral cochlear nucleus (see Fig. 9-1A). These appear to receive primary afferents from the apical part of the cochlea only. In agreement with this, Moushegian, Rupert, and Langford (1967) found that the cells of the medial superior olive are activated mainly by sounds of low frequencies.[6] However, as might be expected, higher centers than the

---

[6] In animals whose ears are adapted for the reception of sounds of high frequencies, as the bat and the porpoise, both the medial superior olive (Irving and Harrison, 1967) and the large spherical cells of the ventral cochlear nucleus (Osen and Jansen, 1965, in the porpoise) are little developed. Not only the cochlear nuclei

superior olive are involved in sound localization. Thus the inferior colliculus appears to play a role in more integrated aspects of sound localization (see Masterton, Jane, and Diamond, 1967). As to the cerebral cortex, Neff, Fisher, Diamond, and Yela (1956) found that in cats bilateral ablation of the primary acoustic cortex (and in some cases the secondary) is followed by impairment in the capacity to localize sound in space. The cortex appears to be essential for the final integration (Masterton, Jane, and Diamond, 1968). As pointed out by Whitfield (1967) behavioral studies are not always conclusive as concerns studies of sensory discrimination. Studies in humans are relatively few and not entirely consistent. Walsh (1957) found that lesions destroying the auditory cortex on one side did not affect the capacity to localize sounds in the horizontal plane (while the localization in the vertical plane may be lost). Sanchez-Longo and Forster (1958), in patients with temporal lobe damage, found impaired accuracy of localization of sounds, especially on the side contralateral to the lesion.

Relatively little is known of the *function of the central acoustic pathways and nuclei in man,* apart from such data as just mentioned. It is reasonable to assume that, in principle, conditions are as in the cat. (However, the different relative developments of certain parts, such as the medial and lateral superior olives, may indicate that there are certain differences.) It is not known where all the acoustic cortical areas defined in the cat are to be sought in man, except that it appears that AI is represented by Brodmann's area 41. It is generally assumed from experiences in man that area 22 in the first temporal gyrus (see Fig. 12-2) is particularly important in the interpretive aspects of hearing (see also Ch. 12). Bailey et al. (1943), using the strychnine method in monkeys and chimpanzees, found this area (and area 42) to be closely related to area 41. The fact that impulses from one ear reach both hemispheres explains that gross hearing defects do not follow unilateral lesions of the temporal cortex in man or unilateral removal of the temporal lobe (Penfield and Erickson, 1941).

Symptomatology in lesions of the acoustic system. Disturbances in the function of the acoustic system in man are, in the overwhelming majority of cases, due to pathological processes affecting the sensory apparatus itself. Since, therefore, these disorders belong to the domain of otology, they will not be treated here. From a neurological point of view it is important to remember the frequency with which diseases of the ear may lead to impaired hearing, and to be careful in attributing too

projections to the medial and lateral superior olive but other of their afferent projections come from particular cell groups or subdivisions of the nuclei (see Osen, 1969b).

505

much diagnostic importance to reduced hearing, before the presence of a local process in the ear is excluded. In the case of diseases of the middle ear, this is, as a rule, not difficult, but with affections of the inner ear it may be impossible in some cases to be sure whether the damage is in the cochlea or in the cochlear nerve, especially since disturbances from the vestibular apparatus or nerve are frequently present at the same time in both types of lesion. The modern methods of analysis of hearing and vestibular functions may, however, enable the otologist, with whom collaboration is recommended in such cases, to obtain valuable information.

Omitting here the symptoms observed in labyrinthitis, otosclerosis, Ménière's disease, professional deafness, and other conditions which affect in some degree the sensorineuronal acoustic apparatus, we will confine ourselves to the symptoms resulting from affections of the intracranial parts of the acoustic system.

Of most practical importance from a neurological point of view are the *symptoms following injury to the cochlear nerve.* On account of the partial crossing of the ascending acoustic fiber systems, lesions of these systems will give few if any symptoms (cf. below). Among the diseases affecting the cochlear nerve, there is one which is far more common than the others and at the same time more important, since surgical therapy is possible, namely, the so-called *acoustic tumor, neurinoma of the VIIIth nerve.* Taking its origin probably from the Schwann cells of the sheath, this tumor, when its slow growth has progressed sufficiently, will exert pressure not only on the cochlear but, also, the vestibular, facial, and intermediate nerves. The symptoms resulting from the damage of the latter nerves are discussed in other chapters (pp. 394 and 408). It will be clear that the deeper in the meatus the tumor starts its growth, the earlier will it be apt to give symptoms, due to compression of the nerves and circulatory disturbances. The symptoms from the cochlear nerve are usually at first subjective, abnormal sensations of hearing of various kinds collectively termed *tinnitus,* and interpreted as due to irritation of the fibers. Eventually the fibers lose their conductive capacity, and an impairment of hearing follows. The tinnitus may occur periodically, but usually is absent when all fibers are interrupted, and the patient is entirely deaf on the affected side. On account of the slow growth of the tumor the patient may have forgotten the initial tinnitus when he seeks medical advice many years later. Since the distance from the internal auditory meatus to the medulla oblongata is very short, a tumor of even a moderate size will soon be able to exert a pressure on the neighboring structures. This will be exerted in a lateral as well as a medial direction. Medially the medulla oblongata will as a rule be pushed aside, without serious symptoms in the beginning. Laterally the continuous pressure on the internal auditory meatus will result in it being slowly widened, and this may be readily recognized in radiograms taken in the appropriate projection. This widening of the meatus is a very valuable localizing symptom in acoustic tumors. If the tumor originally starts in the depth of the meatus, it will cause the same changes, since it will as a rule press itself toward the medial opening of the bony canal. When the tumor grows, eventually pressure effects on the brain usually become apparent. Like other neoplasms in the posterior cranial fossa it will soon give rise to an increased intracranial pressure, betraying itself in headache, vomiting, choked discs, and the other symptoms frequently present when the intracranial pressure is raised. These symptoms may appear earlier than any clear-cut sign of local damage to the central nervous structures, but when such symptoms occur, and occasionally they may appear early, the most conspicuous and regular symptoms point to involvement of the homolateral cerebellar hemisphere. Homolateral ataxia, tremor, and hypotonia appear and may make it difficult to decide if the tumor is a primary cerebellar neoplasm or an acoustic tumor. As a rule, however, the acoustic tumors grow very slowly, and occasionally they may reach an astonishing size before they are diagnosed. The medulla oblongata and pons appear to be able to accommodate themselves to a certain extent to the narrowed space without impairment of their functions.[7]

Far less common than acoustic tumors are other pathological processes affecting the cochlear nerve. Among such conditions may be mentioned *meningeomas of the cerebellopontine angle, syphilitic meningitis, arachnoiditis,* and very infrequently aneurysms of the anterior inferior cerebellar artery. A *cerebellar tumor* in a more advanced stage may give symptoms very similar to those of an acoustic nerve tumor, but the development of the symptoms will be different. On account of the nearness of the nerve to the posterior inferior cerebellar artery changes in this may also lead to cochlear nerve symptoms (see, for example, Stibbe, 1939).

Lesions of the ascending acoustic tracts may occur in all sorts of brain stem lesions, particularly tumors or vascular disorders. The symptoms, consisting of a slightly reduced capacity of hearing in some cases (but apparently not in all), will be an insignificant part of the whole symptom complex.

Lesions of the medial geniculate body or *of the auditory cortex* will not lead to deafness unless they are bilateral. In some cases of temporal

[7] It is generally held that the first symptoms in acoustic neurinomas are those indicating involvement of the eighth cranial nerve. Especially when the tumor arises medially atypical features in the clinical picture, indicating an early affection of the brain stem, are not uncommon (see Sheppard and Wadia, 1956).

lobe tumors a slight reduction in hearing has been observed, and, as referred to above, there may be defects in the capacity to localize sounds. It seems a likely assumption that some impairment of other integrative aspects of hearing will occur in unilateral lesions of the acoustic area, but little appears so far to have been done in this field. Studies of this subject will require the use of elaborate testing methods, and the conclusions which can be drawn will be restricted because the cortical lesions usually extend outside the acoustic cortex.

Subjective acoustic sensations, usually in the form of tinnitus, may occur in temporal lobe lesions involving the acoustic area (particularly in tumors). More infrequently, more complex phenomena result from irritation of the temporal cortex, such as hearing of voices. From the experiences obtained in electrical stimulation of the cortex, it appears that these complex acoustic "hallucinations" are elicited from regions outside the acoustic cortex (see Ch. 12). Epileptic fits, when originating from the temporal lobe, may be preceded by an acoustic aura (frequently combined with vertigo), presumably the expression of irritation of acoustic areas. If a temporal lobe lesion occurs in the left hemisphere of a right-handed person, aphasic disturbances, primarily as concerns interpretation of acoustic symbols, often occur. According to Penfield and Erickson (1941) the middle and inferior temporal gyri can, however, be removed without producing aphasic disorders. (The aphasic disorders are briefly described in Ch. 12.)

It should be stressed that the symptoms from the acoustic areas are not the only ones which may be found in lesions of the temporal lobe (see Ch. 11). On the whole, this is a part of the brain which gives few local symptoms. Particularly if the nondominant hemisphere is affected, auditory disturbances may be entirely absent. Of considerable practical importance is the occurrence of defects in the visual field, which are frequently found on account of the course of the optic radiation (cf. Ch. 8). The so-called uncinate attacks, ascribed commonly to a lesion of the uncus and adjacent part of the gyrus hippocampi (cf. Ch. 10) may occur particularly if the tumor is localized medially. Now and then vestibular disturbances, mainly dizziness, are seen. This fact has been interpreted as indicating the involvement of the cortical area concerned in the reception of vestibular impulses (cf. Ch. 7).

10

The Olfactory Pathways
The Hippocampus
The Amygdala

FROM a clinical point of view the importance of the olfactory system is slight, just as the sense of smell is of relatively minor importance in the normal life of civilized man. However, certain diagnostic information may be obtained from investigations of the sense of smell in clinical cases, particularly when more elaborate test methods are employed. A knowledge of fundamental features in the anatomy of the olfactory connections is, therefore, useful for the neurologist, but no attempts will be made to treat the subject exhaustively. In mammals only part of the amygdaloid nucleus appears to be related to olfaction, and the hippocampus probably has no such relation at all, but for practical purposes both these parts of the brain will be considered here.

The olfactory receptors. The olfactory epithelium is found in the nasal cavity in a limited area on the upper posterior part of the nasal septum and the opposite part of the lateral wall, where it partly covers the superior concha. This part of the nasal mucous membrane has a yellow tint. The slender sensory cells of the olfactory epithelium are kept together by supporting cells. The sensory hairs are situated on a protrusion from the free surface of the sensory cells, an "olfactory rod." This carries 6 to 12 fine hairs which in the electron microscope show the structure of cilia (see de Lorenzo, 1963). The supporting cells are provided with microvilli. The olfactory sensory epithelium differs from other types of sensory cells in the organism (for example hair cells of the inner ear or the rod and cone cells of the retina). From the basal end of each olfactory cell a fine threadlike process transmits the impulses in a central direction. This morphological feature shows that the olfactory epithelium represents the primitive type of sensory cells in the vertebrate phylum, and supports the view that the sense of smell is phylogenetically the oldest and most primitive of all senses. The unmyelinated proximal fibers of the olfactory cells are comparable to axons.

The extent of the olfactory area in the nasal cavity varies greatly in different animals, according to their development of the sense of smell. (In the rabbit there are about 50 million receptors on each side, distributed over about 4.5 cm^2; Allison and Warwick, 1949.) As is well known, humans are able to distinguish a great variety of odors. The odors generally used in tests for the sense of olfaction are arbitrarily selected and do not represent any principal or fundamental types. There is some degree of histological differentiation between the olfactory receptor cells. However, attempts to distinguish particular types on a morphological basis have been unsuccessful in the light microscope (Le Gros Clark, 1956) as well as in the electron microscope (see de Lorenzo, 1963).

Several theories have been suggested to explain how olfactory stimuli can be discriminated, but a final solution has not been achieved.

Amoore and his collaborators (see Amoore and Venstrom, 1967) have produced evidence that there is a strong positive correlation between molecular size and shape and the odor quality of different odorous substances. Substances giving rise to similar subjective olfactory sensations resemble each other with regard to molecular configuration. It was concluded that there are probably seven "primary odors," each corresponding to a particular molecular shape. Complex odors are made up of several "primaries." The interesting suggestion has been ventured that the correlation between odor and molecular configuration ultimately depends on a correspondence between the geometric shape of the molecules and ultramicroscopic slots or hollows in the surface of the receptors. (For a popular presentation of the theory see Amoore, Johnston, Jr., and Rubin, 1964.)

The extremely thin fibers from the olfactory epithelium (about 0.2μ in diameter) unite to form slender bundles which penetrate the cribriform plate of the ethmoid bone to enter the brain in the olfactory bulb. The collection of these olfactory fiber bundles represents the 1st cranial nerve, the *olfactory nerve*.

Some comparative anatomical data. In fishes and amphibians the telencephalon is dominated by afferent fibers carrying olfactory impulses to its pallial part, which betrays no features of a cortex-like structure as seen, for example, in mammals. From comparative anatomical studies it is inferred that the three main regions which can be distinguished within the pallium in amphibians correspond to definite parts which can be recognized in the pallium of higher vertebrates. The medial of these represents the *archicortex* or the anlage of the hippocampus, the lateral the *paleocortex* or the piriform area. Between these is interposed a so-called *dorsal area,* which is considered to correspond to the dorsal cortex or *neopallium,* the *neocortex* of mammals (cf. Fig. 10-1, 1). In reptiles these three divisions become more distinct, although the cortical structure is of a very primitive type (Fig. 10-1, 2). It is only in mammals that the dorsal cortex undergoes a marked development, and increases progressively in the phylogenetic ascent, to reach its peak of development in man, in whom it forms the bulk of the entire pallium (Fig. 10-1, 3 and 4). The distribution of olfactory impulses during this development becomes restricted to the paleo- and archicortex, which on the whole do not undergo further development in higher mammals after they have reached a high degree of differentiation in lower mammals.[1] The archicortex becomes folded, and by the development of the hippocampal fissure will bulge into the medial wall of the lateral ventricle as the *hippocampus.*

With the development of the neopallium or neocortex, the two more primitive areas are finally pushed medially, and in man are found entirely on the medial aspect of the hemisphere, as illustrated in Fig. 10-1, 4. The growth of the neocortex is also responsible for a change in shape of the other areas, since when the occipital pole of the hemisphere is developed, the paleo- and archicortex are drawn posteriorly, and eventually, later on, with the development of a temporal lobe, again anteriorly and ventrally. On this account the representatives of the archicortex and paleocortex in man and most mammals are found as nearly circular structures, extending backward roughly from the region in front of the interventricular foramen, then curving downward and forward, to reach finally the base of the brain below their starting-point. According to this diagrammatic presentation, the archicortex, represented mainly by the hippocampus and the dentate gyrus, should be present along this entire line. However, when the corpus callosum appears in mammals, due to the development of abundant interhemispheral association fibers between the neocortex of the two hemispheres, the part of the archicortex situated at this place becomes much reduced. It is generally held that its homologue here is the

---

[1] When the structure of the cerebral cortex is considered, the neocortex is also designated "isocortex" or "homogenetic cortex," whereas the paleo- and archicortex together are named "allocortex" or "heterogenetic cortex." This differs in some respects from the isocortex (cf. Ch. 12).

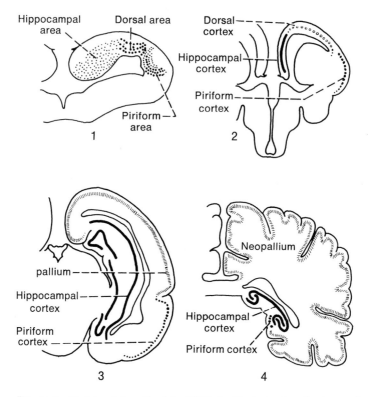

Fig. 10–1 Diagram (after Herrick, 1933) to illustrate the development of the olfactory parts of the brain. In amphibians (drawing 1) a dorsal area is found between the hippocampal area (archipallium) and the piriform area (palaeopallium). In reptiles the dorsal area has the appearance of a cortex (drawing 2); in mammals this develops progressively as the neocortex or neopallium (drawing 3 from opossum) and in man (drawing 4) entirely overshadows the piriform cortex and the hippocampal (archipallial) cortex. (Cf. text.)

induseum griseum. The subcallosal gyrus, beneath the genu of the corpus callosum (cf. Fig. 10-3), is regarded (by some authors) as being the representative of the most anterior part of the hippocampus. The paleopallium develops posteriorly in mammals to form the piriform lobe, in man represented by most of the hippocampal gyrus, and the rest of it is regarded as being present in the form of the cingular gyrus and the retrosplenial cortex, connecting the cingulate with the hippocampal gyrus. However, many authors are of the opinion that the cingulate cortex is really a transitional cortex between the paleo- and neocortex (see below on the "limbic system"). Within the paleo- and archicortex several cytoarchitectonic areas can be distinguished. At this point it is sufficient to draw attention to area 28 of Brodmann in the hippocampal gyrus (Fig. 10-3), the entorhinal area.

The description given above is highly diagrammatic, but it will serve to give an impression of the development of the structures mentioned in phylogenesis. It explains some peculiar features of the fiber connections in mammals and man, such as the long, curved course of the fornix and the stria terminalis. Above all, the comparative anatomical data clearly reveal how the parts of the brain (the paleo- and archicortex), which in lower vertebrates represent the entire hemisphere, become entirely over-shadowed in mammals by the neocortex. The paleo- and archicortical parts of the brain, regarded in lower animals as being first and foremost concerned in olfactory functions in mammals, and particularly higher mammals, have taken over other important functions.

The term *"rhinencephalon"* is often used, but unfortunately, not always in the same sense. On the basis of phylogenetic studies the term is commonly taken to cover the pallial archi- and paleocortex, parts of the basal areas of the telencephalon, such as the septal areas, the olfactory tubercle, tract, and bulb. However, the term has a physiological connotation. An analysis of fiber connections makes clear that in mammals we are not entitled to consider many parts of the so-called rhinencephalon as related especially to smell, as the name would imply. In the author's opinion it is unfortunate to use a term of which it can rightly be said: "From a historical point of view the reader is at present caught up in a morass of terminology, which has led to an almost individual approach to the terminology of that portion of the brain now referred to as the rhinencephalon" (White, Jr., 1965b, p. 28).[2]

Olfactory fiber connections. The centripetal fibers from the olfactory epithelium end in the paired olfactory bulbs, which are parts of the brain, originally evaginated from the telencephalon. From the bulb, situated at the cranial surface of the ethmoid cribriform plate, begin the fiber connections transmitting the olfactory impulses in a central direction. These connections are not yet fully known. In the following only the main features will be considered.

The *olfactory bulb* has much the same structure in all vertebrates (see Allison, 1953b). Broadly speaking, the afferent fibers from the olfactory sensory cells interlock in the so-called glomeruli with the dendrites of second order neurons, the mitral and tufted cells. In addition granule cells are present in large numbers. The structural organization of the olfactory bulb is rather complex. Light microscope observations (Alli-

[2] An impression of the diverse views on the "rhinencephalon" can be gained from a discussion published as a final chapter in *The Rhinencephalon and Related Structures*, 1963.

5 1 3

son and Warwick, 1949; Allison, 1953a) and Golgi studies (Valverde, 1965) have recently been extended and amplified with the electron microscope (Andres, 1965; Rall et al., 1966), and many interesting details in the synaptic organization have been demonstrated, which are of relevance in the interpretation of physiological findings.[3]

In view of the large number of receptor cells it is striking that the numbers of glomeruli and mitral cells are modest, being 1,900 and 48,000, respectively, in the rabbit (Allison and Warwick, 1949). This shows that there is an extensive convergence of impulses from the receptors in the bulb (about 1,000 receptors per mitral cell). In spite of this the discriminative capacity of the sense of olfaction is considerable and presumably depends in part on processes in the olfactory bulb, since ablations of extensive parts of the cortex and of central olfactory nuclei (see below) do not seriously impair simple olfactory discrimination (Allen, 1941). Physiological (Adrian, 1950a) and anatomical studies (Le Gros Clark, 1951) and depth electrode recordings in man (Sem-Jacobsen et al., 1956) indicate some degree of topical localization in the bulb, particular zones being related to special regions of the epithelium and to different odors (see also Le Gros Clark, 1957; Døving, 1967).

In addition to fibers from the olfactory receptors the olfactory bulb receives afferents from the contralateral bulb (see below) and from the brain. The latter were described by Cajal (1909–11), and Kerr and Hagbarth (1955) demonstrated a centrifugal inhibitory influence on the activity of the olfactory bulb on stimulation of various regions of the brain such as the prepiriform cortex and the amygdaloid nucleus. Other authors (Hernández-Peón et al., 1960; Mancia et al., 1962) report that the reticular formation influences the bulbar activity. The presence of *centrifugal fibers in the lateral olfactory tract* (see Fig. 10-3) has been demonstrated experimentally by Cragg (1962), Powell and Cowan (1963), and Price (1968). Some of the fibers have been traced as far as the glomeruli, but their origin is not settled. According to Powell, Cowan, and Raisman (1965) the fibers probably arise in the olfactory tubercle. The above observations emphasize the complexity in the functional organization of the olfactory bulb. They are of general interest since they show that the principle of central control of afferent impulses is valid also for the sense of olfaction. For a recent study see Heimer (1968).

The *central connections from the olfactory bulb,* the axons of the mitral and tufted cells, leave the bulb as the *olfactory tract* (Figs. 10-2 and 10-3). Posteriorly this is flattened and the fiber bundles are found relatively separated as the *lateral and medial olfactory striae* (Fig. 10-3).

[3] For a brief review of the physiology of olfaction see Døving (1967). For further recent data the two symposia on "Olfaction and Taste," 1963 and 1967, should be consulted. For a recent study of the contributions of tufted and mitral cells to the central projections see Lohman and Mentink (1968).

Where the two striae diverge they form a triangular area, the *olfactory trigone*. The striae contribute fibers to several nuclear structures. Following lesions of the olfactory bulb or the olfactory tract, the central connections have been studied in several animal species with the Marchi method and more recently with silver impregnation methods. The results agree on most points. *Some fibers enter the contralateral bulb via the anterior commissure* (Fig. 10-2). There is, however, disagreement among authors concerning the origin of these fibers (see Cragg, 1961; Lohman, 1963; White Jr., 1965a; Powell, Cowan, and Raisman, 1965; Lohman and Mentink, 1968). The commissural fibers to the contralateral bulb have been found to have an inhibitory action (Kerr and Hagbarth, 1955; and others).

The *distribution of the centrally coursing fibers* differs to some extent

FIG. 10–2 A simplified diagram of some of the principal olfactory fiber connections. Some of the connections of the hippocampus, fornix, and stria terminalis are included. (Cf. text.)

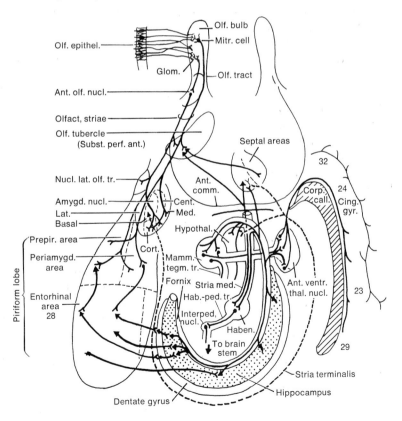

among animals (see Allison, 1953b). In mammals they have been traced in the rat (Ban and Zyo, 1962; White Jr., 1965a; Powell, Cowan, and Raisman, 1965), the guinea pig (Lohman, 1963), the rabbit (Le Gros Clark and Meyer, 1947; Scalia, 1966), the cat (Fox and Schmitz, 1943; Mascitti and Ortega, 1966), and in the monkey (Meyer and Allison, 1949). In spite of minor discrepancies between authors, and leaving out of consideration some minor end stations, it may in summary be stated that fibers from the olfactory bulb, partly with a relay in the *anterior olfactory nucleus* situated at the base of the olfactory tract, pass to the structures indicated in Fig. 10–2 as receiving such fibers, mainly by way of the lateral stria.[4] Some have been traced in animals to the *olfactory tubercle,* which corresponds to the *anterior perforated space* of human anatomy, and is situated immediately behind the olfactory trigone (Figs. 10-2 and 10-3). A fair number of fibers appear to reach the medial, cortical, (and perhaps the central) subnuclei of the amygdaloid nucleus. This is commonly described as part of the corpus striatum (see Ch. 4). but according to its fiber connections part of it is related to the olfactory system. In man it is found in the anterior part of the temporal lobe, beneath the cortex of the hippocampal gyrus, ventral to the lentiform nucleus. The three subnuclei mentioned above belong to what is collectively referred to as the *corticomedial group* of the amygdaloid nucleus (see later). Finally some fibers, in the monkey the great majority according to Meyer and Allison (1949), reach the *cortex of the piriform lobe* (Fig. 10-2), *in the cytoarchitectural areas called prepiriform and periamygdaloid. These areas, then, should represent the primary olfactory cortex.* This is relatively large in some mammals, such as the rabbit, but in man it occupies only a small area on the anterior end of the hippocampal gyrus and uncus, as shown in Fig. 10-3 where an attempt has been made to indicate approximately the extent of this area on the basis of cytoarchitectonic and experimental studies.[5] From a functional point of view this primary olfactory area is to be grouped with the primary cortical areas, such as the striate area, but in contrast to the primary sensory areas for vision, hearing, taste, and somatic sensibility, it is found in the allocortex (cf. Ch. 12). This part of the cortex lacks the typical granular appearance characteristic of the other primary sensory areas. It differs from them also in another respect: its afferent, sensory fibers do not reach it from the interior of the brain after a relay in the thalamus, but arrive from the surface.

[4] Largely corresponding results have been obtained in physiological studies (Fox, McKinley, and Magoun, 1944; and others).

[5] A discussion of these cortical areas may be found in the papers of Brodal (1947b) and Meyer and Allison (1949). See also Allison (1954).

5 1 6

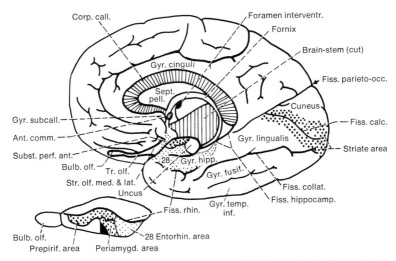

FIG. 10–3 A drawing of the medial aspect of a right human hemisphere, showing some of the olfactory structures. The primary olfactory area is indicated by coarse stippling (like the striate area 17), the entorhinal area by fine stippling. Below to the left a diagram of the basal surface of the rabbit's brain for comparison. The primary olfactory area is indicated according to Rose (1935), and with symbols corresponding to those in the drawing of the human brain.

In view of the confusion over the term "rhinencephalon," mentioned above, it should be emphasized that fibers from the olfactory bulb to the hippocampus, the entorhinal area (see below), and the septal region have not been found in the monkey (Meyer and Allison, 1949) while some authors have described some fibers to the entorhinal area in lower species (for example, White, Jr., 1965a, in the rat). In the rat olfactory fibers have been traced to the hypothalamus, more especially its anterior part (Powell, Cowan, and Raisman, 1963), a finding of interest in connection with observations on the role played by the hypothalamus in the control of reproduction.

It appears from the preceding account that the *primary olfactory cortical region in man is rather restricted*. It may be surmised that this is concerned in the conscious perception of olfactory stimuli, as appears from studies in man (see below). The other terminal regions are presumably related chiefly to reflex activities and behavioral reactions elicited in response to olfactory stimuli. However, second order connections from the primary olfactory cortex and the amygdaloid nucleus must be taken into account as well.

The efferent projections from the primary olfactory cortex have been commented upon by several authors, but in some experimental studies the adjacent cortex or the amygdala has been damaged as well. Following lesions restricted to the piriform cortex in the rabbit, Powell, Cowan, and Raisman (1965), with the Nauta method, traced degenerating fibers to several cell groups. The largest of these are the *mediodorsal thalamic nucleus* (MD), the *basolateral amygdaloid nucleus,* the *entorhinal area,* and the entire rostrocaudal extent of the *hypothalamus.*[6] The fibers to the latter have been described also by Cragg (1961). Since the main efferent projection of the entorhinal area (see Fig. 10-2) goes to the hippocampus, which again projects to the hypothalamus, it appears that olfactory impulses have several routes along which they may influence this region of the brain. Fibers passing directly from the primary olfactory cortex to the hippocampus have, however, not been convincingly demonstrated. By way of fibers to the habenula, the piriform cortex may act on the midbrain.

Impulses arising on olfactory stimulation may influence various parts of the brain along other fiber connections than the routes via the primary olfactory cortex. In recent years these connections and their functions have received much attention and a new concept, "the limbic system," has been created. Before discussing this it seems appropriate to survey the fiber connections and cellular regions concerned. These connections have turned out to be multifarious and complex, but, as in other parts of the nervous system, they are very precisely organized. It is practical to consider them with reference to two important regions, the hippocampus and the amygdaloid nucleus. In the following only the main features will be discussed; for details the original papers quoted should be consulted.

The hippocampus (sometimes called Ammon's horn) has got its name from its resemblance to a sea horse. In man it extends with its main part along the floor of the temporal horn of the lateral ventricle and can be considered as a gyrus of the allocortex, folded inward and covering the hippocampal fissure. Accordingly, the surface facing the ventricle is the deepest layer, and consists of myelinated fibers which collect on its surface as the *alveus,* covered by ependyma. Most of these fibers are efferent and unite to form the *fornix.*[7] While the delimitation of the hippocampus as a gross anatomical structure is fairly clear, its developmental relations to neighboring regions is less obvious. In order to avoid difficulties it is common to speak of a "hippocampal formation" or "hippocampal re-

[6] The hypothalamus in addition may be influenced from the piriform cortex via the basolateral amygdaloid nucleus (see below).

[7] As will appear from the sketch of the development of the brain given above, the hippocampus originally extends in an arch to a region in front of the interventricular foramen. Its most anterior end in man is generally said to be represented by the subcallosal gyrus, from which rudimentary gray masses, the induseum griseum, continue dorsally over the corpus callosum.

gion," including in addition to the hippocampus itself the dentate gyrus and the subiculum (see Fig. 10-4). The *dentate gyrus* accompanies the hippocampus as a narrow band of cortex (for a description see textbooks on neuroanatomy). The cortical areas of the cortex medial to the dentate gyrus are collectively referred to as the *subiculum* (more specifically a distinction may be made between prosubiculum, subiculum, presubiculum, and parasubiculum; see Fig. 10-4). The subiculum occupies part of the hippocampal gyrus, and is contiguous with the area entorhinalis (Brodmann's area 28; see Figs. 10-4 and 12-2) belonging to the paleopallium, and making up part of what in comparative anatomy is often called piriform cortex. (By some authors the entorhinal area is included in the "hippocampal region.") The two fornices are dorsally connected by fibers crossing the midline underneath the corpus callosum. These (largely commissural) fibers are called the *hippocampal commissure* or *psalterium*.

The general principles of organization of the hippocampal formation are simpler than in the neocortex, and for this reason the hippocampal formation has been considered a favorable site for studying general anatomical as well as physiological features of cortical gray matter and for anatomo-physiological correlations. A great many studies performed in recent years have made it clear that the organization of the hippocampal formation is after all rather complex. There are architectonic differences between minor parts.[8] (In the hippocampus, for example, different regions can be distinguished: regio superior or CA 1, a CA 2, a regio inferior or CA 3.) Experimental anatomical mapping of afferents has shown that they are arranged in a very specific manner, fibers from one source ending in restricted laminae within particular architectonic fiones. These differences on many points are reflected in histochemical differences. By correlating light and electron microscopic and electrophysiological studies it has been possible in some instances to determine whether a particular afferent fiber system has excitatory or inhibitory functions. The subdivision into minor regions arrived at on the basis of studies with the methods mentioned above has been shown to be valid when the ontogenetic development is studied by autoradiography (Angevine, 1965). Most of these investigations have been made in animals, especially in the rat. In order to give an idea of the intricate organization it will be sufficient to mention some data from the hippocampus. This is selected as an example because it is so far best known, and because in man it is by far the largest part of the entire hippocampal formation. The following should not be considered as more than a

[8] For accounts and references to the literature, see Blackstad (1956) and Raisman, Cowan, and Powell (1965).

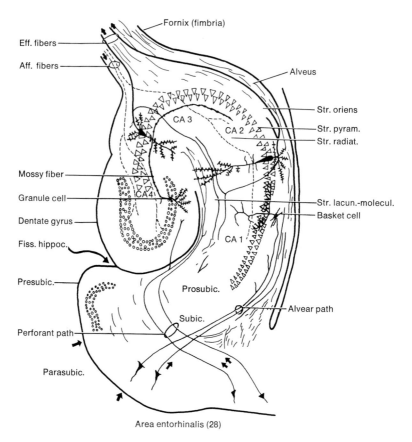

FIG. 10–4 Schematic drawing to illustrate some main features in the organization of the hippocampus. Note that the mossy fibers coming from the granule cells of the dentate gyrus establish contact with the basal parts of the apical dendrites of hippocampal pyramids, while fibers from the entorhinal area (passing in the perforant path) end on the distal arborizations of the apical dendrites. Axons of basket cells in stratum oriens end on the perikarya of pyramidal cells. (Cf. text.)

sketchy outline of a very complicated pattern of organization. The data will be discussed with reference to Fig. 10-4, which is an extremely simplified diagram.

The most impressive cellular elements of the hippocampus are the large *pyramidal cells.* They make up the *pyramidal layer* (stratum pyramidale) and have their base directed toward the surface of the hippocampus with the alveus. Basal dendrites extend in this direction and belong to the *stratum oriens.* From the other end of the pyramids slender apical dendrites extend inward. On account of their regular arrangement the layer harboring the apical dendrites is called the *stratum radiatum*. Distally the apical dendrites branch repeatedly and spread out in the innermost layer, the *stratum lacunosum-moleculare*. The axons of the pyramidal cells give off recurrent collaterals, many of which ascend to the stratum lacunosum-moleculare. Other collaterals are given off to the stratum oriens. While the regular arrangement and shape of the pyramidal cells determine the over-all pattern of the hippocampus, it should be recalled that these cells are not the only ones present. In all layers there are cells of other types (not shown in Fig. 10-4), the axons of which take various courses. Among these cells are the so-called *basket cells,* found in the stratum oriens. They give off axons which ramify between the pyramidal cells, and appear to be the only fibers which end on the perikarya of these cells. The basket and other cells are concerned in the intrinsic activity of the hippocampus. The *efferent fibers* leaving the hippocampus in the fornix are axons of pyramidal cells. *Afferent fibers* to the hippocampus enter it in two bundles coming chiefly from the entorhinal area (the perforant and alvear paths). In addition some afferents pass in the fornix (see below). Fibers from granule cells of the dentate gyrus (see Fig. 10-4) give off so-called *mossy fibers* which pursue a course along the pyramidal cells and make synaptic contacts with the basal parts of the apical dendrites. The above features in the anatomical organization of the hippocampus were clarified by Cajal (1909–11) and supplemented by extensive Golgi studies by Lorente de Nó (1934). More recent experimental anatomical, electron microscopic, histochemical, and electrophysiological studies have brought forward further details.

Experimental tracing of afferent connections by silver impregnation methods shows that the hippocampal commissure contains in part connections between corresponding regions of the two hippocampal formations, in part heterotopic connections, for example, some fibers from the entorhinal area ending in certain parts of the contralateral hippocampus (Blackstad, 1956). The latter fibers are distributed exclusively to the stratum lacunosum-moleculare, while more abundant homotopic commissural fibers end in the stratum oriens and stratum radiatum. Fibers from the ipsilateral lateral entorhinal area end in the upper part of the stratum lacunosum-moleculare and establish contact with the most distal ramifications of pyramidal apical dendrites (Blackstad, 1958; Raisman, Cowan, and Powell, 1965). The recurrent (so-called Schaffer) collaterals of the pyramids end at the distal part of the apical dendrites (in the stratum-lacunosum). Afferents from the cingulum (see below) appear not to end in the hippocampus proper (White, Jr., 1959a; Raisman, Cowan, and Powell, 1965) but only in the presubiculum and the entorhinal area.

Electron microscopic studies have clarified many interesting features concerning *synaptic relations* (for a recent review see Blackstad, 1967). For example, the mossy fibers have giant boutons surrounding the large and ramified spines ("excrescences") of the initial part of the apical pyramidal dendrites (Blackstad and

Kjærheim, 1961; Hamlyn, 1962). Since the various kinds of afferents establish contact at different levels along the apical dendrites the morphology of the synapses of afferents from different sources can be studied with the electron microscope (Westrum and Blackstad, 1962; Hamlyn, 1962, 1963; Blackstad and Flood, 1963; Andersen, Blackstad, and Lømo, 1966). By recording potentials at different depths along the pyramidal cells information on the action of various afferents can be obtained. It appears, for example, that the commissural afferents in the stratum radiatum and stratum oriens exert an excitatory action on the pyramidal cells (Andersen, 1960; Andersen, Blackstad, and Lømo, 1966). The basket cell axons, ending as densely packed boutons on the pyramidal cell bodies (Blackstad and Flood, 1963), have been shown to be inhibitory (Andersen, Eccles, and Løyning, 1964a, 1964b). The recurrent collaterals of the pyramidal cell axons, ending on the apical dendrites, appear to be excitatory (Andersen and Lømo, 1965).

As mentioned above, there are *histochemical differences* between various regions and layers in the hippocampal formation. In the hippocampus acetylcholinesterase is particularly abundant in the stratum oriens and the pyramidal layer (see Storm Mathisen and Blackstad, 1964). It has been suggested that acetylcholine may act as an inhibitory transmitter in the hippocampus (see Andersen, 1966). Other histochemical differences have been found as well (see Green, 1964; Blackstad, 1967; Mellgren and Blackstad, 1967, for some references). A peculiar finding is the selective occurrence of zinc in certain regions (Fleischauer and Horstmann, 1957), particularly in the layers of mossy fibers (von Euler, 1962). Zinc appears to be present only in the boutons of the mossy fibers and not in the postsynaptic excrescences of the basal parts of the apical dendrites as shown in electron microscope studies by Haug (1967). The physiological significance of this is so far not known.

It appears from the studies mentioned above that all fiber systems ending on thin dendrites of the pyramidal cells are excitatory, while those ending on the soma (collaterals of basket cells) are inhibitory. The basket cell will thus be an inhibitory interneuron. On the basis of these findings attempts have been made to interpret the pattern of neuronal activity in the hippocampus (see Andersen, Blackstad, and Lømo, 1966; Andersen, 1966). This activity is influenced by impulses from many sources. Likewise the hippocampus may act on various regions of the brain by way of its efferent fibers. The latter will be considered first.

The *efferent projection from the hippocampus* is made up of the axons of its pyramidal cells (supplemented by some fibers from the subiculum). There seems to be general agreement that the efferents pass in the *fornix*. This massive fiber bundle pursues a characteristic forward course beneath the corpus callosum. Immediately in front of the interventricular foramen (Fig. 10-3) the bundle bends downward and splits into minor components reaching different regions. Some of the fornix fibers descend anterior to the anterior commissure (precommissural fornix); others descend posterior to it (postcommissural fornix). In callosal mammals a minor contingent of hippocampal fibers passes on the dorsal surface of the corpus callosum in the dorsal longitudinal striae of Lancisi (dorsal fornix). Some of these fibers break through the corpus callosum to join fibers from the main fornix. The presence of fornix fibers crossing the midline in the hippocampal commissure was mentioned above. In addition to hippocampal efferents the fornix contains also some fibers coursing in the opposite direction

The fornix contains some 1,200,000 fibers in man (Powell, Guillery, and Cowan, 1957), some 500,000 in the monkey (Daitz and Powell, 1954). Following lesions of the hippocampus the course and sites of termination of the fornix fibers have been mapped by several authors, most recently experimentally with silver impregnation methods [9] by Guillery (1956), Nauta (1956), and Raisman, Cowan, and Powell (1966) in the rat; Nauta (1958) in the cat, and Simpson (1952b) in the monkey.

The findings of various authors agree in all essentials. Fibers of the postcommissural fornix are distributed to the *mamillary body* and the *anterior thalamic nucleus,* but some fibers continue caudally and have been traced to the rostral part of the *periaqueductal gray matter of the mesencephalon* (see Nauta, 1958) and the *pontine nuclei* (Cragg and Hamlyn, 1959). Some of the precommissural fornix fibers likewise reach the mammillary body and anterior thalamic nucleus, while others are distributed to the *preoptic region,* the *lateral hypothalamus,* and the *nuclei of the septum.* The nuclei of the septum are well developed in lower mammals, and according to Stephan and Andy (1962) there is a good correlation between the relative size of these nuclei and the hippocampus. There has been some uncertainty as to the homologue of the septal nuclei in man.[10]

The fibers from different parts of the hippocampus are not distributed diffusely to the various terminal regions. On the contrary, extending observations by previous authors, Raisman (1966a) and Raisman, Cowan, and Powell (1966) demonstrated a very specific pattern within this projection. For example, the anterior part of CA 1 projects chiefly to the anterior thalamic nucleus and the mammillary body, while the fields CA 3 and CA 4 supply the septal nuclei and some associated small nuclei. Within the terminal areas there is likewise a definite pattern. For example, not all subnuclei of the mammillary body receive fibers from the fornix, and there appears to be a spatial correlation between areas of origin in the hippocampus and

[9] The pyramidal cells of the hippocampus do not show retrograde changes following transection of the fornix (see Daitz and Powell, 1954; McLardy, 1955a). This may be due to the abundant recurrent collaterals of the axons.

[10] The septal area, or nuclei, in man does not correspond to the septum pellucidum. By some authors this is considered as part of a postcommissural septum, while the main gray masses representing the precommissural septum are found in front of the anterior commissure at the base of the brain above the olfactory tubercle. It is common to distinguish between a medial and lateral septal nucleus (see Kappers, Huber, and Crosby, 1936).

the terminal area within the mammillary body (Simpson, 1952b; Cragg and Hamlyn, 1959). The projection from CA 3 and CA 4 to the septum appears to reach chiefly the medial septal nucleus. These differences in distribution are of interest when seen in connection with the further projections from the nuclei receiving fibers from the hippocampus and with the afferent connections of the latter (see below).

The nuclei receiving hippocampal impulses may act on other regions. Among these, the *cingulate gyrus* (Figs. 10-2 and 10-3) appears to be especially important. The anterior thalamic nucleus, receiving hippocampal fibers, projects in a topically arranged pattern upon this gyrus. Fibers from various subdivisions of the anterior nucleus [11] appear to supply cortical areas 32, 23, and 24 as well as the retrosplenial areas 29 and 30 (Fig. 10-2). The fibers leave the thalamus in the inferior thalamic peduncle and reach the cortex via the anterior limb of the internal capsule. This projection has been studied experimentally in various animals by mapping retrograde cellular changes in the thalamus following cortical lesions (Le Gros Clark and Boggon, 1933; Lashley, 1941; Bodian, 1942; Rose and Woolsey, 1948; Powell and Cowan, 1954; and others). Studies of human brains, especially from patients subjected to prefrontal leucotomy (see Ch. 12) have been undertaken by Meyer and his collaborators (see Meyer and Beck, 1954) and in recent years especially by Yakovlev and his collaborators, who have in addition made experimental studies in monkeys (see for example, Yakovlev, Locke, Koskoff, and Patton, 1960; Locke, Angevine, and Yakovlev, 1964).[12]

In addition to the above connection there is another route from the hippocampus to the cingulate cortex. Hippocampal efferents end in the mammillary body which projects heavily onto the anterior thalamic nucleus by way of the macroscopically visible *mammillothalamic bundle* (Fig. 10-2). This arises chiefly from the medial mammillary nucleus where most of the fornix fibers end (Simpson, 1952b, in the monkey). There appears to be a topical pattern within the mammillothalamic projection (Cowan and Powell, 1954; Powell and Cowan, 1954; Fry et al., 1963).

The ample connections from the hippocampus to the cingulate cortex

[11] The anterior thalamic nucleus (see Fig. 2-11) is generally subdivided into an anteromedial (AM), an anterodorsal (AD), and an anteroventral (AV) nucleus. In man the latter is best developed, occupies the bulk of the entire nucelus, and produces the anterior tubercle of the thalamus. The AV appears to project chiefly to the anterior areas of the cingulate gyrus.

[12] According to the studies of this group the posterior part of the cingulate gyrus receives a substantial projection from the laterodorsal thalamic nucleus (LD, see Fig. 2-11) which they, therefore, group with the "limbic nuclei of the thalamus." (See also Valenstein and Nauta, 1959.)

discussed above are of special interest since fibers from this part of the cortex have been traced in a posterior direction to the hippocampal formation. These fibers pass in the *cingulum* bundle, running along the cingulate gyrus. (The bundle contains also shorter fibers connecting anterior and posterior parts of the cingulate gyrus.) The fibers from the cingulate gyrus to the hippocampal formation were observed by early neuroanatomists and have later been studied in more detail with silver impregnation methods in the rat (White, Jr., 1959), the rabbit (Adey, 1951; Cragg and Hamlyn, 1959), the macaque (Adey and Meyer, 1952a), and the squirrel monkey (DeVito and White, Jr., 1966). While some of the fibers are described as ending in the hippocampus proper, it appears that in the rat most of them end in the subiculum and parasubiculum, from which there are connections to the hippocampus. Electrophysiological studies in the cat and monkey have given concordant results (White, Jr., Nelson, and Foltz, 1960). This circuit of connections, hippocampus (chiefly CA 1)—anterior thalamus—cingulate gyrus—hippocampus, has received much attention.

In a rather similar way another circuit is established via the *septal nuclei,* in which a fair number of fibers from the hippocampus end (see above). Following lesions of the septal nuclei fibers have been traced to the hippocampus in various mammals (Daitz and Powell, 1954; Cragg, 1965; Raisman, 1966a; DeVito and White, Jr., 1966; and others). According to Raisman (1966a) the fibers end in the hippocampal fields CA 3 and CA 4 and the dentate gyrus. As mentioned above, CA 3 and CA 4 are the main parts of the hippocampus which project onto the septal nuclei. Although the sites of origin of septal efferents to the hippocampus on the whole do not coincide with the septal areas receiving fibers from CA 3 and CA 4 (see Raisman, 1966a, for particulars) there is obviously a definite two-way connection between the posterior part of the hippocampus and the septum.[13] The differences in efferent connections of different regions of the hippocampus strongly indicate that these regions are not functionally similar, and fit in with the presence of differences in the finer structure of the various hippocampal regions.

The *hypothalamic terminations* of fibers of the fornix have been described somewhat differently by students of this subject. Discrepancies appear largely to be due to methodological problems. According to Simpson (1952b) in the monkey these fibers may end chiefly in the ventromedial hypothalamic nucleus (see Ch. 11). Fibers from the hippocampus to the mesencephalon may be more developed in the cat (Nauta, 1958) than in the rat (Nauta, 1956).

---

[13] In physiological studies (Andersen, Bruland, and Kaada, 1961) responses following septal stimulation have been recorded in CA 1.

It is clear from the above that *the hippocampus may act* (*indirectly*) *on the cingulate gyrus and the septum.* Only a modest number of direct connections to the midbrain exist. This direct hippocampal-mesencephalic pathway is, however, supplemented by more indirect routes. From the mammillary body some fibers pass caudally to the midbrain as the *mammillotegmental tract* (Fig. 10-2). Presumably, the fibers end chiefly in the reticular formation.[14] Correspondingly, the hippocampal influence on the hypothalamus may occur not only via direct fibers, but also via the septum, since the septal nuclei give off fibers to the lateral hypothalamus (see Raisman, 1966a).

The hippocampus is acted upon by various regions of the brain by way of *afferent connections.* The fibers from the *cingulum* and from the *septum* were mentioned above. The latter fibers pass in the fornix. This, therefore, is not a purely efferent pathway from the hippocampus, as previously believed. The quantitatively most important group of afferents to the hippocampus comes from the *entorhinal area,* area 28 (Fig. 10-2). This has been known from the early Golgi studies of Cajal and Lorente de Nó and has been studied in more detail experimentally. As referred to previously these fibers enter the hippocampus in the perforant and alvear paths (see Fig. 10-4). The former arise from the lateral part, the latter from the medial part of the entorhinal area. The fibers have been traced experimentally in the rat (Blackstad, 1958; Raisman, Cowan, and Powell, 1965) and in the monkey (Adey and Meyer, 1952b). It appears from these studies that the connections are rather specific, not only with regard to hippocampal areas where they end, but also with regard to the laminae in these fields (see also above). Physiological studies confirm that the entorhinal area markedly influences hippocampal activity (Andersen, Holmqvist, and Voorhoeve, 1966). The commissural connections between the two hippocampal formations were mentioned previously. Some authors advocate projections from the piriform cortex (Cragg, 1961) while others are inclined to deny their existence (Raisman, Cowan, and Powell, 1965; Powell, Cowan, and Raisman, 1965).

Function of the hippocampus. The characteristic gross appearance of the hippocampus and its considerable size in man may in part explain why the question of the function of the hippocampus always has attracted much interest among workers in various fields of neurological research. In attempting to understand the function of the hippocampus one previously had to rely mainly on inferences from comparative anatomical find-

---

[14] Ascending afferents to the mammillary body, making up the *mammillary peduncle,* arise from particular cell groups in the mesencephalon (deep tegmental nucleus, dorsal tegmental nucleus) as studied recently by Cowan, Guillery, and Powell (1964).

ings. In recent years more direct approaches to the question have been made possible due to progress in physiological methods of study.

It will appear from the account given above of the connections of the hippocampus, that it must obviously collaborate very closely with many other regions of the brain. These anatomical features make it clear that it will probably be difficult—and perhaps impossible—ever to define the "function" of the hippocampus as such, and it will certainly be misleading to consider the hippocampus as a "center" for any particular function. The best one can achieve will probably be to identify certain functions in which the hippocampus is concerned to a greater or lesser extent. Moreover, the anatomical and some physiological observations mentioned above leave no doubt that even the hippocampus proper can scarcely be a functional unit, since there are obvious differences between minor parts as regards their structural and functional organization. The technical difficulties involved in stimulating or ablating the hippocampus or parts of it without affecting other regions are considerable. The facts mentioned should be borne in mind in any attempt to study the functions of the hippocampus.

The hippocampus, as mentioned previously, is generally included among the regions of the brain collectively referred to as the "rhinencephalon." Until not very long ago it was accepted that the hippocampus was related to olfactory functions, although it was known that there is no relation between the size of the hippocampus and the development of the sense of smell in various animals. The whales, which are anosmatic or nearly anosmatic, possess a hippocampus (see, for example, Addison, 1915; Ries and Langworthy, 1937), and in some human brains in which the olfactory bulbs and tracts have been absent the hippocampus (as well as the fornix, mammillary body, and cingulate gyrus) has been found to be well developed (see, for example, Stewart, 1939). Microsmatic man has the largest hippocampus of all animals. From a review of the data available in the literature it was clear as early as in 1947 that *any relation between the hippocampus and the sense of smell must be very remote* (see Brodal, 1947b; Allison, 1953b). As mentioned previously the hippocampus does not receive olfactory fibers from the bulb (with the exception of the so-called anterior continuation of the hippocampus, which is rudimentary). Impulses of olfactory nature which may reach the hippocampus could only be transmitted from the piriform lobe. However, hippocampal afferents take origin only from the posterior part of the lobe, the so-called entorhinal area, Brodmann's area 28. (Some of them end in the dentate gyrus which projects to the hippocampus.) The entorhinal area does not receive fibers from the olfactory bulb, but it may be influenced via connections from the primary olfactory cortex by fibers coming from this (Fig. 10-2). Although some authors have reported action potentials in the hippocampus following stimulation of the olfactory bulb in animals (Cragg, 1960; and others) these responses appear to be weak and to be mediated via multisynaptic pathways. While the role of the hippocampus in olfactory function thus appears to be negligible recent studies have brought forward evidence of its involvement in other functions.

The hippocampus has been the subject of a number of electrophysiological studies (for a recent review see Green, 1964). Potentials can be recorded in the hippocampus following stimulation peripherally (visual, acoustic, gustatory, somatosensory, and other kinds of stimuli) or stimulation of the cortex and of various subcortical structures. Conversely stimulation of the hippocampus has been found to give rise to potentials in many other regions of the brain, in agreement with its multifarious efferent connections. Much interest has been devoted to the *electrical activity in the hippocampus* and to factors which may influence it. It is generally agreed that the hippocampal responses are complex, labile, and easily modified by various factors, but as stated by Green (1964, p. 571) ". . . the description of the shape and direction of potentials evoked in the hippocampus available in the literature is utterly confusing." This subject will not be discussed here, but mention should be made of the changes in the spontaneous activity of the hippocampus in various states of consciousness. In situations where the cerebral neocortex becomes "desynchronized" or "activated" (see Ch. 6), the hippocampus shows "synchronization," and presents rhythmic sinusoidal waves of 4 to 7 per second, usually referred to as "theta waves." When the cortex shows synchronization the hippocampal activity is desynchronized. The functional role of this reciprocal relationship is not clearly understood.[15] It appears, however, that both structures are influenced from the reticular formation. As described above there are fiber connections which may mediate such influences, and it has been maintained that the septum may be especially important as concerns the impulse transmission to the hippocampus (Green and Arduini, 1954; and others). This fits in with the results of anatomical studies (see Raisman, 1966a). The hippocampus has a very low seizure threshold and the relation of hippocampal activity to epileptic seizures has attracted considerable interest.

Workers studying the *effects of stimulations or lesions of the hippocampus* have reported changes in several functions, chiefly visceral and endocrine and certain behavioral changes. Many of the latter occur in the field of sexual and reproductive behavior. It appears that the connections with the hypothalamus are especially involved. The hippocampus appears

[15] For a critical review, see Douglas (1967).

further to be related in some way to the release of hormones from the anterior lobe of the pituitary gland (for some references see Green, 1964). Kaada, Jansen, Jr., and Andersen (1953) in unanesthetized cats found that on stimulation of the hippocampus the animals performed quick glancing or searching movements to the contralateral side. Their facial expression indicated "attention," associated with some bewilderment and anxiety. Their reaction to external stimuli was decreased and their attention appeared to be intensely fixed on "something" in the environment which they seemed to experience. Corresponding observations have been made by other authors. The responses are frequently described as betraying "orientation," "hallucinations," "defensive behavior," and "arrest."

Behavioral responses, similar to those mentioned above have been noted also following lesions or stimulations of other parts of the brain, especially regions considered to belong to the "rhinencephalon" (taken in various senses), such as the amygdaloid nucleus (see below). As mentioned previously, when evaluating the findings reported, the complex fiber connections and the difficulties involved in producing isolated lesions or stimulations of the hippocampus should be kept in mind. Green (1964, p. 591) is ". . . tempted to discount many of the results of rhinencephalic lesions and stimulation on the score that they represent spread of activity to other more relevant regions." Nevertheless, the available observations furnish strong evidence that the hippocampus cannot be particularly closely related to any special and relatively simple function. Apparently it is involved in various behavioral reactions to a variety of stimuli, and performs a function of the kind often called "integrative." In recent years this view has received some support from observations which indicate that the hippocampus is involved in processes such as remembering and learning. This is a field where little is known, and where —as usual in such situations—speculations flourish. Semantic difficulties concerning the concepts of "memory" and "learning" contribute to the confusion. Only a few points of clinical relevance will be mentioned here.

Glees and Griffith (1952) reported loss of recent memory and progressive dementia in a patient whose brain at autopsy showed extensive bilateral destruction of the hippocampus and gyrus hippocampi. Since then other cases have been published in which *loss of recent memory has been observed following bilateral lesions or ablations of the hippocampus* with more or less concomitant involvement of neighboring structures (Scoville and Milner, 1957; Victor et al., 1961; Drachman and Arbit, 1966; and others). In most cases studied there has been no loss of old memories or deterioration in personality or general intelligence. The degree of memory deficit was concluded by Scoville and Milner (1957) to vary in proportion to the extent of removal. Some experimental studies in animals have been performed and in general interpreted as supporting the above notion (Kaada, Wulff Rasmussen, and Kveim, 1961; Thompson, Langer, and Rich, 1964, in rats; Stepien, Cordeau, and Rasmussen, 1960; Drachman and Ommaya, 1964, in the monkey; and others). According to Penfield and Milner (1958), in man, unilateral partial temporal lobectomy, including the hippocampus, hippocampal gyrus with the uncus, as well as the amygdaloid nucleus, does not cause any serious psychological impairment if the other temporal lobe is functioning normally. (There may be some difficulty in learning and retention which is specific to verbal material if the dominant temporal lobe is resected.) However, in two of several patients treated in this way for epilepsy, there was a grave and persistent loss of memory for recent events. There is evidence that in these cases there was a destructive lesion in the unoperated temporal lobe, probably due to injury at the time of birth. Victor et al. (1961) suggest that the total amount of destruction of both hippocampi taken together, regardless of whether it is bilateral or unilateral, decides the appearance and degree of loss of recent memory.

Loss of recent memory is a conspicuous and characteristic component in the *Korsakoff syndrome,* also called the "amnestic confabulatory syndrome." In addition to loss of recent memory (for example, the patient does not remember having seen the doctor half an hour ago, what he has had for dinner, etc.) there is often a tendency to confusion and to fabrication. The syndrome is most commonly seen in chronic alcoholism (where deficient supply of thiamine plays an etiological role). It may occur as an element in the so-called Wernicke's polio-encephalitis hemorrhagica superior, or following head injuries, or in cases of tumors at the base of the brain involving the floor of the third ventricle (see Williams and Pennybacker, 1954). In the majority of cases of Korsakoff's syndrome where post-mortem studies have been performed, the mammillary bodies have been found to be affected, showing vascular, inflammatory, traumatic, or degenerative changes according to the disease process (for a brief review see Barbizet, 1963). The regular occurrence of loss of recent memory in Korsakoff's syndrome is of special interest since a large proportion of the hippocampal efferents end in the mammillary bodies. This has been taken to indicate that the hippocampus-fornix-mammillary body are all involved in the processes underlying recent memory.

When evaluating the current view that the hippocampus is essential for recent memory the following facts should be recalled: in none of the human cases described and in no experimental studies has there been isolated damage to the hippocampus, but neighboring regions, especially parts of the hippocampal gyrus, have always been involved. In cases of

Korsakoff's syndrome there are often other changes in addition to those in the mammillary bodies. Some cases of bilateral transection of the fornix in man have been reported in which no defects in recent memory have been found (for references see Victor et al., 1961). Congenital maldevelopment of the hippocampus with absence of the fornix may occur without defects in memory (Nathan and Smith, 1950). While these and other observations do not invalidate the assumption that the hippocampus is concerned in what we call recent memory (see below), there is still no proof that this function is specific to the hippocampus.[16] It has been suggested by some that the ring of connections (hippocampus-mammillary bodies-anterior thalamic nucleus-cingulate gyrus-hippocampus), assumed by Papez (1937) to be part of the basis of emotional processes, may be related to memory mechanisms. Many theories on the mechanisms and the structural basis of memory and learning have been set forth. They will not be considered here (for some references see Green, 1964; Drachman and Arbit, 1966). A few comments on "recent memory" may, however, be appropriate.

The term "recent memory" used above is rather imprecise. In general, loss of recent memory is said to be present when the patient is unable to establish lasting new memories, even if he can remember relatively small amounts of information for seconds or minutes *if he is not distracted* (see Douglas, 1967). It appears as if the patient is unable to "store" the new information, while that stored in the past is retained. This defect prevents learning and as time passes gives rise to a retrograde amnesia of increasing length.[17] Barbizet (1963) in a lucid account describes this as follows (p. 128): "Such patients who no longer fix the present live constantly in a past which preceded the onset of their illness." According to Barbizet the basic disorder in the defect of memorizing "is the impossibility of using present stimuli in a delayed manner so as to memorize them for integration into the whole sum of past acquirements" (loc. cit., p. 132). A similar view is expressed by Douglas (1967). Like several other authors Barbizet is inclined to believe that there are different structures in the brain responsible for the capacity to memorize and the preservation of old memories. The retention of old information seems to require "the integrity of the neuronal, cortical, and subcortical areas which support memorized activities, say praxic, gnostic or motor skill, or to put it in a different way, sensory, intellectual or motor" (loc. cit., p. 133). Among these structures the cerebral cortex is presumably of particular importance. Various regions appear to be predominantly concerned in remembering and learning according to the kind of information involved (visual, acoustic, tactile, etc.). A vast literature has grown up on the subject of learning, but little is so far clear concerning the processes involved

---

[16] Whitty and Lewin (1960) noted a transient Korsakoff syndrome in eight patients following bilateral ablation of the anterior part of the cingulate gyrus (see Ch. 12).

[17] The period of retrograde amnesia following bilateral hippocampal lesions may vary from days to years. The subject of shrinking retrograde amnesia has recently been treated by Benson and Geschwind (1967).

531

and the parts of the brain engaged, except that such processes must engage extensive parts of the brain (see also Ch. 12). In a recent lucid review Douglas (1967) discusses the relation of the hippocampus to behavior and memory and attempts to explain the contradictory observations made in animal studies.

The amygdaloid nucleus, or *nucleus amygdalae,* has got its name from its resemblance to an almond. Its position was mentioned previously. The nucleus has been described in a series of mammals (for references see Brodal, 1947c). In man it is found immediately underneath the uncus (see Fig. 10-2). In all animal species studied the amygdaloid nucleus can be subdivided into a number of cell groups or subnuclei, differing in architecture. The general pattern is similar in all mammals, even if there are differences in details. In a simplified manner a distinction can be made between a *corticomedial* and a *basolateral group of nuclei.* (In addition there are some minor cell groups and transitional areas which will not be considered here.) In the phylogenesis of mammals the basolateral group (containing the basal and lateral nuclei) increases progressively and is especially well developed in man (see Crosby and Humphrey, 1941; Allison, 1954). The corticomedial group (containing the medial, central, and cortical nuclei) is relatively small in man. These differences in size are related to the connections and functions of the two main subdivisions.

The *fiber connections of the amygdaloid nucleus* are rather complex and still insufficiently known. This is true especially as concerns the efferent projections, on account of the difficulties in studying separately the origin of fibers from the various subdivisions. The data available, however, strongly indicates that the various subdivisions of the amygdaloid nucleus have their particular patterns of connections and accordingly are scarcely functionally identical. Only some major features will be considered in the following.

Afferents to the amygdaloid nucleus come from several sources. It has already been mentioned that *fibers from the olfactory bulb* terminate only in the corticomedial group (Fig. 10-2), as determined experimentally (Le Gros Clark and Meyer, 1947; Powell, Cowan, and Raisman, 1965; Scalia, 1966, in the rabbit; Meyer and Allison, 1949, in the monkey; Adey, 1953, in a marsupial). A projection to the central nucleus is questioned (see Lohman, 1963; Cowan, Raisman, and Powell, 1965). It appears likely that the terminal areas are similar in man (Allison, 1954). Physiologically responses to olfactory stimulation have been recorded in the corticomedial group (see Gloor, 1960). The basolateral group has been found to receive fibers from the entire *piriform cortex* (Powell, Cowan, and Raisman, 1965). In this way the basolateral group may be influenced indirectly by olfactory impulses. Other afferents have been

532

reported as well, for example from "nonspecific" thalamic nuclei (Powell and Cowan, 1954), the hypothalamus (Cowan, Raisman, and Powell, 1965) and from certain regions of the neocortex (Whitlock and Nauta, 1956), but many of them are rather uncertain. (Some of these afferents may supply also the medial group.) In physiological studies potentials with relatively short latency have been recorded from the basolateral group of the amygdaloid nucleus following stimulation of various kinds of sensory afferents, somatosensory, auditory, and visual (Machne and Segundo, 1956; Wendt and Albe-Fessard, 1962; and others). The pathways concerned are not known. Wendt and Albe-Fessard (1962) on the basis of electrophysiological studies suggest that the impulses arising on somatosensory stimulation pass via the VPL of the thalamus and the cortical area S II, from which there appear to be projections to the amygdala.

The *efferent projections from the amygdaloid nuclear complex* have been studied by several anatomists, and conclusions as to these connections have been drawn also from physiological studies. It is generally agreed that a fair number of efferent fibers from the amygdala pass anteriorly in the *stria terminalis* (Fig. 10-2), a macroscopically visible fiber bundle which pursues a curved course along the medial surface of the caudate nucleus in the lateral ventricle. Some fibers descend anterior, others posterior to the anterior commissure, and are distributed to *the septal nuclei, the preoptic area, the anterior hypothalamus,* and some minor nuclear groups. Other fibers pass to *the habenula* via the stria medullaris. Not all fibers from the amygdaloid nucleus follow the stria terminalis. Fibers have been described which run medial to *the olfactory tubercle* and neighboring regions or pass to *the thalamus.* Others take a caudal course to *the mesencephalon,* while still others are assumed to pass anteriorly in the longitudinal association bundle of the hemisphere. In a recent experimental study in the monkey by Nauta (1961) the various efferent pathways listed above as not passing in the stria terminalis are collectively referred to as the *ventral amygdalofugal pathways,* and their considerable volume is stressed. Some authors have advocated the existence of fibers from the amygdala to the piriform cortex, temporal cortex, and the cingulate gyrus. Finally there are commissural connections between the nuclei of the two sides.

The above summary gives an impression of the complexity in the efferent projections of the amygdaloid nuclei. It appears likely that the individual subnuclei have their more or less specific projections. However, the reports on this subject in the literature are rather confusing. (Among recent papers may be mentioned those of Ban and Omukai, 1959; Nauta, 1961, 1962; Hall, 1963; Valverde, 1963; Cowan, Raisman, and Powell,

1965.) This presumably is due to difficulties in producing lesions restricted to one nucleus and to the fact that fibers from one subnucleus pass through others. In addition fibers coming from the piriform cortex pass through the amygdaloid complex and will be involved in the lesions.

Some students advocate that the *stria terminalis* originates chiefly from the basal nuclei (Adey and Meyer, 1952b; Nauta, 1961; Hall, 1963), while Fox (1943) concluded that most fibers of the stria come from the corticomedial group. The latter observation agrees with the physiological study of Gloor (1955). According to Cowan, Raisman, and Powell (1965) both groups give off fibers to the stria. These authors as well as Nauta (1961) found that the fibers of the stria supply chiefly the preoptic and anterior hypothalamic region. Fibers in the *ventral amygdalofugal pathway* do not come from the corticomedial group (Cowan, Raisman, and Powell, 1965). The origin of fibers from the amygdaloid nucleus has apparently not been studied by means of the method of retrograde degeneration, except for commissural connections which pass in the anterior commissure.[18] In the rat these fibers were found to come chiefly from the cortical and medial amygdaloid nuclei (Brodal, 1948).

Among the terminations of the projections from the amygdaloid nucleus fibers passing to the *thalamus* have recently attracted particular interest. In the monkey this projection appears to have been observed first by Fox (1949) and confirmed by Nauta (1961). The projection has been described in the cat by Valverde (1963), while it was not seen in this animal by Fox (1943) and Hall (1963) and not found electrophysiologically by Gloor (1955). The fibers from the amygdala have been found to end in the mediodorsal thalamic nucleus (MD). This is generally subdivided into three parts, and according to Nauta (1961) the fibers from the amygdala end in the medial magnocellular part which projects onto the orbitofrontal cortex (Pribram, Chow, and Semmes, 1953, in the monkey). This amygdalo-orbitofrontal pathway may be supplemented by fibers to the hypothalamus since it has been claimed that there is a projection from this onto the medial thalamic nucleus, but the evidence for this appears to be inconclusive.

Even if many features in the connections of the amygdaloid nucleus are still far from clear, there appears on the whole to be some evidence that this nuclear complex (like so many others) has reciprocal connection with the areas to which it sends its fibers. Cowan, Raisman, and Powell (1965) stress the reciprocal amygdalohypothalamic relationships, while Nauta (1962) puts special emphasis on the circuit amygdala-dorsomedial thalamic nucleus-orbitofrontotemporal cortex-amygdala, and

[18] The anterior commissure is a complex fiber system. In addition to the amygdaloid component and the fibers interconnecting the olfactory bulbs, mentioned before, it contains commissural fibers between the piriform cortex, the entorhinal area, the temporal cortex, and some other regions.

upon the less direct relations to the mesencephalon by various neuronal links. These and other circuits have played some role in the attempts to interpret the manifold effects observed following stimulations or lesions of the amygdaloid nuclei, but it must be admitted that this is still a field chiefly for speculations. The various theories and hypotheses set forth will not be considered here, but brief mention will be made of some of the many physiological observations (for a review, see Gloor, 1960).

Function of the amygdaloid nucleus. Numerous experimental studies and some observations on man have yielded some information on this subject, but the literature abounds with conflicting statements (for a review see Gloor, 1960). Following electrical *stimulation* of the amygdaloid nucleus in unanesthetized animals a variety of *responses in the motor and vegetative spheres* have been recorded: arrest of spontaneous ongoing movements ("arrest reaction"); inhibition or facilitation of spinal reflexes and cortically evoked movements; contraversive turning movements of head and eyes; complex rhythmic movements related to eating, such as swallowing, licking, and chewing; changes in respiration and cardiovascular functions; inhibition or activation of gastric motility and secretion; micturition and defecation; uterine contractions; pupillary dilatation; piloerection, etc. Many of these responses appear to be merely components in more complex *behavioral reactions* which can be elicited in unanesthetized animals by stimulation in or near the amygdaloid nucleus. Kaada (1951) and Kaada, Andersen, and Jansen, Jr. (1954), as well as others, in cats, noted the appearance of searching movements to the contralateral side with facial expressions of attention with some bewilderment and anxiety, sometimes fear or anger. This has been called the "attention response." It is accompanied by EEG desynchronization (Ursin and Kaada, 1960). In continued studies it has been shown that the attention response always precedes certain behavior patterns indicating emotional changes which may be obtained on stimulation of the amygdala. These reactions may be of two kinds, generally referred to as fear and anger, respectively. In the "fear response" the searching movements become more rapid, there are anxious glancing movements, the animal becomes restless and finally runs away and hides. In the "anger response" there is growling and hissing and piloerection. The rage or anger seems to be directed toward something imaginary. The former response may perhaps more adequately be referred to as the "flight response," the latter as the "defense reaction" (see Kaada, 1967).

The question whether different neural structures are related to the various kinds of responses has been studied in cats. Kaada, Andersen, and Jansen, Jr. (1954) found that the autonomic responses and chewing, sniffing, licking, as well as tonic and clonic movements were elicited mainly on stimulation of the corticomedial group of nuclei, which receive olfactory fibers. The affective responses and the attention response occurred mainly on stimulation of the basolateral group. In continued studies Ursin and Kaada (1960) and Ursin (1965) outlined topographically separate zones as being more particularly related to either fear (flight) or anger (defense) responses. Other authors, however, found little evidence of a separation of this kind.

The results of isolated *destructions of the amygdaloid nucleus* or parts of it are even less clear-cut than the observations in stimulation experiments (see Gloor, 1960; Kaada, 1967). Most often an increased tameness has been reported to follow destruction of the amygdala (which has to be bilateral). Ursin (1965) found a specific reduction of the flight response without loss of defense behavior following lesions restricted to the "flight zones."

Observations in man which may elucidate the function of the amygdala are relatively scanty and in part contradictory. We will return briefly to this subject when considering the symptoms of damage to the temporal lobe in a following section. However, stimulation of the amygdala in conscious patients (undertaken as a diagnostic procedure in the treatment of epilepsy of temporal lobe origin, "psychomotor epilepsy") has often been observed to give rise to a sensation of fear, as often occurs at the start of an epileptic seizure of this type (see Penfield and Jasper, 1954).

It appears from the observations mentioned above that *the amygdala is functionally related to emotional experiences and reactions. However, it is not alone concerned in these functions.* There is convincing evidence that the hypothalamus is also involved (see Ch. 11); lesions of the septum have been reported to result in aggressive behavior; bilateral ablation of area 24 is said to produce increased tameness and reduced aggressiveness; the mesencephalic gray matter on stimulation may give rage reactions (see Gloor, 1960; Delgado, 1964; Kaada, 1967, for references). As has been described in a previous section, all these regions of the brain are more or less directly interconnected by fibers, making it understandable that they are functionally related. It may perhaps be surmised that the amygdaloid nucleus is more of an integrative center for these functions than the lower ones (see, for example, Fernandez de Molina and Hunsperger, 1962). When evaluating the experimental results it should be recalled that the behavioral reactions elicited from the amygdala are in fact extremely complex processes. Like other behavioral actions they develop over a certain time and consist of sequences of reactions. As emphasized by Delgado (1964, p. 436) in a review: "Electrical stimulation of the brain is a rather crude procedure, and to explain the finesse, co-ordination and drive of many of the evoked reactions, it is necessary

536

to assume the activation of physiological mechanisms." Many behavioral reactions appearing on stimulation of the amygdala and other parts of the brain show considerable flexibility in response to changes in the external circumstances (just as is the case with corresponding reactions in normal animals). This has become especially clear in studies where electrically induced behavioral reactions are produced by implanted electrodes set in action by remote control. The animal can then be watched when free to move under fairly normal circumstances, for instance among fellow animals. Interactions of various kinds between spontaneous and induced behavior have been observed under these circumstances as discussed by Delgado (1964). This author points to the need for precise criteria for definition and classification of behavior and stresses the importance of considering individual variations among animals, anatomically as well as physiologically. A serious difficulty is further presented by the restricted possibilities of performing stimulation of discrete anatomical units without spread of current to neighboring structures or stimulation of passing fibers. Finally a precise anatomical identification of the stimulus site is necessary.

The above considerations apply also to the studies of behavioral changes occurring on stimulation of the amygdaloid nuclei. When different reactions (flight or aggressive behavior) can be elicited preferentially from different regions this does not necessarily mean that there are separate neural substrates. Much work has been devoted especially to identifying structures related to aggressive behavior.[19] Many theories have been set forth. When considered from the anatomical point of view, theories assuming complex actions to be mediated by extensive collaboration of many parts of the brain appear, a priori, most plausible.[20] In fact, all the reactions that can be elicited from the amygdaloid nucleus can be obtained also from other regions of the brain.

The "limbic system."   Reference has been made to this term previously. A perusal of neurological, especially neurophysiological, periodicals from the last fifteen years shows that "limbic system" occurs in the headings of an increasing number of papers. The contents of the term seem to be steadily expanding, but a generally accepted definition of the "limbic system" appears never to have been given.

As far as can be judged from the literature the concept of a "limbic

[19] For some recent data see "Aggression and Defense," 1967.

[20] Delgado (1964) suggests a working hypothesis of fragmental organization of behavior: "Behavioral categories are formed by a series of fragments which have anatomical and functional bases inside the cerebral organization. Single behavioral fragments form part of different behavioral categories and may have a different functional meaning" (loc. cit., p. 437).

system" originates from the term the "limbic lobe," introduced in the nomenclature mainly on the basis of comparative anatomical studies. Unfortunately, there is no unanimously accepted definition of the "limbic lobe." The name is often credited to Broca who in 1878 spoke of *"le grand lobe limbique."* It was conceived of as a ring of gray matter bordering the hemisphere against the central parts of the brain and arranged in a circular manner around the interventricular foramen. The distinction between the "limbic lobe" and "rhinencephalon" is far from clear. (For a historical review see White, Jr., 1965b.) Most authors include in the limbic lobe the following structures: the cingulate gyrus and the induseum griseum, the hippocampus and dentate gyrus, the subiculum, presubiculum, parasubiculum, the entorhinal area, the prepiriform cortex, the septum, the olfactory tubercle, the medial and cortical amygdaloid nucleus, and some minor gray masses. Other authors extend the term to cover in adition other structures, such as the subcallosal gyrus, the posterior orbital cortex in the frontal lobe, the anterior insula, and the temporal polar region, in part on the basis of cytoarchitectonic resemblances to the allocortex. Even if the various regions listed above have in common that they appear early in phylogenesis, their finer structural organization differs considerably. *It is difficult to see that the lumping together of these different regions under one anatomical heading, "the limbic lobe," serves any purpose* (except for illustrating the truth of Goethe's words, quoted in the Preface!).

It is even less justifiable to speak of a "limbic system." This concept is even more diffuse than that covered by the term "limbic lobe." The "limbic system" appears to be a phrase used collectvely for functions attributed to the "limbic lobe," under the tacit assumption that those parts of the brain which have been given a particular collective name by the old anatomists form part of one functional "system." Even if stimulation or ablation of various of these regions have in part given corresponding results, it is becoming increasingly evident, as Kaada (1960, p. 1346) has emphasized, that: ."Recent anatomical and physiological research rather tends to fractionate the 'limbic system' into several units with quite different projections and functional significance." On the other hand, as research progresses it becomes increasingly difficult to separate functionally different regions of the brain. The borderlines between "functional systems" become more and more diffuse. This is in complete accord with the outcome of studies of the fiber connections, and is especially evident from behavioral studies undertaken with modern methods. The "limbic system" appears to be on its way to including all brain functions.[21] As this process continues the value of the term as a useful concept is correspondingly reduced.

[21] See, for example, *Structure and Function of the Limbic System,* 1967.

For the reasons given above it is the author's opinion that *the use of the terms "limbic lobe" and "limbic system" should be abandoned*. For the same reasons no attempt will be made to discuss these subjects here, the more so since correlations of functional observations and anatomical data can only be made to a limited extent. Some of the observations made on particular brain regions belonging to the "system" have been considered in the present chapter; reference to some others has been made occasionally at other places in the text. Several of the general considerations made when discussing data from the hippocampus and the amygdala may be applied to other brain regions which are included as being part of the structural basis of the "limbic system."

Some functional aspects of the central olfactory structures. The regions of the brain considered in this chapter, although all are often listed as parts of the "rhinencephalon" or "limbic system," differ in important respects anatomically and functionally. They are not all related to smell. Several functional aspects have been considered in the preceding sections. Some additional data, particularly with reference to the sense of olfaction will be mentioned.

In fishes and amphibians the sense of smell is of supreme importance. It is essential for informing the animal of approaching enemies as well as in guiding it to its food and mates. With the increasing differentiation of the other senses in the vertebrate phylum, smell loses this supremacy. However, even in man, the capacity to discriminate between smells of different types is a factor of some importance in his reaction to food and drink as well as in his sexual behavior. The widespread use of perfumes in civilized and primitive communities points to the importance of smell for man, and the connoisseurs of perfumes have noted many peculiar relationships between special odors and their psychological effect.

From a clinical point of view the olfactory reflexes are of minor interest. The cortical aspect of olfactory function, however, is of some importance. Animal experiments have given some information on this point. Decorticate cats (i.e. cats in which the entire neocortex has been removed and only the thalamus and striatum are left in connection with the paleo- and archicortex) suffer no marked reduction in their olfactory capacity. They are still in possession of the usual feeding reflexes (Dusser de Barenne, 1933). Even with rather extensive damage to the paleo- and archicortex, highly complicated feeding reflexes are present (Bard and McK. Rioch, 1937). It appears that most of the olfactory reflexes are mediated through subcortical structures. According to Allen's classical studies conditioned positive and negative reactions established to agreeable and disagreeable smells, respectively, are not abolished after bilateral extirpation of the hippocampus (Allen, 1940), but the correct differential response is lost when the piriform cortex is also ablated, although the elementary reflexes persist (Allen, 1941). These findings tend to show that the piriform lobe is essential for the discrimination of smells of different kinds, a finding in harmony with the anatomical features.

On the whole, the relatively sparse data on the human brain is in agreement with experimental observations. In conscious human beings stimulation of the olfactory bulb is followed by olfactory sensations, whereas electrical stimulation of the hippocampus yields no response at all (Penfield and Erickson, 1941). Olfactory sensations occurring in the so-called uncinate fits, to be considered below, appear to be associated with lesions of the uncus and the hippocampal gyrus, but not with lesions of the hippocampus. In patients suffering from epileptic fits a marked cell loss is frequent in the hippocampus, but there is no decisive evidence that these changes are responsible for the disturbances of smell which occasionally may occur in these patients as well as in others.[22]

The examination of the sense of smell.   Before the symptoms following lesions of the olfactory structures of the brain in man are considered, it is appropriate to consider the examination of the sense of smell. Just as in examination of other sensory functions the co-operation of the patient is essential, and the results, therefore, are dependent on his intellectual level, and to a certain extent also his particular familiarity with various odors. It is, therefore, of importance in testing to choose odors which are known by most persons if comparisons have to be made, since it is extremely difficult to describe a particular smell without reference to some object or circumstance commonly associated with it. The patient should not be allowed to recognize the test substances, for example by sight or by feel prior to its application. The odor should be applied to one nostril at a time, and it should always be made certain that local affections of the nasal cavity which interfere with the perception are not present. It is well known that a common cold reduces the olfactory acuity, and this reduction has been shown by Elsberg, Brewer, and Levy (1935) to be present in a decreasing degree for several weeks. The selection of test odors should be made with due consideration of the fact that certain odors have a marked capacity of irritating the mucous membrane and, therefore, are as much trigeminal as olfactory irritants.

In the routine examination smell is usually tested simply by letting the patient inhale vapors of different odor separately by each nostril. This, however, is a rather crude method and as a rule permits only the statement that smell appears normal, or that there is some degree of hyposmia

---

[22] The cell loss is usually found only in part of the hippocampus (Sommer's sector). There has been much discussion of whether these changes are of etiological significance for the epileptic manifestations or whether they are secondary, due to vascular changes occurring during the seizures (see Meyer, 1957).

or that anosmia is present. Several methods have been suggested to obtain a more accurate test. A method worked out by Elsberg and collaborators (Elsberg and Levy, 1935), allows a quantitative determination of olfactory acuity.

Graded quantities of odorous air are injected into the nostrils (monorhinal or birhinal), and the minimal quantity necessary for recognition of the smell is determined. By this "blast injection method" the variable factor of the force of inspiration in sniffing is avoided (the patient holds his breath during the injection), and the quantity of air acting on the olfactory epithelium can be changed at will. The values for the individual odors appear to be approximately the same in different individuals. By applying a continuous stream of odorous air for a certain time, the olfactory fatigue can be determined ("stream injection method"). The method has been used to advantage by others, and its diagnostic value further examined. It is particularly important to be aware of the physiological variations of the threshold values (see Zilstorff-Pedersen, 1964).

If the olfactory epithelium is subjected to a certain smell for a time, as is well known, the individual ceases to perceive it. This fatigue appears to be a central process, since it is increased in central lesions which do not affect the olfactory bulb or tracts (Elsberg, 1935; Elsberg and Spotnitz, 1942). With lesions in the latter parts there is no increased fatigability, but the olfactory acuity is reduced, larger amounts of the odorous substances being required to elicit olfactory impressions. The reduction of olfactory acuity does not necessarily affect the perception of all types of olfactory stimuli, but may be limited to certain qualities of smell.[23] Several other interesting features have also been brought out by these investigations. For example, the olfactory fatigue seen in central lesions is homolateral to the side of the lesion. This tends to show that the bulk of afferent impulses from the olfactory bulb are transmitted to the homolateral half of the brain, and this is in good accord with knowledge of the olfactory pathways.

Olfactory disturbances in lesions of the nervous system. Apart from signs of loss of function of the olfactory structures, irritative symptoms may also occur, but it appears that symptoms of this type have as yet only been observed in the so-called uncinate fits. The more important deficiency symptoms will be treated first.

A *destruction* or a damage leading to interruption of conductive capacity of *the olfactory bulb or tract* may be caused by various processes. *Cranial fractures,* involving the cribriform lamina of the ethmoid bone are not uncommonly responsible for bilateral or unilateral anosmia or hyposmia. The fine olfactory fibers will easily be damaged in their passage

[23] The "fatigue" referred to above may in part be due to adaptation. According to Adrian (1950b) this depends on changes in the olfactory bulb and not in the receptors.

through the bone by the accompanying bleeding or the ensuing scar formation and callus production. It is worth emphasizing, however, that also in cases where no fracture is ascertained, a *closed head injury* may be followed by transient or permanent impairment of smell. The anatomical causes may be traction of the nerve and fibers, or a secondary damage due to bleeding, or even undiagnosed fractures. For a recent extensive account of post-traumatic anosmia see Sumner (1964).

The olfactory bulb and tract will frequently be affected by *tumors* in the anterior cranial fossa. Most consistently this will occur in the *meningeomas arising from the olfactory grove,* in which case unilateral hyposmia or anosmia will be the initial symptom, frequently, however, not noticed by the patient. It is only later on, when the growing tumor causes more alarming symptoms, such as visual disturbances with scotomas and optic atrophy, or when mental changes develop on account of involvement of the frontal lobe, that the disease is discovered. In this stage the anosmia will frequently be bilateral, since the tumor will affect both olfactory lobes or tracts. Other tumors which not infrequently are accompanied by impairment of the sense of smell are the *suprasellar meningeomas,* or those arising from the ala parva of the sphenoid bone. These may give unilateral or bilateral olfactory loss according to their site and size. *Osteomas* from the frontal bone (orbital lamina) may also encroach upon the olfactory bulb or tract. Likewise *diseases of the frontal lobe, gliomas or abscesses,* will sooner or later exert a pressure on these structures. Since the destruction of the frontal lobe may be considerable before clear-cut symptoms are marked, the affection of smell may be a valuable guide in the diagnosis. Finally *hypophyseal tumors* should be remembered, although they will affect the olfactory bulb or tract only when they transcend the sella, and as a rule bilaterally. Occasionally *aneurysms of the internal carotid,* if of the anterior type, may affect the olfactory bulb or tract. In all cases mentioned above there will be a reduction of olfactory acuity, but no increased fatigability, according to Elsberg (1936) (except when the processes affect also the interior of the frontal lobe).

It is not known whether lesions of the anterior perforated space and the adjacent regions are followed by particular olfactory symptoms, but as a rule lesions of these structures will be associated with damage of the olfactory tract. The impairment of smell found in some cases of *increased intracranial pressure* without evidence of local damage to the olfactory structures should be mentioned, although it is difficult to explain satisfactorily. The *hysterical anosmia* should be borne in mind as a source of error. In this case, as a rule, also odors which have a marked trigeminal component are said not to be recognized, whereas a patient suffering from an organic anosmia usually will perceive the trigeminal component.

542

From an analysis of the anatomical and physiological data available, it might be assumed that lesions of the temporal lobe, and more particularly the gyrus hippocampi, would result in defects in olfactory discrimination and interpretation. However, cases sufficiently clear-cut to decide these matters appear not to have been observed.

The most decisive evidence that the cortex of the hippocampal gyrus is concerned in perception or even interpretation of olfactory impressions appears to come from the observation of olfactory "hallucinations" in some cases with lesions of this region. Following the original description by Hughlings Jackson and Beevor in 1890 of a lesion limited to the uncus (see Fig. 10-3) and adjoining parts of the amygdaloid nucleus giving rise to a peculiar disturbance called by Jackson "uncinate fits," a considerable number of similar cases has been observed. The olfactory sensations which the patients experience in these fits are usually of a disagreeable character, and may be accompanied by movements of the lips and tongue (smacking, etc.) and quite frequently also by a so-called "dreamy state," which, however, may ocur without olfactory disturbances in cases of epilepsy. The uncinate fits are regarded as representing a variety of epilepsy; and it appears reasonable to consider the olfactory sensations in the same manner as the other sensory phenomena occurring in epileptic seizures elicited from other sensory areas (visual, acoustic, and sensory) as due to irritation of the olfactory cortex. An uncinate fit may be produced by stimulation of the uncus (Penfield and Kristiansen, 1951).

The "dreamy state" is characterized by the patient having a feeling that things seem unreal as in a dream. He appears to lose contact with his environment. Frequently he tells afterward that during the attack he had the feeling that he had experienced the same situation before, although this cannot have been the case. These psychic phenomena are probably due to the spread of the irritation to other areas of the cerebral cortex (the "highest levels" of Jackson). An uncinate attack may be followed by a generalized seizure, in which case the uncinate attack represents an aura.

Although uncinate fits are most often seen with lesions of the uncus and hippocampal gyrus, they may be observed also in cases where these structures are not directly damaged, but are affected by pressure, for example by tumors in other parts of the temporal lobe.

Symptoms in lesions of the temporal lobe. Some of these have been mentioned previously, for example, homonymous anopsias due to affection of the optic radiation (Ch. 8), the occurrence of an acoustic aura in epileptic fits originating from the superior temporal gyrus and aphasic symptoms, and certain disturbances in auditory functions in affections of this gyrus (Ch. 9). (The disturbances in speech mechanisms will be briefly discussed in Ch. 12.) The uncinate fits were mentioned above.

The bewildering occurrence of ipsilateral hemiparesis in cases of tumors in the temporal lobe should be recalled. When the tumor reaches a certain size, it will push the brain stem to the other side, and the contralateral cerebral peduncle will be compressed against the edge of the tentorium. (Since this takes place above the crossing of the descending fibers in the peduncle the pareses will appear on the side of the lesion.)

Certain disturbances are usually observed only in *bilateral lesions of the temporal lobe.* This is the case with loss of recent memory described above, presumably due to destruction of the hippocampus. Bilateral, more or less symmetrical lesions of the temporal lobe are rare in man. Studies of the consequences of bilateral temporal lobe ablations in experimental animals have, however, been performed by several authors, following the description by Klüver and Bucy (1937, and later) of what is often called, after them, the Klüver-Bucy syndrome.

The Klüver-Bucy syndrome comprises a number of symptoms. There is *visual agnosia:* the animal appears to have lost the ability to recognize and detect the meaning of objects on the basis of visual criteria alone. The animal shows *"oral tendencies,"* a tendency to examine all objects by mouth. There is *"hypermetamorphosis,"* a tendency to pay attention to every visual stimulus. There are changes in *emotional behavior,* an absence of emotional responses. There is a striking increase in *sexual activities* and in the diversity of sexual manifestations. Finally there are conspicuous changes in *dietary habits.* Similar symptoms have been observed in man following bilateral temporal lobectomies (Terzian and Ore, 1955). Since in these lesions the hippocampus, the amygdala, and the hippocampal gyrus, as well as extensive parts of the neocortex are removed it might be surmised that the various symptoms are consequences of the ablation of particular structures. However, as stated by Klüver (1958, p. 177): "Intensive researches along behavioural, clinical, anatomical, and electrophysiological lines during the last twenty years have not settled the question of the particular anatomical structures related to each of the symptoms; they have also not settled the question whether the polysymptomatic picture results from a few fundamental alterations in behaviour or even from only one basic behaviour disturbance." It may perhaps be assumed that the involvement of the amygdala is particularly important in producing the changes in emotional behavior. The results of bilateral stereotaxic amygdalatomy in man (Narabayashi et al., 1963; and others) seem to lend some support to this view. However, following ablations in the monkey of the neocortical parts only of the temporal lobe (sparing the amygdala, gyrus hippocampi, and hippocampus) there develops a partial Klüver-Bucy syndrome, including emotional behavior changes, as shown by Akert et al. (1961). These authors emphasize the presence of connections between the neocortex and the phylogenetically older parts of the temporal lobe. These connections may explain that there are differences in degree only between "rhinencephalic" and "neotemporal" types of the Klüver-Bucy syndrome.

"Temporal lobe epilepsy" has attracted much interest in recent years. Epileptic seizures originating in the temporal lobe are relatively common. There are often special kinds of disturbances in consciousness, as an

initial symptom or during or after the seizure. Reference has been made to the occurrence of acoustic sensations as an aura (Ch. 9) and to olfactory sensations in the "uncinate fits." In other cases complex subjective psychic experiences are described as an aura, and it is common that during the attack the patient is unresponsive, and there is some degree of loss of understanding, even if motor control and reception of sensory stimuli are preserved. The patient may be able to carry out rather elaborate acts during the attack, but following it he has a complete amnesia for what has happened. These types of epileptic seizures are often called "psychomotor attacks," or "automatisms." [24] The accompanying EEG changes are often rather characteristic, and changes may be present between the overt attacks. Operative treatment by partial temporal lobectomy has given favorable results in many cases (see Penfield and Jasper, 1954). Most often the pathological changes appear to be of the atrophic type. The origin or focus eliciting the attacks has been assumed by many to be in the amygdaloid nucleus, and changes have been found in or near this nucleus (Falconer, Serafetinides, and Corsellis, 1964). Others consider changes in the hippocampus to be responsible in most cases (see, for example, Malamud, 1966). In view of the ample interconnections and functional interrelations between the different structures contained in the temporal lobe, it is not astonishing that approximately identical disturbances may result from an abnormal activity starting in almost any of these structures. The initial symptoms may in some instances point to the site of origin (for example olfactory sensations to the uncus). The occurrence of complex psychomotor disturbances especially in epilepsy originating from the temporal lobe, is in agreement with other observations which indicate that this part of the brain is important for some rather complex functions, such as comprehension of verbal symbols (see Ch. 12).

---

[24] Behavioral abnormalities between the attacks are found much more frequently in patients suffering from psychomotor epilepsy than in any of the other types. It has been suggested that this may be due to a continuous state of subictal irritation by the focus (see Gloor, 1960).

11

The Autonomic Nervous System The Hypothalamus

THE autonomic (vegetative or visceral) system is a part of the nervous system which has acquired a large and steadily growing importance in neurology as well as in several other clinical disciplines. Therefore it deserves considerable interest and a rather thorough description. Below, the most important anatomical features will be considered, as well as some of the more fundamental physiological observations, and finally some clinical findings in disturbances of the autonomic system will be dealt with.

Definition. Characteristics of the autonomic nervous system. Originally the concept autonomic or vegetative system comprised only structures found outside the central nervous system, i.e. the sympathetic trunk and the large nervous plexuses in the body cavities. Later the rami communicantes were discovered, and it was ascertained that certain cells of the brain stem and spinal cord sent their axons to the autonomic system. The delimitation of the latter then became less clear, and this was even more the case after the discovery of integrative autonomic centers in the diencephalon. Finally, the discovery that the cerebral cortex also influences the functions attributed to the autonomic system apparently makes any attempt at subdivision into cerebrospinal (somatic) and autonomic (visceral) systems futile. Only more general sweeping definitions of the autonomic system are possible, like that given by Greving (1928): "As autonomic nervous system the entire mass of those nerve cells and fibers is designated which are concerned in the innervation of the internal organs, in so far as these are made up of smooth muscles or belong to glandular organs. They subserve the regulation of processes which usually are not under voluntary influence." From a morphological point of view a feature characteristic of the autonomic nervous system should be emphasized: *The efferent conducting pathway from the central nervous system to the innervated organs is always constituted by two succeeding neurons, one preganglionic with its perikaryon in the central nervous system, and the other postganglionic with its perikaryon outside this.* The nerve cells within the central nervous system which are concerned with autonomic functions as a rule differ also morphologically from those subserving the somatic processes, and frequently are found arranged as definite cell groups or nuclei.

Commonly the autonomic nervous system is subdivided into two major parts, the *sympathetic* or orthosympathetic and the *parasympathetic*. This distinction, introduced by Langley on the basis of physiological studies applies mainly to the efferent components of the autonomic system. Whether a corresponding segregation can be made as concerns the afferent components is doubtful. It is common to speak of visceral afferent fibers and impulses only, thus avoiding the difficulty.

The preganglionic efferent neurons of the sympathetic nervous system in man have their perikarya in the spinal cord, more precisely in all the thoracic and the uppermost two lumbar segments. The preganglionic fibers in the parasympathetic system spring from perikarya situated in certain divisions of the brain stem and in the 3rd and 4th sacral segments of the cord. Synonymous designations for the sympathetic and parasympathetic system therefore are the *thoracolumbar* and *craniosacral* systems.

Another morphological difference between the two divisions of the autonomic system is seen in the position of the postganglionic perikarya. In the sympathetic system these are found in the vertebral and prevertebral ganglia. Those belonging to the parasympathetic are situated either in or on the walls of the organ they supply or in close proximity to it. From the anatomical arrangement of the sympathetic and parasympathetic it is also to be inferred that the former must be involved predominantly as a whole in diffuse reactions affecting the entire organism, whereas in the latter, the structural organization permits more restricted, localized effects. With certain qualifications this holds good.

In many instances these two systems exert an antagonistic influence: where one has a depressing, inhibitory effect on function, the other is stimulating, increasing, accelerating. Certain drugs act preferentially on one of the systems (thus atropine "paralyses" the parasympathetic, pilocarpine stimulates it). Furthermore, the two systems appear to be related to different hormones, noradrenaline being the specific sympathetic hormone, acetylcholine the parasympathetic. Dominated by these facts, conceptions of the autonomic system have shown a tendency to rigid schematization. However, advancing knowledge has made clear that great care must be taken in schematization, in this instance as in most others. The alleged antagonism between the sympathetic and the parasympathetic has especially proved to be far less absolute than originally assumed.[1] Both anatomical and physiological data opposing such a conception is available and a distinction is especially difficult as regards the higher levels of the autonomic centers. It is important to realize that the two divisions of the autonomic system in most instances collaborate, in spite of their partly antagonistic effect on various functions. Both of them take part in the intricate regulation of visceral functions, ensuring a proper adjustment of the functioning of the various organs. This influence is not limited only to adjusting them in regard to each other, but in regard to somatic functions as well. Thus, to take a single example, vasomotor changes, as is well known, are involved in the functional levels of activity of the striated skeletal (somatic) musculature. Correspondingly, the morphological delineation of structures subserving visceral and somatic functions becomes extremely difficult at the higher levels of the central nervous system, where the highest integrative "centers" for the visceral functions cannot be separated from structures involved in somatic integrative functions. Bearing these qualifications in mind, the customary subdivision of the autonomic system into a sympathetic and parasympathetic division may be upheld, and in the following description it will be utilized.

The autonomic preganglionic neurons in the spinal cord and brain stem. *The perikarya of the preganglionic sympathetic neurons,* as already mentioned, are found in all the thoracic and the two upper lumbar segments of the spinal cord.[2] Some authors assume that some of the cervical segments contribute also, but this appears to be a rare exception

---

[1] Particularly as concerns the eye and the bladder the sympathetic innervation appears to play a minor role. The varying parasympathetic tone almost alone determines the autonomic status.

[2] In other mammals upper and lower borders are not always identical with those in man. Confusion has arisen on this point because the number of thoracic, lumbar, and sacral segments of the cord varies in different species, a fact which has not always been considered when delimiting the sympathetic spinal outflow.

according to Wrete (1930), as well as to Pick and Sheehan (1946). Recently, however, Wiesman, Jones, and Randall (1966) have adduced evidence that in the dog and in man preganglionic sympathetic fibers arise in the lower cervical segments. The cells of origin form a distinct group in the lateral horn of the gray matter of the cord, the *intermediolateral cell column* (Fig. 11-1). This nucleus is composed of rather small nerve cells, considerably smaller than the motoneurons in the ventral horns. They are often gathered in small groups and vary in form, being either spindle-shaped or polygonal. The nucleus is relatively large, the nucleolus distinct. The rather scanty cytoplasm contains only finely dispersed tigroid granules. In this respect, also, these cells are clearly different from the motoneurons (cf. Fig. 11-1, a and b). The sympathetic nature of these cells was first suggested by a study of the retrograde changes following transection of the white rami communicantes (cf. below). The results, however, were not clearly convincing, as the cells are small and the difference between normal and changed cells is slight. The definite proof that these cells virtually send their axons through the ventral rami of the spinal nerves was afforded by the direct visualization of this fact in several animals (Bok, 1922; Poljak, 1924). From the ventral rami the axons pass through the white communicant rami, to be described below.

The *preganglionic fibers of the craniosacral, parasympathetic, sys-*

FIG. 11–1 Drawing of a Nissl-stained preparation from the thoracic spinal cord of man. To the right representative cells from the same section drawn with higher magnification. Note the differences between the somatic motoneurons from the ventral horn (*b*) and the visceral efferent cells from the intermediolateral cell column (*a*).

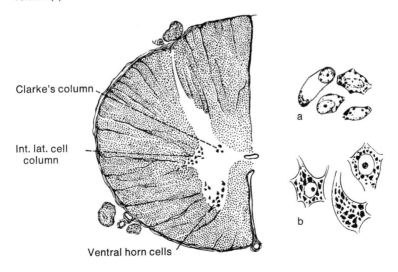

Clarke's column

Int. lat. cell column

a

b

Ventral horn cells

tem take origin from several nuclei in the brain stem and spinal cord. The preganglionic fibers in the *sacral division* come from cells of the same type as those in the intermedio-lateral column, located as a corresponding column in the (2nd), 3rd, and 4th segments.[3] The preganglionic fibers in the *cranial division* of the parasympathetic join some of the cranial nerves, constituting their general visceral efferent components (see Ch. 7). The perikarya of these fibers are groups of cells situated more or less in the proximity of the somatic efferent nuclei of the nerves. Visceral efferent fibers of the parasympathetic type are present in the IIIrd, VIIth, IXth, and Xth cranial nerves (cf. Fig. 11-2). The largest mass of them join the *vagus nerve.* They spring from the *dorsal motor nucleus* of the vagus, situated immediately lateral to the hypoglossal nucleus, under the floor of the 4th ventricle (Figs. 7-2, 7-3, 7-6). Transection of the vagus in the neck causes the cells of the nucleus to undergo retrograde changes. The same is the case with the cells of the nucleus ambiguus, the other effector vagus nucleus. As described in Chapter 7 the cells in the nucleus ambiguus of the same type as the motoneurons, whereas those of the dorsal motor nucleus are similar to the cells in the intermediolateral cell column of the cord, suggesting that the nucleus ambiguus must be concerned in the innervation of the striated muscles supplied by the vagus, the dorsal motor nucleus with the innervation of glands and smooth muscles. Conclusive evidence of a correlation between cell type and function in this case is obtained by the fact that transection of the vagus below the diaphragm, where no striated muscles are supplied by it, leads to retrograde changes only in the dorsal motor nucleus. On closer examination it is found that there are differences in the cell types in different parts of the nucleus in animals as well as in man (Olszewski and Baxter, 1954). Several authors have attempted to decide if various regions of the

[3] Some authors also distinguish other cell groups in the cord as being of parasympathetic nature, e.g. an intermediomedial cell group, placed close to the central canal. Laruelle (1937) has traced this column throughout the cord and has found its rostral end to be continuous with the dorsal motor (visceral efferent) nucleus of the vagus. This column is less developed where the intermediolateral column is distinct, but the cells are of the same type. The two columns are interconnected by transverse fiber bundles, intermingled with some cells. In the sacral division (S_3–S_4) of the cord Laruelle has identified a third cell column placed ventralmost in the ventral horn. The cells of this column are of a type intermediate between the visceral and somatic efferent cells. The axons of these cells leave through the ventral roots, and their perikarya react after section of nerves of the pelvis. Laruelle is inclined to regard these cells as the most important part of the sacral division of the parasympathetic. Their peculiar histological appearance is thought to be an expression of their somatic-visceral function in such processes as emptying of the bladder and bowels and copulation, as here striped as well as smooth muscles are involved.

nucleus are related to the innervation of particular organs, by studying the retrograde cellular changes in the nucleus following transections of branches of the vagus nerve. While Getz and Sirnes (1949) in the rabbit and Mitchell and Warwick (1955) in the monkey found evidence that the fibers to the lungs come largely from other regions than those to the heart and esophagus, other authors (for example Szabo and Dussardier, 1964, in the sheep) found only meager evidence in favor of a somatotopic localization.

The generally accepted notion that the dorsal motor vagal nucleus is the source of the visceral efferent fibers in the vagus has been challenged by Szentágothai (1952b) who failed to find degenerating fibers in the nerve following lesions of the nucleus. Kerr (1967) recently reports that visceromotor effects on stimulation of

FIG. 11–2 Diagram of the craniosacral division of the autonomic nervous system. Preganglionic fibers indicated by heavy lines, postganglionic with light lines. The preganglionic fibers, their endings in the ganglia, and the distribution of the postganglionic fibers are indicated. Modified from Rasmussen (1932).

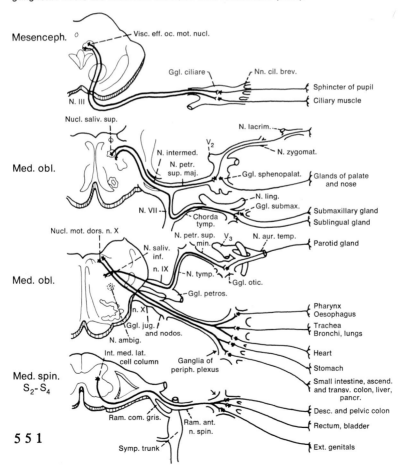

551

the cervical vagus are not altered significantly if the dorsal motor vagal nucleus has been destroyed several weeks previously (leaving time for efferent fibers to degenerate). He, therefore, suggests that the nucleus may possibly give rise only to secretomotor fibers, and that the neurons responsible for vagal visceromotor activity may be found in the vicinity of the nucleus ambiguus. Mitchell and Warwick (1955) argue that the dorsal motor vagal nucleus may be in part sensory, a suggestion which is, however, refuted by Szabo and Dussardier (1964). There are apparently still unsolved problems concerning this nucleus.

The visceral efferent (parasympathetic) nuclei related to the *glossopharyngeal and facial* (intermedius) *nerves* are termed the *inferior* and *superior salivatory nucleus,* respectively (Figs. 7-2 and 11-2), their most important function being the innervation of the salivary glands. They are usually described as forming two small groups of cells of the visceral efferent type, situated in the rostral prolongation of the dorsal motor nucleus of the vagus. The findings in these nuclei following transections of the nerves mentioned have been equivocal. Taking advantage of the modified Gudden method, Torvik (1957c) has been able to show in the cat that the visceral efferent fibers in the glossopharyngeal and vagus nerves come from cells lying rather scattered in certain regions of the reticular formation, and not being collected as clearly delimited nuclei.

The visceral efferent (parasympathetic) fibers, belonging to the *oculomotor* nerve and supplying the sphincter pupillae and the ciliary muscle, come from cells of the same type as those composing the other (general) visceral efferent nuclei, and are grouped with the somatic efferent nuclei innervating the extrinsic ocular muscles, ventral to the aqueduct of the mesencephalon at the level of the superior colliculus, as mentioned in Chapter 7. These cells form the so-called *Edinger-Westphal nucleus,* situated on both sides of the median plane, dorsomedial to the somatic efferent cell groups (Figs. 7-2 and 11-2). From this nucleus preganglionic fibers follow the oculomotor nerve to the ciliary ganglion. The position of the different parasympathetic nuclei is indicated in the diagram in Fig. 11-2 (cf. also Ch. 7).

Terminal nuclei of the afferent autonomic fibers. The efferent nuclei of the sympathetic and parasympathetic fibers differ only in regard to their localization, not in regard to cell type. As concerns the *afferent fibers* of the two divisions of the autonomic system, with one exception it has hitherto not been possible to identify particular cell groups as being especially concerned in the transmission of visceral afferent impulses. The exception is the *nucleus of the solitary tract* (Figs. 7-2, 7-6 and 7-14), described in Chapter 7, forming the terminal station of the visceral afferent fibers of the facial (intermedius), glossopharyngeal, and vagus nerves. As mentioned previously, it receives some trigeminal afferents as well.[4] It is concerned chiefly in the transmission of visceral afferent impressions from the mouth, pharynx, lungs, heart, esophagus, and upper part of the digestive tube with its glands in the abdomen. (In addition it transmits gustatory impulses, see Ch. 7.) These afferent impulses are important mainly in visceral reflexes, but it appears that the afferent vagus fibers especially are also involved in the transmission of certain diffuse sensations, such as nausea and others. Contrary to the afferent fibers in the sympathetic system, they appear not to be concerned with the conduction of pain. The afferent *"sympathetic"* fibers terminate on cells in the dorsal horn and intermediate zone of the spinal cord gray matter, but their precise synaptic relationships are not known. Our knowledge concerning the visceral afferent impulses is still scanty and, as referred to above, it is doubtful if it is appropriate to distinguish between "sympathetic" and "parasympathetic" afferent impulses. The formerly widely accepted fundamental difference between somatic and visceral afferent impulses also appears to be less well founded than formerly believed.

The peripheral parts of the autonomic nervous system. A knowledge of the peripheral parts of the autonomic system [5] is of considerable practical importance, first and foremost for the neurosurgeon. Starting with the *thoracolumbar, sympathetic system,* it has already been mentioned that the axons from the cells of the intermediolateral cell column leave the cord in the ventral roots. However, they soon leave these again and enter the *sympathetic trunk* via the so-called *white rami communicantes.* The sympathetic trunk consists of a paired chain of cell aggregations, situated on the ventrolateral side of the vertebral column, forming the sympathetic, *vertebral ganglia,* and being interconnected by longitudinally arranged bundles of nerve fibers. Transverse connections are also present, in man only below the level of the 5th lumbar vertebra (Pick and Sheehan, 1946). The sympathetic trunk is connected with the spinal nerves by white and gray rami communicantes.

Originally a primordium of a sympathetic ganglion is laid down on each side for each segment of the spinal cord. During development this original pattern is partly lost. Two or more adjacent primordia may fuse, or one may partake in the formation of two ganglia. On account of these and other variations in development there are usually only three ganglia in the cervical sympathetic trunk, the superior, middle (which may be

---

[4] It gives off ascending fibers and the solitariospinal tract, fibers to the reticular formation, and as recently demonstrated by Morest (1967) fibers passing to the dorsal motor vagus nucleus and the nucleus ambiguus, obviously forming links in important reflex arcs.

[5] An exhaustive account of this subject can be found in the monograph of Mitchell (1953).

absent), and inferior cervical ganglion. The inferior is furthermore frequently fused with the 1st or 1st and 2nd thoracic ganglia to form the so-called stellate ganglion. The *superior cervical ganglion* is large, elongated, and placed on the ventral aspect of the transverse processes of the upper two cervical vertebrae in proximity to the nodose ganglion of the vagus. When present the *middle cervical ganglion* is found at the level of the 6th cervical vertebra. *The inferior ganglion,* or the *stellate ganglion,* is situated as a rule behind the subclavian artery. Between the middle and inferior ganglia an intermediate ganglion is commonly present. From this a loop of fibers, forming the *ansa subclavia,* goes around the subclavian artery, and unites the intermediate ganglion with the inferior. There is usually one ganglion for each segment in the thoracic part of the trunk, the first, however, being usually fused in the stellate ganglion. In the lumbar part there may be four or five ganglia, in the sacral part usually four are present, and lastly there is frequently an unpaired coccygeal ganglion. It is of practical revelance that individual variations exist in the number, size, location, and extent of fusion of the sympathetic vertebral ganglia.[6] It is also of considerable interest *that sympathetic ganglion cells* are not confined to the ganglia proper, but that such cells *are constantly found in larger or smaller numbers along the gray rami communicantes as intermediate ganglia,* especially in the cervical and lumbar regions (Wrete, 1935).[7] This is explained by the development, the ganglia arising from cells migrating along the dorsal and ventral roots (Kuntz, 1920). Since the axons from the cells of the intermediolateral column are myelinated, the rami conveying them from the spinal nerve to the sympathetic trunk are whitish, and generally are called *white rami communicantes.* Corresponding to the extension of the intermediolateral cell column in the cord, the spinal autonomic outflow and the occurence of white rami is limited to the segments Th_1-L_2, inclusive (Sheehan, 1941). Some of the preganglionic fibers in the white rami end in the ganglion of the corresponding segment, but other fibers traverse the ganglion without interruption (cf. Figs. 11-3 and 11-4). Some of these preganglionic fibers ascend or descend in the sympathetic trunk, to end in ganglia situated farther cranially or caudally, where they end in synaptic contact with the postganglionic neurons. Other preganglionic fibers which pass through the vertebral ganglia continue in branches

---

[6] Sheehan and Pick (1943) and Pick and Sheehan (1946) have, from studies in monkey and man, stressed the importance of numbering the ganglia not according to their place relative to the level of the vertebral column but according to their connections with the spinal nerves, the gray rami (where separately present) being the most reliable criterion.

[7] For an exhaustive account of the occurrence of intermediate ganglia in man and their clinical importance the monograph of Monro (1959) should be consulted.

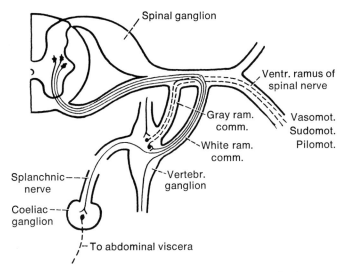

Fig. 11–3 Diagram showing the course of the preganglionic sympathetic fibers (heavy lines) from the spinal cord to a vertebral and a prevertebral ganglion, and the course of the postganglionic fibers (stippled) through the gray rami communicantes back to the spinal nerve.

which pass from the sympathetic trunk to the *prevertebral ganglia* related to viscera. The most important of these latter branches are the *greater and lesser splanchnic nerves.* (It should be noted that these are made up of axons of preganglionic neurons, and correspond to white rami communicantes.) The former arises from branches from the 5th to 6th to the 9th to 10th thoracic ganglia (individual variations are usual), the latter from the (9th) 10th to 11th thoracic ganglia. Both pierce the diaphragm and enter the celiac plexus around the celiac artery, where most of the fibers of the greater splanchnic nerve establish connections with the postganglionic cells of the *celiac ganglion.* The celiac plexus extends along the branches from the abdominal aorta, forming several other plexuses with other ganglia, most conspicuous of which are the *superior and inferior mesenteric ganglia.* The fibers of the lesser splanchnic nerve, following the greater, are mainly distributed to the *renal ganglion,* and partly go to the adrenal medulla. In addition some fibers from the 12th thoracic segment, usually designated the least splanchnic nerve, participate in the innervation of the adrenal. The prevertebral ganglia treated above thus correspond to the vertebral ganglia of the sympathetic system. Both types of ganglia are the terminal station for preganglionic thoraco-lumbar fibers.

5 5 5

In the vertebral and prevertebral ganglia the postganglionic cells of the sympathetic system are found, sending their axons to the organs to be supplied. The postganglionic fibers, being unmyelinated, may behave in two different ways. They may return to the spinal nerves as gray rami communicantes or they may join the arteries and follow these as plexuses of nerve fibers. Gray rami are, in contradistinction to the white, found along the entire sympathetic trunk, connecting the ganglia with the corresponding spinal nerves. Postganglionic sympathetic fibers (mediating vasoconstriction, sweat secretion, and piloarrection) therefore are present in the spinal nerves.[8]

The fibers joining the arteries follow these as plexuses along their course. Thus several postganglionic fibers from the superior cervical ganglion accompany the internal carotid and its branches to supply the structures of the head with sympathetic fibers. Some of these fibers later join several of the cranial nerves (cf. Fig. 11-4). From the stellate ganglion fibers join the subclavian artery to supply the upper extremity (in addition to fibers joining the inferior cervical nerves via gray rami communicantes). Other branches from the cervical ganglia are the *superior, middle, and inferior cardiac nerves,* arising from the corresponding cervical ganglia where the postganglionic neurons are situated. These nerves take part in the formation of the *cardiac plexus,* in combination with postganglionic sympathetic fibers from the upper 4–5 thoracic ganglia and parasympathetic vagus fibers.

From the celiac ganglion and the associated abdominal ganglia, postganglionic sympathetic fibers accompany the branches of the abdominal aorta, as the hepatic, splenic, renal, phrenic and other plexuses. The fibers extend also along the ovarian and testicular arteries, and along the iliac artery and its branches, here being supplemented by fibers from the lumbar and sacral vertebral ganglia, especially in the formation of the (superior) *hypogastric plexus* from which sympathetic fibers are dis-

---

[8] The distinction between white and gray rami has proved to be too schematic. Sheehan and Pick (1943) have emphasized that typical white rami are composed of myelinated fibers of a diameter up to 15μ, whereas the gray rami are of two types, one containing almost entirely small unmyelinated fibers, the other, in addition, many small myelinated fibers (under 3μ in diameter). A few heavier myelinated fibers may also be present in the gray rami. A fourth type of ramus is of a mixed type, one part containing fibers of the type found in the white rami, the rest resembling the gray rami. The medullated fibers in the gray rami are assumed to be at least partly afferent fibers. These anatomical findings (Kuntz and Farnsworth, 1931) are of some practical relevance, since they yield support to the contention of surgeons that white and gray rami cannot be differentiated during operations. The occurrence of mixed rami explains why in some instances only one ramus is found, where theoretically two should be present.

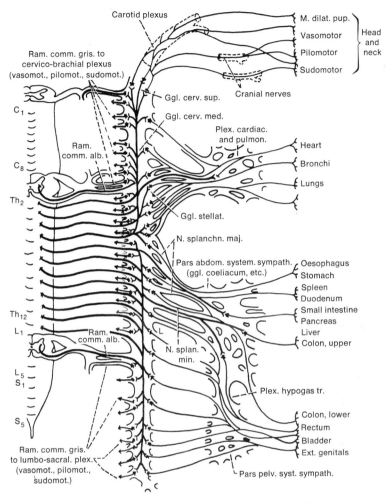

FIG. 11–4 Diagram of the sympathetic division of the autonomic nervous system after the same principle as applied in FIG. 11–2. Modified from Rasmussen (1932).

tributed to most of the pelvic organs. The postganglionic fibers to the intestine arise in the superior mesenteric ganglion for the small intestine and the ascending and transverse colon, in the inferior mesenteric ganglion for the descending and sigmoid colon and rectum. The fibers to the lower extremity are partly derived from plexuses along the arteries (which later join the nerves, cf. below), partly from gray rami from the lumbar and sacral sympathetic ganglia joining the corresponding spinal nerves.

It should be emphasized that, in addition to sympathetic fibers, the

557

plexuses on the visceral arteries also contain parasympathetic fibers, intermingling with the former in the plexuses (cf. below).

In spite of the restriction of the intermediolateral column to only a part of the spinal cord $(Th_1–L_2)$, *all regions of the body are supplied with sympathetic fibers.* This is made possible by the arrangement of the preganglionic sympathetic fibers, some of them traversing the sympathetic ganglia without interruption, to ascend or descend in the sympathetic trunk. Thus many of the fibers originating in the upper thoracic segments end in the superior cervical ganglion, and the sacral vertebral ganglia receive their preganglionic fibers from the lower thoracic and

FIG. 11–5 Diagram of the origin and course of the sympathetic fibers to the upper extremity. The dotted preganglionic fibers are somewhat equivocal. Postganglionic fibers are indicated by broken lines. *S.C.G.:* superior cervical ganglion; *M.G.:* middle cervical ganglion; *S.G.:* stellate ganglion. From Haymaker and Woodhall (1945) after Foerster.

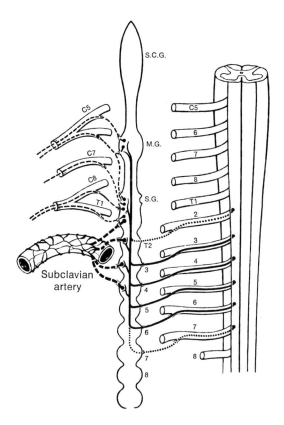

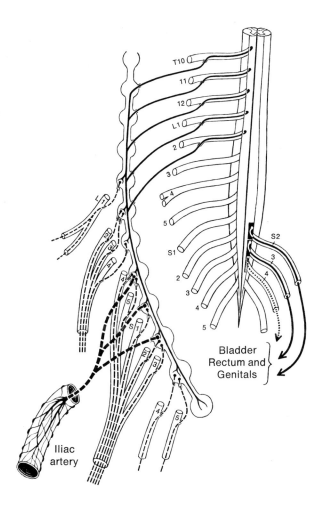

FIG. 11–6 Diagram of the sympathetic supply of the lower extremity after the same principle as in FIG. 11–5. The parasympathetic fibers to the pelvic organs are included on the right side. From Haymaker and Woodhall (1945) after Foerster.

upper two lumbar segments of the cord. This arrangement is diagrammatically represented in Fig. 11-4. This sympathetic innervation of the extremities is not included, but is evident from Figs. 11-5 and 11-6 and is represented also in the table on p. 616. Concerning the segmental sympathetic innervation, see below.

Turning to the *peripheral parts of the parasympathetic system,* it has already been mentioned that the preganglionic fibers of the cranial division join several of the cranial nerves. Contrary to the arrangement in the sympathetic system, the *preganglionic fibers of the parasympathetic system can be followed to the organs to be supplied or close to them,* where the fibers then end in synaptic contact with the postganglionic cells, forming discrete ganglia or more scattered ganglionic plexuses in the walls of the organs.

The *visceral efferent fibers in the oculomotor nerve* accompany the somatic fibers of the nerve to the orbit, where they separate from them and enter the *ciliary ganglion,* behind the eyeball (Fig. 11-2). From here the postganglionic fibers reach the eye as the short ciliary nerves, and terminate in the ciliary muscle and the sphincter of the iris.

The *visceral efferent preganglionic fibers following the facial nerve,* as part of the intermedius, originate from the so-called superior salivatory nucleus (see above) and pursue a complicated course (Fig. 11-2). Some of them leave the nerve in the facial canal, and traverse the tympanic cavity as the chorda tympani which after having left the cranium joins the lingual nerve. In its terminal branches to the *sublingual and submandibular glands* several nerve cells are present, representing the perikarya of the postganglionic neurons and passing to the glandular cells. These cell aggregates are usually termed the *submandibular ganglion.* Other visceral efferent fibers in the intermedius leave the nerve at the geniculate ganglion as the great superficial petrosal nerve, pass through the sphenoid bone (pterygoid canal) to the *sphenopalatine ganglion* in the sphenopalatine fossa. The postganglionic fibers from this ganglion partly pass to the maxillary nerve, and through an anastomosis with the lacrimal nerve reach the lacrimal gland (Fig. 11-2). Other fibers are distributed to the nasal cavity (sphenopalatine nerves) and the oral cavity through the descending palatine nerves.

The *visceral efferent preganglionic fibers of the glossopharyngeal nerve,* arising from the "inferior salivatory nucleus," leave the nerve at the petrous ganglion in the petrous fossa when the nerve has just left the jugular foramen (Fig. 11-2). Forming the tympanic nerve the fibers pierce the floor of the tympanic cavity, ascend on the medial wall, and penetrate the thin roof of the cavity to appear as the lesser superficial petrosal nerve intracranially. This then again leaves the cranial cavity and ends in the *otic ganglion,* medial to the exit of the third division of the trigeminal nerve in the foramen ovale. The postganglionic fibers from this ganglion pass through the auriculotemporal nerve to the *parotid gland.*

By far the most important contingent of preganglionic parasympathetic cranial fibers, however, is contained in the *vagus nerve.* The fibers arise from the dorsal motor nucleus and accompany several of the

560

rami of the nerve (concerning these see Ch. 7). They end in ganglia and plexuses containing ganglion cells in or near the innervated organs (Fig. 11-2). Thus fibers in the *pharyngeal rami* end in relation to ganglion cells in the pharyngeal plexus, from which the glands of the pharynx are innervated. Other fibers are distributed in a similar manner to the *esophagus* (secretory fibers and motor fibers to the smooth muscles). The *heart* receives parasympathetic fibers through the superior, middle, and inferior cardiac branches, which terminate on cells in the cardiac plexus, particularly well developed around the beginning of the aorta and pulmonary artery. This plexus continues also along the coronary arteries.[9] In addition to parasympathetic fibers, the plexuses mentioned above contain sympathetic fibers, as do also the tracheal, bronchial, and pulmonary plexuses, supplied by branches from the vagus. Having pierced the diaphragm the left vagus is distributed mainly on the anterior surface of the stomach, the right on the posterior, and they then take part in the formation of the celiac plexus. Other vagus fibers from the celiac plexus accompany the sympathetic fibers in the plexuses surrounding the arteries and provide parasympathetic fibers to the duodenum, pancreas, small intestine, and large intestine to the left flexure. Fibers to the liver and gall bladder, participating in the hepatic plexus, are derived mainly from the right vagus, and end in relation to postganglionic cells in the hepatic plexus in the porta hepatis and in the wall of the gall bladder and cystic and common bile ducts (Alexander, 1940). In the wall of the stomach a gastric plexus is formed, consisting of fibers and postganglionic cells with short axons. One part of the plexus is found between the muscular layers (plexus myentericus), another in the submucosa (plexus submucosus). Sympathetic fibers are also present in these plexuses which appear to possess a certain degree of local autonomy. Plexuses of a similar type are found also in the other parts of the digestive tube in the abdomen. Collectively they are frequently termed *"enteric plexuses."* The postganglionic fibers of these plexuses are in general secretory and motor.[10]

The *preganglionic fibers belonging to the sacral division of the parasympathetic system* (cf. Fig. 11-2 and Fig. 11-6 to the right) leave the cord in the ventral roots from the 3rd and 4th sacral nerves (occasionally

[9] The innervation of the heart is treated more fully later in this chapter.

[10] According to Kuntz (1938, 1940) there are afferent fibers from these plexuses to the celiac and mesenteric ganglia. Following interruption of all centrally derived afferents to the ganglia, some fibers with intact terminal arborizations are still present in them. The presence of such axons from the enteric plexuses to the prevertebral ganglia might explain the fact that visceral reflex activity, for example, of the stomach, is still possible after the celiac ganglion is separated from the central nervous system. If this is so it will be unnecessary to regard these functions as due to axon reflexes.

561

also S_2 and S_5). They follow the nerves forming the pudendal plexus, and leave them as the pelvic nerves (nervi erigentes) on each side of the rectum. Here they come into contact with the hypogastric plexus and are intermingled with sympathetic fibers. They synapse with post-ganglionic neurons situated within the walls of the bladder, rectum, and genitals; the descending and sigmoid colon also receive their para-sympathetic innervation from the sacral division.

In spite of the restricted origin of the parasympathetic preganglionic neurons, it is seen that at least the majority of the *visceral* organs are supplied by parasympathetic fibers as well as sympathetic. In their pe-ripheral course the fibers of the two divisions of the autonomic system are intermingled, but they retain their functional independence. The principal points of autonomic innervation are summarized in the table on p. 616, in which some functional aspects are also included.

Some physiological aspects. Transmitter substances. Before con-tinuing the account of the anatomy of the autonomic system it will be appropriate to consider some aspects of its physiology. This is a vast field, in which knowledge has increased considerably in recent years. Only some general features will be dealt with here.[11] A few historical remarks may be of interest.

The introduction by Langley of his nicotine method is undoubtedly one of the events which most decisively furthered study in the physiology of the autonomic system. In several now classical papers, dating from about 1890 and later, Langley and his collaborators showed that the application of nicotine (in a solution of a certain concentration) to an autonomic ganglion after a transient facilitation blocked the transmis-sion in the preganglionic-postganglionic synapses, whereas the pre-ganglionic fibers passing through the ganglion were not affected. In other words, nicotine influenced the synapses but not the fibers. In this manner Langley was able to show that stimulation of the uppermost thoracic ventral roots produced dilatation of the pupil when nicotine was painted on the stellate or middle cervical ganglion, but not when it was applied to the superior cervical ganglion. From this the conclusion was drawn that the preganglionic fibers to the eye pass without interruption to the latter ganglion, where the postganglionic neurons begin. In a similar manner the position of the synapses in other efferent autonomic pathways was determined. Furthermore Langley showed that stimulation of the pre-ganglionic sympathetic fibers led to vasoconstriction, piloarrection, and sweat secretion, and that the different body regions are supplied with sympathetic efferents from distinct segments of the spinal cord.

---

[11] References to most of the papers relevant to this section are omitted, since they will be found in comprehensive works on the autonomic system.

A further great step was made with the discovery that certain chemical substances mediate the synaptic transmission in the autonomic nervous system, as was later shown to be the case also in the central nervous system.

In 1921 O. Loewi observed that on stimulation of the vagus nerve in the frog, a substance was liberated in the heart, which when transferred to another animal had the same physiological effect as vagal stimulation. This substance had properties similar to acetylcholine. It is now generally agreed that this vagus substance is *acetylcholine.* Stimulation of the sympathetic was followed by the liberation of a substance very similar to *adrenaline* (Cannon and collaborators) and named *sympathin.* Both substances are set free at the terminal points of the corresponding postganglionic fibers. Sir Henry Dale on this account proposed a distinction between *cholinergic and adrenergic postganglionic fibers,* a nomenclature often used. This mode of distinction, however, does not coincide in all points with the anatomical subdivision into parasympathetic and sympathetic. Thus the postganglionic fibers to the sweat glands, which anatomically are part of the sympathetic system, are cholinergic, in harmony with the long known fact that the sweat glands are susceptible to atropine and pilocarpine (causing inhibition and stimulation, respectively) like parasympathetic fibers in other instances.

Another discovery concerning the humoral side of synaptic transmission also opposes the old customary schematic modes of subdivision. *Synaptic transmission in the autonomic ganglia is accompanied by production of acetylcholine, regardless of whether the ganglion belongs to the craniosacral or thoracolumbar system* (Dale and Feldberg, 1933). Thus acetylcholine is produced at the terminals of all preganglionic fibers in the autonomic ganglia as well as at the terminals of most of the parasympathetic fibers in the organs.

A wealth of new facts has been brought forward in recent years by numerous workers. While confirming the fundamental principles established by the pioneers in the field, many new observations indicate the existence of more specific patterns of functional organization within the autonomic nervous system. Only some points will be mentioned.

Concerning the *transmitter substances,* the problems related to these have turned out to be less simple than originally thought. The *sympathetic transmitter,* originally called sympathin, has been shown to be not adrenaline, but *noradrenaline,* as demonstrated especially by von Euler and his collaborators. (Adrenaline is liberated from the adrenal medulla on stimulation of the splanchnic nerve.) As will be considered later, there appears to be increasing evidence that noradrenaline is related to a particular kind of synaptic vesicles, the so-called dense-core vesicles, seen electron microscopically in sympathetic postganglionic nerve fibers and terminals, and that it is transported along the postganglionic fibers to their terminals, where it is liberated. The mechanisms of its synthesis, storgage, and release have been studied extensively (see von Euler, 1959), as has also the action of the transmitter on the effector cells. This appears to ocur by way of a "receptor substance." Many theories have been set forth to explain the mechanism of the action. A distinction has been made between two kinds of adrenergic receptors, alpha and beta (others have been suggested as well). The different receptors may be selectively blocked by particular drugs. Use is being made of this in medical treatment of some conditions.

As to the other autonomic transmitter substance, *acetylcholine,* less appears to be known concerning its formation and modes of action on the effectors. Just as for noradrenaline much of the liberated transmitter appears to be broken down by enzymatic action, in the case of acetylcholine this happens by means of acetyl cholinesterase.

Mention was made above of the fact that the sweat glands are activated by acetylcholine, in spite of their nervous supply by fibers belonging to the sympathetic system. It appears that this is not the only example of cholinergic fibers in the sympathetic system. The vasodilatation which occurs in skeletal muscle following sympathetic stimulation appears to be a cholinergic mechanism, mediated by sympathetic fibers. These observations are in agreement with the finding (see below) that some cells in the sympathetic ganglia are cholinergic while the majority are adrenergic, and they present another warning against a simplified conception of the autonomic nervous system.

As mentioned previously, *it is generally said that the two divisions of the autonomic system have antagonistic functions:* where stimulation of the parasympathetic results in an increased activity (motility, secretion), stimulation of the sympathetic has the opposite effects, and vice versa. While this is true in general, it is not an absolute rule. The principle is valid for the innervation of the stomach and the gut, where parasympathetic stimulation increases peristalsis and secretion, while sympathetic stimulation has an inhibitory action. In the salivary glands parasympathetic stimulation gives rise to a copious, mucous secretion, while the effect of sympathetic stimulation on secretion appears to be disputed.[12] However, under normal circumstances the two divisions co-

[12] The parasympathetic fibers appear to end on the mucous cells of these glands only. With the fluorescence method (see later) a rich plexus of noradrenergic fibers was found around the serous acini of the submandibular gland, while there were no such fibers in the predominantly mucous sublingual gland (Norberg and Olson, 1965).

operate in an integrated manner, as seen for example in the nervous control of the heart.

In spite of the co-operation between the two divisions, there are certain morphological and functional differences which indicate that the two divisions of the autonomic system are not equivalent. From the anatomical point of view the parasympathetic division is rather clearly fractionated into minor separate cell groups concerned in the regulation of particular functions or organs. This is perhaps most clearly seen in the cranial part, where the Edinger-Westphal nucleus is delegated to the control of the intrinsic ocular muscles only, and the various salivary glands and the lacrimal gland are supplied by particular cell groups. (The syndrome of crocodile tears, described on p. 410, may be taken as an illustration of this.) It appears that segregations of this kind are less marked in the intermediolateral cell column. Supporting evidence comes from comparisons between the number of preganglionic fibers to a ganglion and the number of postganglionic neurons in its two divisions. Billingsley and Ranson (1918) counted more than 120,000 cells in the superior cervical ganglion of the cat, whereas the sympathetic trunk immediately below the ganglion contains only 3,800 myelinated fibers, presumably preganglionic. This gives a ratio of about 32 cells to each preganglionic fiber. Wolf (1941) in similar counts found a ratio of about 15:1, since small unmyelinated fibers were also counted. In the parasympathetic division there appears to be a closer numerical correspondence between preganglionic and postganglionic neurons, as Wolf (1941) in the ciliary ganglion of the cat found a ratio between pre- and postganglionic neurons of only 1:2. Even if these ratios are probably not valid for all sympathetic and parasympathetic ganglia, the differences between them are large enough to suggest an essential dissimilarity between the two divisions of the autonomic system. The anatomical observations are in accord with a number of physiological findings which show that, in general, the parasympathetic has considerable possibilities for influencing local functions, while the sympathetic by way of its more diffuse distribution tends to have widespread and general bodily effects (for example on the cutaneous vessels).

The term *"vegetative tonus"* is sometimes used in clinical language to characterize the conditions within the autonomic system as a whole. This "tonus" is thought to vary from individual to individual and also in the same person at different times. Eppinger and Hess suggested that one could distinguish between vagotonic and sympathicotonic individuals according to whether they present signs of relative dominance of the parasympathetic or sympathetic system, respectively. However, in most persons signs of sympathetic preponderance are coupled with other signs

565

betraying a parasympathetic overaction. Frequently, only one organ reveals a clear-cut parasympathetic or sympathetic dominance (local vagotonia or sympathicotonia). Cannon proposed a more general biological mode of regarding the functions of the autonomic system: Broadly speaking, the parasympathetic functions are protective and serve to maintain and restore the bodily reserves. Thus the parasympathetic protects the retina from excessive light, promotes the secretion of the digestive tract, and is concerned in the emptying of the bladder and rectum. The sympathetic, on the other hand, is mainly brought into play in emergency states, when the bodily reserves are drawn upon, such as physical exertion, fear, rage, and other stress situations. In these the adrenal medulla is activated by way of the splanchnic nerves, and the consequent outflow of adrenaline is important and explains some of the functional changes. In stress situations the sympathetic effects of acceleration of the heart rate, dilatation of the bronchi, elevation of the blood sugar level, but inhibition of gastrointestinal secretion and motility, are all appropriate. It is in keeping with Cannon's views that animals deprived of their sympathetic trunks may live for years in the sheltered conditions of the laboratory, but when exposed to their usual environmental conditions their resistance is reduced and their power of adaptation is impaired. The more easily observed phenomena in stress reactions are only the outward manifestations of numerous extremely complex changes in the organism. These involve also the central nervous system, which has the task of coordinating and controlling the various components of the total reactions. In these functions there are close interrelationships between the nervous and endocrine controlling systems.[13]

Increased knowledge of the role and the chemistry of the transmitter substances has furthered the understanding of the effects of certain drugs on autonomically controlled functions. A rational basis has been found for many well-known observations. On the other hand, progress in neurochemistry and neuropharmacology has shown that these problems are extremely complex and the mechanisms involved very intricate. These matters will not be considered here, but it may be appropriate to mention a few well-known facts, without discussing their pharmacological or chemical basis.

Atropine has long been known to be a parasympathetic inhibiting substance. It appears to act directly on the effector organs. Even if the influence of the vagus on

[13] The roles of noradrenaline and adrenaline (and other biogenic amines such as serotonin) in influencing emotional states has recently attracted great interest because it appears that many drugs used in the psychiatric treatment of patients with affective disorders cause changes in the metabolism and function of various biogenic amines, peripherally and centrally. For a recent review see Schildkraut and Kety (1967).

566

the heart has been abolished by atropine, acetylcholine is still produced on stimulation of the nerve. But the heart muscle is no longer susceptible to the action of acetylcholine. This effect of atropine is utilized in several instances clinically, e.g. in ophthalmology in order to dilate the pupil (homatropine). In bronchial asthma relaxation of the bronchial muscles and reduced secretion result, while in the stomach peristalsis and secretion of gastric juice are reduced. As previously mentioned, sweat secretion is diminished or abolished by atropine, in spite of the sympathetic innervation of the sweat glands.

Pilocarpine has an effect opposite to that of atropine. In general, it stimulates the cholinergically innervated organs and thus produces secretion of salivary, lacrimal, and sweat glands and the glands of the digestive tube and causes contraction of the pupil. The effect is similar to the action of *eserine* (or *physostigmine*), which acts by inhibiting acetylcholinesterase.

A number of other drugs and substances are known today which may influence the synaptic transmission in the autonomic system, such as monoaminoxydase inhibitors and substances known as receptor blockers. In addition the autonomically innervated organs may be subject to the influence of certain hormones such as adrenaline, vasopressin and oxytocin, to changes in the CO_2 level, and ionic alterations in the blood and tissue fluids. Much information on this subject, obtained in animal studies, has been made use of in the treatment of diseases in man.

Sensitization of autonomically denervated organs. It has been known for some time that when the sympathetic innervation of an organ is interrupted by section of the postganglionic fibers or extirpation of the ganglion in which the postganglionic cells are located, the effector organ, in a week or two, usually shows an increased susceptibility to the action of adrenaline (and noradrenaline), whether this be excitatory or inhibitory to the organ in question. For example, following extirpation of the stellate ganglion in Raynaud's disease the immediate effect is a vasodilatation in the head, neck, and arm on the operated side. During the following days, however, this becomes less conspicuous, and a week or so after the operation, a tendency to vasoconstriction is clearly evident on occasions in which an extra output of adrenaline occurs, for example on emotion or exposure to cold. It appears that the effector organ acquires an increased susceptibility to adrenaline, commonly referred to as *sensitization* or *"supersensitivity."* This phenomenon has been observed not only in adrenergically innervated organs, but in cholinergically innervated organs as well (it applies to the pupillary contraction and to sweat secretion in response to acetylcholine). The *postganglionic* neurons can also become sensitized after section of the preganglionic fibers, although clinically the phenomena of sensitization are less marked after preganglionic than after postganglionic ramisection.

The supersensitivity following autonomic denervation appears to be an example of Cannon's "law of denervation." When in a series of efferent neurons one is destroyed, there develops an increased irritability to chemical agents in the isolated structures, most marked in the directly denervated part. (Reference was made in Ch. 3 to the occurrence of sensitization in denervated skeletal muscle.) Several attempts have been made to explain this sensitization, but no generally accepted theory has been set forth (for some data see Hillarp, 1960). The phenomenon is of some clinical interest, not least in surgery on the sympathetic nervous system, although its importance has been questioned by some authors (see Monro, 1959, for some data).

The minute structure of the autonomic ganglia. The nerve cells composing the autonomic ganglia differ in certain respects from those in the central nervous system. Several cell types may be distinguished and there are also structural differences between the various ganglia.[14] In spite of this, however, there are enough common features to allow us to regard these cells as belonging to a fairly uniform group. Reliable criteria which permit a distinction between cells and fibers belonging to the sympathetic and parasympathetic have not been found.

The *autonomic ganglion cells* of the ganglia of the sympathetic trunk and in the peripheral ganglia are usually multipolar and are characterized by possessing numerous and long dendrites (Fig. 11-7). The tigroid substance is finely granular and pigment inclusions are common. The cells, like the spinal ganglion cells, are always surrounded by a capsule with flattened cells, homologous to the glial cells, lying in close contact with the nerve cells (sheath cells). The numerous dendrites may arborize abundantly within the capsule or they may penetrate it. On account of the numerous and long dendrites it is often difficult to identify cell processes which can be designated as axons, but under fortunate circumstances such may be seen. The axon is frequently very thin, and may either spring from the perikaryon or from one of the dendrites. The axons from the postganglionic cells are usually unmyelinated.

Between the ganglion cells an extremely intricate feltwork of fine fibers is present. These fibers are partly dendrites which have pierced the capsules, partly axons and collaterals from preganglionic fibers terminating in the ganglion, and, finally, some of them are fibers passing through the ganglion without interruption. The terminal parts of the preganglionic fibers are frequently unmyelinated or covered with a very delicate myelin investment only, and on this account they cannot, or can only with difficulty, be distinguished microscopically from the dendrites present.

[14] Numerous authors have attempted classifications of autonomic ganglion cells according to size, arrangement of Nissl granules, dendritic arborizations, or other criteria (for some references see Hillarp, 1960). Even if there are some physiological indications that the cells in a ganglion may differ functionally, correlations with morphological differences between cells are so far not possible. The ganglia in man appear to be built as those in animals (for some data see Kirsche, 1958).

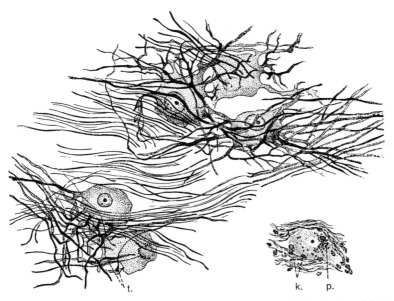

FIG. 11–7 Drawing of cell types from autonomic ganglia. Below to the right a cell from the celiac ganglion in man (autopsy material, modified Cajal method with contrast Safranin staining). The other cells are from a lumbar sympathetic ganglion of man (Bodian's method on autopsy material). *t:* terminal ramifications; *k:* sheath cells; *p:* argentaffine pigment. (Cf. text.) Courtesy of Dr. J. Cammermeyer.

The mode of termination of the axons is highly variable. They may penetrate the capsule surrounding the ganglion cells and end in an intracapsular plexus, or they may end outside the capsules interwoven between dendrites which have penetrated the latter. The axons as well as the dendrites frequently pass in several spirals around the cells, and their course within the ganglia is frequently tortuous and of considerable length. The fibers end with different kinds of terminal formations (ordinary end bulbs, chalyces, pericellular arborizations).

The *nerve bundles interconnecting the autonomic cell groups* are sometimes composed of predominantly myelinated fibers, as, for example, the white rami communicantes and the splanchnic nerves. Sometimes the majority of the fibers are unmyelinated, as is the case with the gray rami communicantes and the plexuses around the arteries. As a general rule it may be said that preganglionic fibers tend to be myelinated, postganglionic not, but there are exceptions. In the vertebral ganglia thicker myelinated fibers take their course through them.

In view of the complicated pictures presented by the autonomic ganglia, it is no wonder that opinions have differed concerning their

569

interpretation. (For reviews see, for example, Hillarp, 1946; Kappers, 1964; Taxi, 1965.) Based on light microscopic studies some authors maintained that it is impossible to distinguish dendrites and axons of these cells and that free nerve endings do not exist, but that the nerve cells form a true syncytium. According to this view the neuron theory should not be valid for the peripheral parts of the autonomic system. However, the evidence to the contrary has gradually become overwhelming. Even before the advent of electron microscopy most authors were convinced that the preganglionic fibers which do not bypass the ganglia are in true synaptic contact with iths cells, as Langley was led to conclude from his physiological experiments. Studies of normal preparations by Cajal and other authors (Kuntz, 1938; and several later students) and experimental data, all supported this conception. Thus transection of the sympathetic trunk in the neck was followed by disappearance of the fibers in the intercellular plexuses in the superior cervical ganglion, whereas the fibers on the internal carotid are not affected (Ranson and Billingsley in dogs, 1918). The fibers in the carotid plexus, therefore, obviously must be axons af cells of the superior ganglion. Other authors reported corresponding results in other ganglia.

The validity of the neuron theory for the autonomic ganglia has been definitely proved in electron microscopic studies, which in addition have given information on other details, for example, the structure of the glial elements. The presence of different kinds of nerve endings, visible in light microscopic preparations, has been confirmed. There is in most points a rather good correspondence with light microscopic pictures, as appears from Taxi's (1965) extensive study. Axosomatic and axodendritic synapses have been seen on the ganglion cells, but there appear to be variations among ganglia and between species with regard to the proportion of the two types. There are also variations with regard to the fine structure of the places of synaptic contact. In general the synaptic structures in the autonomic ganglia correspond to those in the central nervous system (Szentágothai, 1964c; and others; for further references see Grillo, 1966).

Histochemically it has been observed that preganglionic fibers, for example to the ciliary ganglion and the superior cervical ganglion, can be stained with procedures demonstrating the presence of cholinesterases (see for example Szentágothai, Donhoffer, and Raikovits, 1954; Taxi, 1965), and it appears that acetylcholine is present in the fibers and their synaptic endings, although the latter point is not quite settled. Recent histochemical studies in which the method of demonstrating monoamines by making them fluorescent (see below) is used, indicate that many nerve cells in the (vertebral) sympathetic ganglia contain noradrenaline (for a review see Norberg, 1967). It has further been found that the substance made fluorescent by this method is transported along the axons and can be traced to their terminals. Also in the sympathetic ganglia there appear to be some cholinesterase-positive cells (acetyl-cholinesterase). On the whole these histochemical findings are in agreement with conclusions reached in physiological and pharmacological studies which indicate that as a general rule preganglionic and parasympathetic postganglionic neurons are cholinergic, sympathetic postganglionic neurons adrenergic.

It appears from the above that one should be careful not to over-simplify the problems related to the structural and functional organization of the autonomic ganglia and to make generalizations. The synaptic arrangements within the ganglia are far from being fully known. There is reason to believe that the autonomic ganglia are not simple relays, serving only the transmission of impulses from preganglionic to postganglionic neurons (see Hillarp, 1960, for some data). From a functional point of view a question of particular interest is whether there are internuncial cells in the ganglia (with their axon restricted within this and contacting other cells in the ganglion). Small cells which have been interpreted as internuncials have recently been described electron microscopically (Williams, 1967).

The peripheral autonomic fibers.   All organs innervated by the autonomic system contain plexuses of very fine nerve fibers. In microscopical sections these fibers can be demonstrated by the use of various silver impregnation methods and by supravital staining with methylene blue. The details in the organization of the plexuses and in the relations between the nerve fibers and the effector structures (smooth muscles and glandular cells) have been extremely difficult to clarify with the classical methods, and conflicting opinions have been set forth. In recent years studies with the electron microscope have greatly contributed to a better understanding.

On the basis of the studies of silver-impregnated sections, many histologists, Boeke, Støhr, and others, strongly advocated that the terminal nerve fibers form an anastomosing network of extremely thin fibers, a syncytial "terminal" or "preterminal reticulum" or "sympathetic ground plexus." (For a recent brief review see Kappers, 1964.) The terminal fibers of the plexus were held to be continuous with the cytoplasm of the effector cells. The cells found in between the fibers of the plexuses, generally called "interstitial cells," have been the subject of much debate. They have been claimed to be connective tissue elements, supporting cells of the Schwann cell type or nervous elements interposed between the terminal fibers and the effector cells. When electron microscopic studies

5 7 1

became possible several of the controversies were solved. Even if many details remain to be clarified there can be no doubt that the organization of the peripheral autonomic system is, in principle, in agreement with the neuron theory.

In electron microscopic studies the fibers in the peripheral autonomic plexuses have been confirmed to be extremely thin, as small as some 200 Å. (This may explain why they have been misinterpreted in the light microscope as "neurofibrils.") The unmyelinated fibers are covered by the cytoplasm of cells of the Schwann cell type, sometimes called lemmocytes. Within the "cisterns" of these cells there are usually a number of thin axons, a fact which may be of relevance for the conduction of impulses, since depolarization of one axon may influence other axons running in the same cistern (see Ruska and Ruska, 1961). Convincing evidence of a syncytial connection between the lemmocytes has not been obtained. In addition to the lemmocytes the autonomic plexuses contain some other interstitial cells. These differ structurally from the lemmocytes and are most likely connective tissue elements (Richardson, 1958; Taxi, 1965; Rogers and Burnstock, 1966). Anastomoses between individual nerve fibers have not been observed, even if the fibers run in interlocking bundles, together making up the plexus seen in the light microscope. Since the diameters of the postganglionic fibers are very small $(0.3-1.3\mu)$ their conduction velocity is slow, 0.7–2.3 m/sec. Evidence has been produced that the transmitter substance in the sympathetic nervous system, noradrenaline, is present in the thin fibers of the plexuses, as well as in the perikarya of the postganglionic sympathetic neurons (see Norberg, 1967, for a review).

Neuroeffector mechanisms in the autonomic nervous system. How do the impulses in the peripheral fibers of the autonomic system activate the effector elements (smooth muscle and glandular cells) in the autonomically innervated organs? This problem has been far more difficult to solve than the corresponding one for the somatic nervous system (structure and function of the innervation of extrafusal and intrafusal muscle fibers, see Ch. 3). There are still many open questions, and there are divergent views on some points. Below we will consider chiefly what is known of the structural basis of these neuroeffector mechanisms.

As mentioned above, the view that there is a cytoplasmatic continuity between the peripheral autonomic nerve fibers and the effector cells must now be discarded. Again electron microscopic observations have settled an old dispute. Such studies are extremely difficult to perform, and all organs receiving an autonomic innervation have so far not been examined. Most studies have been concerned with the innervation of smooth muscles (see for example Richardson, 1962, 1964;

Taxi, 1965). Some authors have studied glands (Scott and Pease, 1959; and others.) It appears that the situation is not exactly the same in all organs (Taxi, 1965). Most favorable for study are regions with a rich supply of autonomic innervation, for example the vas deferens and the iris. In the vas deferens of the rat, Richardson (1962) could demonstrate that the fine unmyelinated axons pass without a Schwann cell covering between the muscle fibers. At their ends, and in part along their course, the nerve fibers show small swellings which are in close apposition to the muscle fiber membrane—often in a groove on the surface. These swellings contain vesicles and mitochondria and in several respects resemble terminal boutons in the central nervous system. The vesicles are of two kinds. Some contain a dense central granule while others are clear. It appears that all muscle fibers are innervated in this way. Largely corresponding findings have been made in many other organs (for references see Grillo, 1966).

Although in some organs there may be exceptions to the picture briefly outlined above (see Taxi, 1965) the evidence presented permits the conclusion that in autonomically innervated organs there are structures which may be considered as neuroeffector junctions, in agreement with the conclusion of Burnstock and Holman (1961) from physiological studies.[15] The presence of two kinds of vesicles in these and other nerve endings has recently attracted much interest, since there are indications that the granular vesicles (dense-core vesicles) contain catecholamines (see Hillarp, 1960; Norberg, 1967, for references). Accordingly the endings containing such vesicles should belong to the sympathetic (adrenergic) system. As Richardson (1962) mentions, one must be careful in attributing too much importance to these differences in vesicles, and especially in concluding that the clear vesicles are related to the parasympathetic transmitter, acetylcholine. A later observation of relevance to this problem has been made by Richardson (1964) in electron microscopic studies of the iris of the rat. The sphincter, having a rich parasympathetic innervation has nerve endings containing vesicles of the agranular type, while granular vesicles are found in the dilator muscle, supplied by the sympathetic. A method which is claimed to demonstrate monoamines in tissue sections by fluorescence (Falck, 1962) has been extensively used in recent years in order to trace the presence of monoamines in the nervous system. In studies with this method the adrenergic transmitter, noradrenaline, has been concluded to be present in different quantities in a number of autonomically innervated organs. In sections the noradrenergic fibers appear as fine beaded threads, the beads appear-

---

[15] Other possible ways of activation of the effector organs by autonomic fibers have been discussed as well (see von Euler, 1959).

ing to be sites of contact with smooth muscles or glandular cells. As mentioned above, the transmitter appears to be transported along the fibers from the perikaryon to the terminals. Present knowledge in this field has recently been presented in a review by Norberg (1967) to which the reader is referred for particulars.

There seems to be general agreement that as a rule the *autonomic effectors are set in action by chemical transmission* (see von Euler, 1959). As repeatedly mentioned, the transmitter substance in the postganglionic part of the sympathetic system appears to be noradrenaline, in the parasympathetic, acetylcholine. The mode of action of the transmitters on the target cells has been the subject of much discussion. The transmitter appears to be bound to a receptor substance and is involved in complex enzymatic reactions. These problems will not be considered here.

Afferent fibers in the autonomic system. Above, mainly the efferent part of the autonomic system has been dealt with, and only occasionally have afferent fibers been mentioned. These are less well known than the efferent, in spite of their great practical significance. The afferent visceral impulses normally play their most important role in the various visceral reflexes responsible for the preservation of the "internal equilibrium" of the body and the mutual adjustment of the different visceral functions. It should be emphasized that visceral reflexes are not only initiated by visceral afferent impulses, but by somatic impulses as well, even including those from the special sense organs (e.g. vomiting following irritation of the vestibular apparatus). The visceral afferent fibers which are present in some of the cranial nerves (which might be designated as parasympathetic afferents, although objections can be made to this terminology) appear to have their prime importance as afferent links in visceral reflexes. The vagus nerve does not appear to carry pain sensations. Certain visceral afferent impressions mediated through the cranial nerves, however, also reach consciousness, e.g. taste sensations. These afferent visceral fibers leave their perikarya in the ganglia of the cranial nerves in question, those of the vagus predominantly in the nodose ganglion, those of the glossopharyngeal in the petrous ganglion, and those of the intermediate in the geniculate ganglion. These fibers are treated more fully in the chapter on the cranial nerves.

Other visceral afferent fibers enter the spinal cord, follow the efferent sympathetic fibers peripherally, and apparently have the same segmental distribution. They are distributed to the viscera and the blood vessels, where their terminal ramifications act as receptors. Most of these present themselves morphologically as free nerve endings, but other more specialized endings are also found. In the mesentery there are, for example, Pacinian corpuscles. It is now generally agreed that these visceral afferent fibers, like the somatic afferent, have their perikarya in the spinal ganglia. They reach the spinal nerve through the white rami communicantes. In the cervical, lower lumbar, and sacral regions some of them pass through the gray rami to the sympathetic trunk and ascend or descend in this to the thoracic and upper lumbar segments. The visceral afferent fibers from the lower colon, bladder, prostate, and uterine cervix appear to enter the cord in the 2nd–4th sacral nerve, as is corroborated by surgical observations.

Some of the myelinated fibers found in the peripheral sympathetic plexuses are probably afferent. The central course of the visceral afferents is insufficiently known. They probably end in synaptic contact with cells in the dorsal horns of the spinal cord, and apart from being distributed to the sympathetic efferent neurons, some of the impulses ascend in the anterolateral funiculus and may ultimately reach the level of consciousness. We will return to the "sympathetic" afferent impulses when discussing visceral pain.

Central levels of autonomic regulation. The hypothalamus. In the preceding chapters it has been seen that autonomic functions can be influenced from many regions of the brain, among these various parts of the cerebral cortex, the hippocampus, the entorhinal area, parts of the thalamus, basal ganglia, the reticular formation, and the cerebellum. Most of these actions appear to occur by way of the *hypothalamus.* This receives direct or indirect connections from many of the regions mentioned, and appears to be the main part of the brain concerned in the integration of functions in the autonomic sphere. Its influence on such functions is made possible by efferent fibers from the hypothalamus, which are the first links in pathways leading to the preganglionic autonomic neurons located in the brain stem and spinal cord. In addition, the hypothalamus has intimate nervous and vascular relations to the hypophysis which explain much of its influence on the endocrine system. Increasing knowledge of these relations has led to the emergence of a special field of medicine: *neuroendocrinology,* which is steadily expanding.

While the hypothalamus must be considered as probably the "highest" level of the brain concerned in the integration of autonomic functions, for many of them it is not essential. Some regions in the brain stem are able to take care of a fair degree of integration, as exemplified by the fact that cardiovascular and respiratory regulations function rather satisfactorily in animals and humans even following complete interruption of the brain stem above the pontine region. These and other observations demonstrate the presence of integrative "centers" for these functions in the brain stem. As discussed in Chapter 6, certain regions in the medullary, pontine, and mesencephalic reticular formation have been outlined as being concerned in these regulations (see Fig. 6-8), and particular regions appear to be related more specifically to either circulatory pressor or depressor effects and to either inspiratory or expiratory movements. Other "centers" have likewise been described, for example a "vomiting center" and a "center for micturition." As we have seen, there are rather direct pathways from these regions of the reticular formation to the spinal cord, which mediate the effects (even if it appears that reticulospinal fibers do not establish synaptic contact with the cells of the intermediolateral cell column). Under natural circumstances changes in respiration or cardiovascular function scarcely ever occur in isolation, but as parts of a series of functional changes occurring in response to a variety of stimuli. For example, changes in cardiovascular functions accompany such diverse processes as digestion, temperature regulation, muscular exercise, sexual function, and others. The integration of the various changes occurring in the autonomically innervated organs under such circumstances appears to be the task first and foremost of the hypothalamus, as will be discussed later.

In recent years an enormous number of studies have been devoted to the structure and function of the hypothalamus, not least its relations to the hypophysis and its influence on endocrine organs. The latter problems will only be briefly touched upon in the following account, which will mainly be concerned with anatomical data on the hypothalamus and its connections with other parts of the brain and with the hypophysis.

Quantitatively *the hypothalamus* represents only a trifling part of the whole brain, consisting of those parts of the thin-walled 3rd ventricle which are found below the hypothalamic sulcus (Fig. 11-8). Yet this small region is structurally very complicated, made up of several nuclei differing in structure. Anatomically the hypothalamus presents no large-scale variations in different vertebrates, a fact in harmony with the presence within it of centers regulating the autonomic functions which are more or less uniform in different vertebrates.

In Fig. 11-8 a diagram is reproduced, based on the studies of Le Gros Clark, who has undertaken a thorough mapping of the human hypothalamus (1938). Only a simplified presentation of this intricate region will be attempted here. It will be seen that posterior to the optic chiasma emerges the infundibulum, to which the hypophysis is attached. Posteriorly the infundibulum is continuous with a slightly bulging region in the floor of the 3rd ventricle, the *tuber cinereum*. Then the floor increases in thickness at the transition to the mesencephalon below the aqueduct. Here the *mammillary bodies* are found in the interpeduncular fossa, one on each side of the median plane.

576

A microscopic study reveals that the lateral walls and the floor of the 3rd ventricle are made up of gray matter with some minor fiber bundles. Of the larger fiber bundles the *fornix* should be mentioned, passing from the mammillary body forwards and upwards close beneath the ventricular walls, and revealing itself as a curved elevation anterior to the interventricular foramen. The gray matter consists of small nerve cells which extend close to the ependyma lining the ventricle. This *substantia grisea centralis* or central gray matter contains several groups of cells presenting themselves more or less distinctly as separate nuclei. Some of these will be mentioned.

The *supraoptic nucleus* (Fig. 11-8) is one of them. The name refers to its location, above the beginning of the optic tract on both sides. At its most anterior end it is situated above and lateral to the optic chiasma. The cells of the supraoptic nucleus are considerably larger than those composing the central gray matter, being piriform to round in shape, and on account of the arrangement of the tigroid granules and a frequently somewhat peripherally situated nucleus they resemble cells undergoing retrograde changes. Cells of a smilar type are found in another hypothalamic nucleus, the *paraventricular nucleus,* approximately forming a plate immediately beneath the ependyma. In the cells of this nucleus, as well as in those of the supraoptic nucleus, a colloid substance

FIG. 11–8 Diagram of the ventricular surface of the hypothalamus in man, showing the position and extent of the most conspicuous hypothalamic nuclei. (Cf. text.) Slightly modified from Le Gros Clark, Beattie, Riddoch, and Dott (1938).

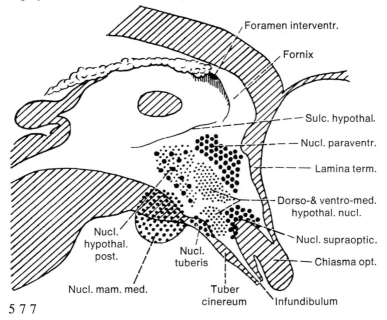

is present (see below). These two nuclei together make up an *anterior group*.

A little distance posterior to the supraoptic nucleus, several small nuclei, usually collectively designated the *nucleus tuberis,* are found (Fig. 11-8). They are situated in the tuber cinereum near its surface, and consist of rather small, multipolar cells. These nuclei are regarded as characteristic primate nuclei by most observers (Ingram, 1940).

Structurally clearly separated from the tuberal nuclei are other nuclear groups exhibiting many features in common. They have been differently named. Le Gros Clark (1938) has designated them the *dorsomedial, ventromedial,* and *lateral hypothalamic nuclei.* Situated above the tuberal nuclei and composed of small and medium-sized nerve cells they form, together with the tuberal nuclei, a *middle nuclear group.* The lateral is especially well developed in anthropoids and man.

A *posterior group* is made up of the nuclei of the mammillary body and a nucleus situated immediately above this. In the mammillary body is found a larger medial small-celled *nucleus mammillaris medialis* and a smaller large-celled *lateral nucleus.* The small-celled part is well developed in anthropoids and man. The other nucleus in the posterior group is the *posterior hypothalamic nucleus,* composed of scattered large cells between a majority of small ones. Apart from the nuclei mentioned, several other nuclear groups are present in the hypothalamus, which will not be considered here.

Other authors have arrived at somewhat different subdivisions of the human hypothalamus. Feremutsch (1955), who discusses the relevant literature, stresses the individual variations in the architecture and is reluctant to consider all the particular cell groups indicated by Le Gros Clark as nuclei. Feremutsch prefers to consider many of these nuclei (except those containing larger cells) as areas representing specializations within the central gray matter. Within this he stresses architectonic differences between the lateral and the periventricular parts. Golgi studies of the hypothalamus of the rat (Szentágothai, Flerkó, Mess, and Halász, 1968) confirm the existence within the hypothalamus of more or less well circumscribed cell groups within a more diffuse conglomerate of cells. These groups differ in part with regard to axonal and dendritic patterns and terminal arborization of afferent fibers. For particulars the reader is referred to the monograph of these authors, which contains also some electron microscopic observations. The authors stress the multifarious interconnections within the hypothalamus, and emphasize certain general differences between the medial and lateral areas. Concerning the former they conclude (loc. cit. p. 56): "Thus a nervous network is established in which, besides the impulses leaving the hypothalamus through the main axons, excitation can spread from a given focus in any direction and can establish an infinite number of closed self-re-exciting chains." The lateral hypothalamic area appears to have fewer local inter-connections. The large neurons present here all appear to project to distant structures. On the other hand, most afferent hypothalamic connections appear to end in this area. This is traversed by fiber bundles of the phylogenetically ancient medial forebrain bundle. Studies on the distribution of cholinesterase and monoamines (including noradrenaline) within the hypothalamus indicate that to some extent these substances are concentrated in particular regions (see Shute and Lewis, 1966, for some data).

The available anatomical information indicates that even if certain cell groups stand out as particular units within the hypothalamus, in much of its territory it is difficult or impossible to draw borders between cell groups. This, as well as the ample interconnections, should be kept in mind in attempts to relate certain regions of the hypothalamus to particular functions. We will return to this question later. For the interpretation of functional observations a knowledge of the connections of the hypothalamus with other regions is important. Unfortunately, most of these connections are so far insufficiently known. In the following discussion the connections of the hypothalamus with other parts of the central nervous system and its relations to the hypophysis will be considered separately.

Fiber connections of the hypothalamus with other regions of the central nervous system. The difficulties involved in making small lesions in the hypothalamus which permit reliable conclusions concerning its efferent fibers are considerable. For this reason precise knowledge on the subject is particularly scanty. The situation is somewhat better as concerns the afferent connections.[16]

The *afferent connections of the hypothalamus* bear evidence that impulses from a number of other regions converge on this part of the brain, as has also been concluded from physiological studies. Information from sensory receptors of different kinds reaches the hypothalamus by more or less direct routes. The existence of *retinal fibers* to the hypothalamus has been claimed by some, but denied by others (see Garey and Powell, 1968, for some data). The recent study of O'Steen and Vaughan (1968), in which the method of autoradiographic tracing of a labeled serotonin precursor was used in rats, provides strong support for the

---

[16] In several anatomical as well as physiological respects the mammillary body differs from the rest of the hypothalamus—being, for example, apparently less closely related to autonomic and endocrine functions. It was considered in Chapter 10 and will be only briefly referred to here.

existence of direct retinohypothalamic fibers. This is relevant to the well-known influence of light on the estrus cycle in many animals.

Some olfactory fibers coming, it appears, largely from the anterior olfactory nucleus, have been claimed to pass directly to the hypothalamus. In addition, as described in Chapter 10, this may be influenced indirectly by olfactory impulses, by way of olfactory projections onto the amygdaloid nucleus and the piriform cortex, both of which give off fibers to the hypothalamus.

In physiological studies potentials have in addition been recorded in the hypothalamus following auditory and cutaneous stimuli and following stimulation of the medial lemniscus (see Cross and Silver, 1966, for references). The anatomical bases for some of these impulse transmissions are not entirely clear. However, hypothalamic afferents have been traced from the *reticular formation* (described in Ch. 6) and may perhaps be involved. Additional influence from the midbrain is possible by way of the connections in the *mammillary peduncle* (see Ch. 10) from the dorsal and deep tegmental nuclei to the mammillary body and to the lateral hypothalamus, and an especially important contribution is established by fibers from the rostral part of the *periaqueductal gray* matter in the mesencephalon (see Nauta, 1958; Szentágothai et al., 1968). There appear to be some fibers from the cerebellum (see Ch. 5).

Several "higher" regions of the brain send fibers to the hypothalamus. There are direct fibers from the *hippocampus* to the hypothalamus, the most massive being the projection to the mammillary body. Secondary connections from the hippocampus may be established via the *septum*. Indirectly the *cingulate gyrus* (via the entorhinal area and the hippocampus, see Ch. 10) may influence the hypothalamus. The *piriform cortex* and probably the amygdala are other sources of hypothalamic afferents. Fibers have been described from the pallidum and from some thalamic nuclei. The presence of hypothalamic afferents from the *neocortex* has been a matter of dispute. In contrast to some previous students, Lundberg (1960) found no evidence for such fibers in an extensive experimental study in the rabbit, nor did Szentágothai et al. (1968) in the cat. Indirect neocortical connections to the hypothalamus have been claimed to exist via the mediodorsal thalamic nucleus (MD, see Fig. 2-11), but the existence of this pathway appears to be doubtful.

The MD is known to project in an orderly topographic manner onto the orbito-frontal cortex (and according to some authors to the lateral surface of the frontal lobe) (Rose and Woolsey, 1948; Roberts and Akert, 1963; Akert, 1964; Narkiewicz and Brutkowski, 1967), and it receives fibers from the frontal cortex, as shown by several authors (for references see DeVito and Smith, 1964; Rinvik, 1968c). In addition the MD receives fibers from the piriform cortex (see Ch. 10). Some authors have advocated the presence of connections from the hypothalamus to the MD as well as of connections passing in the opposite direction. However, as stated by Szentágothai et al. (1968) and Raisman (1966b), the evidence for these connections is not conclusive.

Although far from complete, the above survey clearly demonstrates that the hypothalamus must be influenced—directly or indirectly—from almost all other parts of the brain. It may be conjectured that the various afferents have more or less specific sites of termination within the hypothalamus. Little is known concerning this, however (see Szentágothai et al., 1968, for some data).[17] In a corresponding manner the *efferent connections of the hypothalamus* proceed to many other parts of the brain. Leaving out of consideration the fibers passing to the hypophysis, to be considered in the following section, a summary of our relatively scanty knowledge of the subject is given below (for reviews see Szentágothai et al., 1968; Raisman, 1966b).

To some extent the efferent hypothalamic fiber connections are reciprocal to the afferent ones. Among "ascending" projections the mammillothalamic tract passing to the *anterior thalamic nucleus* (see Ch. 10) is the most massive. Some hypothalamic fibers appear to end in the *amygdala* (see Cowan, Raisman, and Powell, 1965) and in the *septum* (see Raisman, 1966a; Wolf and Sutin, 1966). Of greatest interest are the *pathways by which the hypothalamus may be imagined to act on the preganglionic sympathetic and parasympathetic neurons.* Little is known here either. Hypothalamic efferents descending directly to the parasympathetic cranial nerve nuclei and to the spinal cord have never been convincingly demonstrated anatomically.[18] The descending autonomic pathways must, therefore, be multisynaptic, and only the first link is known with some certainty. Following small lesions in the hypothalamus and using silver impregnation methods, several authors have made largely corresponding findings (see Guillery, 1957; Szentágothai et al., 1968; Wolf and Sutin, 1966; Enoch and Kerr, 1967b). Fibers have been traced consistently to the *mesencephalic periventricular gray* substance. In addition, fibers appear to end in the *pretectal area* and the *superior colliculus*. Fibers traced to the deep tegmental nuclei in the midbrain may possibly be fibers passing through the hypothalamus and coming from other regions (Enoch and Kerr, 1967b). Finally, mention

[17] Among the hypothalamic nuclei the mammillary body appears to be distinguished by more precise and specifically organized connections than the other regions (see Ch. 10).

[18] Recently, Cheatham and Matzke (1966) described descending hypothalamic fibers passing diffusely in the reticular formation to the "dorsolateral visceral gray." The concomitant presence of degenerating corticofugal fibers in their cases appears to invalidate the conclusions.

5 8 1

must be made of the *mammillotegmental tract,* passing from the mammillary body to the midbrain (see Ch. 10). Some fibers have been traced to the raphe nuclei.

The routes along which impulses originating in the hypothalamus are relayed to the medulla and cord from the mesencephalic regions mentioned above are conjectural. It is known that the periaqueductal gray matter gives off a rather massive fanlike projection to almost the entire midbrain and also to the superior colliculus (Nauta, 1958; and others), the "radiatio grisea tegmenti" of Weisschedel (1937). Descending pathways from the mesencephalic reticular formation and the superior colliculus may then conduct further. Physiological studies suggest that the tectospinal tract (situated close to the ventral median fissure in the spinal cord) is scarcely of great importance. Another possibility would be reticulospinal fibers. Since these do not appear to come from the mesencephalon (see Ch. 6) the reticulospinal neurons may be influenced by reticuloreticular fibers from the mesencephalon to the medulla and pons. Certain functional studies in animals and man do not quite fit in with this assumption, however.

Several physiological studies have been undertaken in order to determine the site within the spinal cord of the descending fibers to the autonomic preganglionic neurons. Most often conclusions have been drawn from the effects of partial lesions of the cord on autonomic effects elicited from the hypothalamus or from medullary or pontine regions which influence autonomic functions (the latter regions have been briefly considered in Ch. 6). In a study of this kind in cats and monkeys, in which stimulation of the white matter of the cord was also employed, Kerr and Alexander (1964) tried to locate the pathways mediating vasomotor pressor responses and pressor responses from the urinary bladder (see also Enoch and Kerr, 1967a, 1967b). They concluded that the spinal pathways for the vasomotor pressor responses are situated along most of the surface of the lateral funiculus, while those for vesicomotor as well as pilomotor responses are found in the dorsal part of the same area.[19] In the cervical cord the pupillodilator pathway (passing to the ciliospinal center in C_8–Th_1, see below) was located underneath the surface of the ventral part of the lateral funiculus (Kerr and Brown, 1964).

On account of the practical importance of disturbances in the functions of the urinary bladder following injuries to the spinal cord the

---

[19] It is worthy of notice that the fibers mediating vesicopressor and vasopressor responses appear to pass together in the hypothalamus and midbrain (Enoch and Kerr, 1967b) since the former finally influence the parasympathetic, the latter the sympathetic division of the peripheral autonomic system.

descending pathways concerned in micturition have attracted much interest. In a number of patients subjected to chordotomy Nathan and Smith (1958) found that "a bilateral lesion in the spinal cord which divides the region on an equatorial plane passing through the central canal has an effect upon micturition similar to that produced by a complete transection" (loc. cit. p. 188). It appears that this pathway is involved chiefly in the conscious, voluntary control of micturition, and that the fibers may belong to the corticospinal tract. If so, they apparently do not correspond to the descending vesicopressor fibers studied in animals. We will return to the innervation of the urinary bladder later.

Hypothalamohypophysial relationships. It is an old clinical experience that lesions of the central nervous system, especially of the hypothalamus, may be accompanied by changes in functions which are controlled by the endocrine organs. Of these, only the adrenal medulla receives an inflow of autonomic (sympathetic fibers) of any importance. This explains that the stress-induced increase in adrenal hormone release occurs almost immediately. Most of the other nervous system influences on the endocrine organs evolve much less rapidly. Many of them are now known to be due to the action of hormones from the anterior lobe of the hypophysis on other endocrine organs, such as the gonads, the adrenal cortex, and the thyroid. In recent years the major points in the mechanisms involved in these phenomena have been clarified. It has been shown that the hypothalamus sends abundant nerve fibers to the posterior lobe of the hypophysis, and that there is a vascular link between the hypophysial stalk and the anterior lobe, the hypophysial portal system, which brings the anterior lobe under the control of the hypothalamus. In the following the main anatomical data will be reviewed and some functional observations, related to structure, will be mentioned.[20]

[20] The hypophysis or pituitary gland consists of an anterior lobe or adenohypophysis and a posterior lobe or neurohypophysis. The former is developed embryologically from the epithelium of the primitive pharynx as Rathke's pouch, the latter from the neural tube. The two main lobes may be further subdivided, the most commonly used subdivision being the following: the bulk of the anterior lobe is formed by its pars distalis; dorsally follow the pars tuberalis rostrally and the pars intermedia caudally. The neurohypophysis consists of the median eminence of the tuber cinereum, the infundibular stem caudal to it, and the infundibular process or neural lobe.

The epithelial cells of the adrenohypophysis are of different kinds, and are surrounded by an ample network of sinusoid capillaries. On the basis of their appearance in hematoxylin-eosin stained sections it is common to distinguish between acidophilic (or eosinophilic), basophilic, and neutrophilic (or chromophobe) cells (according to Rasmussen, 1938, about 40, 10, and 50 per cent, respectively). A further subdivision into cell types is possible. There appears to be increasing evi-

Cajal and other early authors described nerve fibers passing from the hypothalamus to the hypophysis in the hypophysial stalk. Knowledge of these connections has since then been considerably extended. The fibers are unmyelinated and numerous, 40,000 in the monkey, some 100,000 in man (Rasmussen, 1940b). Following transection of the stalk in animals retrograde cellular changes and cell loss were observed to a marked degree in the supraoptic and paraventricular nucleus (see Fig. 11-8), the more so the more proximal the section is made. In man likewise a massive cell loss is seen following lesions of the infundibulum (Rasmussen, 1940b). Most of the fibers come from the supraoptic nucleus, in which 80 to 90 per cent of the cells disappear following transection of the stalk (Magoun and Ranson, 1939, in the monkey; O'Connor, 1948, in the rat; and others). As to the paraventricular nucleus, according to O'Connor (1948) and Olivecrona (1957) in the dog and rat, 70 to 80 per cent of its cells give off fibers to the stalk and the posterior lobe. Collectively the fibers from these two nuclei are generally spoken of as the *supraopticohypophysial tract*. The tuberal nuclei likewise give off fibers to the hypophysis, forming the *tuberohypophysial* (or *tuberoinfundibular*) *tract*, but their precise origin has not been experimentally determined. It should be noted that *hypothalamohypophysial fibers have never convincingly been traced to the pars distalis of the anterior lobe*. They are restricted to the posterior lobe (the median eminence, the infundibular stem, and the neural lobe) with a few entering the pars intermedia.

It may now be considered an established fact that the influence of the hypothalamus on the hypophysis occurs by way of a process called *neurosecretion*. Cells which are true nerve cells with axons, dendrites, and Nissl bodies produce substances which are transmitted along the axons and are liberated at their endings. The best known examples of neurosecretory cells are those of the supraoptic and paraventricular

---

dence that there are as many cell types as hormones in the anterior lobe, each type being related to one hormone (see Purves, 1966). Different kinds of basophilic cells are related to the manufacture of the follicle-stimulating (FSH), the luteinizing (LH), and the thyreotrophic (TH) hormone. Two kinds of acidophilic cells produce the growth hormone or somatotrophin (STH) and the lactogenic hormone or prolactin, respectively, while the chromophobe cells are concerned in the production of the adrenocorticotrophic hormone (ACTH). For an exhaustive treatment of the hypophysis see the three-volume monograph: *The Pituitary Gland* (1966).

The main cellular elements in the posterior lobe are the so-called pituicytes. At one time they were believed to be the secretory elements of the neurohypophysis. Presumably they represent a particular kind of glial cell, but their functional role is not yet clear.

nuclei.[21] In these nuclei E. Scharrer in a series of studies from the 1930's described the regular occurrence of what he termed "colloid droplets." They are of various sizes and can be found in the cytoplasm as well as between the cells. Such droplets are found in a number of mammals studied, including man, and also in lower vertebrates (for a comprehensive review see Scharrer and Scharrer, 1954). Scharrer's assumption that these droplets are secretion products, and that the cells are neurosecretory, has been amply confirmed. Using a special method (Gomori's hematoxylin-phloxin stain) Bargmann (1949, and later, see Bargmann, 1954) succeeded in staining the droplets within the cells and could further show that they can be traced along the axons of the hypothalamohypophysial fibers down to the neurohypophysis. In some instances stained droplets were found in the capillaries in the neurohypophysis (Hanström, 1952; and others). Following transection of the hypophysial stalk the stainable substance is found to accumulate above the cut, while it disappears distal to the cut (Hild and Zetler, 1953), and in studies, with the phase-contrast microscope, of tissue cultures from the neurohypophysis, Hild (1954) found evidence that the droplets move along the axons. The relation between the endings of these neurosecretory fibers and the capillaries in the neurohypophysis, where one would assume the substance to enter the blood, has been more difficult to clarify. In silver-impregnated sections from the human neurohypophysis Hagen (1949–50) found that the fibers terminate with small swellings on the capillaries. In the neurohypophysis of the opossum Bodian (1951) observed anatomical features which were favorable for the study of its organization. The neural lobe of the opossum is characterized by a regular subdivision into small lobules. A bundle of nerve fibers enters each of these, and the fibers radiate toward the periphery where they end as palisades of small bulblike swellings against the vascular connective tissue septa surrounding the lobules. The swellings as well as the fibers contain droplets which can be stained with the Gomori method. Following the discovery of the characteristic pattern in the neurohypophysis of the opossum, Bodian (1951) was able to show that in principle the same pattern is present also in man and monkey, although it is less clear.

The neurosecretory material can be stained with other methods than the Gomori stain (see Ortmann, 1960). The so-called *Herring bodies,* rather large, often irregularly shaped, granular or homogeneous bodies visible in ordinary histological sections from the neurohypophysis and noted by the classical anatomists, appear to be particularly large accumulations of neurosecretory material present as swellings at the end of nerve

---

[21] Neurosecretory cells are found also in other locations, in vertebrates as well as invertebrates. For some data see Ortmann (1960).

fibers.[22] From electron microscopic studies it appears that the neuro-secretory material consists of aggregates of granules, 500 to 2000Å in diameter (Bargmann and Knoop, 1957; Palay, 1957; Bodian, 1963, 1966; and others). In addition the palisade terminals contain smaller vesicles of about 300Å in diameter, resembling the synaptic vesicles found elsewhere in nerve endings.[23] Electron microscopic studies have further clarified the relations between the palisade terminals and the capillaries in the neural lobe. Bodian (1963) in the opossum found that the terminals are not separated from the blood vessels by a glial sheath as elsewhere in the brain. The terminals end on the collagen layer, sepa-rated from this only by a basement membrane. Occasionally neuro-secretory granules were seen in the collagen layer. Palay (1955, 1957) observed small pores in the capillary endothelium in the neurohypophy-sis.

On the basis of the findings reviewed above as well as others it ap-pears that the colloid droplets containing the neurosecretory substance are formed in the neurosecretory cells of the nucleus supraopticus and paraventricularis, and that they reach the neurohypophysis by being transported along the fibers of the hypothalamohypophysial tracts. They are finally given off to the blood in the neurohypophysis (see Fig. 11-10). The droplets are assumed to contain the posterior lobe hormones or precursors to them.

This conception is supported by numerous other findings. It was observed rela-tively early in man as well as in experimental animals (Fisher, Ingram, Hare, and Ranson, 1935) that diabetes insipidus follows interruption of the hypophysial stalk as well as destruction of the posterior lobe. In both instances the antidiuretic hor-mone production fails. In attempts to determine the content of posterior lobe hormones [24] in the hypothalamus the hormones have been found in extracts from the supraoptic and paraventricular nuclei but not in extracts from other parts of

[22] Herring bodies have been found in all mammalian neurohypophyses exam-ined. It has been noted by several students that the median eminence and the in-fundibular stem are free of Herring bodies, and according to most authors these regions are also free of Gomori-positive material.

[23] The palisade terminals which can be identified in the median eminence and infundibular stem in the electron microscope contain abundant synaptic vesicles, but only rarely larger granular vesicles (Bodian, 1966). For a detailed electron microscopic study of the median eminence see Rinne (1966).

[24] It seems to be generally agreed that in mammals there are only two such hormones: *oxytocin,* acting chiefly on the smooth muscles of the uterus and the myoepithelial cells of the mammary gland (milk-ejecting factor) and in addition playing a role in parturition and sperm transport in the male and female, and *vasopressin* (corresponding to the former vasopressin and adiuretin) acting particu-larly on smooth muscles in the small arteries and the intestinal tract and on the epithelia of the renal tubules. (There appear to be two kinds of vasopressin, argin-ine and lysine vasopressin.)

the hypothalamus (Hild and Zetler, 1951; and others; see Heller, 1966). In his pioneer studies with implanted electrodes and remote stimulation in rabbits, Harris (1947) demonstrated that stimulation in the region of the supraoptic nucleus or the supraopticohypophysial tract in the course of a few minutes resulted in a reduced diuresis and in animals in estrus in increased uterine contractions. Confirmatory findings have later been made by many authors. Numerous studies have been made of the supraoptic and paraventricular nuclei in animals subjected to thirst for some days. This results in a depletion of stainable neurosecretory substance in the hypothalamus (Hild and Zetler, 1953) as does also the ingestion of massive doses of sodium chloride (Ortmann, 1951). In both cases excessive demands are made on the manufacturing of vasopressin. These and other studies in which cytological details such as changes in nuclear and nucleolar size (see Bargmann, 1954) have been examined, all support the general view of the neurosecretory hypothalamohypophysial system outlined above.

There appears to be increasing evidence that of the two distinct nuclei in the anterior hypothalamus, the supraoptoic nucleus is related especially to vasopressin (adiuretin), the paraventricular to oxytocin. Experimental lesions of the latter nucleus result in a marked decrease in oxytocin in the posterior lobe (Olivecrona, 1957; see also Heller, 1966). This is in keeping with the observation that a differential release of the two hormones may occur under certain conditions; for example, sucking releases preponderantly oxytocin, dehydration chiefly vasopressin.

Some additional observations on the regulation of vasopressin production and release deserve mention. A number of studies have shown that there is in the hypothalamus a region responsible for the regulation of water intake. Following the observations of Andersson (see Andersson, 1957) that drinking can be induced in goats by electrical stimulation of the anterior hypothalamus, several studies have been devoted to the presence of a "thirst center" in the hypothalamus. Fitzsimons (1966) in a recent review concludes that while the hypothalamus is obviously very important in regulating water intake, it is probably part of a more extensive system concerned in regulating food and water intake. Various stimuli (exertion, changes in emotional state, alterations of blood volume, and others) are known to cause increased drinking, but the mechanism by which these stimuli act is not entirely clear. Under several circumstances an increase in the osmotic pressure of the body fluids appears to be the effective stimulus. Verney (1947) demonstrated that the osmolarity of the blood in the carotids influences the release of antidiuretic hormone (vasopressin) and created the term *"osmoreceptors"* for elements in the hypothalamus which are sensitive to osmotic changes. According to Verney the osmoreceptors are found in the anterior part of the hypothalamus, and it was suggested that they are cells situated in or close to the supraoptic nucleus. This assumption receives support from studies of different kinds, recently reviewed by

Joynt (1966). Anatomical data suggests that the cells of the supraoptic nucleus must be especially well suited to acting as osmoreceptors. The supraoptic nucleus and the paraventricular nucleus, especially the former, have an extremely ample blood supply. The capillary density of the supraoptic nucleus exceeds that of any other part of the brain (Finley, 1940; and others). In sections in which the capillaries are stained the two nuclei can be discerned with the naked eye. Furthermore, each cell is surrounded by a network of capillaries without a glial sheath between the capillary and the cell. Occasionally a capillary has even been seen to pass through the cytoplasm of a cell (Scharrer and Gaupp, 1933, in man). Finally it is of interest that the blood supply to the anterior hypothalamus comes directly from the internal carotid or its branches and the circle of Willis (see Dawson, 1958; Daniel, 1966). The situation appears to be essentially the same in man and most other mammals studied.

The cells in the supraoptic nucleus are obviously in an especially favorable situation for reacting to changes in the osmolarity of the blood, increasing osmolarity leading to increased production of antidiuretic hormone (vasopressin).[25] The ways in which the cells are acted upon when diuresis is influenced, for example in emotional changes, are obscure, since little is known of afferent connections to the supraoptic nucleus. In Golgi sections the sparse network of afferents found in the nucleus appears to reach it from above (Szentágothai et al., 1968), but the source of these fibers is unknown.

It appears to be established that the two hormones attributed to the posterior lobe of the hypophysis are not produced there. Substances are formed in the supraoptic and paraventricular nuclei, which are transported along the axons of the cells in the nuclei and enter the blood stream. The question whether the neurosecretory substance seen in light and electron microscopic sections is the hormone, a precursor, or only a carrier substance appears not to be finally settled.[26] Vasopressin appears to be an octapeptide linked in a still unexplained way with a precursor or carrier polypeptide (see Sloper, 1966). Many problems remain unsolved, for example concerning the rate of transportation from the hypothalamus to the neurohypophysis and, not least, concerning the way and form in which the hormones enter the blood in the neurohypophysis. A special functional role for the pituicytes has not yet been found. Some

---

[25] If the osmoreceptors are actually the cells in the supraoptic nucleus, these would then have three functions, since in addition to being osmoreceptors they are responsible for the production of hormone and may produce impulses passing in the supraopticophysial tract.

[26] For some recent data on the neurohypophysis see Farrel, Fabre, and Rauschkolb (1968).

possible relations of these cells to the passage of the hormones into the blood have been suggested by Bodian (1966) on the basis of electron microscopic studies. The function of the "synaptic vesicles" in the palisade nerve endings is another open question.

The problems just discussed concern the antidiuretic hormone, vasopressin, as well as *oxytocin,* apparently produced chiefly in the paraventricular nucleus. The effects of oxytocin, chemically closely related to vasopressin (see Heller, 1966), on the uterine muscles and on the mammary gland have been extensively studied. Some data concerning the latter action may serve to illustrate both mechanisms. As mentioned previously, oxytocin causes the (non-innervated) ectodermal myoepithelial cells surrounding the alveoli of the mammary gland to contract, resulting in emptying of the breast.[27] This is generally referred to as milk let-down. Electrical stimulation of the paraventricular nucleus produces milk let-down, but not when the hypophysial stalk has been transected. A nervous and hormonal reflex is responsible for the milk let-down which occurs during sucking. The afferent part of the reflex arc is nervous, the first link being sensory fibers from the nipple and areola passing to the spinal cord in the intercostal nerves. Along routes which are not fully known the nervous impulses finally act on the paraventricular nucleus, with resulting release of oxytocin. The phenomenon that milk let-down can be influenced from "higher" levels of the nervous system has been demonstrated experimentally, and is well known from daily life. During the period of lactation most mothers observe that milk let-down occurs not only when the baby is sucking. The very thought of putting the baby to the breast may produce some milk let-down.[28] In what way the imagination in this case results in activations of the paraventricular nucleus is not known, but it must occur via nervous connections which ultimately lead to the hypothalamus.

Other *observations in man* are also consistent with the results of experimental studies. *Diabetes insipidus* [29] is met with in tumors which affect the hypothalamus (frequently combined with other hypothalamic

[27] The *secretion* of milk is a complex process in which several anterior lobe hormones are concerned, first and foremost the lactogenic hormone, prolactin, produced presumably by the acidophilic cells.

[28] The concomitant activation of the uterine musculature during sucking illustrates the other main action of oxytocin. It may be imagined that this has a beneficial effect on post-partum involution of the uterus (and serves as one of many arguments in favor of the view that breast feeding of infants should be encouraged!).

[29] The polyuria is the primary feature of the disease, due to deficient reabsorption of water in the renal tubules; the polydipsia is a consequence of the increased elimination of water.

589

symptoms), and sometimes in chronic epidemic encephalitis. Traumatic injuries to the hypothalamus may be followed by diabetes insipidus, but in some cases no explanation for its appearance can be found. Cases of diabetes insipidus have been described in which pathological changes have been found in the anterior part of the hypothalamus, and there appears to be no doubt that also in man diabetes insipidus may be produced by purely hypothalamic as well as by purely hypophysial lesions.

Above, mainly the projections to the hypophysis from the supraoptic and paraventricular nucleus have been considered. In addition there are, as mentioned previously, *fibers from the tuberal region to the neurohypophysis.* Their precise origin has not been experimentally settled, but according to Szentágothai et al. (1968) in Golgi sections they can be seen to come from small cells surrounding the lower part of the third ventricle (particularly from a nucleus called the arcuate nucleus). *These fibers can be traced only to the median eminence and the infundibular stem.* They are often referred to as the tuberohypophysial tract, but as suggested by Szentágothai et al. (1968) a more appropriate name would be the *tuberoinfundibular tract.* These thin fibers end on capillary loops in the median eminence, but in addition a number of endings are aggregated in a so-called palisade zone, situated superficially in the median eminence and the proximal part of the stalk, in immediate contact with the pars tuberalis of the anterior lobe. According to Szentágothai et al. (1968) this zone is essentially a compact system of nerve endings.

As briefly mentioned previously, according to most authors the median eminence and the proximal part of the stalk do not contain neurosecretory material which can be made visible with the Gomori method. When studied with the electron microscope the nerve terminals found here, according to Bodian (1966), contain abundant small vesicles of the "synaptic vesicle" type (about 300Å in diameter), but only rarely are larger vesicles seen. Other authors have found more granular vesicles and a greater variety of vesicles (see Rinne, 1966, for references). The tuberoinfundibular system thus differs in several respects from the supraoptico- and paraventriculo-hypophysial system. The fact that secretory granules of the Gomori-positive type, present in the latter, have not been found by most authors in the tuberoinfundibular system does not, however, exclude the possibility that this too is a neurosecretory system. Lundberg (1957) in a study of human brains described a particular type of Gomori-positive substance, differing in respect to stainability from the usual substance of the supraopticohypophysial system. Granules of this substance (called β-granules by Lundberg) were found in large masses in cells in the tuber region and in their axons (see Rinne, 1966, for particulars concerning the ultrastructure of the median eminence). There is indeed good evidence (see below) that the anterior lobe is dependent for its function on connections with the hypothalamus, and it is generally assumed that the hypothalamic influence occurs by way of neurosecretion. Since hypothalamic fibers do not reach the anterior lobe, this influence was difficult to understand until the discovery of the hypophysial portal vessel system, which provides a vascular link between the median eminence and stalk (where hypothalamic fibers terminate) and the anterior lobe.

The discovery of the *hypophysial portal vessel system* is attributed to Popa and Fielding (1930). In the hypophysial stalk and the median eminence they observed a net of sinusoid capillaries which were connected with vessels entering the anterior lobe as well as with larger vessels of the stalk. Those entering the anterior lobe were connected with the sinuosoids in this. The vessels connecting the two capillary networks (in the stalk and the anterior lobe) were called *portal vessels*.[30] In the following years divergent opinions as to course of the blood flow in these portal vessels were held, but the question could not be decided in purely anatomical studies. By direct observations of the portal vessels in living animals Green and Harris (1949) and others have proved that the blood flow is from above downward, from the stalk and median eminence to the anterior lobe. This fact obviously is essential for the understanding of the functional role of the hypophysial portal vessel system. Before considering this subject, some other observations, extending those mentioned, will be reviewed. This will be done with reference to Fig. 11-9, based on the extensive studies in man by Xuereb, Prichard, and Daniel (1945a, 1945b). These authors, in addition to usual histologic techniques, employed the method of injecting the hypophysial arteries or veins with neoprene latex. When this hardens the tissue is macerated, and casts of the vascular system are obtained.

As seen in Fig. 11-9, the hypophysis is supplied by two sets of arteries, both arising from the internal carotid. The superior hypophysial artery (SHA in Fig. 11-9) runs in a posteromedial direction and forms an arterial ring around the uppermost part of the hypophysial stalk. Some branches from this artery supply the optic chiasma, some pass to the hypothalamus, but the majority enter the upper part of the infundibular stem. From each of the superior arteries a particular branch, the so-called *trabecular artery* of Xuereb et al. (AT in Fig. 11-9), takes off in a

[30] A hypophysial portal system has been found in all vertebrate species studied (see Green, 1951), even in animals in which the anterior and posterior lobe are separated by a well-developed connective tissue septum, as for example in whales (Valsø, 1936; and others).

591

Hypothalamus

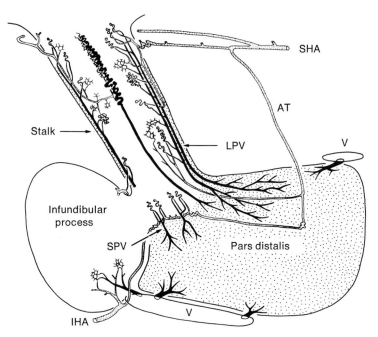

FIG. 11–9 Diagram illustrating the vessels of the hypophysial portal system in man. The portal vessels leading from the sinusoids in the hypophysial stalk to the anterior lobe are shown in black. (Cf. text.) Abbreviations: *IHA* and *SHA:* inferior and superior hypophysial arteries; *AT:* trabecular artery; *LPV* and *SPV:* long and short portal vessels, respectively; *V: veins.* From Adams, Daniel, and Prichard (1965–6).

descending direction and enters the anterior lobe. According to Xuereb, Prichard, and Daniel (1954a) this does not give off branches to the anterior lobe, while other authors maintain that it has a few small end arteries to this (see Stanfield, 1960). There is agreement that the trabecular artery (which has been given different names by other authors) finally enters the hypophysial stalk. The inferior hypophysial arteries (IHA) form a ring around the posterior lobe, from which branches are given off to this as well as to the lower part of the infundibular stem.

The most important finding in these studies is that *the anterior lobe receives all (or practically all) its blood supply via the hypophysial portal vessels.* When the hypophysial arteries enter the hypophysial stalk they break up into a number of coiled and looped sinusoid capillaries. Many of these are arranged in a very complex manner, as clearly shown in the photographs in the papers of Xuereb, Prichard, and Daniel (1954a,

1954b; see also Daniel, 1966). The superior hypophysial artery distributes mainly to a superior net of sinusoids, the inferior to a net in the inferior part of the infundibular stem. Blood from the two nets of sinusoids collects into vessels which pass to the anterior lobe. These are the portal vessels, which after entering the anterior lobe give rise to a second capillary bed in this. A distinction may be made between the long portal vessels (LPV in Fig. 11-9) coming from the superior part of the stem and the short ones (SPV) from the inferior part. The latter supply chiefly the part of the anterior lobe adjacent to the lower infundibular stem. This different distribution is of some interest for the results of operative transection of the hypophysial stalk in man.

This operation has been suggested and in some cases performed as an alternative to hypophysectomy for the treatment of malignant disease, especially mammary cancer, on the assumption that the anterior lobe will be inactivated by the transection. However, a transection of the stalk will interrupt only the blood supply of the anterior lobe coming via the superior portal vessels, while the inferior supply will be spared. In studies of hypophyses from 21 patients subjected to stalk section, Adams, Daniel, and Prichard (1966) found that the territory supplied by the inferior vessels had survived necrosis. Corresponding findings have been made in animals (see Daniel, 1966, for references). The functional activity of the remaining tissue may, however, not be normal. It is well known that the anterior lobe in order to function normally requires intact connections with the hypothalamus. (The hormone production of an autotransplanted hypophysis is much reduced.) In agreement with this, the epithelial cells in the part of the anterior lobe preserved after stalk section are much reduced in size and show other changes as well (see Adams, Daniel, and Prichard, 1966). The posterior lobe also shows changes after some time. Presumably these consequences of stalk section are due to the fact that neurohumors from the hypothalamus no longer act on the still viable part of the anterior lobe and the neural lobe since stalk section interrupts the neurosecretory hypothalamohypophysial fibers (see also below).

As mentioned above, nerve endings of the tuberoinfundibular tract appear to end on the sinusoid capillaries in the loops and nets into which the hypophysial arteries feed when they have entered the median eminence and the infundibular stem. A mechanism similar to that established by the endings of fibers from the supraoptic and paraventricular nuclei on the vessels in the neural lobe would explain that the hypothalamus influences the functions of the anterior lobe: substances transported along the tuberoinfundibular tract would enter the blood in the sinusoids, and via the portal vessels would be transported to the anterior lobe. Here the substances would influence the hormone-producing cells. The hypothalamic control of the anterior lobe would accordingly occur by way of neurosecretion. This view appears now to be generally accepted, and there is, as we have seen, considerable anatomical evidence which is in complete agreement with it, even if many details remain to be clarified, for example the precise origin of the hypothalamic nuclei giving off the fibers, etc.[31]

There is abundant *physiological evidence* that the hypothalamus influences the hormonal activity of the anterior lobe.[32] A few of the earlier studies may be mentioned. Electrical stimulation of the hypothalamus may result in an increased production of gonadotrophic hormones (Markee, Sawyer, and Hollinshead, 1946; Harris, 1948; and others). Stimulation of the posterior hypothalamus with the tuberal region yields secretion of the adrenocorticotrophic hormone, ACTH (de Groot and Harris, 1950; Porter, 1953; and others). From the tuber region ovulation has been induced in rabbits (Harris, 1948). Stimulation of the anterior lobe directly does not have any of these effects. On the other hand, transection of the hypophysial stalk results in cessation of estrus in rabbits (Harris, 1950), and lesions of the posterior hypothalamic regions will abolish the secretion of ACTH which otherwise follows stress stimuli (de Groot and Harris, 1950; and others). A vast number of subsequent physiological studies have on the whole given support to the conclusions drawn by the early workers in the field.

Some particular much-discussed problems in the hypothalamic control of the anterior lobe will be briefly touched upon. One concerns the nature of the neurosecretory substances acting on the cells of the anterior lobe. These are now commonly referred to as *releasing factors* (for a brief review see Harris, Reed, and Fawcett, 1966), and are named according to the hormone they release (corticotrophin, luteinizing hormone, follicle-stimulating hormone, thyreotrophin, somatotrophin, and prolactin releasing factors). Studies of this subject are difficult, and the chemical characterization of the various factors has only begun. It appears that they are peptides. Some of the releasing factors have been found to be present in extracts from the hypothalamus, and in the vessels of the stalk (see McCann, Dhariwal, and Porter, 1968, for references) in agreement with current views on the mode of action of the hypothalamus on the anterior lobe.

Recent research has brought forward a number of observations on the hormones and their action, illustrating the complexities present. The actions of many anterior lobe hormones have turned out to be less specific than formerly believed.

[31] The account of the hypophysial portal system given here is highly simplified. According to studies of Török (see Szentágothai et al., 1968) there are other possible routes for a blood flow from the vascular loops of the hypophysial stalk in addition to the major one to the anterior lobe.

[32] For a fuller treatment of these subjects and references special texts should be considered, for example the monograph of Szentágothai, Flerkó, Mess, and Halász (1968), *The Pituitary Gland* (1966), and the recent review of McCann, Dhariwal, and Porter (1968).

Several have been shown to affect other functions than those related to their main target organs. For example, lactation is known to be influenced by several hormones in addition to prolactin. Many functions in which hypothalamic hormones are involved concern several endocrine as well as other organs. Under normal circumstances such combined effects are produced by a variety of stimuli. The influence of the hormonal level of the target organs on hypothalamic-anterior lobe activity has attracted much interest. It appears to be established, for example, that the level of estrogens in the blood influences the secretion of gonadotrophic hormones (a high level of progesterone reduces the synthesis and release of the luteinizing hormone). Many feedback mechanisms have been demonstrated (for some recent data see McCann, Dhariwal, and Porter, 1968; for an extensive discussion see Szentágothai et al., 1968).

A much debated question related to the hypothalamohypophysial relations concerns a possible correlation between individual anterior lobe hormones or their releasing factors and particular regions of the hypothalamus. This problem has been attacked in different ways.

Changes in the hormone production or hormone-influenced behavior have been searched for following variously placed, isolated lesions of the hypothalamus, following electrical stimulation, and following implants of small quantities of hormones or other substances in the hypothalamus. More indirect methods, studying anatomical and physiological changes in the hypothalamus under various hormonal situations, and morphological changes in the target organs following lesions of the hypothalamus, have also been employed. Studies of these problems meet with a number of difficulties, and there are many sources of error as emphasized recently by Donovan (1966). Apart from difficulties inherent in the physiological methods themselves (types of electrodes, anesthesia, etc.) the anatomical situation in the hypothalamus is extremely unfavorable for studies of these problems.

As we have seen, there are fairly good indications that the paraventricular and supraoptic nucleus are concerned primarily with the production of oxytocin and vasopressin, respectively. As concerns the hypothalamic influence on the anterior lobe hormones the situation is less clear. Different suggestions have been made concerning a functional segregation within the hypothalamus. For example, the gonadotrophin-controlling mechanism has been attributed by some especially to the basal tuberal region, while the anterior hypothalamic region has been claimed to be more particularly related to the control of the thyreotrophic hormone. The situation has been characterized by Donovan (1966, p. 250) as follows: "Strenuous efforts have been made to relate the control of a particular aspect of pituitary function to a particular nucleus or nuclear group, but without great success." Available knowledge of the anatomy of the hypothalamus, although very incomplete, lends little support to the assumption of any marked degree of localization within this part of the nervous system, having chiefly diffuse dendritic, axonal, and terminal ramifications and abundant recurrent collaterals. We will return to this question in the following section. The problems concerning the neuroendocrine relations have turned out to be extremely complex, and their study is beset with great technical difficulties. Many conclusions and current views and opinions must still be considered provisional. There is reason to agree with Cross and Silver (1966, p. 259) when they say: "We shall not be surprised if, ten years hence, views on hypothalamic function have undergone extensive revision." Fig. 11-10 summarizes present concepts of the hypothalamohypophysial relationships.

The *pars intermedia* is a part of the hypophysis which in man appears to be of relatively little importance. In a series of vertebrates it has been known for some time to influence the color of the skin by producing expansion of the melanocytes or dispersion of the melanin granules within their cytoplasm. Its hormone, previously called *intermedin,* now generally referred to as *melanocyte-stimulating hormone* (MSH), has been shown to consist of two components, both peptides. As

FIG. 11–10 Diagram showing the suggested pathways by which nerve cells in the hypothalamus (*H*) transmit neurohumors via their axons into loops of the primary capillary bed (*P*), and thence through the long (*LPV*) and short (*SPV*) portal vessels to control the output of hormone from cells (*C*) in a given area of the pars distalis. The innervation of the capillary bed (*Cap*) in the infundibular process by nerve cells in the hypothalamus is also shown. Compare with FIG. 11–9. From Adams, Daniel, and Prichard (1965–6).

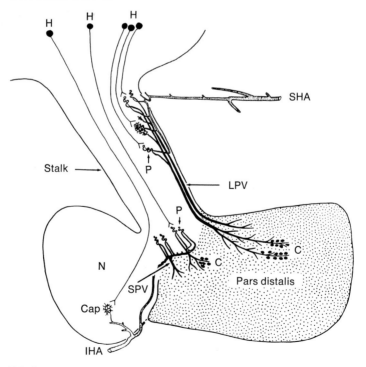

mentioned previously, the pars intermedia receives some nerve fibers from the hypophysial stalk. Their endings, according to most authors, contain neurosecretory granules. Whether the neurosecretory substance acts directly on the cells or by way of the vessels in the poorly vascularized pars intermedia appears uncertain. It has been suggested that in man the hormone may be of some importance for darkening of the skin as protection against sunlight. In patients suffering from adrenocortical insuffiency or some types of pituitary tumors, large amounts of MSH appear to be released and are presumably responsible for the marked darkening of the skin seen in these patients. (For an exhaustive treatment of the intermediate lobe see Volume 3 of *The Pituitary Gland,* 1966.)

Some functional aspects of central levels of autonomic integration. This subject merits some consideration in addition to the scattered data concerning hypothalamoendocrine relations touched on above. It covers a vast field. Many observations have been made, but their interpretation is not easy, and many uncritical suggestions have been set forth. Some of these concern the question of "centers" for the regulation of particular functions influenced by the autonomic system. It is beyond the scope of the present text to treat this subject in any detail. Following a brief presentation of some points, we will chiefly discuss the question of the tenability of the concept of autonomic "centers."

Mention has been made previously of the postulated "centers" in the brain stem (respiratory, cardiovascular, "vomiting," "micturition," and other centers). In the following we shall mainly be concerned with the "centers" assumed to exist in the hypothalamus. As already mentioned, they appear to a large extent to act via the lower "centers," and to serve integration of autonomic functions of a more complex kind than the latter. Changes in a number of functions influenced by the autonomic system have been recorded in experimental animals, following stimulation or destruction of various parts of the hypothalamus. Some information has been obtained from studies in man. It should be noted that many of the effects observed in the autonomic sphere represent fragments of more complex behavior changes.

Cardiovascular functions are influenced on stimulation of the hypothalamus, as noted by early workers in the field. Increase of blood pressure and acceleration of heart rate have been obtained on stimulation of the posterior lateral part of the hypothalamus. Vasodilatation and depressor responses have been seen chiefly from anterior hypothalamic regions.

The hypothalamus appears to play a decisive role in the *regulation of body temperature.* Early workers found that in cats increased loss of heat (which occurs mainly by panting since they only sweat on the pads of the feet) can be elicited by local heating of the anterior hypothalamus, suggesting that in this region there are cells which are susceptible to an increased temperature of the blood. By this mechanism an increase of the temperature of the body above the normal level is prevented. An animal with a bilateral lesion of this region will not start panting and sweating as a normal animal if it is brought into a heated room (Clark, Magoun, and Ranson, 1939), and its body temperature will rise. This reaction, or lack of reaction, is persistent, although some degree of adaptation takes place in the course of some weeks. Conversely, bilateral lesions in the posterior part of the hypothalamus, dorsolateral to the mammillary bodies, are followed by a deficient capacity to adjust to lowered environmental temperatures. Shivering and peripheral vaso-constriction do not occur on exposure to cold.

Further research with more refined methods has extended these early observations (see Cooper, 1966, for a brief survey). The presence of "receptors" in the hypothalamus, sensitive to heating or cooling of the blood, has been confirmed, and several factors involved in the central mechanisms of temperature control have been clarified. Injection of pyrogens in the anterior hypothalamus but not in other regions has been shown to produce fever, but the mechanism by which this occurs is not clear.

Clinical observations indicate that conditions are similar in man. *Postoperative hyperthermia* is not infrequently observed following operations in which the hypothalamus is apt to be injured. This applies particularly to operations for hypophysial tumors and suprasellar meningeomas. In some cases, which have taken a fatal course with death occurring in hyperthermia soon after the operation, lesions in the anterior part of the hypothalamus have been discovered. In the more common cases of moderate and transient postoperative hyperthermia, this is presumably due to a less severe damage to this part of the hypothalamus (edema or minute hemorrhages). Experience obtained in cases of tumors (primary or metastatic) or hemorrhages into the hypothalamus lend further support to the view that the hypothalamus is essential for an effective regulation of body temperature (see for example Davison, 1940; Zimmerman, 1940).[33]

It appears from the available data that the anterior, lateral part of the hypothalamus is a region which is concerned in regulation of the mechanism of heat loss, and in the lateral part of the posterior hypothalamus an area is present which regulates heat production and is able to increase

---

[33] Recent investigations do not support the old conception that the thalamus and the striate body are concerned in the regulation of body temperature. Presumably concomitant injury to the hypothalamus has been responsible for the changes in temperature observed. The antipyretic drugs must be assumed to act mainly on the hypothalamus.

this if necessary. However, none of the areas can be sharply circumscribed, and they apparently do not coincide with definite nuclei.

Some other functions shown to be influenced from the hypothalamus may be mentioned. *Piloarrection* can be elicited on electrical stimulation of several parts of the hypothalamus. The hypothalamus is probably concerned in integrating the activity of the pilomotors with other autonomic functions in which piloarrection is brought into play, as, for example, in temperature regulation and in expressions of rage and fear.

Mention was made previously of the role of the hypothalamus in the regulation of *water metabolism* of the body and of the presence of a "drinking center." Correspondingly, certain regions of the hypothalamus appear to be closely related to the *control of food intake*. Certain medially placed lesions may result in hyperphagia and obesity, while lateral lesions are apt to produce aphagia and consequent emaciation. A lateral "feeding center" and a medial "satiety center" have been postulated. *Growth,* bearing some relation to food intake, may likewise be influenced from the hypothalamus (presumably, in part at least, by way of the somatotrophic hormone from the anterior lobe). These findings are of interest in relation to the frequent occurrence of obesity in hypothalamic lesions in man, and fit in with the view that *dystrophia adiposogenitalis* is due to lesions of the hypothalamus.

Of clinical interest also is the demonstration that the hypothalamus may act on the *digestive organs*. It has been repeatedly demonstrated in animals that stimulation of the anterior hypothalamus produces increase of secretion and peristalsis in the stomach and gut. If the posterior part of the hypothalamus is stimulated, however, these functions are depressed, and symptoms of sympathetic activity occur. Lesions of the hypothalamus in animals have been shown by a number of students to be often followed by ulcerations and hemorrhages in the stomach and gut. Long, Leonard, Chou, and French (1962), making stereotactic hypothalamic lesions in cats, found that anterior lesions often resulted in acute gastric hemorrhage, while posterior lesions were followed either by hemorrhage, or more often, gastric ulceration. Chronic stimulation of the hypothalamus by implanted electrodes is likewise often followed by gastric ulceration or hemorrhage, apparently without reference to any particular localization of the electrode (see Long, Leonard, Story, and French, 1962, for a recent study). Lesions in other parts of the brain have also been shown to result in gastrointestinal hemorrhage and ulceration.

It is well known that melena and hematemesis occasionally may follow intracranial operations. In neurosurgical departments (as in animal laboratories) this is much more frequent after operations in which the hypothalamus is apt to be damaged than after other intracranial procedures. These changes occur very rapidly, in animals as well as in man, and in the course of a few days perforation may induce a fatal course. It has been suggested that the gastrointestinal changes produced by hypothalamic lesions or stimulations result from an imbalance between the two components of the autonomic system. It has been maintained that stress situations are capable of producing gastric ulcers, presumably by influencing the hypothalamic control of the digestive tract. On the basis of experimental and clinical observations it has been suggested that changes in the hypothalamus may play a role in the development of gastric and duodenal ulcers, so frequent in human beings. Although the localization of the ulcers is different (the postoperative ulcerations are usually found on the great curvature or at the cardia or pylorus), it is generally admitted that hypothalamic factors may be of importance in the etiology of ordinary gastric ulcers, even if several factors, not only nervous, but also humoral and mechanical, are involved.

Other functions which appear to be influenced from the hypothalamus are the *sexual functions*. However, little is known regarding details. *Disturbances of sleep* have been observed following affections of the hypothalamus in animals and man as discussed in Chapter 6, and "waking" and "sleeping" centers have been postulated. The role of the hypothalamus in *emotional behavioral reactions* has been much discussed. In this sphere it obviously collaborates with other regions of the brain with which it has fiber connections, not least the amygdaloid nucleus (see Ch. 10).

It should be stressed that a distinction must be made between *emotional expressions and behavior* and *emotions*. The latter must be conceived as being primarily at least conscious feelings of a purely subjective nature. Emotional reactions, which involve autonomic as well as somatic phenomena, do not necessarily occur in emotions but may, at least to a large extent, be suppressed. On the other hand, findings in decorticate animals have shown that emotional *reactions* may be elicited when there can scarcely be any emotions. In animals in which the entire cerebral cortex, the basal ganglia, and the bulk of the thalamus have been removed, leaving only the hypothalamus in connection with the lower parts of the brain, the phenomenon of "sham rage" is observed (Bard, 1928). These animals react with severe expressions of rage, pupillary dilatation, erection of hairs, increased heart rate, scratching, biting, snarling, etc., to various stimuli, even stimuli which normally do not elicit rage. The phenomena have been explained as being due to an outburst of discharges from the posterior hypothalamus, since they cease when this also is removed. In contrast to normal emotionally induced reactions, "sham rage" behavior ceases almost immediately when the stimulation is discontinued.

Lesions of the hypothalamus in man have been observed in several instances to be followed by manic excitement or by depressive states.

In cases in which the hypothalamus has been pressed upon or has been subjected to traction during operations various symptoms have been noted. Anxiety feelings and expressions, flights of ideas and motor hyperactivity and talkativeness, severe depressive feelings, and other phenomena have been repeatedly observed. The emotional changes occurring in chronic epidemic encephalitis, especially in children, have also been claimed to be due to damage to the hypothalamus.

In addition to those mentioned, other functions, such as sweating, urinary secretion, and others, may be influenced from the hypothalamus. In fact, there is scarcely an activity of the body which can not be influenced from this part of the brain. In spite of a number of studies, including recordings of potentials in the hypothalamus following stimulation of various peripheral and central sites and determination of regional variations in the distribution of substances as noradrenaline, acetylcholine, serotonin, and others, we are far from understanding how the hypothalamus is able to perform its remarkably well integrated actions on a diversity of processes. The idea that the two divisions of the peripheral autonomic system are represented in different regions of the hypothalamus is difficult to uphold, even though, as we have seen, there is some evidence concerning certain phenomena that the anterior hypothalamus is related particularly to parasympathetic activity, the posterior to sympathetic. However, so far no clear borders have been defined between these two subdivisions of the hypothalamus, either morphologically or functionally. It should be recalled that it is virtually impossible to destroy or stimulate one of the divisions without involving fiber connections of the other.

"Centers" in the hypothalamus for the control of a number of functions have been postulated; some of them have already been mentioned. The concept of "centers" within the nervous system, i.e. morphologically fairly well circumscribed regions concerned with a particular "function," is becoming less and less attractive and less acceptable as our insight into the organization of the nervous system increases. As concerns the hypothalamus, it is obvious that several of the postulated "centers" should govern extremely complex processes (for example, regulation of body temperature or cardiovascular regulation) many of which involve not only autonomic influences on the target organs, but somatic and often endocrine influences as well (feeding behavior, sexual functions). It seems, *a priori,* to be extremely unlikely that a small spatially restricted collection of cells should be capable of the high degree of integration required for such tasks. The concept of "centers" is made even more dubious since several of them are postulated to have approximately the same location within the hypothalamus. (This indeed would seem to

be a virtue of necessity, since even if each "center" is supposed to be rather small, it would be difficult to accommodate the large number of "centers" described within the small volume of the hypothalamus!)

It appears at present that *the only conclusion which can safely be drawn concerning the hypothalamic "centers" is that they represent areas of the central nervous system which are essential for the proper performance of certain functions.* Damage to these areas results in disturbances of these functions. However, the same functions which are controlled by the hypothalamus can be influenced from other regions of the brain as well, often likewise referred to as "centers." A number of such "centers" have been described, even for fairly elementary functions. For example, as concerns the neural control of sweating, Wang (1964) describes "centers" in the reticular formation, the hypothalamus, the thalamus, and the striopallidum, and mentions the cerebral cortex and the cerebellum as other regions which may influence sweating. In view of the fiber connections of the hypothalamus it is only to be expected that functions which are controlled by it may also be influenced from other parts of the brain. Accordingly it is misleading to consider any of them as "centers." It appears that, in some way which is as yet poorly understood, an intimate collaboration between a number of particular regions of the brain takes place when autonomic functions are influenced, and when these are integrated with each other as well as with somatic and endocrine changes appearing as components in more complex reactions. This does not contradict the assumption that the hypothalamus is a particularly important region for the integration of autonomic functions. From a clinical standpoint the influence of the cerebral cortex on autonomic functions is of particular interest, in view of the obvious relationships between mental activity and autonomic changes, not least those occurring in emotional states. These relationships are far from being understood, in spite of a large body of observations, including those made in behavioral studies of animals and man with lesions of certain parts of the brain. Only a few comments will be made here to indicate the complexity of the problems facing research in the field of behavioral studies (see also comments on pp. 535–537.

The cerebral cortex and autonomic functions. The assumption set forth by some older authors that the cerebral cortex influences autonomic functions has been confirmed. However, no cortical region has been found which can be regarded as influencing autonomic functions only. On the contrary, all evidence available seems to indicate that the "autonomic functions" of the cerebral cortex are taken care of by areas which in addition are concerned in somatic activities. For example, *vasomotor changes* can be elicited on stimulation of areas 4 and 6, most clearly

602

when the animals have been curarized and the somatic motor responses therefore suppressed. (A cortically elicited vasodilatation appears to be accompanied by a constriction of the renal vessels.) Extirpation of the precentral cortex is followed by vasomotor changes, and it is a well-known clinical experience that patients suffering from capsular hemiplegias commonly show vasomotor changes in the paretic extremities. Following stimulation of various cortical areas cardiac acceleration accompanied by increased blood pressure as well as slowing of the heart rate with decrease of arterial tension can be provoked.

Among other symptoms of an autonomic nature which can be elicited from the cortex may be mentioned *pupillary constriction* from area 19 and *pupillary dilatation* from area 8 (cf. Ch. 7). Furthermore, *sweat secretion* and *piloarrection* have been obtained from irritation of area 6 (the former, according to some authors, also from an area of the temporal lobe). The *secretory and motor functions of the stomach* are also influenced from the cortex.

In recent years there has been a tendency to consider the "limbic lobe" and the "limbic system" as especially concerned in the cerebral influence on autonomic functions. The "limbic lobe" has also been named the "visceral brain." Mention has been made previously (see Ch. 10) of some of the observations made on stimulation of various parts of the "limbic lobe." The examples given above of autonomic changes elicited from areas not belonging to the "limbic lobe" cast further doubts on the justification for upholding the concept of the "limbic system," discussed in Chapter 10 (p. 537 ff). The literature on behavioral (including autonomic) changes following stimulation or ablation of certain parts of the brain is overwhelming and rapidly increasing. It abounds with hypotheses, in part mutually incompatible, and is generally rather confusing. At least no over-all tenable hypotheses appear at present to explain the role played by various parts of the brain in most behavioral reactions. The fragments of knowledge cannot yet be put together in a meaningful way. No attempt will be made here to discuss particular data from this literature. Some general points of view may, nevertheless, be ventured.

The anatomical relationships of different parts of the cerebral cortex, and between some of these (especially the phylogenetically older paleo- and archicortex) and subcortical structures as the amygdala and the hypothalamus, indicate that there is a functional collaboration, even if direct connections from the neocortex to the hypothalamus have not been found. We have every reason to believe that what we call mental processes are particularly related to the cerebral cortex. It is well known that psychic activity is accompanied by changes in the autonomic sphere (for example tachycardia and increased blood pressure in anxiety and excitation, salivation evoked by the imagination of palatable food, blushing in shyness and embarrassment). It appears likely that such changes are to a large extent produced by an action of the cortex on the hypothalamus. In a general way this explains that changes in bodily functions may accompany psychic disturbances of many kinds, as is well known to occur, not only in endogenous psychoses, but also in response to psychic influences in mentally normal persons. The occurrence of so-called psychosomatic diseases may be understood from this point of view, even if the brain regions and the connections involved can not be precisely indicated.[34]

Just as various parts of the cerebral cortex may act on the hypothalamus (perhaps to a large extent via the amygdaloid nucleus, as suggested by the fiber connections, among other data), so the hypothalamus acts on the other structures, including the cerebral cortex. Again our knowledge is scanty, but sufficient to permit some general comments. It is a familiar observation that the emotional status of the organism is of importance for the "cortical" functions of the brain, such as abstract reasoning, judgments of events and persons in the past, present, and future. In every conscious mental act our emotions are apt to interfere, thus making a completely objective judgment virtually impossible, at least when the object is of personal interest. That the hypothalamus is involved in some way in this mechanism appears probable, but again it is scarcely the hypothalamic influence alone which is responsible. In this connection it is appropriate to recall that the hormonal status of the organism is probably of importance as well.

The brief outline given in this chapter of functions of the hypothalamus will have made clear that there are still large gaps to be filled in our knowledge of this part of the brain. One fact, however, seems obvious: in the hypothalamus there is evidence of an intimate interrelation between many different functions being involved in a delicately adjusted co-operation to serve the purpose of the organism. A study of the hypothalamus and its functions gives an impression of the immense complexity of the human and animal organism, and emphasizes the danger of violating facts by trying to make them fit into simple schemes.

---

[34] Several bodily effects of mental processes are evidenced by changes in endocrine functions influenced by the hypothalamus via the hypophysis. Mention has been made of the psychic influence on milk let-down. Another well-known example is the cessation of the menstrual cycle following sorrow or other severe psychic stress. In young women even a change of the external milieu, for example when they start education in a new surrounding, may have this effect. The so-called anorexia nervosa is another example.

The peripheral course of autonomic fibers.   As mentioned previously, in the peripheral parts of the autonomic nervous system parasympathetic and sympathetic fibers (coming from the craniosacral and thoracolumbar divisions, respectively) usually run intermingled with each other. The large autonomic plexuses found in the body cavities contain fibers of both kinds, and in between there are usually ganglion cells, belonging in the peripheral plexuses largely to the parasympathetic system; in the upper abdominal plexuses, to the sympathetic. This situation presents considerable difficulties in anatomical and physiological studies and is of importance in surgical interventions on the autonomic system. No systematic description of the peripheral course of autonomic fibers will be given here (see Mitchell, 1953, for a complete account). The subject will be treated in broad outlines only, with emphasis on functional rather than topographical features. Only few references will be given. Since the parasympathetic fibers in the cranial nerves have been dealt with in Chapter 7, we shall here be concerned mainly with the peripheral sympathetic fibers, and the fibers from the sacral division of the parasympathetic.

The sympathetic fibers accompanying the peripheral nerves.   These are postganglionic fibers which reach the nerves from the ganglia of the sympathetic trunk via the gray rami communicantes (cf. Fig. 11-3). These fibers convey impulses to the *arrector pili muscles, the sweat glands, and the peripheral vessels.* Stimulation of these fibers (or the corresponding preganglionic fibers) produces *piloarrection, sweat secretion, and* (with some exceptions, see later) *vasoconstriction.*

It was shown relatively early in animals (Langley; and others) as well as in man (Foerster; André-Thomas; and others) that the *sympathetic fibers supplying the different organs and bodily regions are derived from distinct segments of the spinal cord within the levels between Th_1 and L_2, inclusive.*[35] Electrical stimulation of the ventral roots elicits piloarrection, sweat secretion, and vasoconstriction, and this is localized to the homolateral half of the face and neck when the 2nd to 4th upper thoracic roots are stimulated, and to the upper extremity when the 3rd to 6th thoracic segments are involved (Foerster; André-Thomas maintains the 4th to 8th; White and Smithwick include Th_{2-8}.) The lower extremity is supplied by the 10th thoracic to the 2nd lumbar segment (cf. Figs. 11-5 and 11-6 and table on p. 616). Since fibers from more than one segment of the cord terminate in each ganglion, a single gray ramus communicans will mediate impulses from several spinal cord segments. From this and from what has been said previously it is clear, therefore,

[35] Different authors give somewhat varying limits, and in addition there are individual variations.

that the effect of stimulation of a single ventral root will not be sharply limited to one dermatome, but the resulting changes will be more widespread. However, *a certain segmental distribution is retained,* although not entirely coincident with the somatic. This correspondence is closer in the distribution of the postganglionic fibers.

For example, Guttmann (1940) substantiated and amplified some earlier observations on this point by a study of the areas presenting loss of sweating when the body is exposed to external heat (thermoregulatory sweating) in patients in whom one or more of the cervical ganglia had been extirpated. When the superior cervical ganglion is removed, sweating is abolished in the face and the upper part of the neck corresponding to the dermatomes C_2 and C_3 approximately. When the middle cervical ganglion is extirpated the area also includes the lower part of the neck and the shoulder region (C_4 and part of C_5), and extirpation of the inferior cervical ganglion leads to anhidrosis also of the entire arm, with the exception of its medial aspect which is supplied by the uppermost thoracic nerves. (It is worthy of notice that when an area is thus made anhidrotic a compensatory hypersecretion of sweat is noticed in the adjacent areas.)

Richter and Woodruff (1945) made use of the increased electrical skin resistance which occurs in sympathetic denervated areas. They mapped areas showing increased resistance in a number of patients in whom lumbar and sacral ganglia of the sympathetic trunk had been surgically removed. The sympathetic dermatomes outlined in this way agreed closely with the sensory dermatomes. In previous studies the authors report corresponding findings for the face and trunk. The method has been used by several investigators, for example by Monro (1959) in an extensive study of the results of sympathectomies.

Peripherally, the sympathetic fibers accompany the somatic. *The piloarrection, sweating, and vasoconstriction which appear following irritation of the peripheral nerves after they have taken up the ramus communicans griseus will therefore present a distribution corresponding to the somatic sensory innervation.* In lesions of the plexus they will be of a segmental type, while in lesions of the peripheral nerves they will be found in the territory of the sensory distribution of the nerve in question. Some features of this sympathetic innervation deserve special attention.

The pilomotor impulses and pilomotor reflexes. Stimulation of the sympathetic fibers is followed by erection of the hairs (due to the oblique course of the arrector pili muscles) and the skin presents the well-known appearance of "goose-flesh." An abolition of this aspect of the sympathetic innervation is of little or no importance in man, but the conditions of the pilomotors may give diagnostic information. (In animals piloarrection is a factor in temperature regulation.) Piloarrection may be induced with varying ease in different individuals. The appropriate stimulus is cold, but deep pressure, as well as disagreeable, sharp noises and psychic impressions may also be effective. In the latter cases pathways from the cortex-hypothalamus must be assumed to be involved, but with local, cutaneous stimuli the effect is mediated by *reflexes, having their reflex center in the spinal cord.* Consequently, *lesions of the spinal cord will be followed by changes in the pilomotor reflexes, if the lesion is situated between the 1st thoracic and the 2nd lumbar segment.* The pilomotor reflexes are most easily elicited from the shoulder region (the supraspinous fossa) and the lumbar region. It is typical that this reflexly provoked piloarrection spreads from its starting point in an oral and caudal direction, and that it is confined to the homolateral half of the body. If a transverse lesion of the cord is present, this regular mode of spread will be interrupted, as the damage of the cord prevents the reflex impulses from passing downward or upward. However, it should be remembered that on account of the anatomical conditions (fibers from several segments to each vertebral ganglion) the border of the zone will not correspond exactly to the limit of the sensory changes. Thus, in a transverse lesion of the cord at the 9th thoracic segment, piloarrection elicited from the shoulder region will descend to approximately the 11th or 12th thoracic dermatome, whereas when starting from the lumbar region it will ascend to the 8th or 7th thoracic dermatome. Like other spinal reflexes the pilomotor reflexes cannot be provoked in the initial stages of a transverse lesion of the cord.

Lesions of the rami communicantes and the vertebral ganglia will also be accompanied by changes in the pilomotor reflexes. After extirpation of the stellate ganglion piloarrection will be absent in the face, neck, and arm on the operated side. When a peripheral nerve has been interrupted, a piloarrection progressing regularly will fail to involve the anesthetic area, for example, in a radial nerve lesion the piloarrection will be absent on the dorsal surface of the arm and forearm.[36]

When examining the pilomotor reflexes, care must be taken to avoid sources of error (the influence of room temperature, etc.), and the results obtained must be evaluated critically. There are also *local pilomotor reflexes* which may cause confusion. Such reflexes may occur even in anesthetic cutaneous areas. In many individuals the pilomotor reflexes are weak.

The innervation of the sweat glands. The fibers to the sweat glands, as has been mentioned, accompany the pilomotor fibers, but in contradistinction to these they are *cholinergic.* In lesions of a peripheral nerve an irritation of the nerve will frequently be accompanied by an increased secretion of sweat in its area of distribution, whereas a more severe damage will interrupt the conduction and lead to anhidrosis. This

---

[36] On the dorsum of the hand the arrectores pili are rudimentary, and as will be recalled hairs are absent on the dorsal aspect of the two distal phalanges of fingers and toes, and on the palm of the hand and sole of the foot.

is seen most clearly in lesions of the median nerve which supplies the three radial fingers and the radial half of the fourth finger on the palmar side. The skin will become dry and desquamate in the anesthetic area.[37]

In transverse lesions of the cord it may be observed that reflex sweat secretion behaves in a similar manner to spinal reflex piloarrection. However, spinal sudomotor reflexes cannot be provoked at will. Sweat secretion is an important factor in the regulation of body temperature and appears to be regulated first and foremost by the hypothalamus. Thermoregulatory sweating appears on heating of the body and since it is initiated from the hypothalamus it will be lacking below the transverse lesion, because the descending sudomotor fibers mentioned previously are interrupted. In lesions of the spinal roots or sympathetic ganglia, the anhidrosis will affect the area supplied by them.

The sweat glands considered above are the coiled tubular eccrine glands occurring over most of the body surface. The *apocrine sweat glands,* present in some regions, notably in the axilla, differ from the eccrine sweat glands not only anatomically but also functionally. In the axilla cholinesterase has been identified histologically around the eccrine glands but not around the apocrine glands. The latter are adrenergic and respond to sympathicomimetic drugs. They do not show thermoregulatory sweating but, as is well known, secrete in response to mental stress. It appears that they are influenced humorally by adrenaline. It has been claimed that sympathectomy in man does not abolish sweating from the apocrine glands. For some data see Evans (1957).

Vasomotor fibers and reflexes.   More important than the sudomotor sympathetic fibers are the vasomotor fibers. The vasomotor fibers belonging to the sympathetic system in most instances act as vasoconstrictors. In their peripheral course they follow the pilomotor and sudomotor fibers, and thus like these show an approximate segmental distribution (cf. the table on p. 616). It appears to be settled that the cerebral vessels are also provided with sympathetic nerve fibers (see Krog, 1964).

The sympathetic fibers are distributed to arteries, arterioles, and small veins.[38] It is of some importance that direct fibers from the sympathetic trunk accompany only the larger arteries in their proximal part (in the limbs approximately to the beginning of the brachial and femoral artery respectively). The arteries situated more peripherally in the limbs are supplied with sympathetic fibers by fine branches from the main nerve trunks which usually follow the arteries. Apart from plexuses of nerve fibers encircling the arteries, nerve fibers are present also in the arterial

[37] Guttmann (1940) has drawn attention to the occurrence of lesions of the cervical sympathetic trunk following its violent stretching, without concomitant injury to the spinal nerves or the skeleton. These lesions reveal themselves by local anhidrosis, and the location of this may give information on the site of the lesion.

[38] For an account of the innervation of particular vessels see Mitchell (1953).

608

wall. In the adventitia these fibers are partly myelinated, in the muscular layer they are very fine and unmyelinated. In the adventitial coat of the arteries, furthermore, different types of terminal structures are found, for example some Vater-Pacinian corpuscles. These degenerate after section of the dorsal roots distal to the spinal ganglia. The tiny fibers in the muscular layer of the arteries, on the other hand, degenerate, as do also some of the fine fibers in the adventitia, after interruption of the sympathetic postganglionic supply. Finally, some cells described in the walls of the arteries have been interpreted as peripheral autonomic cells, interpolated between the incoming sympathetic fibers and the smooth muscle cells. They have been assumed to be engaged in the local vasomotor phenomena which may be observed after sympathectomy, but on the whole their significance is doubtful. Normally a local vascular tonus and local vasomotor reflexes are present, but are of little significance.

The *capillaries* are accompanied by very fine nerve fibers, but the nature of these has not been esablished. The sympathetic nervous system and adrenaline appear to have no clear-cut effect on the capillaries, neither has acetylcholine. *The capillaries may change in caliber independently of the arteries and arterioles.* This may be observed, for example, when a fever begins. The skin may be pale (contracted capillaries) but at the same time hot (dilated arterioles). Changes in the caliber of the capillaries have been studied directly under varying circumstances, for example, in the frog in the mesentery or the web of the foot. The opinion held previously by some workers that capillary constriction is produced by contraction of the Rouget-Mayer cells, found close to the wall of the capillaries, appears to be untenable. (See also below.)

Arteriovenous anastomoses, establishing direct communications between arteries and veins, are extremely common. As more careful search for them has been made, they have been found in a large number of organs. They vary in dimensions and complexity, being perhaps most developed in the distal parts of the body, such as the fingers, toes, and ears. Usually they are rather coiled, and the arterial end is abundantly supplied with contractile cells and has an innervation of sympathetic fibers. The arteriovenous anastomoses obviously represent a potent mechanism for changing the pattern of blood flow through the capillary net, according to their variations in caliber. Opening up of the anastomoses in the skin provides an effective means for increasing the blood flow, for example in the external ear or fingers during exposure to cold.[39]

[39] It may be asked whether the role played by the arteriovenous anastomoses has not been unduly neglected in many physiological studies of the peripheral circulation. It is indeed striking that they are still sometimes not mentioned at all in physiological (as well as anatomical) accounts of the vascular system.

The physiology of the peripheral circulation and the many factors, nervous and humoral, which influence it, is a vast and complex field of study. A number of reflexes are involved. Mention was made previously of some data on the central regulation, from which it is seen that vasodilator and vasoconstrictor effects of peripheral vessels can be obtained on stimulation of several regions of the central nervous system, especially the reticular formation of the lower brain stem, the hypothalamus, and certain regions of the cerebral cortex. Ultimately these central controlling and regulating mechanisms act on the peripheral autonomic nervous system.

As mentioned above the *main action of the sympathetic innervation of blood vessels is constrictor.* It appears to be established that the neurotransmitter responsible for this action is *noradrenaline.* In the vessels of the skin and intestine, adrenaline likewise has a pure constrictor effect, while the influence of the latter on the vessels of muscle may be two-fold, depending on the concentration (see Uvnäs, 1960).

The presence of *vasodilator fibers* has been the subject of much debate.[40] It appears to be generally agreed that such fibers are present in the parasympathetic chorda tympani and in the parasympathetic fibers to the external genital organs. The transmitter is assumed to be *acetylcholine.* The observation that vasodilatation may occur following stimulation of nerves led some early workers to postulate the presence of parasympathetic fibers in the peripheral nerves, in opposition to anatomical observations. This controversy is now resolved, since it has been shown, as mentioned previously, that some fibers belonging anatomically to the sympathetic nervous system, are cholinergic. This is the case not only for the sympathetic fibers to the sweat glands, but also for some sympathetic fibers passing to vessels. It has been particularly well demonstrated for skeletal muscle (see Uvnäs, 1960). Whether such fibers are also present in the sympathetic supply of the heart, skin, and intestines has not been finally settled.

On stimulation of a bundle of sympathetic nerve fibers the constrictor effects on the vessels usually predominate and mask the vasodilator effects. The fact that vasodilatation can be clearly demonstrated following stimulation of certain regions of the central nervous system indicates that the two effects presumably may occur separately under normal circumstances. In clinical cases of affections of the peripheral parts of the sym-

---

[40] It should be kept in mind that alterations of the caliber of blood vessels produced by nerve fibers can occur only by variations in a constrictor action. There is no structural mechanism for an *active* dilatation. Accordingly, dilatation of a vessel following changes in its innervation can occur only by a diminishing "tonus" of the constrictor influence which resists the intravascular hydrostatic pressure.

6 1 0

pathetic system the effects on the vasoconstrictors usually dominate the picture.

It was mentioned previously that irritation of the upper thoracic ventral roots is followed by vasoconstriction in the neck and head on the same side. The skin becomes cool and as a rule also pale. (Sweat secretion and piloarrection may appear concomitantly, but it should be pointed out that under normal as well as pathological conditions changes of the vasomotors, sudomotors, and pilomotors may occur independent of each other.) Following extirpation of the stellate ganglion a vasodilatation of face, neck, and lateral part of the arm is observed, betraying itself in an increased temperature and reddening of the skin. This is due to interruption of the vasoconstrictor impulses to the areas mentioned, because they traverse the stellate ganglion. Some of the postganglionic fibers to the head accompany the arteries, but some leave the latter and enter the cranial nerves.

On account of the sensitizing effect of sympathetic denervation, the vasodilatation following an extirpation, for example of the stellate ganglion, is apt to diminish somewhat in the course of a week or two. When instead the sympathetic fibers from the 2nd and 3rd thoracic segments in the white rami are severed, and the sympathetic trunk is divided between the 2nd and 3rd thoracic ganglia, the postganglionic neurons are left intact, sensitization is less pronounced, and the effect is more enduring. A Horner's syndrome is also avoided. Many neurosurgeons, therefore, prefer such *preganglionic* denervation of the upper extremity to extirpation of the stellate ganglion, which represents a postganglionic denervation. The role of sensitization in sympathectomies is still debated (see Monro, 1959, for some data).

In lesions of the peripheral nerves or the brachial or lumbosacral plexuses a paralysis of the vasoconstrictors also appears, but as a rule the increased temperature and reddening of the affected areas are not enduring. In irritative lesions of the peripheral nerves the ensuing vasoconstriction may, however, be rather conspicuous. Lesions affecting a limited part of the intermediolateral cell column will as a rule give no clear-cut symptoms, since each vertebral ganglion receives fibers from more than one segment of the cord.

The *vasomotor reflexes* are of supreme importance for the maintenance of the blood pressure and for the proper distribution of blood to different organs. They will only be briefly touched upon here. Spinal vasomotor reflexes with a transverse reflex arc in the spinal cord are revealed in the well-known phenomenon in which cooling of one hand is usually followed by vasomotor changes in both hands. Other vasomotor reflexes utilize a longitudinal reflex arc, like the pilomotor (cf. above). They may consequently show alterations in transverse lesions of the cord. In the stage of "reorganization" after such lesions (see Ch. 4) the vasomotor reflexes are usually increased below the site of the lesion. The same may be observed in lesions of the brain stem. Lesions of the cord restricted to the region below the 2nd lumbar segment will, however, not be accompanied by vasomotor changes, since the intermediolateral cell column will escape injury.

The caliber of the *capillaries* appears to be controlled mainly by *chemical* means by changes due to local processes in the tissue. Thus an increase in the tension of *carbon dioxide* and a *lowered pH,* due to increased metabolic activity of the tissue, is followed by capillary dilatation, which secures a more abundant circulation of blood to the active tissues. Another substance which provokes a marked capillary dilatation is *histamine.* This phenomenon is closely related to the concept of *axon reflexes* and is of some clinical interest.

Following an intradermal injection of histamine, a conspicuous rubor develops around the place where the injection is made, due to capillary dilatation. This is soon followed by a local edema, changing the reddish spot into an urticarial papule. Surrounding this central spot where the capillaries are maximally dilated and where transudation of fluid from the blood occurs, a zone of active capillary hyperemia with reddening soon appears and has a tendency to widen (Lewis's triple response). The same reaction (but less pronounced) can be observed also after intradermal injection of irritating substances, such as distilled water, weak acids, and other substances. It has been assumed that in these cases the injected substance acts by producing a damage to the local tissue, whereby a substance which was originally thought to be histamine or a histamine-like compound (Lewis's H-substance) is liberated. It appears that the same mechanism underlies the dermographism, usually most pronounced in neurotic individuals. The role played by histamine in the triple reaction is not yet finally settled. Other substances, such as plasmakinins or serotonin, may also be involved.

It is remarkable that the reaction described above as following intradermal injection of histamine does not appear in cutaneous areas in which sensibility is abolished, for example in peripheral nerve lesions. In these cases only the urticarial papule develops. This indicates that nervous factors must be involved. The nerves which are of importance are the cutaneous ones. When a cutaneous sensory nerve is stimulated for a certain time a strong vasodilatation develops in the area of distribution of the nerve. Irritation of a dorsal root yields vasodilatation in the corresponding dermatome.

It appears that the vasodilatation is mediated by fibers which leave the spinal cord in the dorsal roots and travel peripherally in the sensory nerves. It was for some time maintained by some workers that not only afferent, but also some efferent fibers leave the cord in the dorsal roots and that these fibers were specific vasodilators. However, the existence of efferent fibers in the dorsal roots has not been proved. There appears to be decisive evidence that the vasodilator impulses are mediated through the afferent dorsal root fibers, mainly the thinnest unmyelinated ones. Since the vasodilator impulses are transmitted in the opposite direction to the others, they are *antidromic impulses.*

Even if such impulses may arise on artificial irritation of dorsal roots and also may be a factor in the production of the eruption in herpes zoster, these facts do not prove that similar conditions prevail under normal circumstances. It appears that the vasodilatation which is observed following the application of local irritants to the skin, especially painful ones, is mediated by so-called *axon reflexes*. The fine sensory fibers are assumed to branch peripherally. On irritation of the skin, impulses are not only transmitted in a central direction and perceived as pain, but also pass in a peripheral direction through collateral branches. At their terminals histamine or another vasodilator substance (see above) is assumed to be liberated and to produce the capillary dilatation. If this is sufficiently strong, the permeability of the capillaries is increased and a local edema (the urticarial papule) develops. This theory explains why these vasodilator reflexes do not disappear immediately following transection of the dorsal roots distal to the ganglion, but only in the course of several days when the nerve fibers degenerate. It is assumed that the outer zone of vasodilatation which occurs on local application of histamine is due to axon reflexes of this type. When the nerve has degenerated, the usual rubor surrounding the point of injection is, therefore, absent.

It has been concluded by some that axon reflexes play a role within the autonomic nervous system, particularly in the "intrinsic regulation" of autonomic organs. This view is still debated.

The autonomic innervation of some organs. Above, the general aspects of the functions of the autonomic nervous system have been considered. It is appropriate, however, to deal with the innervation of some visceral organs in particular. The problems related to the autonomic innervation of visceral organs have turned out to be far more complex than was assumed a few decades ago. No attempt will be made to discuss this subject exhaustively, but some general and broad statements will be made, with special reference to points of clinical neurological interest. As a general rule the sympathetic and parasympathetic innervation of organs is antagonistic, although exceptions exist.

The autonomic innervation of the *eye* has been treated to some extent in Chapter 7 (see also Fig. 11-2). The parasympathetic fibers, as will be remembered, produce on stimulation contraction of the pupil and of the ciliary muscle (accommodation). The same effect is obtained by certain drugs, such as pilocarpine and eserine. A complete oculomotor palsy results in mydriasis and paralysis of accommodation (in addition to paralysis of most of the extrinsic muscles of the eye). Atropine produces mydriasis. Stimulation of the sympathetic fibers to the eye results in dilatation of the pupil, probably mainly by producing a contraction of the vessels of the iris. An interruption of the sympathetic fibers to the eye, on the other hand, produces a miosis. This will be the case with lesions of the postganglionic fibers, which take origin from the superior cervical ganglion or with lesions of the preganglionic fibers in their course from the 1st and 2nd thoracic segments of the cord through the inferior and middle cervical ganglion and the cervical sympathetic trunk. On this account a lesion of the upper thoracic cord will usually be followed by a miosis in the homolateral eye. The exact region which has to be damaged is the intermediolateral cell column in the 1st and 2nd thoracic segments, and this region is therefore frequently spoken of as the *"centrum ciliospinale."* However, the same result will also follow a lesion of the cervical cord or of the medulla and pons, if it encroaches on the tracts which descend in the lateral part of the medulla and cord to the ciliospinal center. In all cases mentioned a *ptosis* occurs in addition to the *miosis* since the plain tarsal muscle is paralyzed, and frequently an *enophthalmos* is observed: the eyeball appears to be deeper in the orbit than on the other side. The latter phenomenon is usually attributed to a paralysis of the smooth muscles present in the inferior orbital fissure. However, these muscles are very sparse, and can scarcely be assumed to be responsible; furthermore, it appears that, when measurements are made by an exophthalmometer, the difference between the two sides is negligible. The enophthalmos, therefore, appears to be mainly only apparent, due to the ptosis. The combination of miosis, ptosis, and enophthalmos is commonly called *Horner's syndrome.* Its presence indicates a lesion of the structures enumerated above.[41]

If a Horner's syndrome is present, there is usually loss of sweating on the corresponding side of the face. This may be overlooked if not sought for. Occasionally *Raeder's (1924) paratrigeminal syndrome* is found. There is ptosis and miosis but no loss of sweating in the face, indicating that the sympathetic innervation of the eye, but not of the face, is affected. This is usually accompanied by headaches above the eye, often beginning in the morning. Raeder found the syndrome in some cases with head trauma or tumor, and explained it as being due to damage to the sympathetic fibers surrounding the internal carotid artery. Later studies indicate that the syndrome may also be related to migraine (see Ford and Walsh, 1958).

The *lacrimal gland* is supplied by parasympathetic fibers (cf. above and Fig. 11-2) which are secretory. If these fibers are damaged, for instance in fractures of the zygomatic bone, the reflex tear secretion of the corresponding eye is abolished. This reflex is most easily elicited by irritation of the conjunctiva or the nasal mucosa. The afferent path of the reflex arc passes through the trigeminal nerve.

The *digestive organs* on the whole get their secretory and motor impulses through the parasympathetic, their inhibitory through the sympathetic, although the latter statement requires some qualification. The

[41] Some clinicians have utilized the reaction of the pupil to adrenaline instillation into the eye to differentiate between lesions of the pre- and postganglionic sympathetic neurons. If the postganglionic neuron is damaged, i.e. the lesion is peripheral to the superior cervical ganglion, the pupil dilates markedly when adrenaline is applied to the conjunctival sac. If the lesion is central to this, damaging the preganglionic fibers, the pupil reacts approximately normally, namely, very weakly or not at all. The difference is another example of sensitization following lesions of the postganglionic fibers mentioned previously.

course of the parasympathetic fibers to the *salivary glands* has been described previously (cf. Fig. 11-2). On stimulation of the chorda tympani secretion takes place from the submandibular and sublingual glands. The sympathetic fibers appear to be of lesser importance. When the parasympathetic fibers are destroyed, reflex salivation cannot be elicited from the gland in question. Thus there occurs no salivation on olfactory or gustatory stimulation, and the secretion of saliva occurring in response to imagination of palatable food is also abolished. The latter reaction is probably initiated from the cerebral cortex.

The parasympathetic fibers to the *stomach and the gut* are secretory and motor. Thus stimulation of the vagus produces increased peristalsis and secretion of gastric and intestinal juices, whereas the sphincters relax. As will be remembered the rectum and the lower colon (from the splenic flexure) receive their parasympathetic supply from the sacral cord. The sympathetic influence on the digestive tube is, broadly speaking, inhibitory. Stimulation of the sympathetic is followed by reduced peristalsis and secretion and increased tonus of the sphincters. The gastric secretion and peristalsis which occur after psychic, gustatory, and olfactory stimuli are mediated through the vagus. However, quite a considerable secretory and motor activity of the stomach is retained even if both vagi and both splanchnic nerves are cut, and in time it tends to become more normal. It is assumed that this remaining activity is mediated through the nerve cells and plexuses in the wall of the organs (Meissner's and Auerbach's plexuses).

The exocrine glands of the *pancreas* are supplied with secretory fibers from the vagus, although the sympathetic fibers may have some influence in this respect. Nerve fibers have also been traced in the electron microscope to the islands of Langerhans (see Stahl, 1963). In addition, stimulation of the vagus produces increased secretion of insulin. The *liver* appears to receive only sympathetic fibers, but the vagus carries motor fibers to the gall bladder and bile duct, and stimulation of the vagus causes increased flow of bile and relaxation of the sphincter of Oddi. On account of the highly developed local "autonomy" of the digestive organs, symptoms from them will usually not be clearly evidenced in diseases of the autonomic nervous system.

Stimulation of the sympathetic fibers to the *heart* is followed by tachycardia, stimulation of the vagus by bradycardia. In addition such stimulation has other effects, on the cardiac muscle and the coronary vessels (see *Nervous Control of the Heart,* 1965, for some recent data). The distribution of the postganglionic sympathetic and parasympathetic fibers to the heart is still not settled. It appears that the auricle and atrioventricular bundle are supplied with both vagal and sympathetic

THE PRINCIPAL FEATURES OF THE AUTONOMIC INNERVATION OF SOME ORGANS

Organ	SYMPATHETIC			PARASYMPATHETIC		
	Pregangl. neuron	Postgangl. neuron	Action	Pregangl. neuron	Postgangl. neuron	Action
Eye	Th_{1-2}	Sup. cerv. ggl.	Dilatation of pupil	Visc. oc. mot. nucl. n. III.	Ciliary gangl.	Pupillary constriction, accommodation
Lacrimal gland	Th_{1-2}	Sup. cerv. ggl.	?	Sup. saliv. nucl. n. VII	Sphenopalat. gangl.	Secretion of tears
Submandibular and sublingual glands	Th_{1-2}	Sup. cerv. ggl.	Vasoconstriction, secretion (?)	Sup. saliv. nucl. n. VII	Submandib. gangl.	Secretion of saliva, vasodilatation
Parotid gland	Th_{1-2}	Sup. cerv. ggl.	Vasoconstriction, secretion (?)	Inf. saliv. nucl. n. IX.	Otic gangl.	Secretion of saliva, vasodilatation
Heart	$Th_{1-4}(_5?)$	Sup., middle and inf. cerv. ggl., upper thor. ggl.	Acceleration. Dilatation of coronary arteries	Dors. mot. nucl. n. X.	Cardiac plexus	Bradycardia
Bronchi, lungs	$Th_{2-7}(_{2-4}?)$	Inf. cerv. ggl., upper thor. ggl.	Dilatation of bronchi, vasodilatation (?)	Dors. mot. nucl. n. X.	Pulmonary and bronchial plexuses	Constriction of bronchi (secretion?)
Stomach	$Th_{6-10}(_{5-11}?)$ Gr. splanchn. n.	Celiac ggl.	Inhibition of peristalsis and secretion. Contraction of pyloric sph. (?)	Dors. mot. nucl. n. X.	Gastric plexus	Secretion, peristalsis
Pancreas	$Th_{6-10}(_{5-11}?)$ Gr. splanchn. n.	Celiac ggl.	Weak secretion (?)	Dors. mot. nucl. n. X.	Periarterial plexuses	Secretion (pancreatic juice, insulin)
Small intestine, colon asc., transv.	$Th_{6-10}(_{5-11})$ Gr. splanchn. n.	Celiac ggl., sup. mesent. ggl. and other ganglia and plexuses	Inhibition of secretion and peristalsis	Dors. mot. nucl. n. X.	Myenteric and submucous plexuses	Secretion, peristalsis
Colon desc. and sigm., rectum	L_{1-2}	Inf. mesent. ggl., hypogastr. plex. and other ganglia.	Inhibition of secretion and peristalsis	S_{2-4}	Myenteric and submucous plexuses	Secretion, peristalsis
Kidney	$Th_{12}-L_1(Th_{11}-L_2?)$	Celiac ggl., renal plexus	Vasomotor changes	?		
Ureter, bladder	$L_{1-2}(Th_{11-12}?)$	Hypogastr. and other plexuses	Vasoconstriction, contr. of int. sph. in ejaculation	S_{2-4}	Vesical plexus, uret. plexus	Contraction of bladder, (detrusor)
Adrenal medulla	$Th_{11}-L_1(Th_{10}-L_2?)$ Lesser spl. n.	Cells of adrenal medulla	Secretion			
Head, neck (skin, muscles)	$Th_{2-4}(_5?)$	Sup. and middle cerv. ggl.	Vasoconstriction. Sweat secretion. Pilo-arrection	No parasympathetic innervation		
Upper extremity (skin, muscles)	$Th_{3-6}(_{2-8}?)$	Stellate ggl., upper thor. ganglia.				
Lower extremity (skin, muscles)	$Th_{10}-L_2(Th_{11}-L_2?)$	Lower lumbar and upper sacral ganglia.				

fibers, whereas the ventricles are supplied by the sympathetic only. The sinoauricular node is supplied mainly by the right vagus, a finding in harmony with the physiological effect of bradycardia following vagal stimulation. There has been some uncertainty concerning the action of the sympathetic nerves on the coronary vessels. The consensus of opinion has been that their effect is dilator and not constrictor as with other blood vessels. This is in agreement with the needs of the heart muscle under sympathetic stimulation. However, there has been discussion whether the dilator effect of sympathetic stimulation is secondary to changes in the activity of the myocardium. It is important to remember that the sympathetic supply to the heart is derived not only from the cervical sympathetic ganglia (Fig. 11-4 and the table on p. 616), but also from the upper 4-5 thoracic ganglia. Most of the afferent fibers from the heart take the same course as the sympathetic. The afferent fibers from the heart which travel in the vagus nerves appear to be concerned in the mediation of cardiac reflexes such as the aortic reflex and the carotid sinus reflex. (Strictly speaking, however, it is probably mainly the glosso-pharyngeal fibers which are responsible for the carotid sinus reflex, cf. p. 366.)

The *bronchi* and *lungs* are endowed with a rich supply of autonomic fibers, and fine nerve fibers can be traced along the arteries and arterioles up to the respiratory bronchi, where they innervate the smooth muscles. Stimulation of the sympathetic fibers, ultimately derived from the 2nd to 4th thoracic nerves, produces bronchodilatation; stimulation of the vagus results in constriction of the bronchioli and possibly an increased secretion from the bronchial glands. The beneficial effect of adrenaline and atropine in cases of bronchial asthma gives evidence of the action of the two types of autonomic nerves. The afferent fibers from the respiratory organs appear to pass mainly in the vagus, and they influence the reflex activity of the respiratory "centers" in the medulla. There is some uncertainty concerning the action of the nerves on the vessels of the lung, but the sympathetic influence appears to be predominantly vaso-constrictor, although this effect is not as pronounced as in many other organs.

The *kidneys* are supplied by sympathetic fibers which enter the organ with the renal vessels. Section of the splanchnic nerves is said to be followed by an increase of urinary secretion for some weeks, but this is probably due only to the increased blood flow. It is doubtful whether vagal fibers to the kidney exist. The *ureters* receive both sympathetic and parasympathetic fibers, but the peristalsis of the ureters is little influenced if all their nerves are sectioned.

The *autonomic innervation of the bladder* is of some practical impor-

6 1 7

tance to the neurologist. The parasympathetic fibers are derived from the 2nd to 4th sacral segments and are found in the visceral branches of the pudendal plexus, frequently called *nervi pelvici* or *nervi erigentes*. They fuse with the sympathetic fibers from the hypogastric plexus and form a vesical plexus, best developed at the base of the bladder. The preganglionic sympathetic fibers appear to be derived (in man) mainly from the intermediolateral cell column at L_1–L_2, perhaps from Th_{12} and Th_{11} as well (see Fig. 11-4, and the table on p. 616). Some of them descend in the sympathetic trunk to the level of the first four lumbar ganglia from where presumably many of the postganglionic sympathetic neurons to the bladder originate. Others occur scattered in ganglia within the hypogastric plexus. Precise information on this point is not available. Postganglionic parasympathetic neurons are present beneath the serosa and between the muscle bundles of the bladder. *Afferent fibers* from the bladder proceed centrally along the routes taken by the efferents. Structures interpreted as receptors have been described in the bladder wall. The fibers from the stretch receptors, responding to distension of the bladder, are assumed to pass with the pelvic nerves, according to clinical and experimental findings (see Nyberg-Hansen, 1966c, for some references). The afferent fibers following the sympathetic outflow are believed to be concerned mainly with pain sensations.

The external, striated, urethral sphincter is supplied by somatic efferent fibers, being axons of motoneurons in S_{3-4}. They pass via the pudendal nerve.

The *physiology of micturition* is a complex subject, and the nervous factors involved are not yet completely known. It was formerly generally held that the internal sphincter was separate from the main mass of the bladder musculature. The latter is often collectively referred to as the *detrusor*. During micturition a parasympathetically induced contraction of the detrusor was thought to be combined with an inhibitory sympathetic action on the internal sphincter. However, the situation seems to be less schematic. According to later anatomical studies there appears to be no true separate internal sphincter, but only a continuation of the longitudinal detrusor fibers around the bladder outlet, chiefly on its dorsal aspect. It is therefore possible that the opening of the internal urethral orifice on micturition may be achieved simply by the contraction of the detrusor muscle and a separate inhibitory innervation of a sphincter is not necessary (Lapides, 1958). Studies of micturition in humans by "micturition urethro-cystography" (Petersén, Stener, Selldén, and Kollberg, 1962) lend support to this view.

Using the fluorescence method for demonstration of adrenergic nerves and terminals, Hamberger and Norberg (1965) found sympathetic

618

fibers to be restricted to the muscle fibers of the vesical trigone, including the orifices of the ureters and the urethra. (It is of interest in this connection that in contrast to the rest of the bladder which is of entodermal origin, the trigonum vesicae is derived from the mesoderm.)

While there is no dispute that stimulation of the parasympathetic fibers to the bladder produces micturition, the action of the sympathetic has been much debated and opposing views have been held. In discussing the bladder it should be recalled that it has a dual function, that of passive collection of the urine delivered by the ureters, and that of an intermittent active expulsion of its contents. The two functions are related in so far as expulsion is ordinarily elicited when the bladder is filled to a certain point. However, it is not the absolute volume which matters and which is the stimulus for evacuation, but the intravesical tension. When this reaches a certain degree, afferent impulses from the stretch receptors travel centrally, mainly in the pelvic nerves, reach the sacral division of the cord, and by acting on the parasympathetic cells set up contraction of the detrusor muscle. The external sphincter opens later. The bladder wall possesses a certain "tonus" and shows a modest rhythmic contractile activity. While some authors have maintained that "bladder tone" is an intrinsic property of the bladder (see Gjone, 1965, for some references), others have held that it is influenced by the autonomic nervous system. In a recent experimental study in the cat Edvardsen (1967) found that the sympathetic innervation has an inhibitory effect on bladder tone and raises the threshold for micturition, i.e. for the afferent nervous input which via the dorsal sacral roots elicits the micturition reflex by acting on the preganglionic parasympathetic neurons. Sympathicolytic drugs increased bladder tone. Although these observations cannot easily be correlated with the restricted anatomical distribution of sympathetic fibers to the bladder, they are of interest from a clinical point of view, for example with regard to the beneficial effect of ephedrine in some cases of enuresis (see Edvardsen, 1967, for further correlations). The parasympathetic innervation does not appear to play any role in the collecting phase.

All researchers agree that the parasympathetic innervation of the detrusor is essential for micturition. As to the role of the sympathetic in this function of the bladder opinions are divided. Some authors maintain that it is not involved, while others claim that there is a sympathetically controlled functional sphincter mechanism at the outlet of the bladder (Edvardsen, 1967). (The trigonal muscles appear to be operative in the act of ejaculation, mediated by sympathetic fibers to the ductus deferens, by preventing backflow of seminal fluid into the bladder.)

The role of the external sphincter, which can be voluntarily controlled, is mainly to contract in order to stop micturition when this is desirable. The sphincter can be closed very effectively, even if the detrusor contracts. Its opening when micturition begins appears to be reflexly induced. Electromyographic studies of the external sphincter in man by Petersén and his collaborators, and others, have given interesting information, especially when combined with "micturition urethrocystography" (see for example Petersén, Kollberg, and Dhunér, 1961; Petersén et al. 1962).

The act of micturition and presumably also the regulation of "bladder tone" are essentially spinal reflex functions. Like other spinal reflexes, they are subject to *supraspinal influences,* a fact which is well known in man from experiences particularly with lesions of the spinal cord (to be considered later). Like most other autonomic functions those of the bladder have been shown to be influenced from many regions of the brain, often somewhat light-heartedly referred to as "centers for micturition." Both excitation and inhibition of bladder activity have been observed. Among regions giving such effects on electrical stimulation (see Ruch, 1960; Gjone, 1965) may be mentioned: the sensorimotor areas I and II, the orbital gyrus, the cingulate gyrus, the piriform cortex, the amygdaloid nucleus, the hypothalamus, the superior colliculi, and the reticular formation. Inhibition and facilitation have in part been obtained from different points (see Gjone, 1965).[42] Inhibition has further been reported to follow stimulation of the red nucleus, the substantia nigra, subthalamus, certain thalamic nuclei, and the pallidum (Lewin, Dillard, and Porter, 1967). To what extent the results of stimulation at many of these sites are due to stimulation of descending fibers appears to be unsettled, and the significance of the findings is far from clear. *In man* micturition (and defecation) have been observed to be affected following lesions of the superomedial part of the frontal lobe (Andrew and Nathan, 1964). While micturition as such occurs in a normal manner, the "higher control" of it (as well as of defecation) is disturbed with impaired sensation of bladder-filling and extreme urgency of micturition when the patient is awake, with incontinence when he is asleep.

Reference was made previously (p. 582) to the routes followed by descending pathways influencing bladder activity in animals, and to the conclusion by Nathan and Smith (1958) that in the spinal cord of man these fibers are situated in the middle of the lateral funiculus at the level

---

[42] In the amygdala, excitatory responses were obtained chiefly from the basolateral group, inhibitory responses from the corticomedial group (Gjone, 1965). The well-known urge to micturate in situations of fear but not of anger, may have a relation to the observation that fear reactions appear to be elicited most easily from the basolateral amygdaloid region (Ursin and Kaada, 1960).

of the central canal. The ascending fibers, mediating sensation of fullness of the bladder and giving rise to the desire to micturate were located by Nathan and Smith (1951) in the superficial ventral part of the lateral funiculus. Fibers mediating sensations of pain from the bladder and the urethra ascend in the same region. These conclusions were made on the basis of bladder function in a series of patients subjected to chordotomies. The problems related to the central control of the bladder are still far from solved, however. There is reason to believe that the cortical influence may be more important in man than in animals. Most likely it is exerted by way of direct corticospinal fibers. However, a close co-operation must exist between the voluntary control and the influence exerted by other regions of the brain, perhaps first and foremost the hypothalamus.

Lesions of various parts of the nervous connections involved in the normal activity of the bladder may cause disturbances. Bladder disturbances in man are seen most often in lesions of the spinal cord. The symptoms will differ according to the site of the lesion. In lesions above the sacral division voluntary control of the bladder will be abolished if the lesion affects both lateral funiculi. If the conduction of the fibers is completely abolished, control is entirely lost, and the bladder will empty automatically (reflexly) as soon as a certain amount of urine has accumulated. As a rule it will react with smaller quantiies of urine than normal. This is usually interpreted as being due to a decreased supraspinal inhibition. (In the case of a suddenly developing transverse lesion the bladder will at first be entirely paralyzed in the shock stage, as mentioned previously.) In partial lesions the phenomenon of precipitate micturition is common, betraying an imperfect, but not entirely lacking, central control, since the patient is able to suspend micturition for a certain time, although usually very short. This is not infrequently seen in disseminated sclerosis. The symptoms following lesions of the efferent and afferent fibers to the bladder will be considered later, in connection with lesions of the sacral cord.

The autonomic innervation of the *genital organs* is not known in all details. The gonads are supplied by sympathetic fibers following the vessels (the internal spermatic and ovarian arteries respectively). The fibers are derived from the lower thoracic segments of the cord, and are mainly vasomotor. The sympathetic fibers to the seminal vesicles, prostate, and vas deferens are motor and vasoconstrictor. On stimulation of the hypogastric plexus (presacral nerves) ejaculation has been observed. The prostate gland appears, however, to be supplied also by parasympathetic fibers, but the main effect of the parasympathetic innervation is to be found in the vasodilatation of the erectile tissues of the genital organs, which follows stimulation of these nerves. (On account of the erection elicited in this case, the pelvic nerves used to be called the nervi erigentes.) It appears, therefore, that erection is brought about mainly by impulses through the parasympathetic, and on this account an "erection center" has been postulated in the sacral cord. Ejaculation, on the other hand, is initiated through the sympathetic fibers from the lower thoracic and upper lumbar segments, and consequently an "ejaculation center" has been located in this part of the cord.

The motor fibers to the *uterus* appear to be sympathetic, likewise those to the Fallopian tubes. The fibers are distributed mainly to the muscular coat. The presence of a parasympathetic innervation to the uterus is questionable. The action of the sympathetic on the uterus varies according to whether the uterus is pregnant or not, but on the whole the sympathetic innervation appears to be of no great importance. The uterus appears to possess considerable local autonomy. Thus the experimentally completely denervated uterus may still be able to function normally in parturition in animals, and human cases are known in which a normal childbirth has occurred with complete transverse lesions of the cord.

The importance of autonomic fibers to some of the *endocrine* glands is not yet completely understood. The endocrine gland which is most clearly under the influence of the autonomic system is the *adrenal medulla,* which receives an abundant supply of sympathetic fibers through the lesser splanchnic nerve and probably also fibers from the 12th thoracic and 1st lumbar segments. These fibers are, at least to a large extent, preganglionic, and their stimulation is followed by a marked liberation of adrenaline. This is of interest from a functional and clinical point of view, since conditions accompanied by an activity of the sympathetic will be apt to produce a sudden and massive liberation of adrenaline with ensuing symptoms of sympathetic activity. It appears that by this innervation a mechanism is provided for enabling a rapid and widespread sympathetic activity, useful under certain circumstances, particularly in "emergency states."

Visceral sensibility. Referred pain. From a practical point of view the afferent visceral fibers are of no less importance than the efferent. However, our knowledge concerning them is still far from complete. Visceral afferent fibers are first and foremost of importance for the many *visceral reflexes,* some of which have been mentioned previously. However, it appears clear that some of the visceral afferent impulses may be transmitted to higher levels of the nervous system and ultimately reach consciousness. Under normal circumstances these impulses play a minor role and are for the most part not clearly recognized. They mediate impressions of a diffuse nature, such as the feelings of hunger, thirst, fullness of the bladder and bowels, etc. In certain pathological conditions, however, sensory impressions from the viscera are consciously perceived and are clinically important.

Animal experiments have not yielded much information on the question of *visceral sensibility,* although some evidence has been obtained in this manner. Present-day knowledge on this subject has been gained mainly from clinical observations, particularly in recent times when modern neurosurgical techniques have made possible a wide variety of operative procedures on the autonomic nervous system. It has been known for some time that the viscera are themselves insensitive to touch, cutting, cold, and heat, and operations on visceral organs may on this account be performed under local anesthesia. In this type of operation the patients complain of pain or disagreeable sensations only if the parietal peritoneum, pleura, or pericardium are manipulated, or when the mesenteries are stretched. Many diseases of visceral organs, as is well known, are not accompanied by pain (e.g. endocarditis, pulmonary diseases such as tuberculosis, and renal tumors). On the other hand, the violent pains which accompany some diseases of visceral organs clearly demonstrate that these organs are not completely insensitive, but must be endowed with sensory fibers. The conditions giving rise to visceral pain may be grouped under different headings. Most commonly the pain is due to distension of hollow viscera, probably mainly because the distension sets up forcible contractions of the smooth muscles of the walls, usually called "spasms." Of this type are the pains occurring in blockage of the ureter or the bile ducts by concrements ("renal" and "biliary colics" respectively) in which the pains commonly occur in bouts. Another cause of visceral pain is rapid stretching of the capsules of solid organs, such as the liver and the spleen. In the case of the heart a sudden anoxemia may give rise to severe pain and it is probable that the same mechanism may also be responsible in other organs. The pains occurring in some inflammatory diseases of visceral organs may be due to violent contractions of the muscular walls in some cases (thus probably in the case of the pains seen in cystopyelitis), but in other cases they are more probably due to irritation of the peritoneum. The visceral pains have some characteristics in common which distinguish them to some extent from pain in superficial structures. They are as a rule *diffusely localized* by the patient and they have a tendency to *irradiate to cutaneous areas.* On this account they are often assumed by the patient to arise mainly or exclusively in surface regions of the body. This latter pain is termed "referred pain."

As mentioned previously the visceral sensory fibers, like the somatic, have their perikarya in the spinal ganglia and enter the cord in the dorsal roots. Some of these fibers are fine, others are coarse. Several observations allow conclusions to be made concerning the course of the visceral afferent fibers, a point of supreme importance for the surgical treatment of visceral pain. *The bulk of the visceral pain fibers accompany the sympathetic fibers.* Thus transection of the splanchnic nerves or the corresponding communicant rami abolishes pain arising from the upper abdominal viscera, such as the stomach or the gut. Likewise, transection of the dorsal roots of the part of the cord which supplies the organ in question with sympathetic fibers will be effective. For example, the pains of biliary colic may be abolished by section of the dorsal roots of the 4th to 10th thoracic segments as well as by section of the splanchnic nerves. The visceral afferent fibers, at least the majority of them, according to observations of this kind, thus enter the cord through the dorsal roots. However, in some cases section of the dorsal roots has not been entirely successful, and the existence of other afferent pathways has been postulated.

The *only exception* to the rule that visceral pain fibers follow sympathetic fibers appears to be in the case of the fibers from the sigmoid colon and rectum, the neck of the bladder, the prostate, and the cervix of the uterus. These, according to the findings of neurosurgeons (for references see White and Sweet, 1955), enter the cord in the dorsal roots of the 2nd to 4th sacral segments (where the parasympathetic efferents originate). Similarly in their peripheral course these visceral afferent fibers appear to accompany the parasympathetic nerves, being found in the pelvic nerves and the associated plexuses. (The pain fibers from the fundus of the bladder and the fundus of the uterus, however, pass through the hypogastric plexus to the dorsal roots of the 11th thoracic to the 1st lumbar segments.) There has been some dispute as to whether the vagus carries visceral pain fibers. According to surgical experience it apparently does not. Balchum and Weaver (1943) found that pain fibers from the stomach do not pass in the vagus but in the greater splanchnic nerves.

The peculiar phenomenon that visceral disease is frequently accompanied by pain which is referred to definite parts of the body surface, either alone or with concomitant sensation of pain conceived as of visceral origin, has been difficult to explain, and many features of this fact have not yet been clarified. The occurrence of *referred pain* is familiar to clinicians. As examples may be cited the pain in the right scapular region with diseases of the liver or gall bladder, the epigastric pain in gastric ulcer, the inguinal and testicular pain in renal colic. This *parietal pain* is localized quite regularly to definite cutaneous areas in affections of the various organs. In this cutaneous area the skin is frequently hyperesthetic, there may be vasomotor changes, and reflex rigidity of skeletal muscle (*défense,* "guarding") may be observed in the same area. These symptoms may occur also without real pain. The cutaneous areas presenting these changes are commonly termed Head zones, on account of the basic study of these zones by Henry Head. *The cutaneous areas or zones for the various viscera coincide roughly with the segmental distribution of the somatic sensory fibers which take origin from the same segments of the cord as the sympathetic fibers to the viscus in question.* Thus the zone for the stomach corresponds approximately to the dermatomes Th_{5-9}, i.e. the epigastrium, usually mainly on the left side, and within this area the cardiac region appears to be represented most cranially, the pyloric region most caudally. The zone for the liver and gall bladder comprises the dermatomes Th_{7-9} on the right side, that for the appendix and caecum, Th_{10-12}. In angina pectoris the upper thoracic dermatomes are involved, usually only on the left side, namely, the upper parts of the thorax and the ulnar side of the arm. In the case of the viscera which send their pain fibers to the sacral cord (see above) the cutaneous areas coincide with the corresponding sacral dermatomes; they are found extending from the perineum (cf. Ch. 2 on the dermatomes).

The occurrence of these cutaneous zones of Head seems to imply that in one way or another, the visceral impulses must be propagated to the cutaneous sensory fibers or tracts. There appears to be no valid evidence in favor of the view (Dogiel) that this occurs by termination of the visceral afferent fibers on spinal ganglion cells. If the centripetal branches of one or more visceral afferent ganglion cells and one somatic afferent spinal ganglion cell were to terminate on the same nerve cell in the dorsal horn (Ross), it would be expected that painful visceral processes would always be accompanied by parietal pain, but this is not the case. Mackenzie assumed that the abnormally strong visceral impulses occurring in visceral disease produce some sort of increased irritability of the gray matter of the region of the cord where the impulses enter, and on this account reinforce normally subliminal impulses from the somatic structures, and make them perceived. By assuming the presence of an "irritable focus" of this type, the hyperesthesias which are very frequent in the cutaneous zones of referred pain may be explained. An abnormal irritation of the visceral efferent neurons would explain vasomotor, pilomotor, and sudomotor changes in the zone, and the reflex rigidity of somatic musculature might be due to a similar irritation of the ventral horn cells. Hinsey and Phillips (1940) tried to formulate the conceptions of Mackenzie in a more precise manner. They assume that both visceral and somatic afferent fibers are capable of acting on a "common pool" of secondary neurons which are subjected to summation and inhibition.

The phenomenon of referred pain occurs not only in diseases of the viscera. It may be observed in affections of the surfaces of the body cavities, as the pleura and peritoneum ("parietal referred pain"), as well as in injuries or diseases of deep somatic structures, such as muscles, joints, ligaments, and periosteum, and reference of pain from one area of the skin to another is not uncommon. (A particular kind of referred pain is the phantom limb pain, referred to a part of the body which has been removed by amputation.) The many varieties of referred pain have many features in common, suggesting that the basic mechanism involved is essentially the same. Usually the area of reference becomes painful only when the initial pain, localized by the patient more or less precisely to the original focus, has lasted for some time. The referred pain may even persist after the local pain has vanished. The pain as well as the cutaneous changes, such as hyperesthesia, are not always distributed to the expected dermatomes, but may spread over wider areas. In this respect there are individual variations (assumed by some to depend upon anatomical differences in the distribution of sympathetic fibers). These individual differences have been particularly clearly demonstrated by workers (for example Hockaday and Whitty, 1967) who have studied referred pain experimentally in man by injecting irritating substances, such as hypertonic saline solutions in the interspinous ligaments in healthy subjects, as done first by Lewis and Kellgren (1939). Hockaday and Whitty (1967), confirming the findings of other authors, found that anesthetizing the site of the stimulus consistently abolished referred pain and the accompanying changes, such as hyperesthesia and muscle spasm, but anesthetizing the site of reference did not consistently reduce or abolish the referred effects. The latter observations are of interest with reference to the role played by peripheral factors in the appearance of referred pain and especially in the changes accompanying the pain.

It has been held by some that referred pain may be explained by the presence of dichotomizing sensory fibers, one branch passing to the viscus or other organ primarily affected, the other branch to the site of reference (see Sinclair, Weddell, and Feindel, 1948). Although such fibers have occasionally been described, no evidence is available that they exist in higher vertebrates. Lewis assumed that the vascular changes in an area of referred pain are the result of the presence of collaterals of sensory fibers which at their ending liberate a metabolite, presumably histamine (as discussed previously with reference to axon reflexes). The local changes in the skin then give rise to pain impulses. Corresponding local changes may occur in muscles. This theory was expanded by Sinclair, Weddell, and Feindel (1948). While the peripheral alterations occurring at the site of reference may be explained by the theories of Lewis and others, such theories leave many observations unexplained.

The essential factors involved in the mechanism of referred pain must be sought in anatomical and physiological features in the organization of the central nervous system as suggested by Mackenzie. The conclusion can scarcely be avoided that the mechanisms involved are far from simple. Attention should not be restricted to the spinal cord only, even if spinal mechanisms are undoubtedly involved. The descending fibers, influencing the central transmission of afferent messages may play a role, and the recent findings on the finer organization of the sensory pathways and their synaptic stations make it likely that important processes occur at supraspinal levels. Reference was made previously to the recent theory of pain mechanisms, suggested by Melzack and Wall (1965). This is of relevance also for the problems of referred pain, as discussed in their paper, to which the reader is referred. For further comments on referred pain and discussions of possible central mechanisms see White and Sweet (1955), Nathan (1956a), and Noordenbos (1959).

Although the mechanism of "referred pain" cannot yet be adequately explained, it is of considerable importance for the clinician, and not only the neurologist, in the diagnosis of visceral disease. The information which has been obtained concerning visceral sensibility is also of relevance when therapeutic surgical measures are required to cope with pain originating from visceral organs.

In connection with the discussion of visceral pain, a special feature of it, namely, *vascular sensibility,* should be briefly considered. Mention was made previously that the blood vessels are supplied with nerve fibers, some of them sensory, and clinical evidence substantiates this. Thus ligation of an unanesthetized artery is usually painful. Experimental injection of irritating substances (barium chloride, for example) into an artery likewise gives rise to pain and is followed by a general rise of blood pressure, if the nerve plexus of the artery is intact. These nerve fibers accompany the artery for a short distance, but soon leave it to join the main nerve trunks in their central course. The fibers have their perikarya in the spinal ganglia, like other visceral afferent fibers. Clinical experience seems to show that some of the vasosensible and probably also some of the other visceral afferent fibers accompany the arteries during virtually their entire course to finally reach the spinal ganglia via the sympathetic trunk.

Symptoms in lesions of the autonomic system. Lesions of the hypothalamus and brain stem. In view of the incomplete knowledge of the structure and particularly the function of the different parts of the autonomic system, it is no wonder that the clinical aspects of diseases of these structures are insufficiently understood. As a matter of fact, there are as yet not many clear-cut diseases or syndromes which can be unhesitatingly ascribed to lesions of the autonomic system, although there is good reason to believe that the autonomic system is involved in producing some of the symptoms in a multitude of diseases which do not primarily affect the system itself. The intimate interrelation between the hypothalamus and the cortex is worthy of emphasis, and should be especially borne in mind when so-called functional disorders and neuroses are treated.

In the preceding sections reference has repeatedly been made to the clinical aspects of disturbed autonomic functions and to symptoms following lesions of various parts of the autonomic system. The facts already considered will only be briefly mentioned here, and attention will be paid primarily to features which have not been dealt with. No complete account of all the symptoms which belong to this field will be attempted.

The symptoms following lesions of the *hypothalamus* have for the most part already been considered. One or more of the following symptoms are those most commonly observed: *Diabetes insipidus* (when the supraoptic nucleus or the hypophysial stalk is damaged), *disturbances in heat regulation* and *vasomotor disturbances, sleep disturbances* (most frequent as hypersomnia in lesions of the posterior hypothalamus), *dystrophia adiposogenitalis* (region of tuberal nuclei or ventromedial nucleus), *hemorrhages and ulcerations of the alimentary canal.* Furthermore, *Horner's syndrome* and *emotional changes* may occur. On account of the small size and the site of the hypothalamus, lesions of this will very frequently be associated with damage to other neighboring structures, particularly the optic chiasma or tracts and the hypophysis.

The hypothalamus may be affected by *fractures of the base of the skull.* In some of these cases diabetes insipidus develops. *Primary* and *metastatic tumors* may also affect the hypothalamus. Of primary tumors the craniopharyngeomas and the suprasellar meningeomas should be especially recalled (cf. Ch. 8). *Vascular incidents,* on the other hand, very rarely affect the hypothalamus, which has a very rich and efficient blood supply. Occasionally *aneurysms* of the internal carotid or the circulus arteriosus press on the hypothalamus. Far more frequently this region is affected by infections of the central nervous system. The regular involvement of the hypothalamus in *epidemic encephalitis* has been mentioned (cf. also Ch. 4). Another rather common cause of hypothalamic involvement is *syphilitic meningoencephalitis,* and also in *general paresis* symptoms from this part of the brain may occur. In cases of *alcoholic encephalopathy* changes have been described in the hypothalamus, and in the amnestic confabulatory *Korsakoff's psychosis* the pathological alterations are as a rule especially marked in the mammillary body (see Ch. 10). *Progressive leucodystrophy* has been assumed to bear a relation to the hypothalamus. Multiple small hemorrhages, old

628

and recent, have been found in the hypothalamus in cases of *chronic gastric and duodenal ulcers* (Vonderahe, 1940), and in *cancer of the stomach* changes have been described in the mammillary bodies resembling those found in chronic alcoholism (Neubürger, 1937). Baker, Cornwell, and Brown (1952) have drawn attention to the frequent affection of the hypothalamus in *poliomyelitis*. In a clinicopathological study of 115 cases they found clinical evidence of hypothalamic dysfunction (hyperthermia, hypothermia, gastric hemorrhage, and other symptoms) during the acute illness, and slighter changes that could persist for months or even years after recovery.

Lesions of the *pons and medulla oblongata* are apt to interrupt descending fibers to the autonomic preganglionic neurons of the brain stem and spinal cord. This is the case particularly with lesions in the lateral part of the pons and medulla (concerning other symptoms in such lesions see Chs. 2 and 4). Immediately after an acute interruption of the pathways the autonomic reflexes will be abolished below the lesion on the same side, and there will therefore be anhidrosis and lack of piloarrection, and as a rule some vasodilatation in this half of the body. When the initial shock has passed away, Horner's syndrome will become evident, on account of the interruption of the fibers to the centrum ciliospinale. Eventually this, as well as the other symptoms, becomes less conspicuous. Thus the difference in skin temperature and sweating in the two halves of the body will gradually diminish. The pilomotor reflexes are usually increased on the side of the lesion. This as well as other features have been explained as being due to the lack of central regulation of the activity of the spinal autonomic cell groups (Foerster, Gagel, and Mahoney, 1939; List and Peet, 1939).

Lesions of the spinal cord. The conus syndrome. *In lesions of the spinal cord at levels above the 3rd lumbar segment* (stabbing wounds, bullet wounds, compressions due to fractures of the spine or intraspinal tumors, transverse myelitis), the autonomic descending pathways may be interrupted if the lesion involves the lateral funiculus. In these cases the spinal autonomic reflexes will, after some time, increase, just as do the tendon reflexes. The pilomotor reflexes, as has been mentioned, are purely homolateral, whereas the vasomotor and sudomotor reflexes are also mediated by reflex arcs which cross the median plane of the cord. Changes in the latter reflexes may on this account be observed bilaterally even in unilateral lesions of the cord, and their diagnostic value is thus somewhat reduced. It has been mentioned previously that the pilomotor reflexes, especially, may give information on the site of the lesion in such cases, but it should be emphasized that the segmental level of the pilomotor disturbances does not correspond exactly with the level of the somatic symptoms (cf. above). Transverse lesions of the cord will abolish the voluntary control of the bladder.

In addition to producing symptoms due to interruption of the descending antonomic pathways, lesions of the spinal cord between the levels of Th_1–L_2 will as a rule also destroy some of the preganglionic neurons in the intermediolateral cell column. However, symptoms due to such a lesion tend to diminish after some time and, furthermore, an affection of only a limited part of the column will scarcely reveal itself by distinct symptoms.

Lesions in the upper part of the thoracic cord are most likely to produce symptoms due to involvement of preganglionic neurons. If, for example, the *two upper thoracic segments* are affected, a Horner's syndrome will develop on the side of the lesion. If also the following two or three thoracic segments are involved, the vasomotor, sudomotor, and pilomotor reflexes will be abolished not only in the face but also in the homolateral arm. Sweat secretion is abolished in this area, and during the first few days after the lesion has developed, a vasodilatation may be observed. Symptoms of this kind may be met with in *syringomyelia,* which frequently affects the lower cervical and upper thoracic cord. In the beginning, however, signs of sympathetic irritation may be observed, in the form of hyperhidrosis and vasoconstriction. In order for loss of spinal autonomic reflexes to become apparent, several segments have to be affected, since each autonomic ganglion receives fibers from several segments of the cord. If the *lower thoracic and upper two lumbar segments* are affected, symptoms such as those just described will occur in the lower extremity. It has been mentioned previously that loss of the spinal vasomotor and sudomotor reflexes tends to become less distinct after some time, since local autonomic reflexes become exaggerated.

Lesions of the sacral region of the spinal cord deserve particular consideration. The symptom complex which appears in these cases constitutes the so-called *"conus syndrome."* The *somatic* symptoms concern the middle and commonly also the lower sacral dermatomes and myotomes. There will be a *flaccid paralysis* of the muscles of the outlet of the pelvis, including the external anal and vesical sphincters and the ischiocavernosus and bulbocavernosus muscles. *Loss of sensation* will occur in the region of the perineum, around the anal orifice (S_{3-5}) and commonly also some of the posterior aspect of the thigh (S_2), giving the appearance of a so-called *saddle anesthesia.* If the 1st sacral segment is spared, the ankle jerk is usually retained. When pain is present in pure conus lesions it is referred to the sacral dermatomes. The destruction of the preganglionic parasympathetic fibers will result in a *paralysis of the bladder.* The paralyzed bladder will be distended by the accumulating urine, and no automatic emptying occurs. However, when the distension is severe, some overflow will usually occur, with emptying of small quantities of urine at short intervals. This "dribbling incontinence" is not sufficient for emptying the bladder effectively. The voluntary influence on the bladder is, of course, also lost, and contrary to the condition with lesions of the cord at higher levels, which interfere mainly with the voluntary impulses to the bladder, peripheral stimuli will not elicit reflex contraction of the bladder in lesions of the conus. In addition to the paralysis of the bladder, there is also a *paralysis of the rectum and sigmoid colon,* which receive their parasympathetic motor innervation from the sacral cord. Consequently there is *no spontaneous defecation,* but on account of the paralysis of the voluntary, striped, external sphincter of the anus there will be *incontinentia alvi.* However, after some time a certain degree of automatism of the rectum develops, presumably mediated by the peripheral reflex mechanism (cf. above on the local autonomy of the gut). Finally the conus syndrome in the male is characterized by *loss of* the capacity of *erection and ejaculation,* on account of the destruction of the preganglionic parasympathetic neurons, and the somatic motor ventral horn cells. However, emission of semen occurs, since the motor fibers to the ductus deferens and seminal vesicle are sympathetic. (This emission of semen, however, does not occur as in ordinary ejaculation, since in this process the striped, somatic ischio- and bulbocavernosus muscles are also engaged.) During the development of a conus lesion, when some cells are still preserved, priapism may occur, due to irritation of the visceral and somatic motor cells of the sacral cord.[43] If the conus lesion is incomplete, it may also happen that not all symptoms usually included in the syndrome are present. Thus there may be loss of ejaculation and erection, but preserved or only moderately impaired function of the bladder, etc. (dissociated conus syndromes).

In connection with the paralysis of the bladder in lesions of the conus it should be stressed that identical disturbances will occur if the conus is intact, but the *efferent* fibers to the bladder in the pelvic nerves are damaged. On the other hand, a pure lesion of the *afferent* pathways from the bladder, damaging them in the dorsal roots or in the cord, will also prevent reflex evacuation of the bladder and lead to a distended, *atonic* bladder. This is most commonly observed in tabes. From these facts it will be clear that *lesions of the cauda equina* usually will give rise to similar symptoms as the conus lesions. (The deliberations mentioned above concerning the bladder apply also to the rectum and sigmoid colon and the innervation of the genital organs.) However, since a lesion

[43] Priapism may be seen also in acute transverse lesions at higher levels of the cord.

631

of the cauda will be apt to affect not only fibers of the sacral segments of the cord but also a varying number of the lumbar nerves, the sensory and motor losses will as a rule be more extensive and reach higher levels, and furthermore the distribution will usually be more irregular, since some of the roots of the cauda will avoid damage and be merely pushed aside, as in the case of a tumor developing intraspinally.

Brief mention was made previously (p. 621) of the disturbances in bladder function following transverse lesions of the cord above the sacral levels. On account of their frequency (traumatic cord injuries and multiple sclerosis being the most common causes) these disturbances have attracted much interest. Some additional remarks, are therefore, appropriate. (For some recent data see for example *The Neurogenic Bladder,* 1966.) As mentioned previously, following an acute lesion of the cord above the sacral levels, "spinal shock" affects the bladder and there is retention of urine. When the "shock" declines the bladder functions "automatically," the spinal reflex apparatus in the paraplegic patient works without its normal supraspinal control. The micturition reflex is usually more easily elicited than normally and when started, micturition cannot be brought to a stop by voluntary innervation of the external sphincter. Various stimuli below the level of the lesion are apt to elicit the micturition reflex, for example cooling or touching or pricking of the skin of the perineum or the inside of the thigh. This is annoying but may be made use of by the paraplegic patient as a trick to elicit emptying of the bladder.[44] The increased reflex activity often involves the external sphincter. Electromyography has shown that in patients with a spastic paraplegia the external sphincter is often never completely relaxed, and may thus increase the outflow resistance during micturition with a resulting incomplete emptying of the bladder. (Operative interruption of the external sphincter by denervation or division of its fibers may be beneficial.)

In other cases of paraplegia, the bladder may be "overactive" or "uninhibited." This may be counteracted by drugs of the atropine group, which reduce the parasympathetic effect on the detrusor. On the other hand, cholinergic pharmaca are often used with good effect in transitory postoperative retention, and in chronic hypotonic function of the bladder when this is not due to physical obstruction. ("Ganglionic blocking agents" and "polysynaptic inhibitors" may be used with advantage in certain cases of bladder disturbances, as reviewed by Pedersen and

[44] In a number of patients Nathan (1956b) found that even if the spinal cord is completely transected the patient may have a certain awareness of bladder-filling, giving him some control of micturition. It appears that these sensory impulses are transmitted centrally via afferent fibers accompanying sympathetic nerves.

Grynderup, 1966.) As mentioned in a previous section, there is some evidence for a sympathetic influence on micturition. Some slight differences in the symptomatology of the bladder following cord lesions above or below the origin of the sympathetic fibers (but above the level of the sacral outflow) may perhaps be related to the presence or absence of the sympathetic innervation (see Edvardsen, 1967, for some data).

Lesions of the peripheral parts of the autonomic system. Pathological processes affecting the *ganglia of the sympathetic trunk* will produce symptoms identical with those in lesions of the intermediolateral cell column, except that, in pure lesions of the trunk, somatic motor and sensory symptoms will be absent. However, in order to produce symptoms, such lesions have to involve several ganglia at most places, and are therefore not very frequently diagnosed. In the cervical and lumbar part of the trunk, however, even a small lesion will be able to interrupt fibers to ganglia situated cranially or caudally, respectively (cf. Fig. 11-4). Most common among lesions of peripheral parts of the sympathetic are perhaps lesions of the upper thoracic ganglia and inferior cervical ganglion or the stellate ganglion. As has been mentioned, these lesions are followed by abolished sweat secretion and piloarrection of the head and arm on the side of the lesion, accompanied by a vasodilatation. If the inferior cervical ganglion is included, Horner's syndrome is usually the most enduring symptom. Causes of such lesions include stabbing or gunshot wounds, most commonly seen in wartime, mediastinal tumors, aneurysms of the aorta, glandular abscesses of the neck, and operative lesions. If the lesion develops gradually, irritative symptoms commonly mark the beginning, betraying themselves by vasoconstriction, sweat secretion, and piloarrection.

Interruption of the sympathetic innervation of the *abdominal and thoracic viscera* as a rule does not yield clear-cut symptoms, regardless of whether the vertebral ganglia or more peripheral structures are involved.

It has been remarked previously that *lesions of the plexuses of the spinal nerves or the peripheral nerves* themselves will be followed by disturbances of sympathetic nature which present a distribution corresponding to the arrangement of the somatic sensory fibers. In lesions of the plexuses, for example the brachial, a segmental vasodilatation, anhidrosis, and abolished piloarrection may be observed. In irritative lesions the symptoms may be more conspicuous, betraying the affection of the sympathetic fibers by the presence of vasoconstriction, increased sweating, and not infrequently also trophic disturbances even of the bones. In cases of polyneuritis irritative symptoms may occur together with deficiency symptoms. However, it is a peculiar circumstance that in some cases of lesions of the peripheral nerves with a complete anesthesia in the area of distribution, a certain diffuse, uncharacteristic sensibility may be retained. As a rule this sensibility is most clearly demonstrated by pinching or deep pressure. In some cases even the slightest touch or a slight pressure may give rise to severe pain, as in cases of causalgia. It has been assumed that this sensibility must be mediated through the sensory fibers which accompany the vessels.

No disease is known which can be attributed to a selective lesion of the *peripheral autonomic plexuses.* However, on the basis of animal experiments and findings made in operations on these structures in man, there is reason to believe that disturbances of the visceral innervation may be responsible for some symptoms seen in various diseases.

Operations on the autonomic nervous system. Most of these operations were originally made on the basis of theoretical speculations in cases where the etiology of the disease was unknown. Operations on the sympathetic system have been performed in nearly all types of diseases. The results have been of varying value. A considerable proportion of the operative procedures have as their principal aim the relief of otherwise intractable pain.

An interruption of the sympathetic pathways can be achieved by operations of various kinds. A *periarterial sympathectomy* (periarterial neurectomy) consists essentially in removing the periarterial sympathetic plexus of a part of an artery after it has been exposed. The adventitia is stripped off the artery for a certain length. Most neurosurgeons have found that the ensuing vasodilatation peripheral to the sympathectomized part of the artery is only transient and the effect on pain has not been convincing. This may perhaps be due to the fact, mentioned previously, that apart from the main arterial trunks of the proximal extremities, the vessels obtain their sympathetic fibers from the nerves in their immediate vicinity (see also Stürup and Carmichael, 1935).

A complete interruption of sympathetic impulses to a certain region of the body can be accomplished by removing all the ganglia of the sympathetic trunk through which the impulses pass. This procedure is commonly called *ganglionectomy* (or sometimes sympathectomy). The same effect will be obtained also by cutting the white rami communicantes to the region in question. This *ramisection,* however, is a more delicate operation, and as a rule it will not be possible to cut only the white rami, the gray being also included. It will be understood that a ganglionectomy will in some cases represent an interruption mainly of the *preganglionic* fibers. This is the case, for instance, when the upper lumbar ganglia are removed in sympathectomy for the lower extremity (as a rule the 2nd to 4th ganglia are removed; the 1st should be spared in order to avoid sterility in the male by paralyzing the ductus deferens). In this case the postganglionic neurons in the lowest lumbar and sacral ganglia of the trunk will not be affected. When the stellate ganglion is removed in order to obtain a sympathetic denervation of the arm, this, on the other hand, involves removing the *postganglionic* neurons. (In order to be effective the upper two thoracic ganglia have been included in the extirpation, since frequently the 2nd thoracic ganglion contains some postganglionic neurons to the arm.)

Following sympathectomies it has been noted by many neurosurgeons that some areas of the body are not sympathetically denervated. This subject has been thoroughly studied by Monro (1959). In a number of patients he tested the effect of sympathectomies by means of the electrical skin resistance method. Following cervicodorsal sympathectomy (which includes the stellate and 2nd thoracic ganglion) there is an "escape area" in the central region of the face. Following a thoracolumbar sympathectomy (which includes the 4th thoracic to the 3rd lumbar ganglion) there is an area with retained sudomotor activity which comprises the 1st and 2nd lumbar dermatomes and often even extends above and below these dermatomes. In addition the perineum is an "escape area." On the basis of careful clinico-anatomical investigations and anatomical studies of normal material Monro (1959) concludes that the lumbar "escape area" following thoracolumbar sympathectomies is due to the presence of intermediate ganglia associated with the nerve roots of L_1 and L_2 whose connections have remained intact. The intermediate ganglia associated with the nerve roots of L_4 and L_5 will not cause sweating, because their preganglionic fibers have been sectioned below the lower level of the sympathetic outflow. (Monro found this to be at L_3 in 85 per cent of his patients.) No satisfactory explanation can be given for the occurrence of the "escape areas" in the face and perineum. Monro's monograph (1959) contains a wealth of observations of clinical interest. He discusses the fact that results are usually more satisfactory following thoracolumbar than cervicodorsal sympathectomies.

Before an operation is undertaken a *diagnostic injection of procaine* into the ganglia in question is usually made. This procaine block is effective in interrupting the conduction of the fibers, and if the results of it are unsatisfactory not much benefit can be expected from an operation.[45] On the other hand, sometimes the effect (for example on pain)

---

[45] As mentioned previously, the area of temporary sympathetic denervation produced by the block may be judged by determining the distribution of anhidrosis in tests of thermoregulatory sweating or by mapping the distribution of increased electrical skin resistance.

of a procaine block is more enduring than should be expected, and in some cases repeated injections of procaine have been followed by complete relief. It is generally assumed that procaine in these cases acts by breaking a "vicious circle."

A similar effect to that obtained on extirpation of sympathetic ganglia may be achieved by *alcohol or phenol injections* into the ganglia. Although a minor procedure, this has in some cases a less enduring effect, and damage to neighboring structures cannot always be avoided. Thus damage of the intercostal nerves in injections into the stellate ganglion may give rise to neuralgias after some time.

Of other operative procedures may be mentioned *section of the splanchnic nerves, resection of the hypogastric plexus* (presacral neurectomy), and resections of the superior and inferior mesenteric plexuses.

In the first period of enthusiasm, surgery on the autonomic system was attempted in a variety of diseases. As more experience was gained operations of this kind have been limited to conditions where the results are generally satisfactory. In some instances advances in pharmacotherapy have abolished or minimized the need for surgical interventions, for example in the treatment of essential hypertension. In the following, reference will be made to some conditions where surgery on the autonomic nervous system has been found to be of benefit, even if in some of these disorders such operations are rarely performed nowadays. (For complete accounts see White and Smithwick, 1942; White and Sweet, 1955.)

Sympathetic denervation of one or more extremities has been frequently employed in diseases in which there is reason to believe that at least one factor responsible for the symptoms is an abnormal state of contraction of peripheral vessels. The most clear-cut disease of this type is the so-called *Raynaud's disease.*

This disorder occurs more frequently in women than in men, and is characterized mainly by vasomotor changes in peripheral parts of the body, most commonly fingers or toes, accompanied by pain. Cooling as well as emotional factors are apt to provoke the attacks, during which the fingers and hands or toes and feet become cold and frequently at the same time cyanotic. The cooling is due to constriction of the arterioles, the cyanosis to the slow circulation of the blood in the capillaries which are dilated. Sometimes the capillaries are contracted and the skin accordingly pale. The pain is dull, deep, and may be accompanied by paresthesias. When the attack recedes, the affected parts grow warm and red, and this vasodilatation is usually followed by a severe burning pain. In long-lasting cases permanent changes are apt to develop. Necroses of the skin, particularly on the finger tips, and ulcerations and eventually atrophic changes in the subcutaneous tissues and the bones are not uncommon in long-lasting cases.

The etiology of the disease is not known. Probably several factors are responsible. That the sympathetic innervation of the blood vessels is of importance seems to be clear from the beneficial results obtained in sympathectomies. However, in this respect there is as concerns the upper extremity a marked difference between the postganglionic procedures applied previously and the preganglionic methods now commonly used. In the former cases the sensitization which developed in a week or two was responsible for the transient effect, and following the operation attacks were usually induced by slighter stimuli than before, although they were less severe and the patient had the benefit of being relieved of his pain. Those having experience with the preganglionic operative method have on the whole obtained satisfactory results in cases of Raynaud's disease (see, for example, White and Smithwick, 1942). For an evaluation of sympathectomy in vascular diseases see Boguslawski, Banach, and Dabrowski (1960).

Whether sympathectomies are of any use in peripheral vascular disorders appears to depend mainly on whether there is a component of vasospasm involved in the production of the symptoms. When organic changes in the vessels have advanced to a certain degree no relief is, as a rule, to be expected. Among conditions which in some cases have benefited from sympathetic denervation may be mentioned *endarteritis obliterans* (Bürger's disease). In senile and diabetic gangrene some surgeons have tried sympathectomy, and some have found that demarcation is favored and that healing takes place more rapidly. The same holds good in some cases of chronic ulcers of the extremities, in cases in which there is reason to believe that the circulation is impaired by vasospasm.

Before the advent of modern hypotensive drugs, attempts were made to treat *essential hypertension* by extensive sympathetic denervation, and several authors reported favorable results, for example, following resection of the splanchnic nerves.

Resection of the splanchnic nerves is not followed by definite symptoms from the abdominal viscera. This is in accord with other findings which have shown that these viscera possess a considerable degree of local autonomy. When disturbances in the functions of the abdominal viscera are present, removal of their sympathetic innervation has been attempted in some cases as a therapeutic measure, with most success in disorders in which there is reason to assume that overactivity of the sympathetic is responsible for abnormal states of contraction of smooth muscles. Such operations have been performed, for example in cases of cardiospasm and as a treatment for pylorospasm.

Although pain of visceral origin may be abolished by section of the appropriate dorsal roots or by chordotomy, it is obviously preferable to cope with visceral pain without producing loss of somatic sensibility. As a rule, therefore, visceral pain is treated by operative procedures involving the autonomic nervous system, even if in some cases the other methods have to be resorted to. Some conditions in which operations on

637

the sympathetic nervous system have been employed to alleviate pain will be mentioned.

The pain of *angina pectoris,* which, as has been seen, must be assumed to travel via the afferent fibers from the heart, and which follow the sympathetic fibers, has been relieved by operations on the sympathetic, by alcohol injections in vertebral ganglia, or by ganglionectomy. It is essential that not only the stellate ganglion be removed, but that the upper two or (better) three thoracic ganglia are also included. Some recommend removing also the 4th thoracic ganglion (see White and Sweet, 1955). When the operation was first performed the stellate ganglion alone was ablated, and the results were not satisfactory. The reason for this is clear since afferent fibers from the heart may reach the cord as low as the 4th (and in some cases probably even the 5th) thoracic ganglion.

There appears to be no alteration in the function of the heart after the operation. Some authors have warned against the operation, claiming that when the pain impulses from the heart are abolished, the patient loses his warning signal. However, some diffuse feeling, sufficient to warn the patient of an attack, remains, such as a feeling of oppression, or palpitations (see, for example, Lindgren and Olivecrona, 1947). Since many patients suffering from angina pectoris are poor operative risks, paravertebral alcohol injections were employed in many cases, but on account of the neuritis which is apt to appear and other complications, the operative treatment is preferred if the patient is able to stand it. A diagnostic procaine block is of particular interest in cases of angina pectoris, since if injection is made during an attack of anginal pain, the pain will be abolished.

Dysmenorrhoea has been treated by interruption of the sympathetic supply of the uterus. This is done by removing the sympathetic plexus descending from the aorta to the pelvis as the hypogastric plexuses or "presacral nerves." The operation is, therefore, commonly called "*presacral neurectomy.*"

Presacral neurectomy has also been performed in some cases of painful disorders of the bladder and prostate. However, the results have not been very satisfactory, as can be explained on the basis of the innervation of these organs (cf. above). In cases of malignant tumors, relief from pain can only be expected as long as the tumor has not infiltrated the surroundings, since somatic fibers will then be involved in addition.

Attempts to relieve the pain of *trigeminal neuralgia* by operations on the cervical sympathetic, particularly by removal of the superior cervical ganglion, have been made by some. There appears to be no sound basis for the view that the sympathetic is involved in producing the pain of trigeminal neuralgia, and the operation is not used any more.

Painful disorders of the extremities have been treated with operations on the sympathetic supply in many cases. The symptom complex called *causalgia* (meaning burning pain) by Weir Mitchell occurs in some cases of penetrating wounds with lesions of peripheral nerves, most often bullet wounds. As a rule the nerve is not entirely interrupted. Most frequently the symptoms are seen following injury to the median or sciatic nerves.

Causalgia or a closely similar clinical picture may, however, also be observed in irritative nerve lesions of other types. The symptoms often appear immediately after the injury or during the process of healing of the wound. The distressing pain, which is of a burning type, is localized in the area of distribution of the nerve peripheral to the lesion, and is often exaggerated by heat and diminished by cold. The affected area is extremely hyperesthetic, and the slightest stimulus of the skin is liable to provoke severe pain, as is also movement of the extremity, and in sensitive persons psychic stimuli may also start an attack of pain. In the hyperesthetic area, which frequently exceeds the cutaneous area of the nerve, thermal stimuli and deep pressure may also provoke pain. In typical cases objective alterations occur in the affected area. The skin is often hot and red, and may be glossy. A marked sweating may occur.

The pathogenesis of the syndrome is unknown. Many hypotheses have been set forth, but none of them is entirely satisfactory. According to Richards (1967) who reviews the literature, the most likely explanation for the appearance of the symptoms, especially the burning pain, is an abnormal interaction at the site of injury between efferent sympathetic and afferent sensory fibers.

In those cases of causalgia in which spontaneous recovery does not occur, several types of operations and treatment have been attempted. Intraneural injection of alcohol above the place of the lesion, resection or crushing of the nerve, periarterial sympathectomy, and other procedures have been tried without much success. The only satisfactory results are seen following interruption of the sympathetic nerve supply of the affected limb, by removal of the appropriate sympathetic ganglia, in the case of the upper limb cervicothoracic ganglionectomy. According to reports in the literature the results of such operations have been excellent in 77 per cent of the cases, good in 19 per cent, and poor in 4 per cent (Richards, 1967).

Other disorders in which pain occurs in the extremities, and in which there is reason to believe that disturbance in the autonomic innervation is an important factor have also been more or less successfully treated by surgical procedures (see White and Sweet, 1955). However, little is known of the nature of these disorders, which commonly develop following closed traumatic injuries of an extremity, and are designated post-traumatic dystrophies, post-traumatic painful osteoporosis, etc. The distinction between these conditions and typical causalgia is not always clear.

Recent advances in pharmacotherapy have gradually lessened the need for surgical interventions on the autonomic nervous system, and further advances are to be expected in this field in the future.

12

The Cerebral Cortex

THE CEREBRAL CORTEX has been touched upon repeatedly in the preceding chapters. It will, however, be appropriate to consider the structure and function of the cortex more thoroughly, and to give a brief review of symptoms following lesions of the cortex apart from those already mentioned.

The cerebral cortex is developed from the telencephalon, forming the rostral part of the prosencephalon. However, the cortex cerebri is neither structurally nor functionally an entity. Some regions primarily have connections with fibers from the olfactory bulb, directly or through relay stations. These phylogenetically oldest parts of the cortex are often loosely called *the "rhinencephalon."* In lower vertebrates such as amphibians and reptiles, these parts constitute a considerable proportion of the telencephalon as has been described in Chapter 10. The other divisions of the cortex first undergo a marked progressive development in mammals, in the phylogenetic scale. The parts of the hemisphere appearing at this stage are usually called *neocortex* or *neopallium*. In the higher mammals and man the neocortex increases enormously in size. Its surface area, relatively, becomes increasingly greater than its volume, a condition made possible by the appearance of fissures and convolutions, necessary to accommodate the growing brain within the skull.

Structure of the cerebral cortex. Cytoarchitecture and areal parcellation. The general principles of structure of the neocortex are similar in all mammals, despite the progressive differentiation which reaches its

640

peak in man. Some of the phylogenetical features will be touched upon below, after the description of the neocortex in man.

The neocortex is frequently also designated *isocortex* (O. Vogt) or *homogenetic cortex* (Brodmann) since its different parts develop in the same manner during ontogenesis. This isocortex, which makes up the bulk of the cerebral cortex in man, presents several minor differences in various parts of the brain, to be discussed below, but with some modifications all regions can be made to fit into a general scheme of a six-layered cortex when examined in preparations stained for nerve cells. This is depicted in Fig. 12-1, the left column showing the cells as they appear in Golgi preparations, where axons and dendrites are made visible, the center column representing the picture seen in Nissl-stained sections. The separate layers are as follows:

I. *The molecular or zonal layer,* immediately beneath the pia, is rich in fibers but poor in cells. Scattered small nerve cells are present, the horizontal cells of Cajal, orientated with their longest axes parallel to the surface of the cortex. The fibers form a dense tangentially running plexus.

II. *The external granular layer* is composed of densely packed small cells, some of a pyramidal type, others round or star-shaped. The pyramidal cells in this layer, as in the other layers containing pyramids, have their apices directed towards the surface.

III. *The pyramidal layer* consists predominantly of pyramidal cells of medium size. The largest ones are found in the deeper parts of the layer.

IV. *The internal granular layer* is dominated by small cells lying close together, most of them star-shaped, whereas some are of the pyramidal type. This layer contains abundant horizontally directed fibers (the outer band of Baillarger, cf. below).

V. *The ganglionic layer* is composed mainly of pyramidal cells, mostly medium-sized and large. Like the other pyramidal cells, these have long apical dendrites, directed toward the molecular layer, and a generous amount of basal dendrites, leaving the cells at their bases and running more or less horizontally.

VI. *The multiform layer* contains predominantly spindle shaped cells. It is frequently subdivided into an outer part VI*a* and an inner VI*b,* the latter at most places fusing gradually with the white matter of the hemisphere.

On closer examination it becomes apparent that, in spite of features common to all cortical regions, clear-cut differences can be ascertained between various smaller parts. This recognition is comparatively recent. The fundamental investigations in this field we owe to Campbell (1905), Brodmann (1909), and von Economo (1927). The cortex presents not only a varying thickness in different parts (ranging from 4.5 mm to 1.3 mm), but also microscopical differences. In cell-stained sections it is clearly seen that the different layers exhibit varying thicknesses, varying densities of cells, and also differences in regard to the sizes and types of cells which they contain. On the basis of these differences in structure, *the cytoarchitecture,* several more or less distinct small *areas* may be discerned within the cerebral cortex. Brodmann distinguished some fifty different areas, von Economo nearly twice this number.

Fig. 12-2 reproduces the cytoarchitectural map of the human cortex as worked out by Brodmann. Each area has been designated by a different figure. Von Economo employed other symbols in his map, but in the principal features the subdivisions of Brodmann and von Economo coincide. Since Brodmann's labeling is most extensively employed and more simple than that of von Economo, the latter will not be considered in more detail. A glance at the map of Brodmann will reveal that the borders

FIG. 12–1 Diagram of the structure of the cerebral cortex. To the left, from a Golgi preparation; center, from a Nissl preparation; to the right, from a myelin sheath preparation. I: lamina zonalis; II: lamina granularis externa; III: lamina pyramidalis; IV: lamina granularis interna; V: lamina ganglionaris; VI: lamina multiformis. After Brodmann and O. Vogt.

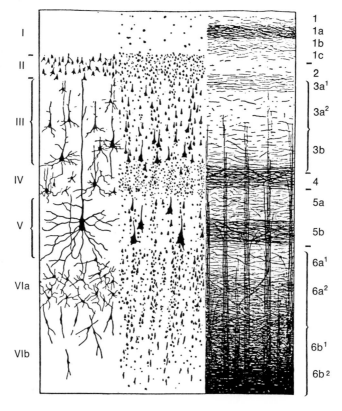

between the different cortical areas to a large extent do not coincide with the sulci on the cerebral surface. Microscopically the limits between adjacent areas are also not quite sharp everywhere.

C. and O. Vogt have elaborated Brodmann's map in a somewhat more detailed manner, and proposed a further subdivision of some of Brodmann's areas.

FIG. 12–2 Brodmann's cytoarchitectural map of the human brain. The various areas are labeled with different symbols and their numbers indicated by figures.

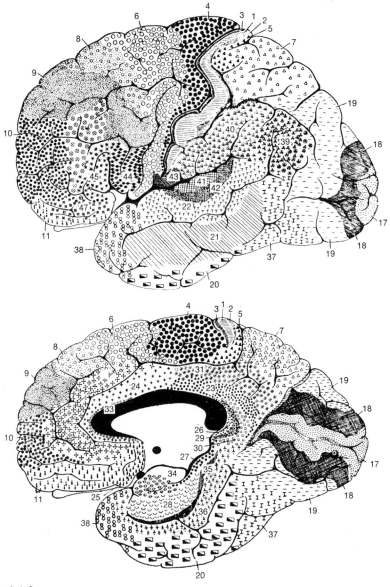

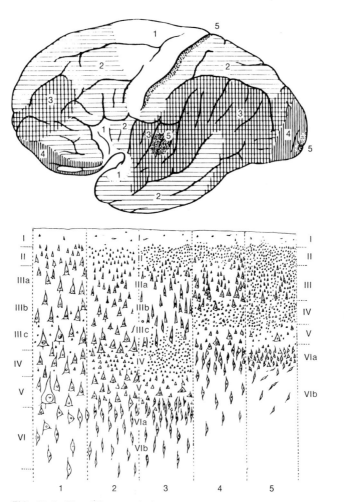

FIG. 12–3 The different principal types of cortex (below) and their distribution in the hemisphere (above). 1: agranular cortex; 2: frontal type of cortex; 3: parietal type; 4: polar type; 5: granular cortex, koniocortex. (Cf. text.) After von Economo from Kornmüller and Janzen (1939).

The parcellation derived by the Vogts in the monkey was transferred to the human brain by Foerster and employed by him in his presentation of clinical experiences in electrical stimulation of the cortex. However, objections may be raised to this, and although the Vogt–Foerster map was extensively employed by experimenters upon the cerebral cortex, recent research tends to show that a minute parcellation like that of the Vogts is not always justified.

Common features of several cytoarchitectural fields makes it possible to collect some of them in larger groups. Von Economo arranges the

644

different areas in five fundamental groups, as shown in Fig. 12-3. The cortical types labeled 2, 3, and 4 in the lower diagram of the figure contain the six typical layers, described above, although not all of them are developed to the same degree in the different types. These types are *homotypical* on this account, contrary to the *heterotypical* cortical types 1 and 5, in which six layers cannot be clearly discerned when the cortex is fully developed. (During fetal life, however, this heterotypical cortex, according to Brodmann, also passes a six-layered stage. On this account it belongs to the homogenetic cortex or isocortex.)

It will be seen from the figure that the cortex of fundamental type no. 1 is distinguished by its lack of distinct granular layers (II and IV), whereas layers III and V are well developed. This *agranular cortex,* as will be seen from the upper drawing, is found first and foremost in the posterior parts of the frontal lobe, from the central sulcus forward. Areas 4 and 6 belong to this type, likewise part of areas 8 and 44. In addition the same type of cortex is found on the medial surface of the hemisphere in the paracentral lobule, the anterior half of the gyrus cinguli, and anterior to the lamina terminalis, and in part of the hippocampus and uncus (the latter regions belong to the *allocortex,* cf. Ch. 10). A particular type of agranular cortex is found in area 4, where between the larger pyramids in the Vth layer the giant pyramids of Betz are found (cf. Ch. 4). Fig. 8-7a is a photomicrograph from area 4 showing some of the principal features. The more massive efferent projection systems take origin preponderantly from agranular cortex. *The agranular cortex, therefore, with certain qualifications, can be considered the prototype of "motor" cortex.*

The other type of heterotypical cortex is labeled 5 in Fig. 12-3. This type is characterized by its richness in granular cells and the strongly developed granular layers II and IV. The layers III and V, on the other hand, are only poorly developed. Areas belonging to this type of cortex are found (cf. Fig. 12-3) in the anterior part of the postcentral convolution, along the calcarine fissure (only the dorsalmost end of this area is visible in Fig. 12-3, see also Fig. 10-3), in a limited part of the upper surface of the first temporal convolution, and finally in restricted parts of the hippocampal gyrus (not visible in Fig. 12-3). Cortex of this type, *granular cortex* or *koniocortex, is characteristic of those cortical areas which receive the primary afferent sensory systems.* The most elaborate type of such koniocortex is found in the area striata, where as will be remembered the fibers of the optic radiation end. The number of granular cells is exceedingly high, and the granular layers are thick, the inner granular layer (IV) being in addition subdivided into two sublayers, IVa and IVc (see Fig. 8-7c). Layer IVb represents the intermediate layer, being poor in cells but abundant in myelinated fibers, which, as has been mentioned, form the line of Gennari or Vicq d'Azyr (cf. Fig. 8-6).

From Fig. 12-3 it is seen that cortex of type 2 is found in the frontal lobe anterior to the distribution of cortex of the agranular type, but in addition it occupies parts of the parietal and temporal lobes. The pyramidal cells of layers III and V are well developed, making the cortex resemble in certain respects that of the agranular type. On the other hand, the parietal type (3 in Fig. 12-3) has less massive pyramidal layers and more elaborate granular layers. The lamination is distinct in this type, which, however, is not limited to the parietal lobe. The last type, the polar, no. 4, is characterized *inter alia* by its thinness and high content of granular cells.

Just as a parcellation of the cerebral cortex can be made on the basis of differences in the amount, type, and pattern of distribution of the nerve cells, so detailed scrutiny of the myelinated fibers allows for a parcellation. The *myeloarchitectural areas* delimited in this way coincide fairly well with the cytoarchitectural areas.

In a myelin sheath stained section through the cerebral cortex of man (Fig. 12-1, right column) a wealth of myelinated fibers are seen. Some of these fibers ascend perpendicular to the surface of the cortex, more or less distinctly aggregated in radial bundles. Other fibers run parallel to the surface. In most parts of the cortex they are concentrated in three zones. The most superficial is found in the lamina zonalis or molecularis, the other two are situated more deeply, forming the so-called outer and inner lines or bands of Baillarger (4 and 5b in Fig. 12-1, to the right). Studies of myeloarchitecture have been particularly extensively performed by C. and O. Vogt and their pupils. The various areas present differences in the amount of fibers in the various layers as well as in the thickness of the fibers, their course, and terminal distribution. Following this line of investigation a parcellation of the cortex even more detailed than the cytoarchitectural has been found.

It has further been shown, particularly by Pfeifer (1940), that there also exist in the cortex regional variations in the vascular supply. The density of the capillaries, their arrangement, caliber, and other features differ in various layers and various parts of the cortex. In many respects this *angioarchitectural parcellation* is in accord with the results obtained from the other methods of areal subdivision of the cortex. In a corresponding manner the distribution and arrangement of the *glial cells* differs in different areas, but the details have not yet been completely elucidated. In recent years some studies have been made on the *chemoarchitecture* of the cortex. It turns out that there are differences between areas and between layers as concerns chemical composition as well as amounts of different enzymes present. (For a recent brief review, see Pope, 1967.) Such studies have been made in man as well as in animals, and attempts have been made in this way to gain information on pathological processes in the cortex, for example in certain types of presenile dementia (see Pope, Hess, and Lewin, 1964). This field of research seems promising but is still in its beginning.

Studies of the chemical differences between minor parts of the cortex can be made with histochemical methods. More precise data can, however, be obtained by excising small cylinder-shaped vertical blocks from the cortex by biopsy or from autopsy material. The block is immediately frozen and subsequently serially sectioned. Alternate sections are used for cytoarchitectonic identifications and for microchemical determinations. The intracortical distribution of chemical constituents can then be related to cytoarchitecture.

The discovery that the cerebral cortex could be subdivided into structurally different areas highly influenced the views on the problem of cerebral localization. The adherents to the view that the cerebral cortex contains "centers" for different specific functions, found in this fact a solid foundation for their hypotheses concerning cerebral function. However, many facts are known which give clear evidence that a mutual interdependence exists between different areas. We will return later to this subject.

The total number of nerve cells in the human cerebral cortex is enormous. Several workers have made calculations of this figure, and values up to 14×10^9 (von Economo and Koskinas, 1925) have been reported. Most workers have not taken into consideration the shrinkage of the brain occurring during the histological procedures. Pakkenberg (1966), considering this, found a total number of 2.6×10^9 (2.6 billions) nerve cells in the brain of a young adult. The considerable variations in the numbers calculated by different authors may in part be due to technical factors. However, it does not seem unlikely that there may well be quite considerable individual variations among human brains in this respect.[1]

In recent years much valuable information has been obtained on the organization, structural and functional, of the neocortex. Before considering this subject it will be appropriate to review briefly some main features of the fiber connections of the cerebral cortex.

The fiber connections of the cerebral cortex. Many of these connections have been described in previous chapters. Here only some principal features will be summarized. The fiber connections of the cerebral cortex may be subdivided in a schematic way into four groups: (1) corticofugal or efferent projection fibers; (2) corticopetal or afferent

---

[1] It appears to be established that the number of cortical neurons decreases with advancing age. See Brody (1955) for particulars.

647

fibers; (3) association fibers, connecting different regions of the same hemisphere; and (4) commissural fibers, interconnecting the two hemispheres.

Among *corticofugal projection fiber systems,* in man one of the largest appears to be *the pyramidal tract.* Its fibers arise in various cortical areas but most of them in the pre- and postcentral gyrus (see Ch. 4). Other efferent fiber systems are *the corticopontine tracts,* likewise well developed in man (see Ch. 5). The topically arranged projection from rather extensive cortical areas to *the caudate nucleus* and *the putamen* as well as corticofugal fibers to *the red nucleus* and to *the reticular formation* have been considered in Chapter 4. Minor contingents end in *the dorsal column nuclei* (see Ch. 2), *the inferior olive* (see Ch. 5), *the substantia nigra,* and *the subthalamic nucleus* (see Ch. 4). Other corticofugal fibers, especially from the occipital lobe, pass to *the colliculi* and *the optic tectum.* Finally, mention should be made of the abundant topically organized *corticothalamic fibers.* These largely pass to the thalamic nucleus from which the cortical area emitting them receives its thalamic afferents. When analyzing the various efferent fiber systems it becomes apparent that a considerable number of the long corticofugal fibers take origin from the central region (areas 4, 3, 1, 2, and, in part, 6).[2] It is further to be noticed that there are relatively few subcortical gray masses (for example the pallidum and the vestibular nuclei) which do not receive projections from the cortex. This reflects the importance of the cortical influence on a number of functions (including the central transmission of sensory impulses, see Ch. 2).

In a corresponding manner *afferent fibers* appear to reach extensive regions of the neocortex. Most, if not all, of these fibers are derived from *the thalamus.* (The presence of direct cortical afferents from some other regions, such as the hypothalamus and the reticular formation, is disputed.) In general the thalamocortical projections are topically organized, a particular cortical area receiving its fibers from a particular subdivision of the thalamus, as described in Chapter 2. To the thalamocortical projection belong also the cortical projections from *the lateral and medial geniculate bodies* (Chs. 8 and 9, respectively).

According to classical teaching the final links of the great sensory pathways (somatosensory, optic, and acoustic) end in cortical areas of the granular type (areas 3, 1 and 2, 17 and 41, respectively). However, as has been described in Chapters 2, 8, and 9, these projections are not restricted to granular cortex (type 5 in Fig. 12-3) only. For example, the lateral geniculate body sends fibers to areas 17, 18, and 19, and the

---

[2] It is not known to what extent different cells give rise to fibers passing to the various destinations listed. Certainly many fibers passing to a more distant place give off collaterals to nuclei situated along their course.

thalamic nuclei receiving the somatosensory pathways project not only onto areas 3, 1, and 2, but to agranular cortex in front of the central sulcus as well. In spite of this the proportion of the total cortex receiving sensory information fairly directly from various kinds of receptors is rather restricted. Other cortical regions can be outlined as the projection areas of thalamic nuclei which receive more or less well defined afferent connections (for example the VL from the cerebellum, the VA from the pallidum, the anterior thalamic nucleus from the mammillary body, the MD from the amygdaloid nucleus). As to other thalamic nuclei projecting onto the cortex, especially the pulvinar and the lateral nucleus (LP and LD, see Fig. 2-11), their afferents are little known. The cortical projection areas of such nuclei, covering chiefly parts of the temporal and parietal cortex, were formerly often included among the so-called *cortical association areas,* on the assumption that they are less influenced from other regions of the nervous system than the other parts of the cortex. These areas, as well as the thalamic nuclei projecting onto parts of them, increase in phylogenesis and are particularly well developed in man. Their main task was considered to be the association and integration of impulses reaching other parts of the cortex from various subcortical stations. Accordingly, they were assumed to be involved chiefly in more complex functions, not least in processes related to mental activity. While this view still seems to be generally valid, it has become apparent that in the highest integrative processes occurring in the brain the cortex collaborates in a complex way with a number of subcortical structures as well as with regions belonging to the archi- and paleocortex (for example the thalamus, the hippocampus, the amygdaloid nucleus) as must indeed be concluded from the extensive fiber connections interrelating the cortex and these regions. Integration of impulses from various sources occurs also in subcortical regions. The superior colliculus, for example, receives optic fibers, fibers from the visual and other areas of the cortex, fibers belonging to the somatosensory system, and probably some fibers of the acoustic pathways (see Garey, Jones, and Powell, 1968, for particulars).

A correlation of the activity of different cortical areas may occur by way of the *association fibers*. Such fibers are present in large numbers in the cerebral cortex. Some of the association fibers are very short and pass entirely within the gray matter of the cortex. Others are somewhat longer and course in the white matter from one gyrus to another. Finally there are some longer fibers, making up bundles which appear to interconnect more distant regions of a hemisphere. These bundles were in part identified by the old anatomists by dissection, but it is doubtful whether all fibers in some of these bundles are really association fibers and long ones. Presumably the fibers in a bundle may differ with regard to their sites of origin and terminations.[3] Experimental studies are necessary to trace the cortical association fibers.

It is becoming more and more obvious that in spite of their ubiquitous occurrence, the association fibers are arranged in an orderly manner, presumably yielding evidence of the more or less close functional relationship between various areas. Grossly speaking, it appears that those areas which have the closest functional interrelations are most closely linked by association fibers, as appeared from early studies with the Marchi method (Polyak, 1927b; Mettler, 1935; Jansen, 1937). Thus the bulk of association fibers from area 6 goes to area 4. Area 4 appears to be particularly well provided with incoming association fibers.

In recent years the association fibers have been studied in more detail with the use of silver impregnation methods, especially the fibers interconnecting the visual areas 17, 18, and 19 (described in Ch. 8) and association fibers of the somatosensory areas (see Ch. 2 and especially Jones and Powell, 1968a). *Long association fibers* have been traced from the peristriate regions to the inferior convexity of the temporal lobe (see Kuypers et al., 1965) and from the frontal to the temporal lobe (see Nauta, 1964). Information has also been obtained from physiological studies in which the strychnine method of Dusser de Barenne [4] has been used (see for example, McCulloch, 1944). The recent studies on the visual and somatosensory areas strongly indicate that in general the different areas have their specific patterns of associational pathways. Much remains to be done in this field. Investigations of the cortical associational fibers require the utmost care and precision in placing the small lesions which are needed as well as in determining the sites of termination of the degenerating fibers.

The commissural connections between the two cerebral hemispheres are extensive. The vast majority of these fibers pass in the corpus callosum (Fig. 10-3), others in the hippocampal commissure and the anterior commissure. Those in the hippocampal commissure appear to be derived

[3] It is customary to distinguish several long bundles. One is the cingulum, passing in the cingulate gyrus and mentioned in Chapter 10. The superior longitudinal fasciculus passes from the frontal to the occipital region; the inferior longitudinal fasciculus passes from the occipital lobe to the temporal pole; the uncinate fasciculus connects the temporal and frontal lobes. Other bundles have been described as well.

[4] A small amount of strychnine is placed in or on a nervous structure. The strychnine blocks postsynaptic inhibition and thus enhances the activity of the nerve cells (it acts only where synapses are present), and this activity is evidenced electrically by the appearance of large potential changes, usually termed "strychnine spikes" at the sites where the axons of the excited cells end. The name "physiological neuronography" has been applied to this method. However, the assumption that strychnine-evoked potentials never traverse a synapse requires some qualifications.

only from the paleo- and allocortex, as described in Chapter 10. Such fibers also utilize the anterior commissure, but this in addition carries (in its posterior limb) a fair number of commissural fibers from the temporal neocortex in the rat (Brodal, 1948) and probably in the monkey (Akert et al., 1961). (The massa intermedia, which may be absent, contains interthalamic fibers.)

The corpus callosum develops in proportion to the neocortex and reaches its greatest development in man.[5] Almost all information on the course of its fibers comes from animal studies. It appears that even if the majority of its fibers interconnect homotopic regions in the two hemispheres, there are also heterotopic connections. The callosal connections have so far been most precisely determined for the visual areas and the somatosensory areas as described in Chapters 8 and 2, respectively. Some areas of the neocortex do not receive commissural fibers, for example area 17, and the hand and foot regions of the somatosensory cortex. The total distribution of commissural fibers has been studied recently by Ebner and Myers (1965) in the cat and the racoon. Largely corresponding findings have been made in the monkey, as seen from Fig. 12-4, which shows that there are clear regional variations with

[5] The development of the cerebral commissures has been studied by a number of authors, most recently by Rakic and Yakovlev (1968). The number of callosal fibers is enormous. In the cat each square millimeter contains some 700,000 fibers (Myers, 1959). Not all fibers are commissural, however. Some pass to the striatum and other destinations.

FIG. 12–4 The dotted areas show the regions of the left hemispheres of the monkey receiving commissural fibers from the opposite hemisphere. Note that the striate area in the occipital cortex and the hand region of the first somatosensory area in the postcentral gyrus are free from commissural connections. From Myers (1965).

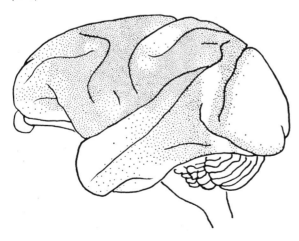

regard to the distribution of commissural afferents. In general, anatomical and physiological studies have given concordant results concerning the distribution pattern of callosal fibers (see Heimer, Ebner, and Nauta, 1967, for references), but there are still lacunae in our knowledge. The problem of the topography of callosal connections has aroused renewed interest in recent years on account of new views on the function of the corpus callosum (see below). The very specific patterns in these connections are well illustrated by the findings of Jones and Powell (1968b) in their study of the commissural connections of the somatosensory areas S I and S II.

Intrinsic organization and synaptology of the cerebral cortex. When attempting to arrive at an understanding of the function of the cerebral cortex, we must avoid the pitfall of regarding the cortex cerebri simply as a two-dimensional sheet of mutually interconnected, structurally different areas. It would indeed be strange if the lamination, the regular arrangement of the cells in layers (varying in details from area to area), should have no functional meaning. What is, for example, the functional reason for the extraordinary development of granule cells and granular layers in the areas receiving the "direct" sensory systems? Why are the "effector regions," to employ a somewhat unprecise designation, particularly rich in large pyramidal cells? The conclusion was drawn quite early by investigators in this field, that there must be some correlation between "sensory" function and the development of the granular layers, between "motor" function and pyramidal layers, particularly the Vth layer. Evidence of several kinds has been brought forward to confirm this. Nissl in 1908 demonstrated in the rabbit that if the connections of the cerebral cortex with deeper structures are interrupted soon after birth, the deeper cortical layers ultimately become profoundly atrophied (the efferent fibers being cut) but the superficial layers continue to develop almost normally. The so-called "laminar thermocoagulation" introduced by Dusser de Barenne has given supporting results. By applying a heated metal surface onto the cortex, a varying deleterious effect on the cortex can be achieved by altering the temperature and the duration of application. In this way it was shown that thermocoagulation of the three superficial layers of the motor cortex does not interfere with its capacity to react to electrical stimulation. If, however, the Vth layer is also destroyed, the cortex loses this capacity. These and other findings led to the statement that the outer layers of the cortex, layers I to IV, have predominantly receptive and associative functions, whereas the effector functions of the cortex are taken care of by the deeper layers V and VI. This statement could be no more than a rough approximation as long as the details concerning the course and ramifications of the axons and dendrites within the cerebral cortex were not completely known. A clari-

652

fication of these features and the so-called *synaptology* requires minute studies by means of different methods. Lorente de Nó (1949) attacked these problems in systematic investigations with the Golgi method, supplementing and extending the now classical work of Cajal in this field. A summary of his results serves as a useful basis for the presentation of more recent data on the subject.[6]

According to the behavior of their axons, Lorente de Nó distinguishes between four fundamental types of nerve cells in the cerebral cortex (cf. Fig. 12-5). One type sends its axon toward the white matter where it eventually continues as a projection fiber to deeper structures (1-5 in Fig. 12-5). Another type has only a very short axon, which arborizes in the immediate vicinity of the perikaryon (8, 9, 10 in Fig. 12-5). A third type of cell sends its axon toward the surface, and the axon and its collaterals are distributed to one or more cortical layers (11 in Fig. 12-5). The last type consists of cells with axons taking a horizontal course (12 in Fig. 12-5). The nervous impulses to the cortical cells are derived from axons and collaterals of cells in the thalamus, partly from cells situated in other parts of the cortex on the same side (association fibers), or from the contralateral side (commissural fibers), and finally also from cortical cells in the immediate vicinity.

Fig. 12-5 represents some of the principal features in the intracortical arrangement of axons and dendrites in a very simplified fashion. Only a few of the numerous dendrites and collaterals of each cell are included in order to simplify the picture. On the extreme left in the figure are seen afferent fibers entering the cortex. According to Lorente de Nó the bulk of the fibers from the thalamus, forming part of the direct sensory pathways, end with huge plexuses of terminal ramifications in the internal granular lamina, lamina IV (fibers a and b in Fig. 12-5). These "specific afferent fibers," as is seen, do not give off collaterals in their passage through the deeper layers. Other thalamocortical fibers behave as represented by the fiber c in the figure. They can be followed to the molecular lamina I and send some collaterals to several layers. Afferents of this type are often called "nonspecific" (cf. Ch. 2). In a similar manner association fibers from other cortical areas pass through all layers, but most of their collaterals are found ending on cells in the upper four layers, particularly layers II and III (d in Fig. 12-5).

Among cells sending their axons out of the gray matter of the cortex, some give origin to projection fibers traveling to remote nuclear masses, for example in the pyramidal tract. This holds true particularly of the cells in the Vth layer (1 in Fig. 12-5). The axons of other cells course as association fibers to other cortical areas in the same hemisphere, or as

[6] The studies of Lorente de Nó do not include the frontal lobe. Presumably, however, conditions are similar to those found in the other three lobes.

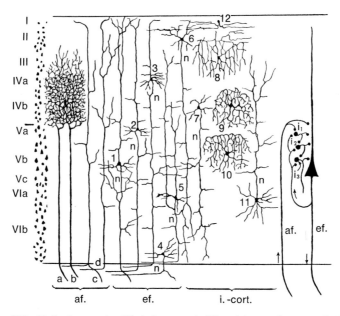

FIG. 12–5 A very simplified diagram of different types of neurons in the cerebral cortex, with axons, dendrites, and collaterals. *af.:* axons of afferent fibers; *a, b,* and *c:* fibers from the thalamus, *d:* association fibers; *ef.:* neurons sending their axons out of the cortex, from the cell labeled 1 as a projection fiber, from cells 2–5 as association fibers; *i.-cort.:* cells whose axons arborize intracortically, those of cells 6 and 7 in the deeper layers, of cells 8 to 10 mainly in their own layer, cell 11 with its axon to more superficial layers and cell 12 with a horizontal course of the axon. Cf. text. To the right a simplified diagram of the passage of impulses within the cortex. *af.* and *ef.:* afferent and efferent fibers; i_1, i_2, and i_3: intercalated neurons. Redrawn and simplified from diagrams of Lorente de Nó (1949).

commissural fibers to the opposite hemisphere (2-5 in Fig. 12-5). Cells of this type are found particularly in layers III, V, and VI. It will be seen from the figure that the axons of all the latter cells have numerous collaterals which are given off during their course in the cortex and thus must be able to influence the nerve cells in the deeper layers through which the axons pass. The fiber plexuses of the Vth layer are, to a considerable extent, composed of collaterals from these efferent axons. Some of the cells in the deeper layers in addition send recurrent collaterals to the more superficial layers of the cortex (cell 5 in Fig. 12-5). The "effector" cells of layers V and VI will therefore be able to influence cells in more superficial layers.

Within all layers of the cortex there are cells whose axons and collaterals are only distributed within the cortex itself. Particularly abundant are cells of the second type of Golgi, often called stellate cells, (cells 8, 9, 10 in Fig. 12-5). The axon arborizes extensively in the close vicinity of the perikaryon. All layers in addition contain cells (labeled 11 in Fig. 12-5) whose axons are directed toward the surface, where they are distributed to one or, more frequently, several layers. This implies that when cells in the deeper layers of the cortex are brought into action, they will be able to send impulses toward the surface, to the more superficial layers. Intracortical neurons with horizontal axons dominate in layer I (12 in Fig. 12-5).

It appears from these investigations that the afferent impulses to the cerebral cortex are, roughly speaking, distributed first and foremost to the superficial cortical layers. Particularly the IVth layer seems to be the terminal station for the direct sensory projection systems (the systems of the medial lemniscus, the spinothalamic tracts, and the brachium conjunctivum, optic, and acoustic systems). The other thalamocortical fibers and the incoming association fibers, on the other hand, exert their effect not only on the superficial layers but also on the deep ones. The findings support the idea that the deeper layers, particularly the Vth, are the most important sources of the efferent projection. The association fibers likewise spring predominantly, although not exclusively, from the two deepest layers.

It is, however, equally clear from these investigations that functionally the deeper layers cannot be regarded as effector, the superficial as receptor, without qualifications. This is evidenced by the large number and variety of cells whose fibers arborize entirely within the cortex itself, some of which are provided with ascending axons, others with descending axons (6 and 7 in Fig. 12-5), whereas others are endowed with amply arborizing axons within their own layer. Every impulse reaching the cerebral cortex, by influencing these intracortical neurons, will be able to act upon cells in all cortical layers. Another feature contributing to this is the collaterals given off by the efferent neurons themselves.

An extremely simple path of a nervous impulse reaching the cortex may be imagined to be as shown in the diagram to the extreme right of Fig. 12-5. The afferent impulse entering through the fiber labeled af. is transmitted not only to an effector cell, sending its axon for example in the pyramidal tract, but will also reach the intracortical neuron i_1. The latter cell when discharging will not only be able to add another stimulus to the effector cell, but will also act on another association cell i_2, which in turn excites a third cell i_3, both the latter in turn influencing the effector cell. Finally the activity of these intercalated neurons will be influenced by the discharge of the effector cell through its recurrent collaterals.

A closer scrutiny of the mutual arrangement of the nerve cells in the cortex and the distribution of their dendrites, axons, and collaterals,

655

makes it clear that there must be almost unlimited possibilities for variations in the impulse transmissions within the cortical gray matter. The interplay between excitatory and inhibitory influences on the individual cells will play a decisive role in the route taken by the impulses. Much work has been devoted to obtaining information on how the cerebral cortex performs its function, but this is an extremely difficult problem to solve. It has been approached from several angles, but so far only some rather general hypotheses have been formulated.

Actual *recording of the activity of cortical nerve cells* has become possible by the use of microelectrodes, and a number of such investigations have been made since the 1950's (for reviews see Amassian, 1961; Eccles, 1966b; Creutzfeldt, Lux, and Watanabe, 1966). One of the limitations of this method is that it can so far only be used for large cells. Another is that the cells studied can be identified only in instances where they can be activated antidromically by stimulation of their axons. This requires that the axons be stimulated separately, a condition fulfilled almost only by the corticospinal fibers (by stimulation of the pyramid). Most of the studies of this kind have therefore been made on the Betz cells contributing to the corticospinal tract. With regard to their functional properties these cells appear in most respects to resemble the motoneurons of the spinal cord. The influence of afferent impulses on such cells has been investigated. Certain differences in their reaction to stimulation, for example, of "specific" and "nonspecific" thalamic nuclei, have been observed, but the interpretation of the potential changes is made difficult on account of our incomplete knowledge of the exact sites of termination and synaptic relations of the "specific" and "nonspecific" fibers, respectively. (In addition, as has been described in Ch. 2, there is no clear relation between "specific" and "nonspecific" afferents and "specific" and "nonspecific" thalamic nuclei.) Whether some of the purely intracortical neurons are inhibitory appears to be disputed. The contribution of the potentials occurring in single cells to the composite changes recorded in the electroencephalogram (EEG) is still a disputed question.[7]

In most of the studies alluded to above electrical stimulation of afferents has been used. In studies where discrete natural stimuli are used some information of interest concerning the organization of the cortex has been obtained. The observations of Mountcastle and his collaborators on single units in the first somatosensory area (see Ch. 2) and of Hubel and Wiesel on units in the visual areas (see Ch. 8) point to the existence of a *columnar functional organization in the cortex* as do also findings in the "motor" cortex (see Ch. 4). In cell-stained sections cut perpendicularly to the surface of the cortex a columnar arrangement of the cells is

[7] This subject will not be discussed here. The recording and interpretation of the EEG has developed into a particular branch of neurology which requires special training and insight also in general electrophysiology. Apart from the use of EEG as a tool in the diagnosis and prognosis of diseases of the nervous system, the study of the EEG under various conditions has given valuable information on questions of basic neurophysiological interest.

easily seen in most cortical regions (see Fig. 8-7a and 8-7c). Since the afferent and efferent cortical fibers are to a large extent arranged in radially running bundles (Fig. 12-1, right column), the columnar organization of the cortical nerve cells might be simply a consequence of this fiber arrangement. This, however, is not the only reason. As mentioned above, many of the cortical nerve cells extend their dendrites and give off axons preferentially perpendicular to the surface (Fig. 12-5). Colonnier (1966, 1967) has drawn attention to the frequent occurrence of a particular type of intracortical neuron, described by Cajal (1909–11) and named *"cellule fusiforme à double bouquet dendritique."* This cell (not shown in Fig. 12-5) gives off two dense bunches of dendrites, one extending toward the surface, the other toward the depth. The thin axons of these cells, present in layers II, III, and IV, pass vertically in either direction, give off a number of short, fine collaterals, and may extend throughout all layers of the cortex. Their number is considerable, especially in man. By studying Golgi sections cut parallel to the cortical surface, Colonnier (1964, 1966, 1967) further found the lateral distribution of the dendrites of most cortical nerve cells to be rather restricted. Except for the cells in layer I (12 in Fig. 12-5) there is only one other type of cell whose axon spreads in the tangential direction. This is found in layers III and IV and has been likened to the basket cells in the cerebellum (Fig. 5-3) and in the hippocampus (Fig. 10-4). It appears from these observations that *there is a structural basis for a functional columnar organization within the cortex,* since there are particularly close interconnections in the radial direction between the nerve cells of different layers. Interaction between different columns may occur by way of cells with tangentially oriented axons and dendrites as well as by axons passing to the white matter and entering neighboring regions.[8] On the basis of such findings some ideas about the "working machinery" of the neocortex may be formulated, but they must remain very generalized until much more is known of the details in the anatomical organization, such as the synaptic relations between the various elements and the precise distribution of axons of intrinsic cells and of afferent fibers. Some observations on these subjects have been forthcoming in recent years.

On the basis of studies of silver-impregnated sections it has been doubted whether there are true terminal boutons in the neocortex, since such structures were seen only occasionally. Improved methods have made it possible to clarify many points in the *synaptology of the cerebral cortex* and have demonstrated that synaptic contacts in the cortex as elsewhere are established by means of terminal boutons. In electron

[8] Physiological evidence for an horizontal correlation between columns in the striate area has recently been presented by Hubel and Wiesel (1968).

microscope studies, Gray (1959) found axosomatic as well as axodendritic synapses on cortical cells. This has been shown also by means of the method of Armstrong, Richardson, and Young (1956) for staining of boutons (Colonnier, 1967). There are differences in the size, density, and distribution of boutons in the different layers and between cytoarchitectonic areas. The number of synapses is enormous. Cragg (1967) in an electron microscope study estimated the numbers of neurons and the numbers of synaptic contacts in the motor and striate areas in the mouse and the monkey. In the motor area he found on an average 60,000 synapses per neuron in the monkey, 13,000 in the mouse; in the striate area the figures were 5,600 and 7,000, respectively, for the two species.[9] Even if it is likely that one afferent fiber establishes synaptic contact with a particular cell by means of several boutons (see also below), these figures make it clear that a single cell must be subject to the influence of numerous others. Using rather conservative estimates Cragg (1967) figures that some 600 *intracortical* neurons may contact a cell in the motor cortex of the monkey, 65 in the striate area. Another indication of the multitude of possible interconnections is found in the Golgi studies of the motor and striate area in the cat (Sholl, 1953) since the dendrites of one stellate cell extend over an area which contains 2,000 to 4,000 perikarya. Conversely, the branches of one afferent fiber encompass a territory which may contain 5,000 neurons (see Sholl, 1956).[10]

These figures give an impression of the wealth of possible interconnections in the cortex, but more specific information is needed. Some has been obtained in Golgi, electron microscopic, and experimental studies. As to the afferents to the cortex it appears to be generally agreed that the type called "specific" (fibers *a* and *b* in Fig. 12-5) supply mainly layer IV with some branches to layer III (see Colonnier, 1967), while association fibers extend to all layers (*d* in Fig. 12-5). The dendrites of cortical nerve cells are amply provided with spines (formerly often thought to be artifacts, see Ch. 1). This is the case for the apical dendrites of the pyramidal cells. The number of spines increases exponentially with the distance from the cell body (Valverde, 1967). Running

---

[9] The marked increase in the number of synapses in the motor cortex when passing from the mouse to the monkey is correlated with a reduction in neuronal density. The neuronal density is even less in man than in the monkey (see Sholl, 1956; Cragg, 1967), indicating that still more of the space is taken up by axonal and dendritic branches.

[10] On the basis of an extensive material Sholl (1956) studied in addition other quantitative aspects of cortical cells in the cat. Applying statistical methods in the evaluation of the observations and probability theory in the formulation of their interpretation Sholl suggested certain principles of organization of the cortex, with particular reference to problems concerning processes of learning and memory.

along the apical dendrites there are fine axons which in Golgi sections appear to make series of synaptic contacts with the spines of the dendrite along its course. This has been described also in the human brain (Marin-Padilla, 1968). These "climbing fibers" have been held to belong to collaterals of pyramidal cells, commissural afferents, association fibers from other cortical areas, and from intracortical cells in the vicinity.

It has been observed that the spines on the apical dendrites of the pyramidal cells are reduced in number in mice which have been reared in complete darkness since birth (Valverde, 1967) and in rabbits (Globus and Scheibel, 1967a) and mice (Valverde, 1968) after eye enucleation or lesions of the lateral geniculate body. The lack of visual stimuli, normally transmitted to the striate area, thus produces morphological changes in its cells (as is known from previous studies). The disappearance of the spines on the central parts of the apical dendrites might indicate that the thin axons contacting the apical dendrites are fibers from the geniculate body, which terminate in layer IV and, in part, in III. However, following enucleation, there are also specific variations in the orientation of the dendrites of stellate cells in layer IV (Valverde, 1968). The changes in the spines of the pyramidal cells may therefore be secondary.

Following transection of the corpus callosum in rabbits at birth, Globus and Scheibel (1967b) found loss of about one third of the spines on the oblique branches only of the apical dendrites of the pyramidal cells in the parietal cortex. This suggests that callosal afferents are distributed to these regions (i.e. laminae IV and III). Authors using the Nauta method (see for example Ebner and Myers, 1965) found a somewhat more extensive distribution of callosal fibers (chiefly to laminae VI to IV), while Heimer, Ebner, and Nauta (1967), using the silver impregnation method of Fink and Heimer (1967), conclude that callosal afferents supply all layers.

There are thus still open questions concerning the precise synaptic relations of thalamic and callosal afferents to the cortex. Even more difficult is it to obtain information on the synaptic relations of the numerous intracortical neurons.

Attempts to elucidate the terminations of intracortical cells have been made by studying the structure in pieces of cortex which have been isolated from the underlying white matter for a longer period, so that afferent endings will have degenerated. The undercutting of the cortex may also be made between layers. From light and electron microscope studies of this kind Szentágothai (1965b) concludes that the tangential fibers in layer I are mainly derived from cells in the deeper layers, as has been concluded also from Golgi studies. The axons of intracortical cells appear to end mainly on the perikarya, and to take part in the pericellular baskets found around the perikarya of the pyramidal cells (see also Colonnier, 1967). The recurrent collaterals of the latter cells appear to establish mainly axodendritic contacts.

Many questions concerning the synaptic relationships in the cerebral cortex are still unanswered. The relatively scanty data available suggests that terminals of different kinds of fibers, extracortical and intracortical, may differ with regard to the cells with which they establish synaptic contact, and that axons from different sources may contact different regions of, for example, the pyramidal cells (apical dendrite, side branches of this, perikaryon, etc.). As described in Chapter 10, a situation of this kind is found in the hippocampus, and may probably be an illustration of a general principle, which is valid also for the neocortex. The analogy may not be complete, however.

It seems precocious to conclude that the axons "climbing" along the apical dendrites of the pyramidal cell in the neocortex are excitatory because the synapses on the apical dendrites of hippocampal pyramids and Purkinje cells appear to be of this kind, and to consider the tangentially oriented "basket" cells in layers II and IV as inhibitory because they morphologically resemble the presumably inhibitory basket cells in the hippocampus and cerebellar cortex. Hypothetical schemes of the neuronal arrangement and the synaptic mechanisms in the neocortex, based upon the assumptions metioned above, have been set forth (see Colonnier, 1966; Eccles, 1966b). Other authors maintain that it is not necessary to postulate the presence of inhibitory neurons in the cerebral cortex to explain the electrophysiological observations (see Creutzfeldt, Lux, and Watanabe, 1966). In view of the very complex structural arrangement of the neocortex and the limited possibilities of studying particular kinds of cells electrophysiologically, all hypotheses to explain the functional arrangements in the cortex should be taken with a grain of salt.

The cerebral cortex in phylogenesis. The higher an animal is in the phylogenetic scale, the more elaborate the transmission of nervous impulses in the cortex appears to be. The percentage of association cells, and particularly of intracortical neurons, increases markedly during phylogenesis. In man such cells make up a considerable part of the entire cell content of the cerebral cortex (Lorente de Nó). The cerebral cortex in mammals presents an increasing degree of cytoarchitectural and myeloarchitectural differentiation in phylogenesis. Although some of the more elementary areas can be recognized to be fairly uniform throughout the mammalian scale, for example the area striata, there can be little doubt that in the higher mammals a progressive differentiation of many areas has taken place. In the anthropoid apes and man, areas have been recognized which are missing in lower mammals. Particularly those areas of the cortex which are presumed to function as "association areas" show a progressive development in man. The parietal and temporal lobes appear to be particularly rich in areas of this type.[11] On the other hand, the areas giving rise to or receiving projection fibers do not increase

[11] In this connection some findings on the ontogenetical development of the human cortex are of interest. Conel (1939) has shown that in newborn children area 4 is the area which has progressed farthest in differentiation. Least developed are the areas in the anterior part of the frontal lobe. The terminal areas of the large sensory projection systems are also rather well differentiated at birth. For some further data on cortical ontogenesis see Holloway (1968).

correspondingly, and therefore occupy a *relatively* smaller part of the entire cerebral surface. Various aspects of cortical evolution have been critically reviewed by Holloway (1968).

Functions of the cerebral cortex. On account of the elaborate differentiation of the cerebral cortex in phylogenesis physiological experiments in animals can only to a certain extent give information concerning the function of the cortex in man. In general the results of experimental studies are in fairly good accord with observations in man, if allowance is made for the different development of the structures in question. Examples of this have been mentioned repeatedly in preceding chapters when discussing the results of stimulation or destruction of several cortical areas, especially of the sensorimotor, the visual and the acoustic areas. As far as these and some other cortical areas are concerned it seems reasonable to conclude that they are related predominantly to particular functions.[12] On the whole the cortical regions delimited by physiological methods as functionally different fields coincide fairly well with certain cytoarchitectural areas, even if the old notions that the area striata alone represents the visual cortex, areas 41 (and 42?) the acoustic cortex, areas 3, 1, and 2 the somesthetic cortex, and area 4 the cortical motor area are no longer tenable. These questions have been considered in Chapters 8, 9, 2, and 4, respectively, to which the reader is referred.

Even if the regions of the cortex related more specifically to fairly well defined and relatively elementary functions occupy a much greater part of the entire neocortex than previously assumed, extensive cortical regions are left. The functions of these regions appear to be more complex than those of the other areas and are difficult to investigate, especially since they are related to processes which in a loose manner may be characterized as "mental" (of various complexities) and which can, therefore, be properly studied only in man. (Many of these faculties are probably almost specific for man.) The functional observations concerning these parts of the neocortex will be considered briefly here, since they can be correlated with our present-day anatomical knowledge only to a very limited extent. To a certain degree it is possible to indicate certain regions of the cortex as related to particular, although rather complex functions. Following a consideration of the frontal lobes we will turn to the regions related to language and other so-called "psychosomatic" functions, and finally discuss some recent observations on the corpus callosum.

The frontal lobe. This is generally said to undergo an extensive differentiation in monkeys and particularly in man. This assumption may,

---

[12] The term function is here used in a purely colloquial manner. See also the last section of this chapter.

however, be questioned (see Holloway, 1968). It has been generally assumed that the frontal lobe must be concerned in some of the higher mental functions. Animal experiments as well as clinical findings have given some information about functions which appear to be dependent on intact frontal lobes, or more specifically the so-called *prefrontal areas,* a (somewhat unfortunate) term applied to the part of the frontal lobe which is situated in front of areas 4, 6, and 8. Stimulation of these areas yields no motor responses. The functional aspects of the posterior parts of the frontal lobe, areas 4, 6, and 8, have been considered elsewhere (Chs. 4 and 7, respectively).

All experimenters agree that unilateral removal of the anterior areas of the frontal lobe produces little or no change while bilateral ablations are followed by characteristic symptoms. In monkeys the most conspicuous feature is a "hyperactivity," which is betrayed by the restless walking of the animal in its cage (Kennard, Spencer, and Fountain, Jr., 1941; and others).

Ruch and Shenkin (1943) concluded that ablation of the posterior orbital cortex is responsible for the motor hyperactivity. In chimpanzees, Jacobsen and collaborators (1935, and later) in addition observed an increased distractibility, weakened memory, and a reduced capacity for solving problems (as, for example, when they have to connect together several sticks in order to reach a piece of food). It has been suggested that the hyperactivity represents a release phenomenon, due to removal of a normally present inhibitory influence on motor activity by this part of the cortex (see Kaada, 1951, 1960).

On stimulation of the posterior orbital cortex a series of responses have been observed in cats and monkeys, such as inhibition of spontaneous and cortically and reflexly induced movements and inhibition or acceleration of respiratory movements, autonomic responses from the cardiovascular and digestive systems, and emotional reactions in the form of "arrest reaction," "attention" or "arousal" (see Kaada, 1960, for a review). As mentioned in Chapter 10 the posterior orbital cortex is usually included as part of the morphological basis of the "limbic system." Largely similar symptoms have been observed following stimulation of the anterior part of the cingulate gyrus (containing area 24), likewise generally considered as part of the "limbic system" (see Kaada, 1951, 1960). Bilateral ablation of the anterior cingulate cortex has been reported by several authors to result in an increased tameness and "social indifference" (Smith, 1944b; Ward, 1948; Glees, Cole, Whitty, and Cairns, 1950; and others). Other authors have found that the operation may result in a temporary increase in aggressiveness (Mirsky, Rosvold, and Pribram, 1957). Some authors noted some hyperactivity. The data mentioned above suggests that even if the posterior orbital cortex and the anterior cingulate cortex in many respects are functionally rather similar, they are not identical. In recent years several authors have undertaken extensive behavioral studies with complex tests of monkeys subjected to ablations of the anterior frontal areas (and in human patients) (for some reports see "The Frontal Granular Cortex and Behavior," 1964). On the whole it appears that little is so far definitely known. Among the views set forth on the basis of these recent studies may be mentioned that the hyperactivity described by previous students may be a hyperreactivity rather than hyperactivity. Special deficits have been noted in tasks which require a rapid shift from one way of solving a problem to another.

In man several symptoms have long been recognized as being to a certain extent characteristic of lesions of the frontal lobe (the motor symptoms, including forced grasping, have been described in Ch. 4 and are due to lesions of the precentral and supplementary motor cortical areas). Most authors hold that also in man the lesion must be bilateral if the symptoms are to become distinct. However, Rylander (1939) in a study of the symptoms following unilateral partial ablations of the frontal lobe in thirty-two patients, found distinct postoperative changes in all these cases.

The symptoms most commonly described as following bilateral damage to or removal of the prefrontal areas in man are frequently grouped under two headings: reduction of intellectual ability and of ethical standards. The patients present signs of complacency and self-satisfaction, and frequently also of boastfulness. Their powers of concentration, their initiative, and their endurance are reduced, and they are more distractible than normal. Often they are in high spirits, in a somewhat puerile manner. Memory for recent events suffers, and their capacity of solving problems requiring intellectual effort is reduced, particularly as regards abstract problems. Their power of judging their own situation is impaired, and the patient's horizon is narrowed to the present and his own person. In syphilitic general paresis, where conspicuous anatomical changes are usually found in the cortex of the frontal lobe, and also in cases of *Pick's disease* with the same localization, similar symptoms are frequent.

Additional information concerning the functions of the prefrontal areas in man has been obtained from cases where a *frontal lobotomy* or a *prefrontal leucotomy* has been performed on patients suffering from mental disorders. Introduced by Egaz Moniz in 1936, this operation was for some years much used. The principle of the operation is to cut the fiber connections of the frontal "association areas." This is done by inserting an instrument through a burr hole and moving it in a coronal plane. Some surgeons preferred to make an open leucotomy, i.e. with the frontal lobe exposed by a craniotomy. As a rule these operations were performed bilaterally. Although they were made on patients suffering from one sort or another of mental disorder (schizophrenia, obsessions, etc.), the postoperative changes occurring in behavior and mind following a prefrontal leucotomy closely resembled those observed in cases of diseases of the frontal lobe. Most prominent appeared to be changes in the emotional sphere, whereas there was some dispute as to whether purely intellectual functions suffer. However, the patient's capacity of judging the future consequences of his actions was as a rule reduced.

After the introduction of the potent so-called *psychopharmaca* in the treatment of mental illness, prefrontal leucotomies are only rarely performed. However, studies of the many patients subjected to this operation gave rise to a number of publications, and some valuable information on the function of certain parts of the brain was obtained. Some of this data may be mentioned. Particularly the clear-cut influence of leucotomy on the emotional sphere attracted much interest. Freeman and Watts (1942) and others drew attention to the fact that delusions or obsessive ideas frequently do not disappear after operation, but they do not disturb the patient any more. Still more striking was the observation (see Freeman and Watts, 1946) that patients who have been subjected to leucotomy on account of unbearable pain of somatic origin are not troubled by the pain, even if it is present.

Attempts were soon made to find out whether less drastic surgical procedures than the classical leucotomy could be employed.[13] Attention was focused on two regions, the cingulate gyrus and the orbitofrontal cortex with their connections, in part on the basis of the observations in animals mentioned above. A question of special importance was whether a *selective orbital leucotomy* or a *cingulotomy* (or *cingulectomy,* ablation of the anterior part of area 24 in the cingulate gyrus) would prove to be most effective in the treatment of special types of mental

---

[13] The fortuitous nature of the anatomical effects of leucotomy was convincingly demonstrated by Meyer and Beck (1945) in a study of nine brains from patients subjected to leucotomy. The place of the section in the brain varied greatly. This is to be expected in view of the considerable individual variations which exist within human brains and in addition between the brain and the surface markings of the skull which have to be relied upon when a leucotomy is performed. Furthermore, it was evident that the depth and localization of the section also varied, even if the same technique was employed. Still more important, perhaps, is the fact that extensive secondary changes were found in certain of the cases, such as large cysts, probably due to intracerebral bleedings. Secondary changes (for example, bleedings) may be found far from the place of the cut.

disturbances. Definite answers to this question have scarcely yet been given, even if favorable results have been reported following both kinds of operation.[14] Lewin (1961), reviewing the results of cingulectomies and selective orbital leucotomies in more than one hundred patients, found that some mild personality changes occur following both kinds of operation. From his material it appears that operations of the orbital cortex are to be preferred for symptoms of anxiety and depression, while cingulectomy is likely to be of greater benefit for obsessional disorders. Reduction of intellectual function was not seen following orbital leucotomy in Lewin's material. It appears that "the more the superolateral surface of the frontal lobe is involved the greater the chance of intellectual deficit" (Lewin, 1961, p. 44).

A number of difficulties are met with in attempts to evaluate and correlate the psychological, neurological, and anatomical effects of leucotomies (for a thorough treatment of these subjects see the monograph *Selective Partial Ablation of the Frontal Cortex,* 1949). It is scarcely surprising, therefore, that it has not been possible to relate certain parts of the frontal lobe to particular functions. It appears, however, from the results of selective leucotomies as well as from studies in animals that even if the anterior cingulate gyrus and the orbital cortex have some functional properties in common, they differ in other respects (see for example Le Beau and Petrie, 1953; Lewin, 1961). Further support for this assumption can be found in differences in their fiber connections.

As described in Chapter 10 the anterior cingulate gyrus receives its thalamic afferents from the anterior thalamic nucleus, which again receives a large number of afferents from the mammillary body. To this comes a heavy projection from the hippocampus.[15] This in addition sends some fibers directly to the anterior thalamic nucleus. The orbitofrontal cortex receives thalamic afferents from the mediodorsal thalamic nucleus MD (see Ch. 11). This receives fibers from the piriform cortex and probably the amygdaloid nucleus, possibly also from the hypothalamus. These connections point to rather close functional relations of the cingulate gyrus with the hippocampus, of the orbitofrontal cortex with the amygdaloid nucleus, relations which are probably of functional importance.

The observation (Freeman and Watts, 1942, 1946) that a prefrontal leucotomy may alter the patient's conscious appreciation of pain and

[14] From a study of the brains of 102 patients subjected to prefrontal leucotomy Meyer and Beck (1954) concluded that for a successful result destruction of the mid-central, orbital, and cingulate sectors of the frontal lobe were most important. However, the amount of cortex removed or cut off from its connections appears also to be of importance.

[15] As is seen from the account in Chapter 10 the pathway from the hippocampus to the cingulate gyrus may perhaps go mostly to the middle and posterior parts of the cingulate gyrus, not so much to area 24.

his reactions to it has been repeatedly confirmed. It has been claimed that cingulectomies are particularly effective. On the assumption that the important factor in this operation is the transection of the cingulum bundle, cingulumotomy has been performed with equally good results (Foltz and White, Jr., 1962).

The changes following prefrontal leucotomy must be a consequence of an interruption of the connections of the anterior parts of the frontal lobe. In posterior lesions, or when the fibers from areas 4 and 6 are interrupted, a contralateral hemiplegia develops as described in Chapter 4. Before leaving the frontal lobe mention must be made of another symptom, *motor aphasia,* seen in lesions of the dominant hemisphere involving the regions immediately in front of the cortical motor face area. This region is often called Broca's area, since it was first drawn attention to by Broca in 1861. Motor aphasia is briefly characterized by the patient's being incapable of expressing his thoughts in words. The peripheral apparatus involved in speech, the laryngeal, facial, and lingual muscles, are not paralyzed and can be used properly in other acts. There is, for example, no dysarthria. It is the *integration* of the movements necessary for performing articulate speech which is defective. In some cases of motor aphasia the patient has in addition lost the capacity to write, a condition called *agraphia,* in spite of his fingers not being paralyzed or paretic and being used normally in other performances. Motor aphasia is only one type of disturbances of the language functions which may be seen in lesions of the brain. Before discussing these it will be appropriate to consider the question of cerebral dominance.

Cerebral dominance. The term cerebral dominance refers to the fact that one of the cerebral hemispheres is the "leading" one in certain functions, the difference being most marked as concerns the complex language functions. The notion of a "leading hemisphere" appears to have been put forward by Hughlings Jackson in 1869 (see Zangwill, 1960) on the basis of the frequent occurrence of motor (and other kinds of) aphasia in right-handed persons when they suffer a hemiplegia of the right limbs, while a left-sided hemiplegia in such persons usually is not accompanied by aphasia. In left-handed individuals the situation is often said to be the reverse (a lesion of the right hemisphere, but not of the left, being likely to result in aphasia). It is generally assumed that cerebral dominance is largely genetically determined. Numerous observations have shown that in the overwhelming number of persons, being right-handed, the left hemisphere is the dominant one. However, this is no absolute rule. Also in left-handed persons quite often the left hemisphere may be the dominant one. It appears likely that cerebral dominance is a graded characteristic, varying individually with regard to its degree. According to Zangwill (1960, p. 27), likewise: "Handedness must be regarded as a graded characteristic; left-handedness, in particular, being less clear-cut than right-handedness and less regularly associated with the dominance of either hemisphere." This conclusion is based on studies of the incidence of language disorders in left-handed patients who had sustained a strictly unilateral injury to the brain.[16] Corresponding conclusions have been made by Penfield and Roberts (1959) and others.

These results are of practical interest, for example in surgical therapy involving cortical excisions, particularly in the operative treatment of epilepsy. In recent years a method introduced by Wada in 1949 (see Wada and Rasmussen, 1960) has made it possible to identify the dominant hemisphere in patients before they undergo operation. A solution of amylobarbital sodium is injected into one common carotid artery. The injection produces an immediate and temporary loss of function of the cerebral structures supplied by the artery.[17] Thus there ensues a transient contralateral hemiplegia. If the affected hemisphere is the dominant one, aphasia develops, as can be ascertained by various verbal and other tests. This method is now widely used. The results confirm that cerebral dominance cannot be judged on handedness alone. For example, Serafetinides, Hoare, and Driver (1965) found that of 12 patients who by this test had a left dominant hemisphere for speech, 8 were right-handed, 2 left-handed, and 2 were ambidextrous. Three left-handed patients had a right cerebral dominance, while three had no exclusively unilateral representation of speech.

There appears to be little doubt that so far as the perception of language and the performance of speech are concerned, in most persons one hemisphere is dominant. There are some reports that the two hemispheres differ in their influence on other functions as well. Injection of amylobarbital on the side of the dominant hemisphere has been accompanied by depressive emotional reaction, injection on the nondominant side by an euphoric reaction (Perria, Rosadini, and Rossi, 1961; and others). Serafetinides, Hoare, and Driver (1965) even suggest that there is a "cerebral dominance for consciousness," but Rosadini and Rossi (1967) failed to find support for this view.

In recent years many studies have been devoted to the problems re-

[16] The above observations are of interest for attempts to explain the occurrence of "congenital word blindness" in children (see Zangwill, 1960).

[17] Occasionally, however, even a unilateral injection may give bilateral clinical signs as well as bilateral changes in the EEG (see Perria, Rosadini, and Rossi, 1961). In such cases the test permits no conclusions as to cerebral dominance.

lated to "cerebral dominance." Information obtained in studies of patients in whom the corpus callosum has been transected and corresponding experimental studies have greatly furthered our understanding of how the two hemispheres collaborate, and have shed light on the question whether certain functions are related to one hemisphere only. Piercy (1967, p. 119) concludes: "Specialization for particular functions appears to occur in both hemispheres, although it is perhaps fair to say that this is more extreme and occurs for a wider range of functions in the left hemisphere." In a general way the left hemisphere is particularly related to verbal skills, while nonverbal skills depend more on the right hemisphere. The parts of the hemispheres showing these differences are first and foremost the lower part of the parietal lobe and the adjoining temporal cortex. These regions, as has been mentioned above, belong to the "association" areas of the cortex. So far little evidence for anatomical differences between the two hemispheres has been produced. Geschwind and Levitsky (1968) report left-right asymmetries in the temporal speech region.

The cerebral cortex and language functions. Mention was made above of the fact that disturbances in language functions occur in lesions of the dominant hemisphere only (if there is a clear dominance). These disturbances are usually called *aphasias* and have attracted much interest by clinicians, psychologists, and linguists. The literature dealing with disturbances of speech and the perception of language (spoken or written) is enormous, and crowded with classifications and designations. It is just as crowded with hypotheses, presenting to one unfamiliar with the matter a veritable jungle, difficult to penetrate even to a limited extent.[18] A variety of aphasic disturbances which may be seen have been given particular names. A crude distinction is often made between disorders in which the production of speech suffers while the understanding of spoken and written language is intact (motor aphasia, see preceding section), and aphasias where primarily the receptive functions suffer (sensory aphasia and alexia). The defects in understanding in these cases may result in difficulties in expression. The two groups are also referred to as *expressive* and *receptive* aphasias, respectively. The era of classifications of aphasias into a number of different specific kinds or types appears now to have passed. It seems to be generally agreed that when patients suffering from one or another "type" of aphasia are closely examined, one never encounters the pure types. In all cases

[18] Of works dealing with the problems of aphasia a few may be mentioned: Weisenburg and McBride (1935); Nielsen, 1946; Penfield and Roberts, 1959; Brain, 1961, 1965; "Disorders of Language," 1964; "Brain Mechanisms Underlying Speech and Language," 1967.

features are present which, according to classical schemas, are peculiar to other types of aphasia. Scarcely two patients show identical symptoms. The disturbances in the language functions appear to be determined not only by the site and size of the lesion, but also by the premorbid personality of the person, his intellectual standard, his sphere of knowledge, etc. In their now classical monograph on aphasia Weisenburg and McBride (1935, p. 442) state: "A study of the essential nature of the aphasic disorder shows individual differences which are so great that no single hypothesis will account for the changes."

The study of aphasias has several aspects, psychological, physiological, and anatomical. The latter aspect concerns the question whether a lesion of a particular part of the brain will result in language disturbances and whether differently situated lesions give rise to different aphasic phenomena. At one time it was customary to assign particular locations to different types of aphasic disturbances, and to speak of "speech areas" in the cortex, on the assumption that the different "types" of aphasia were caused by affections of rather circumscribed parts of the cerebral cortex, and that these areas were "centers" for particular components of the complex language functions. In keeping with the realization that pure types of aphasia scarcely exist, these classical detailed "psychoanatomical" correlations have had to be discarded. This has become clear from careful investigations of the speech disorders occurring in cases of controlled surgical ablations of parts of the cortex and from post-mortem studies of aphasic patients whose language performances have been carefully studied prior to death. Additional valuable information has been produced in studies of the results of electrical stimulations of the "speech areas" in conscious patients. Such studies, performed especially by Penfield and his collaborators, have given information of other aspects of the psychophysical functions of the brain as well. Some of these observations will be briefly mentioned. Most of the observations have been made in patients suffering from temporal lobe epilepsy.

On stimulation of the temporal lobe the patient may experience what Penfield has called an *experiential response* (see Penfield and Perot, 1963). This may be visual, auditory, combined visual and auditory, or more difficult to classify. The patient on stimulation recalls a scene from his past: hears a familiar voice, sees some of his relatives, etc.[19] Responses of these kinds were obtained only from the temporal lobe, the great majority from the superior temporal gyrus. They tend to occur more often on stimulation of the nondominant temporal lobe than of the dominant lobe. Other phenomena were also noted, collectively designated as

[19] Corresponding phenomena may occur during spontaneous seizures in these cases (then called "experiential hallucinations"). In the experiential response the patient is fully aware of his present situation.

"interpretive responses," or "interpretive illusions" (see Mullan and Penfield, 1959). The sounds heard may seem louder or fainter; things seen may seem clearer, blurred, larger, or smaller; present experience may seem familiar (*déjà vue* sensation), stronger, altered, or unreal. Other sensations also occurred. The visual responses were obtained from the temporal lobe, predominantly of the nondominant hemisphere, the acoustic responses from the superior temporal gyrus on either side. Stimulation of other parts of the cortex does not give rise to such phenomena.

From the findings, briefly summarized above, it is concluded that the temporal lobe, especially the first or superior temporal gyrus, plays a particular role in the recall of perceptions from the past (chiefly auditory and visual) and in the interpretation of acoustic and visual signals. For these reasons this cortical region is called by Penfield the *"interpretive cortex."* It is stressed that this cortex *is separate from the cortical areas which appear to be concerned in language mechanisms.*

These are influenced by stimulation of rather extensive regions of the cortex (Fig. 12-6). An anterior region covers approximately Broca's area, destruction of which would give rise to motor aphasia. A posterior region occupies the inferior and posterior parts of the parietal lobe and the adjoining posterior part of the temporal lobe, except the first temporal gyrus (see above). This region covers approximately the area described long ago by Wernicke as the area whose destruction resulted in "sensory aphasia." In addition, changes in speech may be obtained from a third, superior region covering the supplementary motor area.

On electrical stimulation of the brain two kinds of effects on speech may be obtained (see Penfield and Roberts, 1959). Electrical stimulation may produce vocalization, or it may result in inability to vocalize or to use words properly. Vocalization, in the form of a sustained or interrupted vowel cry, can be elicited from the face subdivisions of the first and the supplementary motor areas in both hemispheres. These effects are presumably due to interference with the motor control of the organs of speech.

Arrest of speech or inability to vocalize spontaneously follow stimulation of the "motor areas," but may also be seen on stimulation of more extensive cortical areas, particularly those outlined in Fig. 12-6. From these areas in addition other effects have been observed: slurring of speech, distortion and repetition of words and syllables, confusion of numbers while counting, inability to name objects, with retained ability to speak. Occasionally other effects, such as difficulty in reading, have been observed. No significant differences have been found between the results of stimulation of the anterior, posterior, and superior area. Several of the effects listed above, which are obtained from the dominant hemisphere (usually the left) regardless of handedness, can scarcely be interpreted as due to disturbances in the control of muscles used in

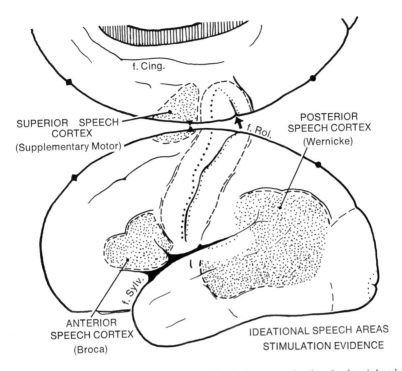

FIG. 12–6 Map of the cortex showing (dots) the areas in the dominant hemisphere of man from which interference with speech has been obtained on electrical stimulation. Note that the anterior part of the superior temporal gyrus is not
included. (Cf. text.) From Penfield and Roberts (1959).

speech. The observations strongly suggest that the areas are involved in
more integrated aspects of speech and language functions. This is in
agreement with the studies of the consequences of cortical lesions involving these regions.

This subject has been studied most extensively by Penfield and his
collaborators, and has been discussed in some detail by Penfield and
Roberts (1959). It appears from their material that transient aphasic
disturbances may follow upon excision of various parts of the cortex.
Persistent aphasia or dysphasia will result only when the removal involves
the areas which on stimulation give disturbances in language functions
(see Fig. 12-6). These areas are all assumed to be concerned in the
"ideational mechanism of speech." The posterior area is considered indispensable to normal speech, the superior is the least important. No
conclusive evidence that particular regions of the posterior area are related to different aspects of language functions could be produced, al-

though there are some indications that lesions of the posterior parts are more likely to give rise to aphasic disorders most pronounced in the visual sphere. On the whole, corresponding results have been reported by Hécaen and Angelergues (1964) in a study of patients with local brain damage.

Even if there appears to be convincing evidence that certain regions of the dominant cerebral hemisphere (see Fig. 12-6) are particularly closely related to the complex functions involved in understanding and using language, some important qualifications should be borne in mind. In the first place, these areas do not function in isolation but in collaboration with other parts of the brain (the "interpretive cortex" of Penfield in the superior temporal gyrus may be especially important). Aphasic disturbances may indeed be seen with lesions outside these parts of the cortex.[20] Secondly, we have no reasons to assume that particular aphasic disturbances can be more precisely linked with certain regions of these areas. Finally, it should be realized that when a certain type of speech disturbance is observed following a circumscribed cerebral lesion, this does not mean that the destroyed region is a "center" for a certain component of the mechanism of speech. What is observed is really quite another thing, namely, to what extent the remaining intact parts of the brain are able to perform such functions.

Lord Brain in a review of "the neurology of language" (1961, p. 164) expresses his views as follows: "We have seen that the physiological organizations upon which speech depends are of great complexity, extend over considerable areas of the brain, and are organized in time as well as in space. These serve psychological functions, but the breakdown of a physiological schema does not necessarily, or indeed usually, disturb speech in a way that corresponds to a single type of psychological defect. Moreover, the anatomical organization of the schemas means that only rarely will a single type of schema be disturbed in isolation from others."

The *anatomical connections of the cortical areas related more closely to speech* are insufficiently known. Associational connections with neighboring regions are presumably well developed. In monkeys the corresponding regions receive (in part) abundant commissural connections (see Fig. 12-4). Of particular interest is the fact that these cortical

---

[20] It should also be remembered that language functions are closely related to the emotional conditions of the person at the moment. This may be even more true for musical faculties. From an extensive clinical study of patients suffering from amusia, Ustvedt (1937) arrives at the conclusion that also subcortical centers (hypothalamus, thalamus, and corpus striatum) are important for the musical functions, particularly for the more emotional components of them.

regions receive most of their thalamic afferents from the pulvinar (especially well developed in man) since this appears not to be played upon by afferents from more "specific" subcortical regions (for some data on the connections of the pulvinar, see footnote on p. 67). Conversely the pulvinar receives cortical fibers. These relations to the pulvinar make it extremely likely that it is functionally closely related to the posterior cortical "speech region." Some evidence for this is indeed available. Penfield and Roberts (1959, p. 215) describe a patient with a small hemorrhagic lesion in the pulvinar of the dominant hemisphere, who had a severe aphasia. Following stimulations or stereotactic lesions involving the pulvinar in man aphasic disturbances have been reported by several authors, most recently by Ojemann, Fedio, and van Buren (1968). These authors observed anomia (failure to name objects correctly) on stimulation of the left pulvinar and also on stimulation of the white matter in both parietal lobes, presumably due to activation of commissural fibers.

The parietal lobe. Since particular symptoms have been correlated with lesions of the parietal lobe, this will be considered under a separate heading. In Chapter 2 the *sensory symptoms* resulting from irritation or lesions of the anterior parts of the parietal lobe (the postcentral gyrus and the superior parietal lobule) were discussed at some length. Among other symptoms which may be seen in lesions of the parietal lobe (considered fully in Critchley's monograph, 1953) mention is made of the occurrence of *muscular wasting in the contralateral half of the body.* Usually the atrophy is most marked in the upper limb. It may occur in slowly developing lesions (tumors, atrophies) and in acute cerebrovascular affections. There may be an accompanying paresis with some spasticity, which is often explained as being due to concomitant involvement of the precentral region. No satisfactory explanation of the muscular atrophy following lesions of the parietal lobe has so far been given, but its appearance may be of some diagnostic value. *Ataxia* of "sensory" type is often seen as a consequence of parietal lobe lesions.

Symptoms indicating derangement of more complex functions, involving somatic as well as psychic elements, have often been observed following lesions of the parietal lobe, especially the right. The literature on this subject is almost as confusing and the terminology as manifold as is the case for aphasia. Some of these disturbances are collectively designated as *agnosias* (lack of awareness), and a number of different types have been described. The common feature is a defective recognition of sensory impressions.

In *visual agnosia* the vision of the patient may be intact, but he fails to recognize known objects or persons. In *tactile agnosia* the patient lacks the power of synthesizing and associating the sensations experienced, for example, when handling an object with his eyes closed. In spite of normal sensation and absence of asterognosia (the patient is, for example, able to decide if the object is rough or smooth), he cannot realize which object he is holding. More rarely so-called *finger-agnosia* is seen. Here the patient is unable to name his fingers or to indicate individual fingers on request and often has difficulties in distinguishing right from left. Even stranger is a condition called *anosognosia* (lack of awareness of disease) where the patient, for example, does not recognize that his limbs (usually the left) are paralyzed, or denies that he is blind (Anton's syndrome). Relatively common in affections of the parietal lobe is apraxia. Different types have been described. One is a condition called *constructional apraxia,* where in its simplest form the patient has difficulties "in putting together one-dimensional units so as to form two-dimensional figures or patterns" (Critchley, 1953, p. 172). This may become evident when the patient tries to copy a drawing.[21] Many kinds of this disorder have been described, and by many it is considered to be closely related to agnostic disturbances. Constructional apraxia as well as agnostic disorders have been considered also as elements in a disturbance of the *"body scheme"* or *"body image."* These terms refer to the individual's awareness of his own body and of his spatial relationships to the surroundings. The patient may have difficulties in route-finding and orientation. It scarcely needs stressing that the study of these complex functions requires special and often rather complex tests, if conclusive results are to be obtained.

The above list of disturbances which may be seen in lesions of the parietal lobe is far from complete. There has been much discussion of whether the particular symptoms and symptom constellations are variants of disturbances of a common basic function or represent separate entities. For example, it has been held by many that finger-agnosia, being a component of Gerstmann's syndrome [22] is a specific disturbance caused by a lesion of the angular gyrus of the parietal lobe. This view appears to be based on very meager evidence (see Critchley, 1966). Further points of discussion have been the relations between agnostic and aphasic disorders, and the question whether the symptoms mentioned above occur only with lesions of the right parietal lobe (in the nondominant hemisphere) as advocated by some authors. In several agnostic disorders there is obviously a defect in symbolic thinking, closely related to language functions. In general it appears that disorders of "spatial thought," such as anosognosia and constructional apraxia are most often observed following affections of the right parietal lobe. (Finger-agnosia, however, appears to occur with almost equal frequency in lesions of the left and right parietal lobes.) From a detailed study of 17 patients sub-

[21] The term *apractognosia* appears to be somewhat more extensive and to cover defects in practical tasks (dressing, etc.) as well as ideational difficulties.

[22] A fully developed Gerstmann's syndrome as generally defined includes in addition to finger-agnosia, also dysgraphia, dyscalculia and right-left disorientation (see Critchley, 1966).

jected to localized ablations of the parietal lobe Hécaen, Penfield, Bertrand, and Malmo (1956) concluded that agnosia of various kinds (including apractognosia) and disturbances in the body scheme appeared only when the ablation involved the lower and posterior parts of the parietal lobe and the upper part of the temporal lobe. The area coincides approximately with the "posterior speech area" (see Fig. 12-6), but while the latter is regularly found in the dominant (usually the left) hemisphere, the other disturbances are most often observed following ablations of the right parietal lobe. They are then contralateral. However, according to Hécaen et al., corresponding ablations of the left parietal lobe are followed by bilateral disturbances in gnostic functions and topographical relationships (body scheme), in addition to aphasic disturbances. It has been argued by some that the preponderance of such disturbances observed in patients with right parietal lesions is due to the fact that a present aphasia in left-sided lesions will obscure agnostic disturbances or at least make them difficult to notice, unless especially searched for. This view receives some support from a study of Weinstein, Cole, Mitchell, and Lyerly (1964), who further found that in lesions of the left parietal lobe there is usually an inverse relationship between the degree of aphasia and anosognosia.

The many and complex questions touched upon are far from solved. It may seem a likely assumption that if the neural mechanisms related to language (with all what this involves in the use of symbols, etc.) "occupy" parts of the dominant hemisphere only, the corresponding tissue in the other hemisphere should be available for other functions. However, the data briefly discussed above, as well as other data, makes the idea of a strict functional segregation between the two hemispheres as concerns more complex "psychosomatic functions" seem less convincing than before. The distinction between a dominant (major) and a nondominant (minor) hemisphere appears to be less definite than formerly believed.[23] The observations available may suggest that a collaboration between the two hemispheres, particularly between the parietal lobes, is of major importance for the functions. Further support for this view comes from recent studies of the functional importance of the commissural connections of the cerebral cortex.

Function of the corpus callosum. As described in a previous sec-

---

[23] Even if cerebral dominance, as mentioned above, appears to be to some extent genetically determined (cf. inheritance of left-handedness) it seems likely that it is only by being used preferentially in certain functions that one hemisphere comes to be the "leading" one. This may perhaps occur already in the first years of life (see Penfield and Roberts, 1959). Environmental factors presumably play a role in the development of cerebral dominance.

tion the corpus callosum is the main commissural connection between the two neocortices. The phylogenetic increase of the neocortex in mammals is followed by a parallel increase in the size of the corpus callosum. It seems a likely assumption that the main function of this great fiber mass would be to secure a co-operation between the two cerebral hemispheres, and that this function should be especially important in man, but until recently little was known of the function of the corpus callosum. It has been known for a long time that in some individuals the corpus callosum is not developed (agenesis of the corpus callosum). This condition can now be diagnosed during life by air encephalography. Although in some such cases there is evidence of other developmental deficits, usually there are no neurological symptoms. In patients who have had their corpus callosum sectioned in attempts to treat spread of epileptic convulsions no marked behavioral deficits were observed (see for example Smith and Akelaitis, 1942; Bridgman and Smith, 1945). Observations of these kinds lead some to believe that the corpus callosum could scarcely be of great importance for the functioning of the human brain. It is now clear that the reason for the negative findings is that appropriate tests were not employed to unravel the function of the corpus callosum.[24]

The first conclusive evidence of the functional role of the corpus callosum came from the *experimental studies* in cats and monkeys by Myers, Sperry, and others and concerned visual functions. Advantage was taken of the presence of crossed as well as uncrossed connections in the visual pathways (see Ch. 8). Following transection of the optic chiasm, visual impulses from one eye will be transmitted to the ipsilateral striate area only. With one eye occluded the cats were trained to discriminate between different figures, for example, a square and a circle (Myers, 1956). This discrimination must be due to processes occurring in the hemisphere ipsilateral to the eye used. If this eye is then covered, and the other eye used, the animals can discriminate equally well, even if the sensory input is then only to the other hemisphere which had so far not been used. Obviously, there must be a highly developed transmission of visual experiential information between the two hemispheres. If, in a cat with transected optic chiasm, the corpus callosum and anterior commissure in addition are transected the situation is completely different. The animal is not able to recall through one eye the tasks learned through the other eye. If it is trained subsequently to use the second eye, no evidence of benefit from the previous training of the first eye is found.

---

[24] For some data see "Interhemispheric Relations and Cerebral Dominance," 1962; "Functions of the Corpus Callosum," 1965. A complete account of all published cases of agenesis of the corpus callosum and of 33 of their own cases has been published by Unterharnscheidt, Jachnik, and Gött (1968).

Obviously, the commissural connections have been responsible for transmitting the information related to visual pattern discrimination from the hemisphere receiving the information to the other. Similar results have been obtained in studies of visually guided behavior in monkeys with transection of the commissures and the optic chiasm (Downer, 1959).

The importance of the corpus callosum for information transmission has been demonstrated also in other spheres. Myers and Henson (1960) studied tactuokinesthetic learning in chimpanzees. A chimpanzee with its corpus callosum and anterior commissure transected is taught to solve a latch box problem by using only one of its hands. If the same problem is later presented to it in a situation which requires that it use the other hand for sensory information the chimpanzee does not know how to solve the problem. In contrast, under the same conditions a normal animal will immediately solve the problem equally well with the other hand. Again it appears that the information of the test situation has not been transmitted to the opposite hemisphere. A number of studies on "split-brain" monkeys have been performed in recent years in order to get a better understanding of the interhemispheric transfer. Other approaches have been tried as well. By making use of the inactivation of the cortex produced by "spreading cortical depression," blocking of one hemisphere during training can be obtained. From studies of this kind in rats, Russell and Ochs (1963) concluded that a memory trace may be restricted to the "trained" hemisphere for two weeks or more. Transfer to the other hemisphere occurred, however, if the animal was allowed one reinforced response with bilateral cortical function.

In agreement with what is known of the anatomy of the commissural connections, different regions of the corpus callosum are involved in the transfer of visual and somatosensory information. The fibers responsible for transfer of information of visual experience are found posteriorly. Section of the posterior part of the corpus callosum in cats prevents the transfer, while following section of the anterior part the animals react as normal ones in these tests (Myers, 1959). Concerning the cortical regions involved it is of relevance to recall the anatomical distribution of the commissural fibers (see Fig. 12-4). The striate area, the hand region, and to a lesser extent the foot region, of the primary sensorimotor area and the primary acoustic area appear to be devoid of commissural connections. Thus, the transfer must occur between other areas, presumably first and foremost those adjoining the specific sensory areas, assumed to be concerned in more complex perceptual processes. Information is most complete concerning the visual areas (see Ch. 8). Area 18 is amply interconnected with its partner on the opposite side, while area 19 appears to be more sparsely supplied with commissural fibers. Area 17 sends numerous association fibers to areas 18 and 19, which are also interconnected. It appears a likely assumption, however, that the interhemispheric "cross talk" involves other commissural fibers in addition to those from the areas immediately surrounding the specific sensory areas. This receives some support from other experimental findings as well as from observations in man (see Geschwind, 1965).

Possibilities for the study of *interhemispheral relationships in man* have been greatly increased following the introduction of transection of the corpus callosum as a therapeutic measure in certain cases of epilepsy. Several investigations on such patients have been performed in recent years. In addition to confirming the findings in animals, human studies have given some new information of problems concerning the function of the cortex in language mechanisms and on the relative role played by the right and left hemispheres in these functions. Studies of this kind require very elaborate tests, and conclusions must be drawn with caution. Only a few data will be mentioned. Gazzaniga, Bogen, and Sperry (1965), studying two patients with complete transection of the commissures, concluded that "activities that involved speech and writing were well preserved, but only in so far as they could be governed by the left hemisphere" (loc. cit. p. 236). In a further study Gazzaniga and Sperry (1967) found, in agreement with the above statement, that sensory information which entered the left hemisphere could be reported through speech and writing without difficulty. But the patients were totally unable to give accurate spoken or written reports for even the simplest kind of sensory information reaching the right hemisphere. They were, for example, unable to name objects palpated with the left hand. These studies thus are in agreement with conclusions made from stimulation and ablation experiments of the parietal lobe, that *verbal expression* is a matter almost exclusively of the left hemisphere. The same appears to be the case for calculation. As concerns *comprehension of language,* Gazzaniga and Sperry (1967) found evidence for its being related to both hemispheres, in contrast to observations by others. For other interesting observations the reader is referred to their paper.

There seems to be agreement among those studying the subject that sectioning of the corpus callosum is not followed by changes in intellect, behavior, or emotions. The condition is briefly characterized as follows by Sperry (1966, p. 299): "Everything we have seen so far indicates that the surgery has left these people with two separate minds, that is, two separate spheres of consciousness. What is experienced in the right hemisphere seems to be entirely outside the realm of awareness of the left hemisphere. This mental division has been demonstrated in regard to perception, cognition, volition, learning, and memory. One of the hemispheres, the left, dominant or major hemisphere, has speech and is normally talkative and conversant. The other, the minor hemisphere, however, is mute or dumb, being able to express itself only through nonverbal reactions."

The question whether each hemisphere in these split-brain patients "has its own consciousness" is likely to interest philosophers. It appears from the studies undertaken that in daily life there is only rarely evidence of conflict between the two hemispheres. Experimental situations may, however, be arranged where this can be observed. Animal studies have likewise shown that the two hemispheres may learn different tasks, which may be performed simultaneously under appropriate experimental conditions. In the normal brain it appears that any information reaching one hemisphere is regularly communicated to the other, largely to corresponding regions. Some of the findings made in patients with transected commissures indicate that the distinction between the two hemispheres in regard to language functions and body scheme may not be as marked as previously assumed. Some of the aphasic disturbances may perhaps be easier to understand in the light of the new findings. Geschwind (1965) who discusses these problems stresses the importance of intracortical connections between the cortical regions involved in these functions, in addition to the commissural ones. He has coined the name "disconnection syndromes" as a common denominator for "the effects of lesions of association pathways, either those which lie exclusively within a single cerebral hemisphere or those which join the two halves of the brain" (loc. cit. p. 242). More knowledge of the anatomy of the connections is highly needed. Even with present knowledge, however, it appears from the analysis of Geschwind (1965) that an explanation may be found for the occurrence of similar functional disturbances with lesions differently situated.

The findings made in split-brain animals and man are of great interest for the understanding of several aspects of brain functions, such as the learning of language as well as other kinds of learning and behavior. A vast literature has grown up on these subjects, which will not, however, be considered here. Several symposia have been devoted to discussion of these problems,[25] but much is still conjectural. It should not be overlooked in the treatment of these subjects that the cortex must collaborate with many other parts of the nervous system. Particularly one should not minimize the emotional aspects of the functions, betrayed in everyday language by terms such as interest, motivation, etc.

Evaluation of clinical findings in lesions of the cerebral cortex. It

[25] See, for example, "Brain Mechanisms and Learning," 1961; "Brain and Conscious Experience," 1966.

will appear from the preceding account that lesions of the cerebral cortex in man may result in a multitude of different symptoms: motor, sensory, autonomic, behavioral, and purely mental. Lesions of various parts of the cortex give rise to fairly characteristic symptoms, and from a knowledge of the anatomical and functional organization of the cortex the site of the lesion can in many cases be determined quite accurately. If a proper and careful examination of the patient is made this might be expected to be a relatively simple affair. Unfortunately, this is often not the case. Several circumstances contribute to this, some of which will be mentioned below.

A tumor may cause widespread secondary changes in other parts of the brain, which may even progress after the tumor has been removed. In the case of the surgical removal of a malignant tumor it is difficult to exclude the possibility that some of the mass is left and that this may be responsible for some of the symptoms. Secondary, even remote bleedings, may occasionally occur, and damage may be inflicted on subcortical structures. At operation it is not always easy to be sure which gyri are removed and which have been left, on account of the deformation of the convolutional pattern, edema, and dislocation of the brain which so frequently occur. With regard to mental changes, their evaluation is invalidated by the fact that, as a rule, comparable data from the patient's normal life before the onset of disease are lacking. Some information may be gained only concerning major behavioral features. These factors urge that the utmost care should be taken in interpreting certain symptoms as due to removal of a particular part of the cortex. For the same reason anatomical inferences—often too lightheartedly drawn from clinical observations—should be evaluated very critically. If reliable conclusions are to be made a complete post-mortem examination of the brain is essential. Hebb (1945) stresses these facts, and points particularly to the possibility of failure arising from the effect which the presence of a pathological process in the brain may have on the function of other parts. On the basis of the findings in a patient in whom the anterior third of both frontal lobes were removed on account of epilepsy following traumatic injury (Hebb and Penfield, 1940) and who showed moderate postoperative clinical changes, Hebb maintains that the presence of a pathological process in the brain may affect the mental state of a patient more than the absence of a part of the brain.

As has been mentioned at several occasions in other chapters, a pathological process as a rule will not be limited to certain structural and functional "units" (in so far as such are present at all), but it will affect several structures. However, it is fortunate that some diseases show a marked predilection for occurring in or affecting predominantly certain regions of the brain. This is the case for many of the tumors. This circumstance may allow the experienced clinician to determine not only the site of the lesion, but to calculate with a fair degree of accuracy also the nature of the disease, apart from information which the case history may yield on this point. On the other hand, it should be remembered that the lesion may be found in other places than expected. One of the classical examples is the occurrence of a frontal lobe tumor which clinically imitates a cerebellar tumor (see Ch. 5). Indeed, "false localizing signs" are not uncommon, as appears from the exhaustive account of Gassel (1961) based on observations in a series of 250 patients with intracranial meningeomas. Diffuse processes may cause diagnostic difficulties, since they may give rise to focal symptoms, in spite of being widespread. Thus some cortical atrophies may simulate the presence of a tumor (see, for example, Jackson, 1946; Fleminger, 1946). When a process starts in the so-called "mute regions" it may be without focal symptoms for a considerable time, making diagnosis difficult. It is, on the whole, important to bear in mind the frequent occurrence of secondary changes in order to avoid overestimation of "focal" signs.

The above considerations refer mainly to the problems encountered in clinical examinations of the patients. Many of the difficulties mentioned can be overcome or at least reduced when use is made of ancillary methods, as X-ray investigations, pneumoencephalography, ventriculography, angiography, electroencephalography, or other procedures (localization of certain tumors by intravascular injections of radiocative isotopes, and other methods). However, even with the use of all available methods there are still cases where a precise diagnosis of the type and site of a cerebral lesion cannot be made.

Cortical localization. This subject has been repeatedly touched upon in the present chapter. In concluding the account of the cerebral cortex it will be appropriate to consider whether any conclusions can be reached concerning the problem of cortical localization.[26] Is it legitimate to assume, as those who adhere to the theory of extreme localization do, that the various cytoarchitectural areas each subserve a special function? Or does the cerebral cortex always function as a whole, as the most ardent opponents of the theory of cortical localization maintain?

Before proceeding it is essential to devote some thought to *the concept of "function."* In the first place we should not overlook the fact

[26] A vast literature has grown up on this subject. The comments made in the following do not pretend to be more than a brief statement of some principal points of view. On this account definition of the many terms employed, such as localization, activity, etc., which should rightly precede any discussion of a subject like this, is omitted.

that the classification of events and processes in the organism into various "functions" is arbitrary. When we speak of movements, secretion, sensory perception, etc., as functions, this is a convention adopted for practical purposes. In the living organism activity is scarcely ever restricted to one of these "man-made" categories of function. Even the slightest movement of a finger is accompanied by, for example, vascular alterations in it, and by stimulation of sensory receptors. At the other extreme, in behavioral reactions a multitude of different functions are always integrated, such as motor, secretory, cardiovascular, respiratory, alterations in the sensitivity of sensory mechanisms, etc. As one passes from more elementary functions to the more complex ones it becomes increasingly impossible to relate a particular part of the nervous system (a nucleus or a fiber tract) to a particular function. Examples of this have been mentioned in several chapters of this book, and the fallacies inherent in considering a particular region of the central nervous system as a "center" for one or another "function" have repeatedly been emphasized. The fact that the stimulation or ablation of a brain region gives rise to alterations in certain functions should not induce us to forget that what it is possible to observe in the experimental situation are only fragments of the totality of changes which actually take place. These must of necessity be intimately linked in order to secure an integrated reaction from the organism, adapted to the incessant changes in the organism itself and in its surroundings.

As concerns the cerebral cortex we have seen that *the classical conception of a clear-cut functional localization cannot be upheld.* For example, no clear distinction can be made between "motor" and "somatosensory" cortical areas. The striate area is not purely sensory, since it gives rise to pathways which mediate ocular movements. Damage to rather extensive cortical regions may result in disturbances of the extremely complex language functions. Particular cortical areas cannot be related to specific "functions," when this word is taken in the usual sense. On the other hand, certain cortical areas are more or less closely related to some of the functions. Indeed, recent research has made it clear that the functional role of, for example, the three somatosensory cortical regions is not identical; areas 17, 18, and 19 are not equivalent in the function of vision.

The parcellation of the cerebral cortex into a number of cytoarchitecturally different areas has been criticized severely by many students (see for example, Lashley and Clark, 1946), and it may probably rightly be said that the parcellations have been overdone by some. It is further obvious that the borders between areas (with a few exceptions, the striate area being the most notable) are not sharp. With these qualifications, however, the principle of a parcellation of the cortex into minor regions which differ structurally in certain respects, is sound. The cyto-architectonic differences between areas parallel other structural features, as described previously in this and other chapters. Where recent studies of fiber connections of the cortex have been performed accurately, they have demonstrated the correctness of this view, with the above qualification that the borders are not sharp. As examples of this, one may mention the afferent and efferent projections of the first sensorimotor region considered in Chapters 2 and 4, of the visual areas 17, 18, and 19 (Ch. 8), and of the thalamocortical and corticothalamic projections.[27] With increasingly precise studies more and more details are brought to light supporting the validity of the concept of a cortical morphological parcellation. It was mentioned in a preceding section of this chapter that the internal organization of the radially oriented cortical "units" differs between areas, and that the total number of boutons differs. Regional differences in the intracortical distribution pattern of callosal afferents have been noted (Heimer, Ebner, and Nauta, 1967). The presence of chemical differences should also be mentioned. On almost every point where the problem has been investigated, even neighboring cortical areas have also been found to differ in certain respects physiologically (for example areas 3, 1, and 2 in the sensorimotor cortex).

When taken together the available anatomical information, although far from complete, strongly supports the idea that *the various cortical areas differ with regard to their finer structural organization,* even if they all present variations of a common pattern. This leads to the assumption, supported by an increasing number of physiological observations, that the cortical areas have different tasks, or different functions, provided one takes care not to use the word function in the usual sense (movement, sensation, etc.). In any of the latter functions in which the cortex is involved, a number of cortical areas must participate in an extensive mutual collaboration, and they must collaborate with subcortical structures. If considered in this way, and if regard is taken to the different connotations of the word "function," there appears to be no real incompatibility between the view that the cortex is a mosaic of units, each with its particular function, and the holistic view of the cortex and the brain functioning as a whole. The problem, as so many others, is reduced to one of semantics.

[27] There are differences between areas as to the sources of their afferent fibers, destinations of their efferent fibers, in calibers of fibers, and concerning other features.

Epilogue
Some General
Considerations

THE READER who has had the patience to follow the account given in the preceding twelve chapters may have been impressed, overwhelmed, and perhaps frustrated by the amount of anatomical detail presented in the text, even though in many places the anatomical features have been treated rather summarily. Some questions have probably arisen in the minds of many readers: Do we need all this detailed anatomy? What is the use of it? Can it help us in the diagnosis and treatment of disorders of the nervous system? Some general comments bearing on these questions may be appropriate.

As we have seen, by combining various methods of study it is today possible to determine the anatomical organization of the brain in rather great detail, but in spite of considerable advances in recent years there are still vast areas of the brain which are insufficiently known. As progress has been made one feature has become increasingly clear, and will have struck any student of the subject: *In the anatomical organization of the central nervous system there is an extremely high degree of order. This is true even with regard to the most minute structural features.* Many examples have been described in the text. A particular cell type

684

may present a regular topographic distribution as well as a highly specific arrangement with regard to its dendritic and axonal processes. Strict topographical localization is found in the interconnections between many nuclei as well as in the associational and commissural connections of the cerebral cortex. Somatotopical patterns have been demonstrated in fiber projections where they were previously unknown. The various contingents of afferent fibers to a nucleus may show a differential and precisely organized distribution within this. Afferents from different sources may establish synaptic contacts at different sites of the dendrites or perikarya of a category of nerve cells. Many varieties of synaptic structures are known, and different presynaptic formations have been shown to belong to afferent fibers of different origin. Even regions generally considered as being rather diffusely organized, such as the reticular formation and the "nonspecific" thalamic nuclei, have been shown to possess a fair degree of specificity in their anatomical organization and further research may well produce further evidence in support of this. There can be little doubt that if sufficiently meticulous studies are made in the future more and more data will be brought forward and will demonstrate the extremely precise and orderly anatomical arrangements existing in the central nervous system.

The recent data alluded to above leads us to *consider the central nervous system as being composed of a multitude of minor units, each with its particular structural organization, specific as regards its finer intrinsic organization as well as its connections with other units.* Scarcely two regions are identically organized. If the structure of living matter is related to its function, an axiom which is generally accepted, it follows that *there are in the nervous system as many minor functional units as there are structural ones.* Provided that the term functional is not applied to "function" ("sensory," "motor," etc.) as discussed in the consideration of cortical localization (p. 681), there is nothing to contradict this view. In fact, wherever anatomical information is precise enough and sufficiently detailed physiological analyses have been performed, evidence in support of it has been found, as for example in the studies of the somatosensory fiber systems, of the vestibular nuclei, the visual system, and in other places. Studies of single unit potentials especially have in many instances shown a complete agreement with anatomical data, as concerns for example the behavior of units in response to afferent impulses from different sources. In some instances chemical and pharmacological studies have demonstrated differences between minor subdivisions of a structure, but on the whole evidence of this kind is so far relatively sparse, because a sufficiently close correlation of the findings with the structural organization has not been possible or has not been performed.

For the total behavior of the organism collaboration of the many structural and functional "units" of the nervous system is essential. This collaboration occurs by way of fiber connections between the "units." The more precisely these connections are studied, the more obvious it is that there are far more connections than previously assumed, and that they are much more multifarious and complex than was believed some decades ago. In fact, it is possible to envisage connections which may—via more or less circuitous routes—lead from almost any "unit" to almost any other "unit." While this does not permit the conclusion that these connections are all always utilized when a "unit" is active, it demonstrates the *possibilities* for a widespread and varied impulse conduction under different circumstances. In a general way it explains the well-known variability of responses to a particular stimulus, depending on the concomitant activity of other parts of the nervous system than those immediately activated by the stimulus, produced by other external or internal stimuli. Other features influencing the response are the chemical and hormonal conditions in the organism at the moment. The above considerations apply generally, even to "simple" spinal reflexes, but are especially relevant with regard to more complex behavioral and mental responses to a variety of stimuli, as is well known to everyone from experiences in daily life.

The more we know of the structural and functional organization of the central nervous system, the more obvious its extreme complexity becomes. So tremendous is this complexity that there may be reason to doubt that the human brain is good enough to fully understand the human brain. Attempts have been made to make models of parts of the brain, of particular systems or fragments of it, and to apply cybernetic principles and computer analysis. While such attempts may throw light on certain aspects, it would be naïve to believe that they can really tell us much, for the very reason that they are yet too simple. They suffer from the disadvantage that a number of factors, at work in the living brain, are left out of consideration. The important aspect of the collaboration between "units" is unduly oversimplified, in part because too little is known of the structure and function of the parts included in the model, and in part because taking all relevant parts into consideration would amount almost to making a model of the entire brain, an obviously impossible undertaking. Attempts to analogize the human brain with electronic computers has induced some, particularly nonbiologists, to adopt a rigid mechanistic view of the brain.

Even if our prospects of really understanding our most complex organ are indeed small, there is no doubt that we may advance much further than we have so far. It is important to be aware, however, that if progress is to be made, studies of the nervous system have to be concerned with the most minute details of its function and structure. It is only by knowing these that we may hope to put bits of evidence together and to increase our understanding. As Whitfield (1967, p. 192) phrases the problem: "Each time we examine a yet smaller sub-unit of the nervous system we find it to consist of some more interconnected 'black-boxes,' and always we find that a behavioural model of the black-box makes little contribution to our understanding of the mechanism. There is no substitute for taking the lid off."

It may be added that *the investigation of the structure of the nervous system in all its detail is a prerequisite for progress in studies of its function.* Every function is carried out by a structure, and conclusions about functions without reference to the structures involved will remain incomplete and easily may lead us astray.

The view of the nervous system outlined above may seem pessimistic and may be particularly disheartening to the clinical neurologist, since it obviously runs counter to the traditional tendency to correlate a particular clinical symptom to damage to—or dysfunction of—a certain part or "system" of the brain. It is well known to critical clinical neurologists that more often than not, the symptoms observed in a patient do not correspond to the traditional schematic presentations in the textbooks. But all too often features in the clinical picture which do not fit the schema are disregarded as being of little importance. In the preceding chapters of this book numerous examples have been mentioned of symptoms which according to traditional concepts are considered as specific to involvement of one or another part of the brain, but which have turned out to be far from "specific," the so-called pyramidal tract syndrome being perhaps the most impressive. The complexity and multitude of interconnections in the central nervous system may help us to understand the remarkable degree of functional restitution or "compensation" which is often seen in lesions of the brain. An understanding of the complexities in the organization of the nervous system will relieve the neurologist of the "moral obligation" to make his findings fit preconceived traditional conceptions. It will encourage him to penetrate deeper in his analysis of the particular case. Even if he will often have to admit that a final conclusion as to the site and nature of the disturbance may not be possible, it will make clinical neurology more fascinating and engaging. An approach to the subject in this way will encourage observations which may increase our understanding of disturbances of the nervous system of man. The story of medicine contains many examples of how careful investigation of a single patient has given more information of value than a collective analysis of a number of cases showing (apparently) identical symptoms. If clinical neurological work in the future is to bring results of value, it is essential that the neurologist understand the major principles in the organization of the nervous system, and that he have a fair knowledge of its structure and function. In particular a knowledge of the lines of communication between the "units" of the nervous system is essential. It is also essential that improved and precise methods for the study of functional disturbances of the nervous system in man be developed. As has been seen, in recent years considerable advances have been made in this field, and additional work along this line should be encouraged.

The reader will have realized that in spite of all the research devoted to the nervous system, our knowledge is still rather limited. On almost all points there are unsolved problems. Our present-day concepts are still to a large extent based upon assumptions and hypotheses, built upon a modest body of factual knowledge. If further progress is to be made, it is important to be aware of this situation, and to make every effort to distinguish between observations and interpretations. Working hypotheses are important and necessary tools in research, but, as the history of science shows, they have a tendency to become accepted as truths and to hamper instead of promoting progress. The author has done his best to stress the relatively weak foundations upon which many of our present concepts of the central nervous system are built. Accordingly, few final conclusions can be found in this text, perhaps to the disappointment of some students who would like to have clear-cut and final statements. It is the author's hope that the present book, by emphasizing many unsolved problems, may contribute to making the reader aware of the challenge and fascination of the study of the nervous system, and to fostering a fruitful and rewarding approach to the problems which face the clinical neurologist in his daily work.

References

ADAL, M. N., and D. BARKER (1965). Intramuscular branching of fusimotor fibres. *J. Physiol.* (*Lond.*) *177,* 288–299.

ADAMS, J. H., P. M. DANIEL, and M. M. L. PRICHARD (1965–66). Observations on the portal circulation of the pituitary gland. *Neuroendocrinology 1,* 193–213.

ADAMS, J. H., P. M. DANIEL, and M. M. L. PRICHARD (1966). Transection of the pituitary stalk in man: anatomical changes in the pituitary glands of 21 patients. *J. Neurol. Neurosurg. Psychiat. 29,* 545–555.

ADAMS, R. D., D. DENNY-BROWN, and C. M. PEARSON (1962). *Diseases of Muscle. A Study in Pathology,* 2nd ed. Paul B. Hoeber, New York.

ADDISON, W. H. F. (1915). On the rhinencephalon of *Delphinus delphis. J. comp. Neurol. 25,* 497–522.

ADES, H. W. (1944). Midbrain auditory mechanisms in cats. *J. Neurophysiol. 7,* 415–424.

ADES, H. W., and R. FELDER (1942). The acoustic area of the monkey (*Macaca mulatta*). *J. Neurophysiol. 5,* 49–54.

ADEY, W. R. (1951). An experimental study of the hippocampal connexions of the cingulate cortex in the rabbit. *Brain 74,* 233–247.

ADEY, W. R. (1953). An experimental study of the central olfactory connections in a marsupial (*Trichosurus vulpecula*). *Brain 76,* 311–330.

ADEY, W. R., and M. MEYER (1952a). An experimental study of hippocampal afferent pathways from prefontal and cingulate areas in the monkey. *J. Anat.* (*Lond.*) *86,* 58–74.

ADEY, W. R., and M. MEYER (1952b). Hippocampal and hypothalamic connexions of the temporal lobe in the monkey. *Brain 75,* 358–384.

689

ADIE, W. J. (1932). Tonic pupils and absent tendon reflexes: A benign disorder *sui generis;* its complete and incomplete forms. *Brain 55,* 98–113.

ADIE, W. J., and M. CRITCHLEY (1927). Forced grasping and groping. *Brain 50,* 142–170.

ADLER, A. (1934). Zur Topik des Verlaufes der Geschmackssinnsfasern und anderer afferenter Bahnen im Thalamus. *Z. ges. Neurol. Psychiat. 149,* 208–220.

ADRIAN, E. D. (1941). Afferent discharges to the cerebral cortex from peripheral sense organs. *J. Physiol. (Lond.) 100,* 159–191.

ADRIAN, E. D. (1943). Afferent areas in the cerebellum connected with the limbs. *Brain 66,* 289–315.

ADRIAN, E. D. (1950a). Sensory discrimination. With some recent evidence from the olfactory organ. *Brit. med. Bull. 6,* 330–332.

ADRIAN, E. D. (1950b). The electrical activity of the mammalian olfactory bulb. *Electroencephal. clin. Neurophysiol. 2,* 377–388.

Advances in Stereoencephalotomy, III (1967). Third International Symposium on Stereoencephalotomy, Madrid (E. A. Spiegel and H. T. Wycis, eds.) *Confin. neurol. (Basel) 29,* 65–282.

Aggression and Defense. Neural Mechanisms and Social Patterns, Brain Function, Vol. V (1967) (C. D. Clemente and D. B. Lindsley, eds.) Univ. of California Press, Berkeley and Los Angeles, California.

AGNEW, R. F., J. B. PRESTON, and D. G. WHITLOCK (1963). Patterns of motor cortex effects on ankle flexor and extensor motoneurons in the "pyramidal" cat preparation. *Exp. Neurol. 8,* 248–263.

AITKEN, J. T., and J. E. BRIDGER (1961). Neuron size and neuron population density in the lumbosacral region of the cat's spinal cord. *J. Anat. (Lond.) 95,* 38–53.

AJMONE MARSAN, C. (1965). The thalamus. Data on its functional anatomy and on some aspects of thalamocortical integration. *Arch. ital. Biol. 103,* 847–882.

AKERT, K. (1964). Comparative anatomy of frontal cortex and thalamofrontal connections. In *The Frontal Granular Cortex and Behavior* (J. M. Warren and K. Akert, eds.), pp. 372–394. McGraw-Hill Book Co., New York.

AKERT, K. (1965). The anatomical substrate of sleep. In *Sleep Mechanisms, Progress In Brain Research,* Vol. 18 (K. Akert, C. Bally, and J. P. Schadé, eds.), pp. 9–19. Elsevier Publishing Co., Amsterdam.

AKERT, K., and B. ANDERSSON (1951). Experimenteller Beitrag zur Physiologie des Nucleus caudatus. *Acta physiol. scand. 22,* 281–298.

AKERT, K., R. A. GRUESEN, C. N. WOOLSEY, and D. R. MEYER (1961). Klüver-Bucy syndrome in monkeys with neocortical ablations of temporal lobe. *Brain 84,* 480–498.

ALBE-FESSARD, D. (1968). Central nervous mechanisms involved in pain and analgesia. In *Pharmacology of Pain,* Vol 9. Proceedings 3rd International Pharmacological Meeting 1966, pp. 131–168. Pergamon Press, Oxford—New York.

ALBE-FESSARD, D., G. ARFEL, and G. GUIOT (1963). Activités électriques caractéristiques de quelques structures cérébrales chez l'homme. *Ann. Chir. 17,* 1185–1214.

ALBE-FESSARD, D., G. ARFEL, G. GUIOT, P. DEROME, and G. GUILBAUD (1967). Thalamic unit activity in man. *Electroenceph. clin. Neurophysiol. Suppl. 25,* 132–142.

ALBE-FESSARD, D., G. ARFEL, G. GUIOT, P. DEROME, E. HERTZOG, G. VOURC'H,

690

References

H. Brown, P. Aleonard, J. de la Herran, and J. C. Trigo (1966). Electrophysiological studies of some deep cerebral structures in man. *J. neurol. Sci. 3,* 37–51.

Albe-Fessard, D., and D. Bowsher (1965). Responses of monkey thalamus to somatic stimuli under chloralose anaesthesia. *Electroenceph. clin. Neurophysiol. 19,* 1–15.

Albe-Fessard, D., and J. Delacour (1968). Notions anatomo-physiologiques sur les voies et les centres d'intégration des messages douloureux. *J. Psychol. norm. path. 65,* 1–44.

Albe-Fessard, D., G. Guiot, Y. Lamarre, and G. Arfel (1966). Activation of thalamocortical projections related to tremorogenic processes. In *The Thalamus* (D. P. Purpura and M. D. Yahr, eds.), pp. 237–249. Columbia Univ. Press, New York.

Albe-Fessard, D., and J. Liebeskind (1966). Origine des messages somato-sensitifs activant les cellules du cortex moteur chez le singe. *Exp. Brain Res. 1,* 127–246.

Albe-Fessard, D., J. Massion, R. Hall and W. Rosenblith (1964). Modifications au cour de la veille et du sommeil des valeurs moyennes de réponses nerveuses centrales induites par des stimulations somatiques chez le Chat libre. *C. R. Acad. Sci. (Paris) 258,* 353–356.

Alema, G., L. Perria, G. Rosadini, G. F. Rossi, and J. Zattoni (1966). Functional inactivation of the human brain stem related to the level of consciousness. *J. Neurosurg. 24,* 629–639.

Alema, G., and G. Rosadini (1964). Données cliniques et EEG de l'introduction de'amytal sodium dans la circulation encephalique concernant l'état de conscience. *Acta Neurochir. 12,* 240–257.

Alexander, L. (1942a). The vascular supply of the strio-pallidum. *Res. Publ. Ass. Res. nerv. ment. Dis. 21,* 77–132.

Alexander, L. (1942b). The fundamental types of histopathological changes encountered in cases of athetosis and paralysis agitans. *Res. Publ. Ass. Res. nerv. ment. Dis. 21,* 334–493.

Alexander, R. S. (1946). Tonic and reflex functions of medullary sympathetic cardiovascular centers. *J. Neurophysiol. 9,* 205–217.

Alexander, W. F. (1940). The innervation of the biliary system. *J. comp. Neurol. 72,* 357–370.

Alksne, J. F., T. W. Blackstad, F. Walberg, and L. E. White, Jr. (1966). Electron microscopy of axon degeneration: A valuable tool in experimental neuroanatomy. *Ergebn. Anat. Entwickl.-Gesch. 39,* 1–32.

Allen, W. F. (1940). Effect of ablating the frontal lobes, hippocampi and occipito-parieto-temporal (excepting pyriform areas) lobes on positive and negative olfactory conditioned reflexes. *Am. J. Physiol. 128,* 754–771.

Allen, W. F. (1941). Effect of ablating the pyriform-amygdaloid areas and hippocampi on positive and negative olfactory conditioned reflexes and on conditioned olfactory differentiation. *Am. J. Physiol. 132,* 81–91.

Allen, M. W. Van (1967). Transient recurring paralysis of ocular abduction. A syndrome of intracranial hypertension. *Arch. Neurol. (Chic.) 17,* 81–88.

Allison, A. C. (1953a). The structure of the olfactory bulb and its relationship to the olfactory pathways in the rabbit and the rat. *J. comp. Neurol. 98,* 309–353.

Allison, A. C. (1953b). The morphology of the olfactory system in the vertebrates. *Biol. Rev. 28,* 195–244.

ALLISON, A. C. (1954). The secondary olfactory areas in the human brain. *J. Anat.* (*Lond.*) *88*, 481–488.

ALLISON, A. C., and R. T. T. WARWICK (1949). Quantitative observations on the olfactory system of the rabbit. *Brain 72*, 186–197.

ALNÆS, E., J. K. S. JANSEN, and T. RUDJORD (1965). Fusimotor activity in the spinal cat. *Acta physiol. scand. 63*, 197–212.

ALPERS, B. J. (1942). Partial paralysis of upward gaze. *Confin. neurol.* (*Basel*) *5*, 1–12.

ALTMAN, J. (1962). Some fiber projections to the superior colliculus in the cat. *J. comp. Neurol. 119*, 77–95.

ALTMAN, J., and M. B. CARPENTER (1961). Fiber projections of the superior colliculus in the cat. *J. comp. Neurol. 116*, 157–178.

AMASSIAN, V. E. (1961). Microelectrode studies of the cerebral cortex. *Int. Rev. Neurobiol. 3*, 67–136.

AMASSIAN, V. E., and R. V. DE VITO (1954). Unit activity in reticular formation and nearby structures. *J. Neurophysiol. 17*, 575–603.

AMOORE, J. E., J. W. JOHNSTON JR., and M. RUBIN (1964). The stereochemical theory of odor. *Scientific Amer. 210*, 42–49.

ı.MOORE, J. E. and D. VENSTROM (1967). Correlations between stereochemical assessments and organoleptic analysis of odorus compounds. In *Olfaction and Taste II*. Proceedings Second International Symposium Tokyo 1965, pp. 3–17. Pergamon Press, Oxford.

ANDERSEN, P. (1960). Interhippocampal impulses. IV. A correlation of functional and structural properties of the interhippocampal fibres in cat, rabbit and rat. *Acta physiol. scand. 48*, 329–351.

ANDERSEN, P. (1966). Correlation of structural design with function in the archicortex. In *Brain and Conscious Experience* (J. C. Eccles, ed.), pp. 59–84. Springer-Verlag, Berlin.

ANDERSEN, P., and S. A. ANDERSSON (1968). *The Physiological Basis of the Alpha Rhythm.* Appleton-Century-Crofts, New York.

ANDERSEN, P., T. W. BLACKSTAD, and T.LØMO (1966). Location and identification of excitatory synapses on hippocampal pyramidal cells. *Exp. Brain Res. 1*, 236–248.

ANDERSEN, P., C. McC. BROOKS, J. C. ECCLES, and T. A. SEARS (1964). The ventro-basal nucleus of the thalamus: Potential fields, synaptic transmission and excitability of both presynaptic and post-synaptic components. *J. Physiol.* (*Lond.*) *174*, 348–369.

ANDERSEN, P., H. BRULAND, and B. R. KAADA (1961). Activation of the field CAI of the hippocampus by septal stimulation. *Acta physiol. scand. 51*, 29–40.

ANDERSEN, P., J. C. ECCLES, and Y. LØYNING (1964a). Location of postsynaptic inhibitory synapses on hippocampal pyramids. *J. Neurophysiol. 27*, 592–607.

ANDERSEN, P., J. C. ECCLES, and Y. LØYNING (1964b). Pathway of postsynaptic inhibition in the hippocampus. *J. Neurophysiol. 27*, 608–619.

ANDERSEN, P., J. C. ECCLES, R. F. SCHMIDT, and T. YOKOTA (1964a). Depolarization of presynaptic fibers in the cuneate nucleus. *J. Neurophysiol. 27*, 92–106.

ANDERSEN, P., J. C. ECCLES, R. F. SCHMIDT, and T. YOKOTA (1964b). Identification of relay cells and interneurons in the cuneate nucleus. *J. Neurophysiol. 27*, 1080–1095.

ANDERSEN, P., J. C. ECCLES, and T. A. SEARS (1964a). Cortically evoked de-

References

polarization of primary afferents fibers in the spinal cord. *J. Neurophysiol. 27,* 63–77.

ANDERSEN, P., J. C. ECCLES, and T. A. SEARS (1964b). The ventro-basal complex of the thalamus: types of cells, their responses and their functional organization. *J. Physiol. (Lond.) 174,* 370–399.

ANDERSEN, P., B. HOLMQVIST, and P. E. VOORHOEVE (1966). Excitatory synapses on hippocampal apical dendrites activated by entorhinal stimulation. *Acta physiol. scand. 66,* 461–472.

ANDERSEN, P., and T. LØMO (1965). Excitation of hippocampal pyramidal cells by dendritic synapses. *J. Physiol. (Lond.) 181,* 39–40P.

ANDERSON, F. D. (1963). The structure of a chronically isolated segment of the cat spinal chord. *J. comp. Neurol. 120,* 279–316.

ANDERSON, F. D., and C. M. BERRY (1959). Degeneration studies of long ascending fiber systems in the cat brain stem. *J. comp. Neurol. 111,* 195–229.

ANDERSSON, B. (1957). Polydipsia, antidiuresis and milk ejection caused by hypothalamic stimulation. In *Neurohypophysis* (H. Heller, ed.), pp. 131–140. Butterworths Scientific Publications, London.

ANDERSSON, S. A. (1962). Projection of different spinal pathways to the second somatic sensory area in cat. *Acta physiol. scand. 56, Suppl. 194,* 1–74.

ANDERSSON, S., and B. E. GERNANDT (1954). Cortical projection of vestibular nerve in cat. *Acta oto-laryng. (Stockh.) Suppl. 116,* 10–18.

ANDERSSON, S., and B. E. GERNANDT (1956). Ventral root discharge in response to vestibular and proprioceptive stimulation. *J. Neurophysiol. 19,* 524–543.

ANDRES, K. H. (1961). Untersuchungen über morphologische Veränderungen in Spinalganglien während der retrograden Degeneration. *Z. Zellforsch. 55,* 49–79.

ANDRES, K. H. (1965). Der Feinbau des Bulbus olfactorius der Ratte unter besonderer Berücksichtigung der synaptischen Verbindungen. *Z. Zellforsch. 65,* 530–561.

ANDREW, J., and P. W. NATHAN (1964). Lesions of the anterior frontal lobes and disturbances of micturition and defæcation. *Brain 87,* 233–262.

ANGAUT, P., and A. BRODAL (1967). The projection of the "vestibulocerebellum" onto the vestibular nuclei in the cat. *Arch. ital. Biol. 105,* 441–479.

ANGEL, R. W., and W. W. HOFMANN (1963). The H reflex in normal, spastic, and rigid subjects. *Arch. Neurol. (Chic.) 8,* 591–596.

ANGEVINE, J. B., JR. (1965). Time of neuron origin in the hippocampal region. An autoradiographic study in the mouse. *Exp. Neurol. Suppl. 2,* 1–70.

ANGEVINE, J. B., JR., S. LOCKE, and P. I. YAKOVLEV (1962). Limbic nuclei of thalamus and connections of limbic cortex. IV. Thalamocortical projection of the ventral anterior nucleus in man. *Arch. Neurol. (Chic.) 7,* 518–528.

ANGEVINE, J. B., JR., E. L. MANCALL, and P. I. YAKOVLEV (1961). *The Human Cerebellum. An Atlas of Gross Topography in Serial Sections.* J. & A. Churchill, Ltd., London.

APPELBERG, B., and I. Z. KOSARY (1963). Excitation of flexor fusimotor neurons by electrical stimulation in the red nucleus. *Acta physiol. scand. 59,* 445–453.

APTER, J. T. (1945). Projection of the retina on superior colliculus of cats. *J. Neurophysiol. 8,* 123–134.

APTER, J. T. (1946). Eye movements following strychninization of the superior colliculus of cats. *J. Neurophysiol. 9,* 73–86.

AREY, L. B., and M. GORE (1942). The numerical relation between the ganglion cells of the retina and the fibers in the optic nerve of the dog. *J. comp. Neurol. 77,* 609–617.

ARING, C. D. (1944). Clinical symptomatology. In *The Precentral Motor Cortex* (P. C. Bucy, ed.), pp. 409–423. Univ. of Illinois Press, Urbana, Illinois.

ARING, C. D., and J. F. FULTON (1936). Relation of the cerebrum to the cerebellum. II. Cerebellar tremor in the monkey and its absence after removal of the principal excitable areas of the cortex (areas 4 and 6a, upper part). III. Accentuation of cerebellar tremor following lesions of the premotor area (area 6a, upper part). *Arch. Neurol. Psychiat. (Chic.) 35,* 439–463.

ARMSTRONG, J., K. C. RICHARDSON, and J. Z. YOUNG (1956). Staining neural end feet and mitochondria after postchroming and carbowax embedding. *Stain Technol. 31,* 263–270.

ARTHUR, R. P., and W. B. SHELLEY (1959). The peripheral mechanism of itch in man. In *Pain and Itch. Nervous Mechanisms.* Ciba Foundation Study Group, No. 1 (G. E. W. Wolstenholme and M. O'Connor, eds.), pp. 84–95. J. & A. Churchill, London.

ASANUMA, H., and H. SAKATA (1967). Functional organization of a cortical efferent system examined with focal depth stimulation in cats. *J. Neurophysiol. 30,* 35–54.

ASCHAN, G. (1958). Different types of alcohol nystagmus. *Acta oto-laryng. (Stockh.) Suppl. 140,* 69–78.

ASCHAN, G. (1964). Nystagmography and caloric testing. In *Neurological Aspects of Auditory and Vestibular Disorders* (W. S. Fields and B. R. Alford, eds.), pp. 216–246. Charles C Thomas, Springfield, Illinois.

ASCHAN, G., M. BERGSTEDT, and L. GOLDBERG (1964). Positional alcohol nystagmus in patients with unilateral and bilateral labyrinthine destructions. *Confin. neurol. (Basel) 24,* 80–102.

ASCHAN, G., M. BERGSTEDT, and J. STAHLE (1956). Nystagmography. Recording of nystagmus in clinical neuro-otological examinations. *Acta oto-laryng. (Stockh.) Suppl. 129,* 1–103.

ASCHAN, G., L. EKVALL, and G. GRANT (1964). Nystagmus following stimulation in the central vestibular pathways using permanently implanted electrodes. International Vestibular Symposium, Uppsala, 1963. *Acta oto-laryng. (Stockh.) Suppl. 192,* 63–77.

Aspects of Cerebellar Anatomy (1954). (J. Jansen and A. Brodal, eds.). Johan Grundt Tanum Forlag, Oslo.

BACH, L. M. N. (1952). Relationships between bulbar respiratory, vasomotor and somatic facilitatory and inhibitory areas. *Amer. J. Physiol. 171,* 417–435.

BACH-Y-RITA, P., and F. ITO (1966). Properties of stretch receptors in cat extraocular muscles. *J. Physiol. (Lond.) 186,* 663–688.

BAILEY, P., G. VON BONIN, H. W. GAROL, and W. S. McCULLOCH (1943). Functional organization of temporal lobe of monkey (*Macaca mulatta*) and chimpanzee (*Pan satyrus*). *J. Neurophysiol. 6,* 121–128.

BAILEY, P., and H. CUSHING (1925). Medulloblastoma cerebelli: a common type of midcerebellar glioma of childhood. *Arch. Neurol. Psychiat. (Chic.) 14,* 192–223.

BAKER, A. B., S. CORNWELL, and I. A. BROWN (1952). Poliomyelitis. VI. The hypothalamus. *Arch. Neurol. Psychiat. (Chic.) 68,* 16–36.

BAKER, A. B., H. A. MATZKE, and J. R. BROWN (1950). Poliomyelitis. III. Bulbar

References

poliomyelitis, a study of medullary function. *Arch. Neurol. Psychiat. (Chic.)* 63, 257–281.

BAKER, G. S., and F. W. L. KERR (1963). Structural changes in the trigeminal system following compression procedures. *J. Neurosurg. 20,* 181–184.

BALCHUM, O. J., and H. M. WEAVER (1943). Pathways for pain from the stomach of the dog. *Arch. Neurol. Psychiat. (Chic.) 49,* 739–753.

BALLESTEROS, M. L. F., F. BUCHTHAL, and P. ROSENFALCK (1965). The pattern of muscular activity during the arm swing of natural walking. *Acta physiol. scand. 63,* 296–310.

BALTHASAR, K. (1952). Morphologie der spinalen Tibialis- und Peronaeus-Kerne bei der Katze: Topographie, Architektonik, Axon- und Dendritenverlauf der Motoneurone und Zwischenneurone in den Segmenten L$_6$-S$_2$. *Arch. Psychiat. Nervenkr. 188,* 345–378.

BAN, T., and F. OMUKAI (1959). Experimental studies on the fiber connections of the amygdaloid nuclei in the rabbit. *J. comp. Neurol. 113,* 245–279.

BAN, T., and K. ZYO (1962). Experimental studies on the fiber connections of the rhinencephalon. I. Albino rat. *Med. J. Osaka Univ. 12,* 385–424.

BARBIZET, J. (1963). Defect of memorizing of hippocampal-mammilary origin: a review. *J. Neurol. Neurosurg. Psychiat. 26,* 127–135.

BARD, PH. (1928). A diencephalic mechanism for the expression of rage with special reference to the sympathetic nervous system. *Amer. J. Physiol. 84,* 490–515.

BARD, PH., and D. McK. RIOCH (1937). A study of four cats deprived of neocortex and additional portions of the forebrain. *Bull. Johns Hopk. Hosp. 60,* 73–147.

BARGMANN, W. (1949). Über die neurosekretorische Verknüpfung von Hypothalamus und Neurohypophyse. *Z. Zellforsch. 34,* 610–634.

BARGMANN, W. (1954). *Das Zwischenhirnhypophysensystem.* Springer-Verlag, Berlin.

BARGMANN, W., and A. KNOOP (1957). Elektronenmikroskopische Beobachtungen an der Neurohypophyse. *Z. Zellforsch. 46,* 242–251.

BARKER, D. (1948). The innervation of the muscle-spindle. *Quart. J. micr. Sci. 89,* 143–186.

BARKER, D. (1962). The structure and distribution of muscle receptors. In *Symposium on Muscle Receptors* (D. Barker, ed.), pp. 227–240. Hong Kong Univ. Press; Oxford Univ. Press, London.

BARKER, D. (1966). The motor innervation of the muscle spindle. In *Nobel Symposium I: Muscular Afferents and Motor Control* (R. Granit, ed.), pp. 51–58. Almqvist & Wiksell, Stockholm; John Wiley & Sons, New York.

BARNARD, J. W. (1936). A phylogenetic study of the visceral afferent areas associated with the facial, glossopharyngeal and vagus nerves, and their fiber connexions. The efferent facial nucleus. *J. comp. Neurol. 65,* 503–602.

BARNARD, J. W. (1940). The hypoglossal complex of vertebrates. *J. comp. Neurol. 72,* 489–524.

BARNARD, J. W., and C. N. WOOLSEY (1956). A study of localization in the cortico-spinal tracts of monkey and rat. *J. comp. Neurol. 105,* 25–50.

BARNARD, J. W., C. N. WOOLSEY, and R. A. LENDE (1953). Localization in the cortico-spinal tract. (Abstract.) *Anat. Rec. 115,* 279.

BARNES, W. T., H. W. MAGOUN, and S. W. RANSON (1943). The ascending auditory pathway in the brain-stem of the monkey. *J. comp. Neurol. 79,* 129–152.

BARNHART, M., R. RHINES, J. C. McCARTER, and H. W. MAGOUN (1948). Distribu-

695

tion of lesions of the brain stem in poliomyelitis. *Arch. Neurol. Psychiat. (Chic.) 59*, 368–377.

BARRIS, R. W. (1936). A pupillo-constrictor area in the cerebral cortex of the cat and its relationship to the pretectal area. *J. comp. Neurol. 63*, 353–368.

BARRIS, R. W., W. R. INGRAM, and S. W. RANSON (1935). Optic connexions of the midbrain and thalamus of the cat. *J. comp. Neurol. 62*, 117–153.

BARRON, D. H. (1936). A note on the course of the proprioceptor fibers from the tongue. *Anat. Rec. 66*, 11–15.

BATES, J. A. V. (1953). A comparison between movements produced by stimulation of the motor cortex and the internal capsule in the same individual. *J. Physiol. (Lond.) 123*, 49–50P.

BATES, J. A. V. (1957). Observations on the excitable cortex in man. *Lect. sci. Basis Med. 5*, 333–347.

BATES, J. A. V. (1960). The individuality of the motor cortex. *Brain 83*, 654–667.

BATES, J. A. V. (1963). The significance of complex motor patterns in the response to cortical stimulation. *Int. J. Neurol. (Montevideo) 4*, 92–99.

BATES, J. A. V., and G. ETTLINGER (1960). Posterior biparietal ablations in the monkey. Changes to neurological and behavioral testing. *Arch. Neurol. (Chic.) 3*, 177–192.

BATINI, C., F. MAGNI, M. PALESTINI, G. F. ROSSI, and A. ZANCHETTI (1959). Neural mechanisms underlying the enduring EEG and behavioral activation in the midpontine pretrigeminal cat. *Arch. ital. Biol. 97*, 13–25.

BATINI, C., G. MORUZZI, and O. POMPEIANO (1957). Cerebellar release phenomena. *Arch. ital. Biol. 95*, 71–95.

BATINI, C., and O. POMPEIANO (1958). Effects of rostro-medial and rostro-lateral fastigial lesions on decerebrate rigidity. *Arch. ital. Biol. 96*, 315–329.

BEATTY, R. A., O. SUGAR, and T. A. FOX (1968). Protrusion of the posterior longitudinal ligament simulating herniated lumbar intervertebral disc. *J. Neurol. Neurosurg. Psychiat. 31*, 61–66.

BECK, E. (1950). The origin, course and termination of the prefronto-pontine tract in the human brain. *Brain 73*, 368–391.

BECK, E., and A. BIGNAMI (1968). Some neuro-anatomical observations in cases with stereotactic lesions for the relief of Parkinsonism. *Brain 91*, 589–618.

BENDER, M. B., and E. A. WEINSTEIN (1944). Effects of stimulation and lesion of the medial longitudinal fasciculus in the monkey. *Arch. Neurol. Psychiat. (Chic.) 52*, 106–113.

BENJAMIN, R. M. (1962). Some thalamic and cortical mechanisms of taste. In *Olfaction and Taste*. Proceedings First International Symposium Wenner-Gren Center 1962 (Y. Zotterman, ed.), pp. 309–329. Pergamon Press, Oxford.

BENJAMIN, R. M., and K. AKERT (1959). Cortical and thalamic areas involved in taste discrimination in the albino rat. *J. comp. Neurol. 111*, 231–259.

BENJAMIN, R. M., R. EMMERS, and A. J. BLOMQUIST (1968). Projection of tongue afferents to somatic sensory area I in squirrel monkey *(Saimiri sciureus)*. *Brain Research 7*, 208–210.

BENJAMIN, R. M., and W. I. WELKER (1957). Somatic receiving areas of cerebral cortex of squirrel monkey *(Saimiri sciureus)*. *J. Neurophysiol. 20*, 286–299.

BENSON, D. F., and N. GESCHWIND (1967). Shrinking retrograde amnesia. *J. Neurol. Neurosurg. Psychiat. 30*, 539–544.

BERGMANS, J., and S. GRILLNER (1968). Monosynaptic control of static α-motoneurones from the lower brain stem. *Experientia (Basel) 24*, 146–147.

References

BERKE, J. J. (1960). The claustrum, the external capsule and the extreme capsule of *Macaca mulatta. J. comp. Neurol. 115,* 297–331.

BERNHARD, C. G., E. BOHM, and I. PETERSEN (1953). Investigation on the organization of the cortico-spinal system in monkeys. *Acta physiol. scand. 29,* 79–103.

BERTRAND, C., and S. N. MARTINEZ (1962). Localization of lesions, mostly with regard to tremor and rigidity. *Confin. neurol. (Basel) 22,* 274–282.

BERTRAND, G. (1956). Spinal efferent pathways from the supplementary motor area. *Brain 79,* 461–473.

BERTRAND, G., H. JASPER, and A. WONG (1967). Microelectrode study of the human thalamus: Functional organization in the ventro-basal complex. *Confin. neurol. (Basel) 29,* 81–86.

BESSOU, P., and Y. LAPORTE (1962). Responses from primary and secondary endings of the same neuromuscular spindle of the tenuissimus muscle of the cat. In *Symposium on Muscle Receptors* (D. Barker, ed.), pp. 105–119. Hong Kong Univ. Press; Oxford Univ. Press, London.

BETTAG, W., and T. YOSHIDA (1960). Über stereotaktische Schmerzoperationen. *Acta neurochir. (Wien) 8,* 299–317.

BILLINGSLEY, P. R., and S. W. RANSON (1918). On the number of nerve cells in the ganglion cervicale superius and of nerve fibers in the cephalic end of the truncus sympathicus in the cat, and on the numerical relations of preganglionic and postganglionic neurons. *J. comp. Neurol. 29,* 359–366.

BISHOP, P. O. (1953). Synaptic transmission. An analysis of the electrical activity of the lateral geniculate nucleus in the cat after optic nerve stimulation. *Proc. roy. Soc. B 141,* 362–392.

BJÖRK, A., and E. KUGELBERG (1953a). Motor unit activity in the human extraocular muscles. *Electroenceph. clin. Neurophysiol. 5,* 271–278.

BJÖRK, A., and E. KUGELBERG (1953b). The electrical activity of the muscles of the eye and eyelids in various positions and during movement. *Electroenceph. clin. Neurophysiol. 5,* 595–602.

BJÖRKMAN, A., and G. WOHLFART (1936). Faseranalyse der Nn. oculomotorius, trochlearis und abducens des Menschen und des N. abducens verschiedener Tiere. *Z. mikr.-anat. Forsch. 39,* 631–647.

BLACKSTAD, T. W. (1956). Commissural connections of the hippocampal region in the rat, with special reference to their mode of termination. *J. comp. Neurol. 105,* 417–537.

BLACKSTAD, T. W. (1958). On the termination of some afferents to the hippocampus and fascia dentata. *Acta anat. (Basel) 35,* 202–214.

BLACKSTAD, T. W. (1967). Cortical grey matter. A correlation of light and microscopic data. In *The Neuron* (H. Hydén, ed.), pp. 49–118. Elsevier Publishing Co., Amsterdam.

BLACKSTAD, T., A. BRODAL, and F. WALBERG (1951). Some observations on normal and degenerating terminal boutons in the inferior olive of the cat. *Acta anat. (Basel) 11,* 461–477.

BLACKSTAD, T. W., and P. R. FLOOD (1963). Ultrastructure of hippocampal axosomatic synapses. *Nature (Lond.) 198,* 542–543.

BLACKSTAD, T. W., and Å. KJAERHEIM (1961). Special axo-dendritic synapses in the hippocampal cortex: Electron and light microscopic studies on the layer of mossy fibers. *J. comp. Neurol. 117,* 133–159.

BLAKESLEE, G. A., I. S. FREIMAN, and S. E. BARRERA (1938). The nucleus lateralis medullae. An experimental study of its anatomic connections in *Macacus rhesus. Arch. Neurol. Psychiat. (Chic.) 39,* 687–704.

BLOMQUIST, A. J., R. M. BENJAMIN, and R. EMMERS (1962). Thalamic localization of afferents from the tongue in squirrel monkeys (*Saimiri sciureus*). *J. comp. Neurol. 118,* 77–87.

BLOMQUIST, A. J., and C. A. LORENZINI (1965). Projection of dorsal roots and sensory nerves to cortical sensory motor regions of squirrel monkey. *J. Neurophysiol. 28,* 1195–1205.

BODIAN, D. (1937). An experimental study of the optic tracts and retinal projection of the Virginia opossum. *J. comp. Neurol. 66,* 113–144.

BODIAN, D. (1942). Studies on the diencephalon of the Virginia opossum. III. The thalamocortical projection. *J. comp. Neurol. 77,* 525–575.

BODIAN, D. (1946). Spinal projections of brainstem in rhesus monkey, deduced from retrograde chromatolysis. (Abstract.) *Anat. Rec. 94,* 512–513.

BODIAN, D. (1947). Nucleic acid in nerve-cell regeneration. In *Nucleic Acid, Symp. Soc. exp. Biol. (N.Y.) 1,* 163–178.

BODIAN, D. (1949). Poliomyelitis: Pathologic anatomy. In *Poliomyelitis. Papers and Discussions Presented at the First International Poliomyelitis Conference,* pp. 62–84. J. B. Lippincott Co., Philadelphia.

BODIAN, D. (1951). Nerve endings, neurosecretory substance and lobular organization of the neurohypophysis. *Bull. Johns Hopk. Hosp. 89,* 354–376.

BODIAN, D. (1963). Cytological aspects of neurosecretion in opossum neurohypophysis. *Bull. Johns Hopk. Hosp. 113,* 57–93.

BODIAN, D. (1964). An electron-microscopic study of the monkey spinal cord. I. Fine structure of normal motor column. II. Effects of retrograde chromatolysis. III. Cytologic effects of mild and virulent poliovirus infection. *Bull. Johns Hopk. Hosp. 114,* 13–119.

BODIAN, D. (1966). Herring bodies and neuro-apocrine secretion in the monkey. An electron microscopic study of the fate of the neurosecretory product. *Bull. Johns Hopk. Hosp. 118,* 282–326.

BODIAN, D., and R. C. MELLORS (1944). Phosphatase activity in chromatolytic nerve cells. *Proc. Soc. exp. Biol. (N.Y.) 55,* 243–245.

BOGAERT, L. VAN, and I. BERTRAND (1932). Étude anatomo-clinique d'un syndrome alterne du noyau rouge avec mouvements involontaires rythmés de l'hémiface et de l'avant-bras. *Rev. neurol. 1,* 38–45.

BOGUSLAWSKI, S., S. BANACH, and M. DABROWSKI (1960). Clinical and statistical evaluation of the results obtained by sympathectomy in 285 cases of various peripheral vascular diseases. *J. Neurosurg. 17,* 824–829.

BOHM, E. (1953). An electro-physiological study of the ascending spinal anterolateral fibre system connected to coarse cutaneous afferents. *Acta physiol. scand. 29, Suppl. 106:8,* 1–35.

BOHM, E., and R. R. STRANG (1962). Glossopharyngeal neuralgia. *Brain 85,* 371–388.

BOK, S. T. (1922). Die Entwicklung von Reflexen und Reflexbahnen. II. Die Ontogenese des Rückenmarkreflexapparates mit den zentralen Verhältnissen des Nervus sympathicus. *Psychiat. neurol. Bl. (Amst.) 26,* 174–233.

BOLK, L. (1906). *Das Cerebellum der Säugetiere.* De Erven F. Bohn, Haarlem; G. Fischer, Jena.

BONIN, G. VON (1944). Architecture of the precentral motor cortex and some adjacent areas. In *The Precentral Motor Cortex* (P. C. Bucy, ed.), pp. 7–82. Univ. of Illinois Press, Urbana.

BONNEVIE, K. (1943). Hereditary hydrocephalus in the house mouse. I. Manifestation of the *hy*-mutation after birth in embryos 12 days old or more. *Skr. Norske Vidensk.-Akad., I. Mat.-nat. Kl.* No. 4.

BONNEVIE, K., and A. BRODAL (1946). Hereditary hydrocephalus in the house mouse. IV. The development of the cerebellar anomalies during foetal life with notes on the normal development of the mouse cerebellum. *Skr. Norske Vidensk.-Akad., I. Mat.-nat. Kl.* No. 4.

BOTTERELL, E. H., and J. F. FULTON (1938). Functional localization in the cerebellum of primates. *J. comp. Neurol. 69,* 31–46, 47–62, and 63–87.

BOWSHER, D. (1957). Termination of the central pain pathway in man: The conscious appreciation of pain. *Brain 80,* 606–622.

BOWSHER, D. (1958). Projection of the gracile and cuneate nuclei in Macaca mulatta: an experimental degeneration study. *J. comp. Neurol. 110,* 135–156.

BOWSHER, D. (1961). The termination of secondary somatosensory neurons within the thalamus of *Macaca mulatta:* An experimental degeneration study. *J. comp. Neurol. 117,* 213–227.

BOWSHER, D. (1962). The topographical projection of fibres from the anterolateral quadrant of the spinal cord to the subdiencephalic brain stem in man. *Psychiat. et Neurol. (Basel) 143,* 75–99.

BOWSHER, D., and P. ANGAUT (1968). Ascending projections from the red nucleus in the decerebellate cat. *Experientia (Basel) 24,* 262–263.

BOYD, I. A. (1962). The structure and innervation of the nuclear bag muscle fibre system and the nuclear chain muscle fibre system in mammalian muscle spindles. *Phil. Trans. B 245,* 81–136.

BOYD, J. D. (1937). Observations on the human carotid sinus and its nerve supply. *Anat. Anz. 84,* 386–399.

BOYD, J. D. (1941). The sensory component of the hypoglossal nerve in the rabbit. *J. Anat. (Lond.) 75,* 330–344.

BRADLEY, P. B., B. N. DHAWAN, and J. H. WOLSTENCROFT (1964). Some pharmacological properties of cholinoceptive neurones in the medulla and pons of the cat. *J. Physiol. (Lond.) 170,* 59–60P.

BRADLEY, P. B., and J. H. WOLSTENCROFT (1962). Excitation and inhibition of brain-stem neurones by noradrenaline and acetylcholine. *Nature (Lond.) 196,* 840 and 873.

BRAIN, R. (1961). The neurology of language. *Brain 84,* 145–166.

BRAIN, R., and M. WILKINSON (1959). Observations on the extensor plantar reflex and its relationship to the functions of the pyramidal tract. *Brain 82,* 297–320.

BRAIN, W. R. (1965). *Speech Disorders. Aphasia, Apraxia, and Agnosia,* 2nd. ed. Butterworths, London.

Brain and Conscious Experience (1966). (J. C. Eccles, ed.). Springer-Verlag, Berlin.

Brain Mechanisms and Consciousness (1954). CIOMS Symposium (J. F. Delafresnaye, ed.). Blackwell Scientific Publ., Oxford.

Brain Mechanisms and Learning (1961). CIOMS Symposium (J. F. Delafresnaye, ed.). Blackwell Scientific Publ., Oxford.

Brain Mechanisms Underlying Speech and Language (1967). Proceedings of a conference held at Princeton, New Jersey, November 9–12, 1965 (C. H. Millikan and F. L. Darley, eds.). Grune and Stratton, New York.

BRAITENBERG, V., and R. P. ATWOOD (1958). Morphological observations on the cerebellar cortex. *J. comp. Neurol. 109,* 1–33.

BREIG, A. (1960). *Biomechanics of the Central Nervous System. Some Basic Normal and Pathologic Phenomena.* The Year Book Publishers, Inc., Chicago, Illinois.

BREMER, F. (1935a). Cerveau isolé et physiologie du sommeil. *C. R. Soc. Biol. (Paris) 118,* 1235–1242.

BREMER, F. (1935b). Le cervelet. In *Traité de physiologie normale et pathologique,* Vol. *10: Physiologie nerveuse* (G. H. Roger and L. Binet, eds.), pt. 1–2. Masson & Cie., Paris.

BREMER, F., and R. S. DOW (1939). The acoustic area of the cerebral cortex of the cat. A combined oscillographic and cyto-architectonic study. *J. Neurophysiol. 2,* 308–318.

BRIDGMAN, C. S., and K. U. SMITH (1945). Bilateral neural integration in visual perception after section of the corpus callosum. *J. comp. Neurol. 83,* 57–68.

BRINDLEY, G. S., and P. A. MERTON (1960). The absence of position sense in the human eye. *J. Physiol. (Lond.) 153,* 127–130.

BRION, S., and G. GUIOT (1964). Topographie des faisceaux de projection du cortex dans la capsule interne et dans le pédoncule cérébral. Étude des dégénérescences secondaires dans la sclérose latérale amyotrophique et la maladie de Pick. *Rev. neurol. 110,* 123–144.

BROCKLEHURST, R. J., and F. H. EDGEWORTH (1940). The fibre components of the laryngeal nerves of *Macaca mulatta. J. Anat. (Lond.) 74,* 386–389.

BRODAL, A. (1939). Experimentelle Untersuchungen über retrograde Zellveränderungen im unteren Olive nach Läsionen des Kleinhirns. *Z. ges. Neurol. Psychiat. 166,* 624–704.

BRODAL, A. (1940a). Modification of Gudden method for study of cerebral localization. *Arch. Neurol. Psychiat. (Chic.) 43,* 46–58.

BRODAL, A. (1940b). Experimentelle Untersuchungen über die olivo-cerebellare Lokalisation. *Z. ges. Neurol. Psychiat. 169,* 1–153.

BRODAL, A. (1941). Die Verbindungen des Nucleus cuneatus externus mit dem Kleinhirn beim Kaninchen und bei der Katze. Experimentelle Untersuchungen. *Z. ges. Neurol. Psychiat. 171,* 167–199.

BRODAL, A. (1943). The cerebellar connections of the nucleus reticularis lateralis (nucleus funiculi lateralis) in the rabbit and the cat. Experimental investigations. *Acta psychiat. (Kbh.) 18,* 171–233.

BRODAL, A. (1945). Defective development of the cerebellar vermis (partial agenesis) in a child. *Skr. Norske Vidensk.-Akad., I. Mat.-nat. Kl.* No. 3.

BRODAL, A. (1947a). Central course of afferent fibers for pain in facialis, glossopharyngeal, and vagus nerves. Clinical observations. *Arch. Neurol. Psychiat. (Chic.) 57,* 292–306.

BRODAL, A. (1947b). The hippocampus and the sense of smell. A review. *Brain 70,* 179–222.

BRODAL, A. (1947c). The amygdaloid nucleus in the rat. *J. comp. Neurol. 87,* 1–16.

BRODAL, A. (1948). The origin of the fibers of the anterior commissure in the rat. Experimental studies. *J. comp. Neurol. 88,* 157–205.

BRODAL, A. (1949). Spinal afferents to the lateral reticular nucleus of the medulla oblongata in the cat. An experimental study. *J. comp. Neurol. 91,* 259–295.

References

BRODAL, A. (1952). Experimental demonstration of cerebellar connexions from the peri-hypoglossal nuclei (nucleus intercalatus, nucleus praepositus hypoglossi and nucleus of Roller) in the cat. *J. Anat. (Lond.) 86,* 110–129.

BRODAL, A. (1953). Reticulo-cerebellar connections in the cat. An experimental study. *J. comp. Neurol. 98,* 113–154.

BRODAL, A. (1956). Anatomical aspects of the reticular formation of the pons and medulla oblongata. In *Progress in Neurobiology.* (J. Ariëns Kappers, ed.) pp. 240–255. Elsevier Publishing Co., Amsterdam.

BRODAL, A. (1957). *The Reticular Formation of the Brain Stem. Anatomical Aspects and Functional Correlations.* The Henderson Trust Lecture. Oliver and Boyd, Edinburgh.

BRODAL, A. (1962). Spasticity—Anatomical aspects. *Acta neurol. scand. 38, Suppl. 3,* 9–40.

BRODAL, A. (1963). Some data and perspectives on the anatomy of the so-called "extrapyramidal system." *Acta neurol. scand. 39, Suppl. 4,* 17–38.

BRODAL, A. (1964a). Anatomical organization and fiber connections of the vestibular nuclei. In *Neurological Aspects of Auditory & Vestibular Disorders* (W. S. Fields and B. R. Alford, eds.), pp. 107–145. Charles C Thomas, Springfield, Illinois.

BRODAL, A. (1964b). Anatomical points of view on the alleged morphological basis of consciousness. *Acta neurochir. (Wien) 12,* 166–186.

BRODAL, A. (1965a). Experimental anatomical studies of the corticospinal and cortico-rubro-spinal connections in the cat. *Symp. Biol. Hung. 5,* 207–217.

BRODAL, A. (1965b). *The Cranial Nerves. Anatomy and Anatomico-Clinical Correlations,* 2nd ed. Blackwell Scientific Publ., Oxford.

BRODAL, A. (1967a). Anatomical studies of cerebellar fibre connections with special reference to problems of functional localization. In *The Cerebellum, Progress in Brain Research,* Vol. 25 (J. P. Schadé, ed.), pp. 135–173. Elsevier Publishing Co., Amsterdam.

BRODAL, A. (1967b). Anatomical organization of cerebello-vestibulo-spinal pathways. In *Myotatic, Kinesthetic and Vestibular Mechanisms.* Section III. Vestibular Mechanisms: Nervous Pathways. Ciba Foundation Symposium (A. V. D. de Reuck and Julie Knight, eds.), pp. 148–166. J. & A. Churchill, Ltd., London.

BRODAL, A., and P. ANGAUT (1967). The termination of spinovestibular fibres in the cat. *Brain Research 5,* 494–500.

BRODAL, A., S. BØYESEN, and A. G. FRØVIG (1953). Progressive neuropathic (peroneal) muscular atrophy (Charcot-Marie-Tooth Disease). *Arch. Neurol. Psychiat. (Chic.) 70,* 1–29.

BRODAL, A., and P. A. DRABLØS (1963). Two types of mossy fiber terminals in the cerebellum and their regional distribution. *J. comp. Neurol. 121,* 173–187.

BRODAL, A., and A. C. GOGSTAD (1954). Rubro-cerebellar connection. An experimental study in the cat. *Anat. Rec. 118,* 455–486.

BRODAL, A., and A. C. GOGSTAD (1957). Afferent connexions of the paramedian reticular nucleus of the medulla oblongata in the cat. An experimental study. *Acta anat. (Basel) 30,* 133–151.

BRODAL, A., and G. GRANT (1962). Morphology and temporal course of degeneration in cerebellar mossy fibers following transection of spinocerebellar tracts in the cat. An experimental study with silver methods. *Exp. Neurol. 5,* 67–87.

BRODAL, A., and E. HAUGLIE-HANSSEN (1959). Congenital hydrocephalus with

7 0 1

defective development of the cerebellar vermis (Dandy-Walker syndrome). *J. Neurol. Neurosurg. Psychiat. 22,* 99–108.

BRODAL, A., and B. HØIVIK (1964). Site and mode of termination of primary vestibulocerebellar fibres in the cat. An experimental study with silver impregnation methods. *Arch. ital. Biol. 102,* 1–21.

BRODAL, A., and J. JANSEN (1941). Beitrag zur Kenntnis der spino-cerebellaren Bahnen beim Menschem. *Anat. Anz. 91,* 185–195.

BRODAL, A., and J. JANSEN (1946). The ponto-cerebellar projection in the rabbit and cat. Experimental investigations. *J. comp. Neurol. 84,* 31–118.

BRODAL, A., and O. POMPEIANO (1957). The vestibular nuclei in the cat. *J. Anat. (Lond.) 91,* 438–454.

BRODAL, A., and O. POMPEIANO (1958). The origin of ascending fibres of the medial longitudinal fasciculus from the vestibular nuclei. An experimental study in the cat. *Acta morph. neerl.-scand. 1,* 306–328.

BRODAL, A., O. POMPEIANO, and F. WALBERG (1962). *The Vestibular Nuclei and their Connections. Anatomy and Functional Correlations.* The Henderson Trust Lectures. Oliver and Boyd, Edinburgh.

BRODAL, A., and B. REXED (1953). Spinal afferents to the lateral cervical nucleus in the cat. An experimental study. *J. comp. Neurol. 98,* 179–212.

BRODAL, A., and G. F. ROSSI (1955). Ascending fibers in brain stem reticular formation of cat. *Arch. Neurol. Psychiat. (Chic.) 74,* 68–87.

BRODAL, A., and L. F. SAUGSTAD (1965). Retrograde cellular changes in the mesencephalic trigeminal nucleus in the cat following cerebellar lesions. *Acta morph. neerl.-scand. 6,* 147–159.

BRODAL, A., T. SZABO, and A. TORVIK (1956). Corticofugal fibres to sensory trigeminal nuclei and nucleus of solitary tract. An experimental study in the cat. *J. comp. Neurol. 106,* 527–556.

BRODAL, A., E. TABER, and F. WALBERG (1960). The raphe nuclei of the brain stem in the cat. II. Efferent connections. *J. comp. Neurol. 114,* 239–259.

BRODAL, A., and A. TORVIK (1954). Cerebellar projection of paramedian reticular nucleus of medulla oblongata in cat. *J. Neurophysiol. 17,* 484–495.

BRODAL, A., and A. TORVIK (1957). Über den Ursprung der sekundären vestibulocerebellaren Fasern bei der Katze. Eine experimentell-anatomische Studie. *Arch. Psychiat. Nervenkr. 195,* 550–567.

BRODAL, A., F. WALBERG, and T. BLACKSTAD (1950). Termination of spinal afferents to inferior olive in cat. *J. Neurophysiol. 13,* 431–454.

BRODAL, A., F. WALBERG, and E. TABER (1960). The raphe nuclei of the brain stem in the cat. III. Afferent connections. *J. comp. Neurol. 114,* 261–281.

BRODAL, P. (1968a). The corticopontine projection in the cat. I. Demonstration of a somatotopically organized projection from the primary sensorimotor cortex. *Exp. Brain Res. 5,* 212–237.

BRODAL, P. (1968b). The corticopontine projection in the cat. II. Demonstration of a somatotopically organized projection from the second somatosensory cortex. *Arch. ital. Biol. 106,* 310–332.

BRODAL, P., J. MARSALA, and A. BRODAL (1967). The cerebral cortical projection to the lateral reticular nucleus in the cat, with special reference to the sensorimotor cortical areas. *Brain Research 6,* 252–274.

BRODMANN, K. (1909). *Vergleichende Lokalisationslehre der Grosshirnrinde.* J. A. Barth, Leipzig.

702

References

BRODY, H. (1955). Organization of the cerebral cortex. III. A study of aging in the human cerebral cortex. *J. comp. Neurol. 102,* 511–556.

BROOKE, R. N. L., J. DE C. DOWNER, and T. P. S. POWELL (1965). Centrifugal fibres to the retina in the monkey and cat. *Nature (Lond.) 207,* 1365–1367.

BROUWER, B., and W. P. C. ZEEMAN (1926). The projection of the retina in the primary optic neuron in the monkey. *Brain 49,* 1–35.

BROUWER, B., W. P. C. ZEEMAN, and A. W. HOUWER (1923). Experimentell-anatomische Untersuchungen über die Projektion der Retina auf die primären Opticuszentren. *Schweiz. Arch. Neurol. Psychiat. 13,* 118–138.

BROWN, J. R. (1949). Localizing cerebellar syndromes. *J. Amer. med. Ass. 141,* 518–521.

BROWN, J. W. (1967). Physiology and phylogenesis of emotional expression. *Brain Research 5,* 1–14.

BRUESCH, S. R. (1944). The distribution of myelinated afferent fibers in the branches of the cat's facial nerve. *J. comp. Neurol. 81,* 169–191.

BRUESCH, S. R., and L. B. AREY (1942). The number of myelinated and unmyelinated fibers in the optic nerve of vertebrates. *J. comp. Neurol. 77,* 631–665.

BUCHTHAL, F. (1961). The general concept of the motor unit. In *Neuromuscular Disorders, Res. Publ. Ass. nerv. ment. Dis. 38,* 3–30.

BUCHTHAL, F. (1962). The electromyogram. Its value in the diagnosis of neuromuscular disorders. *Wld Neurol. 3,* 16–34.

BUCHTHAL, F. (1965). Electromyography in paralysis of the facial nerve. *Arch. Otolaryng. 81,* 463–469.

BUCHWALD, N. A., and C. D. HULL (1967). Some problems associated with interpretation of physiological and behavioral responses to stimulation of caudate and thalamic nuclei. *Brain Research 6,* 1–11.

BUCY, P. C. (1944a). Effects of extirpation in man. In *The Precentral Motor Cortex* (P. C. Bucy, ed.), pp. 353–394. Univ. of Illinois Press. Urbana, Illinois.

BUCY, P. C. (1944b). Relation to abnormal involuntary movements. In *The Precentral Motor Cortex* (P. C. Bucy, ed.), pp. 395–408. Univ. of Illinois Press, Urbana, Illinois.

BUCY, P. C. (1957). Is there a pyramidal tract? *Brain 80,* 376–392.

BUCY, P. C., and J. E. KEPLINGER (1961). Section of the cerebral peduncles. *Arch. Neurol. (Chic.) 5,* 132–139.

BUCY, P. C., J. E. KEPLINGER, and E. B. SIQUEIRA (1964). Destruction of the "pyramidal tract" in man. *J. Neurosurg. 21,* 385–398.

BUCY, P. C., and H. KLÜVER (1955). An anatomical investigation of the temporal lobe in the monkey (*Macaca mulatta*). *J. comp. Neurol. 103,* 151–252.

BUCY, P. C., R. LADPLI, and A. EHRLICH (1966). Destruction of the pyramidal tract in the monkey. The effects of bilateral section of the cerebral peduncles. *J. Neurosurg. 25,* 1–20.

BURANDT, D. C., G. M. FRENCH, and K. AKERT (1961). Relationships between the caudate nucleus and the frontal cortex in *Macaca mulatta. Confin. Neurol. (Basel) 21,* 289–306.

BUREN, J. M. VAN, and M. BALDWIN (1958). The architecture of the optic radiation with the temporal lobe in man. *Brain 81,* 15–40.

BÜRGI, S. (1957). Das Tectum Opticum. Seine Verbindungen bei der Katze und seine Bedeutung beim Menschen. *Dtsch. Z. Nervenheilk. 176,* 701–729.

BURNSTOCK, G., and M. E. HOLMAN (1961). The transmission of excitation from autonomic nerve to smooth muscle. *J. Physiol. (Lond.) 155,* 115–133.

BUSCH, H. F. M. (1961). *An Anatomical Analysis of the White Matter in the Brain Stem of the Cat.* Van Gorcum & Co. N. V., Assen.

BUSER, P. (1966). Subcortical controls of pyramidal activity. In *The Thalamus* (D. P. Purpura and M. D. Yahr, eds.), pp. 323–347. Columbia Univ. Press, New York.

BUSKIRK, C. VAN (1945). The seventh nerve complex. *J. comp. Neurol. 82,* 303–333.

BUTLER, R. A., I. T. DIAMOND, and W. D. NEFF (1957). Role of auditory cortex in discrimination of changes in frequency. *J. Neurophysiol. 20,* 108–120.

BUXTON, D. F., and D. C. GOODMAN (1967). Motor function and the corticospinal tracts in the dog and raccoon. *J. comp. Neurol. 129,* 341–360.

BÖRNSTEIN, W. S. (1940). Cortical representation of taste in man and monkey. II. The localization of the cortical taste area in man and a method of measuring impairment of taste in man. *Yale J. Biol. Med. 13,* 133–156.

CAIRNS, H. R. (1952). Disturbances of consciousness with lesions of the brainstem and diencephalon. *Brain 75,* 109–146.

CAJAL, S. RAMON Y (1909–11). *Histologie du Système Nerveux de l'Homme et des Vertébrés.* Maloine, Paris.

CAJAL, S. RAMON Y (1954). *Neuron Theory or Reticular Theory?* (W. U. Purkiss and C. A. Fox, trans.). Consejo Superior de Investigaciones Cientificas Instituto "Ramon y Cajal," Madrid.

CALNE, D. B., and C. A. PALLIS (1966). Vibratory sense: A critical review. *Brain 89,* 723–746.

CAMMERMEYER, J. (1960). The post-mortem origin and mechanism of neuronal hyperchromatosis and nuclear pyknosis. *Exp. Neurol. 2,* 379–405.

CAMMERMEYER, J. (1962). An evaluation of the significance of the "dark" neuron. *Ergebn. Anat. Entwickl.-Gesch. 36,* 1–61.

CAMMERMEYER, J. (1963). Peripheral chromatolysis after transection of mouse facial nerve. *Acta neuropath. (Berl.) 2,* 213–230.

CAMPBELL, A. W. (1905). *Histological Studies on the Localisation of Cerebral Function.* Cambridge Univ. Press, Cambridge.

CARLI, G., K. DIETE-SPIFF, and O. POMPEIANO (1967a). Responses of the muscle spindles and of the extrafusal fibres in an extensor muscle to stimulation of the lateral vestibular nucleus in the cat. *Arch. ital. Biol. 105,* 209–242.

CARLI, G., K. DIETE-SPIFF, and O. POMPEIANO (1967b). Mechanisms of muscle spindle excitation. *Arch. ital. Biol. 105,* 273–289.

CARMAN, J. B., W. M. COWAN, and T. P. S. POWELL (1963). The organization of the cortico-striate connexions in the rabbit. *Brain 86,* 525–562.

CARMAN, J. B., W. M. COWAN, and T. P. S. POWELL (1964a). The cortical projection upon the claustrum. *J. Neurol. Neurosurg. Psychiat. 27,* 46–51.

CARMAN, J. B., W. M. COWAN, and T. P. S. POWELL (1964b). Cortical connexions of the thalamic reticular nucleus. *J. Anat. (Lond.) 98,* 587–598.

CARMAN, J. B., W. M. COWAN, T. P. S. POWELL, and K. E. WEBSTER (1965). A bilateral cortico-striate projection. *J. Neurol. Neurosurg. Psychiat. 28,* 71–77.

CARMEL, P., and A. STARR (1963). Acoustic and nonacoustic factors modifying middle-ear muscle activity in waking cats. *J. Neurophysiol. 26,* 598–616.

CARMICHAEL, E. A., M. R. DIX, and C. S. HALLPIKE (1954). Lesions of the cerebral hemispheres and their effects upon optokinetic and caloric nystagmus. *Brain 77,* 345–372.

References

CARMICHAEL, E. A., M. R. DIX, and C. S. HALLPIKE (1965). Observations upon the neurological mechanism of directional preponderance of caloric nystagmus resulting from vascular lesions of the brain stem. *Brain 88,* 51–74.

CARMICHAEL, E. A., and H. H. WOOLLARD (1933). Some observations on the fifth and seventh cranial nerves. *Brain 56,* 109–125.

CARNEY, L. R. (1967). Considerations on the cause and treatment of trigeminal neuralgia. *Neurology (Minneap.) 17,* 1143–1151.

CARPENTER, D., A. LUNDBERG, and U. NORRSELL (1963). Primary afferent depolarization evoked from the sensorimotor cortex. *Acta physiol. scand. 59,* 126–142.

CARPENTER, M. B. (1957). The dorsal trigeminal tract in the rhesus monkey. *J. Anat. (Lond.) 91,* 82–90.

CARPENTER, M. B. (1960). Experimental anatomical-physiological studies of the vestibular nerve and cerebellar connections. In *Neural Mechanisms of the Auditory and Vestibular Systems* (G. L. Rasmussen and W. Windle, eds.), pp. 279–323. Charles C Thomas, Springfield, Illinois.

CARPENTER, M. B. (1961). Brain stem and infratentorial neuraxis in experimental dyskinesia. *Arch. Neurol. (Chic.) 5,* 504–524.

CARPENTER, M. B. (1964). Ascending vestibular projections and conjugate horizontal eye movements. In *Neurological Aspects of Auditory and Vestibular Disorders* (W. S. Fields and B. R. Alford, eds.), pp. 150–189. Charles C Thomas, Springfield, Illinois.

CARPENTER, M. B., G. M. BRITTIN, and J. PINES (1958). Isolated lesions of the fastigial nuclei in the cat. *J. comp. Neurol. 109,* 65–89.

CARPENTER, M. B., and C. S. CARPENTER (1951). Analysis of somatotopic relations of the corpus Luysi in man and monkey. *J. comp. Neurol. 95,* 349–370.

CARPENTER, M. B., W. GLINSMANN, and H. FABREGA (1958). Effects of secondary pallidal and striatal lesions upon cerebellar dyskinesia in the rhesus monkey. *Neurology (Minneap.) 8,* 352–358.

CARPENTER, M. B., and G. R. HANNA (1961). Fiber projections from the spinal trigeminal nucleus in the cat. *J. comp. Neurol. 117,* 117–131.

CARPENTER, M. B., and G. R. HANNA (1962). Lesions of the medial longitudinal fasciculus in the cat. *Amer. J. Anat. 110,* 307–332.

CARPENTER, M. B., and R. E. MCMASTERS (1964). Lesions of the substantia nigra in the Rhesus monkey. Efferent fiber degeneration and behavioral observations. *Amer. J. Anat. 114,* 293–320.

CARPENTER, M. B., and F. A. METTLER (1951). Analysis of subthalamic dyskinesia in the monkey, with special reference to ablations of agranular cortex. *J. comp. Neurol. 95,* 125–158.

CARPENTER, M. B., and N. L. STROMINGER (1964). Cerebello-oculomotor fibers in the rhesus monkey. *J. comp. Neurol. 123,* 211–230.

CARPENTER, M. B., and N. L. STROMINGER (1965). The medial longitudinal fasciculus and disturbances of conjugate horizontal eye movements in the monkey. *J. comp. Neurol. 125,* 41–66.

CARPENTER, M. B., and N. L. STROMINGER (1966). Corticostriate encephalitis and paraballism in the monkey. *Arch. Neurol. (Chic.) 14,* 241–253.

CARPENTER, M. B., and N. L. STROMINGER (1967). Efferent fibers of the subthalamic nucleus in the monkey. A comparison of the efferent projections of the subthalamic nucleus, substantia nigra and globus pallidus. *Amer. J. Anat. 121,* 41–72.

CARREA, R. M. E., and F. A. METTLER (1947). Physiologic consequences following extensive removals of the cerebellar cortex and deep cerebellar nuclei and effect of secondary cerebral ablations in the primate. *J. comp. Neurol. 87,* 169–288.

CARREA, R. M. E., M. REISSIG, and F. A. METTLER (1947). The climbing fibers of the simian and feline cerebellum. Experimental inquiry into their origin by lesions of the inferior olives and deep cerebellar nuclei. *J. comp. Neurol. 87,* 321–365.

CARRERAS, M., and S. A. ANDERSSON (1963). Functional properties of neurones of the anterior ectosylvian gyrus of the cat. *J. Neurophysiol. 26,* 100–126.

CAUNA, N. (1954). Nature and functions of the papillary ridges of the digital skin. *Anat. Rec. 119,* 449–468.

CAUNA, N., and G. MANNAN (1958). The structure of human digital Pacinian corpuscles (*Corpuscula lamellosa*) and its functional significance. *J. Anat. (Lond.) 92,* 1–20.

CAWTHORNE, E. A., G. FITZGERALD, and C. S. HALLPIKE (1942). Studies in human vestibular function. II. Observations on directional preponderance of caloric nystagmus ('Nystagmusbereitschaft') resulting from unilateral labyrinthectomy. *Brain 65,* 138–160.

CELESIA, G. G. (1963). Segmental organization of cortical afferent areas in the cat. *J. Neurophysiol. 26,* 193–206.

CELESIA, G. G., R. J. BROUGHTON, T. RASMUSSEN, and C. BRANCH (1968). Auditory evoked responses from the exposed human cortex. *Electroenceph. clin. Neurophysiol. 24,* 458–466.

CERF, J. A., and L. W. CHACKO (1958). Retrograde reaction in motoneuron dendrites following ventral root section in the frog. *J. comp. Neurol. 109,* 205–219.

CHACKO, L. W. (1948). The laminar pattern of the lateral geniculate body in the primates. *J. Neurol. Neurosurg. Psychiat. 11,* 211–224.

CHAMBERS, W. W. (1947). Electrical stimulation of the interior of the cerebellum in the cat. *Amer. J. Anat. 80,* 55–93.

CHAMBERS, W. W., and C-N. LIU (1957). Cortico-spinal tract of the cat. An attempt to correlate the pattern of degeneration with deficits in reflex activity following neocortical lesions. *J. comp. Neurol. 108,* 23–55.

CHAMBERS, W. W., C-N. LIU, G. P. McCOUCH, and E. D'AQUILI (1966). Descending tracts and spinal shock in the cat. *Brain 89,* 377–390.

CHAMBERS, W. W., and J. M. SPRAGUE (1955a). Functional localization in the cerebellum. I. Organization in longitudinal cortico-nuclear zones and their contribution to the control of posture, both extrapyramidal and pyramidal. *J. comp. Neurol. 103,* 105–130.

CHAMBERS, W. W., and J. M. SPRAGUE (1955b). Functional localization in the cerebellum. II. Somatotopic organization in cortex and nuclei. *Arch. Neurol. Psychiat. (Chic.) 74,* 653–680.

CHANG, H.-T., and T. C. RUCH (1947). Topographical distribution of spinothalamic fibres in the thalamus of the spider monkey. *J. Anat. (Lond.) 81,* 150–164.

CHASE, M. H., Y. NAKAMURA, C. D. CLEMENTE, and M. B. STERMAN (1967). Afferent vagal stimulation: neurographic correlates of induced EEG synchronization and desynchronization. *Brain Research 5,* 236–249.

CHATRIAN, G. E., L. E. WHITE, JR., and C. M. SHAW (1964). EEG pattern resembling wakefulness in unresponsive decerebrate state following traumatic brain-stem infarct. *Electroenceph. clin. Neurophysiol. 16,* 285–289.

CHEATHAM, M. L., and H. A. MATZKE (1966). Descending hypothalamic medullary pathways in the cat. *J. comp. Neurol. 127,* 369–379.

CHOW, K. L. (1950). A retrograde cell degeneration study of the cortical projection field of the pulvinar in the monkey. *J. comp. Neurol. 93,* 313–340.

CHOW, K. L., and K. H. PRIBRAM (1956). Cortical projection of the thalamic ventrolateral nuclear group in monkeys. *J. comp. Neurol. 104,* 57–75.

CLARK, D. A. (1931). Muscle counts of motor units: a study in innervation ratios. *Amer. J. Physiol. 96,* 296–304.

CLARK, G., H. W. MAGOUN, and S. W. RANSON (1939). Hypothalamic regulation of body temperature. *J. Neurophysiol. 2,* 61–80.

CLARK, G., and J. W. WARD (1948). Responses elicited from the cortex of monkeys by electrical stimulation through fixed electrodes. *Brain 71,* 332–342.

CLARK, W. E. LE GROS (1926). The mammalian oculomotor nucleus. *J. Anat. (Lond.) 60,* 426–448.

CLARK, W. E. LE GROS (1936a). The termination of ascending tracts in the thalamus of the macaque monkey. *J. Anat. (Lond.) 71,* 7–40.

CLARK, W. E. LE GROS (1936b). The thalamic connections of the temporal lobe of the brain in the monkey. *J. Anat. (Lond.) 70,* 447–464.

CLARK, W. E. LE GROS (1937). The connections of the arcuate nucleus of the thalamus. *Proc. roy. Soc. B 123,* 166–176.

CLARK, W. E. LE GROS (1941a). Observations on the association fibre system of the visual cortex and the central representation of the retina. *J. Anat. (Lond.) 75,* 225–235.

CLARK, W. E. LE GROS (1941b). The laminar organisation and cell content of the lateral geniculate body in the monkey. *J. Anat. (Lond.) 75,* 419–433.

CLARK, W. E. LE GROS (1942). The cells of Meynert in the visual cortex of the monkey. *J. Anat. (Lond.) 76,* 369–375.

CLARK, W. E. LE GROS (1951). The projection of the olfactory epithelium on the olfactory bulb in the rabbit. *J. Neurol. Neurosurg. Psychiat. 14,* 1–10.

CLARK, W. E. LE GROS (1956). Observations on the structure and organization of olfactory receptors in the rabbit. *Yale J. Biol. Med. 29,* 83–95.

CLARK, W. LE GROS (1957). Inquiries into the anatomical basis of olfactory discrimination. *Proc. roy. Soc. B 146,* 299–319.

CLARK, W. E. LE GROS, J. BEATTIE, G. RIDDOCH, and N. M. DOTT (1938). *The Hypothalamus. Morphological, Functional, Clinical, and Surgical Aspects.* Oliver and Boyd, Edinburgh.

CLARK, W. E. LE GROS, and R. H. BOGGON (1933). On the connections of the anterior nucleus of the thalamus. *J. Anat. (Lond.) 67,* 215–226.

CLARK, W. E. LE GROS, and R. H. BOGGON (1935). The thalamic connections of the parietal and frontal lobes of the brain in the monkey. *Phil. Trans. B 224,* 313–359.

CLARK, W. E. LE GROS, and M. MEYER (1947). The terminal connexions of the olfactory tract in the rabbit. *Brain 70,* 304–328.

CLARK, W. E. LE GROS, and D. W. C. NORTHFIELD (1937). The cortical projection of the pulvinar in the macaque monkey. *Brain 60,* 126–142.

CLARK, W. E. LE GROS, and G. G. PENMAN (1934). The projection of the retina in the lateral geniculate body. *Proc. roy. Soc. B 114,* 291–313.

CLARK, W. E. LE GROS, and T. P. S. POWELL (1953). On the thalamo-cortical connexions of the general sensory cortex of Macaca. *Proc. roy. Soc. B 141*, 467–487.

CLARKE, A. M. (1967). Effect of the Jendrassik maneuvre on a phasic stretch reflex in normal human subjects during experimental control over supraspinal influences. *J. Neurol. Neurosurg. Psychiat. 30*, 34–42.

CLARKE, W. B., and D. BOWSHER (1962). Terminal distribution of primary afferent trigeminal fibers in the rat. *Exp. Neurol. 6*, 372–383.

CLEMENTE, C. D., and M. B. STERMAN (1963). Cortical synchronization and sleep patterns in acute restrained and chronic behaving cats induced by basal forebrain stimulations. *Electroenceph. clin. Neurophysiol. Suppl. 24*, 172–187.

COËRS, C., and A. L. WOOLF (1959). *The Innervation of Muscle. A Biopsy Study.* Blackwell Scientific Publ., Oxford.

COGAN, D. G. (1966). *Neurology of the Visual System.* Charles C Thomas, Springfield, Illinois.

COHEN, B., K. GOTO, S. SHANZER, and A. H. WEISS (1965). Eye movements induced by electrical stimulation of the cerebellum in the alert cat. *Exp. Neurol. 13*, 145–162.

COHEN, B., J.-I. SUZUKI, and M. B. BENDER (1964). Eye movements from semicircular canal nerve stimulation in the cat. *Ann. Otol. (St. Louis) 73*, 153–169.

COHEN, D., W. W. CHAMBERS, and J. M. SPRAGUE (1958). Experimental study of the efferent projections from the cerebellar nuclei to the brain stem of the cat. *J. comp. Neurol. 109*, 233–259.

COHEN, L. A. (1961). Role of eye and neck proprioceptive mechanisms in body orientation and motor coordination. *J. Neurophysiol. 24*, 1–11.

COHEN, M. J., S. LANDGREN, L. STRØM, and Y. ZOTTERMAN (1957). Cortical reception of touch and taste in the cat. A study of single cortical cells. *Acta physiol. scand. 40, Suppl. 135*, 1–50.

COLLIER, J., and E. F. BUZZARD (1901). Descending mesencephalic tracts in cat, monkey and man; Monakow's bundle; the dorsal longitudinal bundle; the ventral longitudinal bundle; the ponto-spinal tracts, lateral and ventral; the vestibulo-spinal tract; the central tegmental tract (centrale Haubenbahn); descending fibres of the fillet. *Brain 24*, 177–221.

COLLINS, W. F., JR., F. E. NULSEN, and C. T. RANDT (1960). Relation of peripheral nerve fiber size and sensation in man. *Arch. Neurol. (Chic.) 3*, 381–385.

COLONNIER, M. (1964). The tangential organization of the visual cortex. *J. Anat. (Lond.) 98*, 327–344.

COLONNIER, M. L. (1966). The structural design of the neocortex. In *Brain and Conscious Experience* (J. C. Eccles, ed.), pp. 1–18. Springer-Verlag, Berlin.

COLONNIER, M. (1967). The fine structural arrangement of the cortex. *Arch. Neurol. (Chic.) 16*, 651–657.

COLONNIER, M., and E. G. GRAY (1962). Degeneration in the cerebral cortex. In *Electron Microscopy. Fifth International Congress for Electron Microscopy.* Vol. 2, U-3 (S. S. Breese, Jr., ed.). Academic Press, New York.

COLONNIER, M., and R. W. GUILLERY (1964). Synaptic organization in the lateral geniculate nucleus of the monkey. *Z. Zellforsch. 62*, 333–355.

COMBS, C. M. (1956). Bulbar regions related to localized cerebellar afferent impulses. *J. Neurophysiol. 19*, 285–300.

References

CONEL, J. LE ROY (1939). *The Postnatal Development of the Human Cerebral Cortex*, Vol. I. The Cortex of the Newborn. Harvard Univ. Press, Cambridge, Massachusetts.

COOK, A. W., and E. J. BROWDER (1965). Function of posterior columns in man. *Arch. Neurol. (Chic.) 12*, 72–79.

COOK, W. H., J. H. WALKER, and M. L. BARR (1951). A cytological study of transneuronal atrophy in the cat and rabbit. *J. comp. Neurol. 94*, 267–292.

COOKE, P. M., and R. S. SNIDER (1953). Some cerebellar effects on the electrocorticogram. *Electroenceph. clin. Neurophysiol. 5*, 563–569.

COOPER, I. S. (1959). Dystonia musculorum deformans alleviated by chemopallidectomy and chemopallidothalamectomy. *Arch. Neurol. (Chic.) 81*, 5–19.

COOPER, I. S. (1965a). Clinical and physiologic implications of thalamic surgery for disorders of sensory communication. Part 1. Thalamic surgery for intractable pain. *J. neurol. Sci. 2*, 493–519.

COOPER, I. S. (1965b). Clinical and physiologic implications of thalamic surgery for disorders of sensory communication. Part 2. Intention tremor, dystonia, Wilson's disease and torticollis. *J. neurol. Sci. 2*, 520–553.

COOPER, I. S., L. L. BERGMANN, and A. CARACALOS (1963). Anatomic verification of the lesion which abolishes Parkinsonian tremor and rigidity. *Neurology (Minneap.) 13*, 779–787.

COOPER, K. E. (1966). Temperature regulation and the hypothalamus. *Brit. med. Bull. 22*, 238–242.

COOPER, S. (1929). The relations of active and inactive fibres in fractional contraction of muscle. *J. Physiol. (Lond.) 67*, 1–13.

COOPER, S. (1953). Muscle spindles in the intrinsic muscles of the human tongue. *J. Physiol. (Lond.) 122*, 193–202.

COOPER, S. (1960). Muscle spindles and other muscle receptors. In *Structure and Function of Muscle*, Vol. I. Structure (G. H. Bourne, ed.), pp. 381–420. Academic Press, New York.

COOPER, S., and P. M. DANIEL (1949). Muscle spindles in human extrinsic eye muscles. *Brain 72*, 1–24.

COOPER, S., and P. M. DANIEL (1963). Muscle spindles in man; their morphology in the lumbricals and the deep muscles of the neck. *Brain 86*, 563–586.

COOPER, S., P. M. DANIEL, and D. WHITTERIDGE (1951). Afferent impulses in the oculomotor nerve from the extrinsic eye muscles. *J. Physiol. (Lond.) 113*, 463–474.

COOPER, S., P. M. DANIEL, and D. WHITTERIDGE (1953a). Nerve impulses in the brainstem of the goat. Short latency responses obtained by stretching the extrinsic eye muscles and the jaw muscles. *J. Physiol. (Lond.) 120*, 471–491.

COOPER, S., P. M. DANIEL, and D. WHITTERIDGE (1953b). Nerve impulses in the brainstem of the goat. Responses with long latencies obtained by stretching the extrinsic eye muscles. *J. Physiol. (Lond.) 120*, 491–513.

COOPER, S., P. M. DANIEL, and D. WHITTERIDGE (1955). Muscle spindles and other sensory endings in the extrinsic eye muscles; the physiology and anatomy of these receptors and of their connexions with the brain-stem. *Brain 78*, 564–583.

CORAZZA, R., E. FADIGA, and P. L. PARMEGGIANI (1963). Patterns of pyramidal activation of cat's motoneurons. *Arch. ital. Biol. 101*, 337–364.

CORBIN, K. B. (1940). Observations on the peripheral distribution of fibers arising in the mesencephalic nucleus of the fifth cranial nerve. *J. comp. Neurol. 73,* 153–177.

CORBIN, K. B., and F. HARRISON (1940). Function of mesencephalic root of the fifth cranial nerve. *J. Neurophysiol. 3,* 423–435.

CORDEAU, J. P., A. MOREAU, A. BEAULNES, and O. LAURIN (1963). EEG and behavioral changes following microinjection of acetylcholine and adrenalin in the brain stem of cats. *Arch. ital. Biol. 101,* 30–47.

COURVILLE, J. (1966a). Rubrobulbar fibres to the facial nucleus and the lateral reticular nucleus (nucleus of the lateral funiculus). An experimental study in the cat with silver impregnation methods. *Brain Research 1,* 317–337.

COURVILLE, J. (1966b). The nucleus of the facial nerve; the relation between cellular groups and peripheral branches of the nerve. *Brain Research 1,* 338–354.

COURVILLE, J. (1966c). Somatotopical organization of the projection from the nucleus interpositus anterior of the cerebellum to the red nucleus. An experimental study in the cat with silver impregnation methods. *Exp. Brain Res. 2,* 191–215.

COURVILLE, J., and A. BRODAL (1966). Rubrocerebellar connections in the cat. An experimental study with silver impregnation methods. *J. comp. Neurol. 126,* 471–485.

COWAN, W. M., L. ADAMSON, and T. P. S. POWELL (1961). An experimental study of the avian visual system. *J. Anat. (Lond.) 95,* 545–563.

COWAN, W. M., R. W. GUILLERY, and T. P. S. POWELL (1964). The origin of the mamillary peduncle and other hypothalamic connexions from the midbrain. *J. Anat. (Lond.) 98,* 345–363.

COWAN, W. M., and T. P. S. POWELL (1954). An experimental study of the relation between the medial mammillary nucleus and the cingulate cortex. *Proc. roy. Soc. B 143,* 114–125.

COWAN, W. M., and T. P. S. POWELL (1955). The projection of the midline and intralaminar nuclei of the thalamus of the rabbit. *J. Neurol. Neurosurg. Psychiat. 18,* 266–279.

COWAN, W. M., and T. P. S. POWELL (1963). Centrifugal fibres in the avian visual system. *Proc. roy. Soc. B 158,* 232–252.

COWAN, W. M., and T. P. S. POWELL (1966). Striopallidal projection in the monkey. *J. Neurol. Neurosurg. Psychiat. 29,* 426–439.

COWAN, W. M., G. RAISMAN, and T. P. S. POWELL (1965). The connexions of the amygdala. *J. Neurol. Neurosurg. Psychiat. 28,* 137–151.

COWEY, A. (1964). Projection of the retina on to striate and prestriate cortex in the squirrel monkey, *Saimiri sciureus. J. Neurophysiol. 27,* 366–393.

COXE, W. S., and W. M. LANDAU (1965). Observations upon the effect of supplementary motor cortex ablation in the monkey. *Brain 88,* 763–772.

CRACCO, R. Q., and R. C. BICKFORD (1968). Somatomotor and somatosensory evoked responses. *Arch. Neurol. (Chic.) 18,* 52–68.

CRAGG, B. G. (1960). Responses of the hippocampus to stimulation of the olfactory bulb and of various afferent nerves in five mammals. *Exp. Neurol. 2,* 547–572.

CRAGG, B. G. (1961). Olfactory and other afferent connections of the hippocampus in the rabbit, rat, and cat. *Exp. Neurol. 3,* 588–600.

CRAGG, B. G. (1962). Centrifugal fibers to the retina and olfactory bulb, and

710

composition of the supraoptic commissures in the rabbit. *Exp. Neurol. 5,* 406–427.

CRAGG, B. G. (1965). Afferent connexions of the allocortex. *J. Anat. (Lond.) 99,* 339–357.

CRAGG, B. G. (1967). The density of synapses and neurones in the motor and visual areas of the cerebral cortex. *J. Anat. (Lond.) 101,* 639–654.

CRAGG, B. G., and L. H. HAMLYN (1959). Histologic connections and electrical and autonomic responses evoked by stimulation of the dorsal fornix in the rabbit. *Exp. Neurol. 1,* 187–213.

CRAVIOTO, H., J. SILBERMAN, and I. FEIGIN (1960). A clinical and pathologic study of akinetic mutism. *Neurology (Minneap.) 10,* 10–21.

CREUTZFELDT, O., and H. AKIMOTO (1958). Konvergenz und gegenseitige Beeinflussung von Impulsen aus der Retina und den unspezifischen Thalamuskernen an einzelnen Neuronen des optischen Cortex. *Arch. Psychiat. Nervenkr. 196,* 520–538.

CREUTZFELDT, O. D., H. D. LUX, and S. WATANABE (1966). Electrophysiology of cortical nerve cells. In *The Thalamus* (D. P. Purpura and M. D. Yahr, eds.), pp. 209–230. Columbia Univ. Press, New York.

CRILL, W., and T. T. KENNEDY (1967). Inferior olive of the cat: Intracellular recording. *Science 157,* 717–718.

CRITCHLEY, M. (1953). *The Parietal Lobes.* Edward Arnold, London.

CRITCHLEY, M. (1966). The enigma of Gerstmann's syndrome. *Brain 89,* 183–198.

CROSBY, E. C. (1953). Relations of brain centers to normal and abnormal eye movements in the horizontal plane. *J. comp. Neurol. 99,* 437–480.

CROSBY, E. C., and J. W. HENDERSON (1948). The mammalian midbrain and isthmus regions. Part II. Fiber connections of the superior colliculus. B. Pathways concerned in automatic eye movements. *J. comp. Neurol. 88,* 53–92.

CROSBY, E. C., and T. HUMPHREY (1941). Studies of the vertebrate telencephalon. II. The nuclear pattern of the anterior olfactory nucleus, tuberculum olfactorium and the amygdaloid complex in adult man. *J. comp. Neurol. 74,* 309–352.

CROSBY, E. C., R. C. SCHNEIDER, B. R. DEJONGE, and P. SZONYI (1966). The alterations of tonus and movements through the interplay between the cerebral hemispheres and the cerebellum. *J. comp. Neurol. 127, Suppl. 1,* 1–91.

CROSS, B. A., and I. A. SILVER (1966). Electrophysiological studies on the hypothalamus. *Brit. med. Bull. 22,* 254–258.

CROWE, S. J., S. R. GUILD, and L. M. POLVOGT (1934). Observations on the pathology of high-tone deafness. *Bull. Johns Hopk. Hosp. 54,* 315–379.

CURZON, G. (1967). The biochemistry of dyskinesias. *Int. Rev. Neurobiol. 10,* 323–370.

CUSHING, H. (1904). The sensory distribution of the fifth cranial nerve. *Bull. Johns. Hopk. Hosp. 15,* 213–232.

CUSHING, H. (1922). The field defects produced by temporal lobe lesions. *Brain 44,* 341–396.

Cutaneous Innervation. Advances in Biology of Skin, Vol. 1 (1960). (W. Montagna, ed.). Pergamon Press, Oxford—New York.

DAHLSTRÖM, A., and K. FUXE (1964). Evidence for the existence of monoamine-containing neurons in the central nervous system. *Acta physiol. scand. 62, Suppl. 232,* 1–55.

DAITZ, H. M., and T. P. S. POWELL (1954). Studies of the connexions of the fornix system. *J. Neurol. Neurosurg. Psychiat. 17,* 75–82.

DANIEL, P. (1946). Spiral nerve endings in the extrinsic eye muscles of man. *J. Anat. (Lond.) 80,* 189–193.

DANIEL, P. M. (1966). The blood supply of the hypothalamus and pituitary gland. *Brit. med. Bull. 22,* 202–208.

DARIAN-SMITH, I. (1965). Presynaptic component in the afferent inhibition observed within trigeminal brain-stem nuclei in the cat. *J. Neurophysiol. 28,* 695–709.

DARIAN-SMITH, I. (1966). Neural mechanisms of facial sensation. *Int. Rev. Neurobiol. 9,* 301–395.

DARIAN-SMITH, I., J. ISBISTER, H. MOK, and T. YOKOTA (1966). Somatic sensory cortical projection areas excited by tactile stimulation of the cat: A triple representation. *J. Physiol. (Lond.) 182,* 671–689.

DAVIS, H. (1961). Some principles of sensory receptor action. *Physiol. Rev. 41,* 391–416.

DAVISON, C. (1940). Disturbances of temperature regulation in man. *Res. Publ. Ass. nerv. ment. Dis. 20,* 774–823.

DAVISON, C. (1942). The rôle of the globus pallidus and substantia nigra in the production of rigidity and tremor. A clinico-pathological study of paralysis agitans. *Res. Publ. Ass. nerv. ment. Dis. 21,* 267–333.

DAWSON, B. H. (1958). The blood vessels of the human optic chiasma and their relation to those of the hypophysis and hypothalamus. *Brain 81,* 207–217.

DEKABAN, A. (1953). Human thalamus: An anatomical developmental and pathological study. *J. comp. Neurol. 99,* 639–683.

DELGADO, J. M. R. (1963). Effect of brain stimulation on task-free situations. *Electroenceph. clin. Neurophysiol. 24,* 260–280.

DELGADO, J. M. R. (1964). Free behavior and brain stimulation. *Int. Rev. Neurobiol. 6,* 349–449.

DELL, P., M. BONVALLET, and H. HUGELIN (1961). Mechanisms of reticular deactivation. In *The Nature of Sleep.* Ciba Foundation Symposium (G. E. W. Wolstenholme and M. O'Connor, eds.), pp. 86–102. J. & A. Churchill, Ltd., London.

DE LORENZO, A. J. D. (1963). Studies on the ultrastructure and histophysiology of cell membranes, nerve fibers and synaptic junctions in chemoreceptors. In *Olfaction and Taste* (Y. Zotterman, ed.), pp. 5–17. Pergamon Press, Oxford.

DEMPSEY, E. W., and R. S. MORISON (1942). The production of rhythmically recurrent cortical potentials after localized thalamic stimulation. *Amer. J. Physiol. 135,* 293–300.

DEMEYER, W. (1959). Number of axons and myelin sheaths in adult human medullary pyramids. Study with silver impregnation and iron hematoxylin staining methods. *Neurology (Minneap.) 9,* 42–47.

DENNY-BROWN, D. (1962). *The Basal Ganglia and Their Relation to Disorders of Movement.* Oxford Univ. Press, London.

DE ROBERTIS, E. (1967). Ultrastructure and cytochemistry of the synaptic region. *Science 156,* 907–914.

DESMEDT, J. E. (1962). Auditory-evoked potentials from cochlea to cortex as influenced by activation of the efferent olivo-cochlear bundle. *J. acoust. Soc. Amer. 34,* 1478–1496.

References

DESMEDT, J. E. (1966). Presynaptic mechanisms in myasthenia gravis. *Ann. N.Y. Acad. Sci. 135,* 209–246.

DeVITO, J. L. (1967). Thalamic projection of the anterior ectosylvian gyrus (somatic area II) in the cat. *J. comp. Neurol. 131,* 67–78.

DeVITO, J. L., and O. A. SMITH, JR. (1964). Subcortical projections of the prefrontal lobe of the monkey. *J. comp. Neurol. 123,* 413–424.

DeVITO, J. L., and L. E. WHITE, JR. (1966). Projections from the fornix to the hippocampal formation in the squirrel monkey. *J. comp. Neurol. 127,* 389–398.

DIAMANTOPOULOS, E., and P. Z. OLSEN (1967). Excitability of motor neurones in spinal shock in man. *J. Neurol. Neurosurg. Psychiat. 30,* 427–431.

DIAMOND, I. T., and J. D. UTLEY (1963). Thalamic retrograde degeneration of sensory cortex in opossum. *J. comp. Neurol. 120,* 129–160.

DIERSSEN, G., L. BERGMANN, G. GIONI, and I. S. COOPER (1962). Surgical lesions affecting parkinsonian symptomatology: A clinico-anatomical discussion of two cases. *Acta Neurochir. (Wien) 10,* 125–133.

DIETE-SPIFF, K., G. CARLI, and O. POMPEIANO (1967). Comparison of the effects of stimulation of the VIIIth cranial nerve, the vestibular nuclei or the reticular formation on the gastrocnemius muscle and its spindles. *Arch. ital. Biol. 105,* 243–272.

DIMITRIJEVIC, M. R., and P. W. NATHAN (1967a). Studies of spasticity in man. 1. Some features of spasticity. *Brain 90,* 1–30.

DIMITRIJEVIC, M. R., and P. W. NATHAN (1967b). Studies of spasticity in man. 2. Analysis of stretch reflexes in spasticity. *Brain 90,* 333–358.

Disorders of Language (1964). A Ciba Foundation Symposium (A. V. S. de Reuck and M. O'Connor, eds.). J. & A. Churchill, Ltd., London.

DODT, E. (1956). Centrifugal impulses in rabbit's retina. *J. Neurophysiol. 19,* 301–307.

DOMINO, E. F. (1958). A pharmacologic analysis of some reticular and spinal cord systems. In *Reticular Formation of the Brain* (H. H. Jaspers, et al., eds.), pp. 285–312. Little, Brown and Co., Boston.

DONOVAN, B. T. (1966). Experimental lesions of the hypothalamus. *Brit. med. Bull. 22,* 249–253.

DOUGLAS, R. J. (1967). The hippocampus and behavior. *Psychol. Bull. 67,* 416–442.

DOW, R. S. (1936). The fiber connections of the posterior parts of the cerebellum in the cat and rat. *J. comp. Neurol. 63,* 527–548.

DOW, R. S. (1938a). Efferent connections of the flocculo-nodular lobe in *Macaca mulatta*. *J. comp. Neurol. 68,* 297–305.

DOW, R. S. (1938b). The effects of unilateral and bilateral labyrinthectomy in monkey, baboon and chimpanzee. *Amer. J. Physiol. 121,* 392–399.

DOW, R. S. (1938c). Effects of lesions in the vestibular part of the cerebellum in primates. *Arch. Neurol. Psychiat. (Chic.) 40,* 500–520.

DOW, R. S. (1939). Cerebellar action potentials in response to stimulation of various afferent connections. *J. Neurophysiol. 2,* 543–555.

DOW, R. S. (1942a). The evolution and anatomy of the cerebellum. *Biol. Rev. 17,* 179–220.

DOW, R. S. (1942b). Cerebellar action potentials in response to stimulation of the cerebral cortex in monkeys and cats. *J. Neurophysiol. 5,* 121–136.

DOW, R. S. (1969). Cerebellar syndromes including vermis and hemispheric syndromes. In *Handbook of Clinical Neurology,* Vol. 2 (P. J. Vinken and G. W. Bruyn, eds.) [In press.] North-Holland Publishing Co., Amsterdam.

Dow, R. S., and G. Moruzzi (1958). *The Physiology and Pathology of the Cerebellum. Univ. of Minnesota Press,* Minneapolis, Minnesota.

Downer, J. L. de C. (1959). Changes in visually guided behaviour following midsagittal division of optic chiasm and corpus callosum in monkey (*Macaca mulatta*). *Brain 82,* 251–259.

Downman, C. B. B., C. N. Woolsey, and R. A. Lende (1960). Auditory areas I, II and Ep: Cochlear representation, afferent paths and interconnections. *Bull. Johns Hopk. Hosp. 106,* 127–142.

Drachman, D. A., and J. Arbit (1966). Memory and hippocampal complex. II. Is memory a multiple process? *Arch. Neurol (Chic.) 15,* 52–61.

Drachman, D. A., and A. K. Ommaya (1964). Memory and the hippocampal complex. *Arch. Neurol. (Chic.) 10,* 411–425.

Druckman, R. (1952). A critique of "suppression," with additional observations in the cat. *Brain 75,* 226–243.

Druga, R. (1968). Cortico-claustral connections. II. Connections from the parietal, temporal and occipital cortex to the claustrum. *Folia morph. (Praha) 16,* 142–149.

Dubner, R. (1967). Interaction of peripheral and central input in the main sensory trigeminal nucleus of the cat. *Exp. Neurol. 17,* 186–202.

DuBois, F. S., and J. O. Foley (1937). Quantitative studies of the vagus nerve in the cat. II. The ratio of jugular to nodose fibers. *J. comp. Neurol. 67,* 69–87.

Duensing, F., and K.-P. Schaefer (1957a). Die Neuronaktivität in der Formatio reticularis des Rhombencephalons beim vestibulären Nystagmus. *Arch. Psychiat. Nervenkr. 196,* 265–290.

Duensing, F. and K.-P. Schaefer (1957b). Die "locker gekoppelten" Neurone der Formatio reticularis des Rhombencephalons beim vestibulären Nystagmus. *Arch. Psychiat. Nervenkr. 196,* 402–420.

Duensing, F., and K.-P. Schaefer (1958). Die Aktivität einzelner Neurone im Bereich der Vestibulariskerne bei Horizontalbeschleunigungen unter besonderer Berücksichtigung des vestibulären Nystagmus. *Arch. Psychiat. Nervenkr. 198,* 225–252.

Duensing, F., and K.-P. Schaefer (1959). Über die Konvergenz verschiedener labyrinthärer Afferenzen auf einzelne Neurone des Vestibulariskerngebietes. *Arch. Psychiat. Nervenkr. 199,* 345–371.

Dusser de Barenne, J. G. (1933). 'Corticalization' of function and functional localization in the cerebral cortex. *Arch. Neurol. Psychiat. (Chic.) 30,* 884–901.

Dusser de Barenne, J. G., H. W. Garol, and W. S. McCulloch (1941). The 'motor' cortex of the chimpanzee. *J. Neurophysiol. 4,* 287–303.

Dusser de Barenne, J. G., H. W. Garol, and W. S. McCulloch (1942). Physiological neuronography of the cortico-striatal connections. *Res. Publ. Ass. nerv. ment. Dis. 21,* 246–266.

Dusser de Barenne, J. G., and W. S. McCulloch (1938). Functional organization in the sensory cortex of the monkey (*Macaca mulatta*). *J. Neurophysiol. 1,* 69–85.

Duvoisin, R. C., M. D. Yahr, M. D. Schweitzer, and H. H. Merritt (1963). Parkinsonism before and since the epidemic of encephalitis lethargica. *Arch. Neurol. (Chic.) 9,* 232–236.

Døving, K. B. (1967). Problems in the physiology of olfaction. In *Chemistry and*

References

Physiology of Flavors. Symposium on Foods (H. W. Schultz, E. A. Day, and L. M. Libbey, eds.), pp. 52–94. Avi Publishing Co., Westport, Connecticut.

EAGER, R. P. (1963a). Efferent cortico-nuclear pathways in the cerebellum of the cat. *J. comp. Neurol. 120,* 81–103.

EAGER, R. P. (1963b). Cortical association pathways in the cerebellum of the cat. *J. comp. Neurol. 121,* 381–394.

EAGER, R. P. (1966). Patterns and mode of termination of cerebellar cortico-nuclear pathways in the monkey (*Macaca mulatta*). *J. comp. Neurol. 126,* 551–565.

EAGER, R. P., and R. J. BARRNETT (1966). Morphological and chemical studies of Nauta-stained degenerating cerebellar and hypothalamic fibers. *J. comp. Neurol. 126,* 487–510.

EARLE, K. M. (1952). The tract of Lissauer and its possible relation to the pain pathway. *J. comp. Neurol. 96,* 93–111.

EBNER, F. F., and R. E. MYERS (1965). Distribution of corpus callosum and anterior commissure in cat and raccoon. *J. comp. Neurol. 124,* 353–365.

ECCLES, J. C. (1957). *The Physiology of Nerve Cells.* The Johns Hopkins Press, Baltimore.

ECCLES, J. C. (1964). *The Physiology of Synapses.* Springer-Verlag, Berlin.

ECCLES, J. C. (1966a). Functional organization of the cerebellum in relation to its role in motor control. In *Muscular Afferents and Motor Control.* First Nobel Symposium, Stockholm, Sweden, 1965 (R. Granit, ed.), pp. 19–36. Almqvist and Wiksell, Stockholm; John Wiley & Sons, New York.

ECCLES, J. C. (1966b). Cerebral synaptic mechanisms. In *Brain and Conscious Experience* (J. C. Eccles, ed.), pp. 24–50. Springer-Verlag, Berlin.

ECCLES, J. C., R. M. ECCLES, I. IGGO, and A. LUNDBERG (1960). Electrophysiological studies on gamma motoneurons. *Acta physiol. scand. 50,* 32–40.

ECCLES, J. C., R. M. ECCLES, and A. LUNDBERG (1957). The convergence of monosynaptic excitatory afferents on to many different species of alpha motoneurons. *J. Physiol. (Lond.) 137,* 22–50.

ECCLES, J. C., R. M. ECCLES, and A. LUNDBERG (1960). Types of neurone in and around the intermediate nucleus of the lumbosacral cord. *J. Physiol. (Lond.) 154,* 89–114.

ECCLES, J. C., M. ITO, and J. SZENTÁGOTHAI (1967). *The Cerebellum as a Neuronal Machine.* Springer-Verlag, Berlin.

ECCLES, J. C., O. OSCARSSON, and W. D. WILLIS (1961). Synaptic action of group I and II afferent fibres of muscle on the cells of the dorsal spinocerebellar tract. *J. Physiol. (Lond.) 158,* 517–543.

ECCLES, J. C., and C. S. SHERRINGTON (1930). Numbers and contraction-values of individual motor-units examined in some muscles of the limb. *Proc. roy. Soc. B 106,* 326–357.

ECCLES, R., and A. LUNDBERG (1959). Synaptic actions in motoneurons by efferents which may evoke the flexion reflex. *Arch. ital. Biol. 97,* 199–221.

ECONOMO, C. VON (1927). *Zellaufbau der Grosshirnrinde des Menschen.* Julius Springer, Berlin.

ECONOMO, C. VON (1929). *Die Encephalis lethargica, ihre Nachkrankheiten und ihre Behandlung.* Urban & Schwarzenberg, Berlin.

ECONOMO, C. VON, and G. N. KOSKINAS (1925). *Die Cytoarchitektonik der Hirnrinde des erwachsenen Menschen.* Springer-Verlag, Berlin.

EDGAR, M. A., and S. NUNDY (1966). Innervation of the spinal dura mater. *J. Neurol. Neurosurg. Psychiat. 29,* 530–534.

EDVARDSEN, P. (1967). Nervous control of urinary bladder in cat. A survey of recent experimental results and their relation to clinical problems. *Acta neurol. scand. 43,* 543–563.

EHNI, G., and H. W. WOLTMAN (1945). Hemifacial spasm. Review of one hundred and six cases. *Arch. Neurol. Psychiat. (Chic). 53,* 205–211.

EISENMAN, J., S. LANDGREN, and D. NOVIN (1963). Functional organization in the main sensory trigeminal nucleus and in the rostral subdivision of the nucleus of the spinal trigeminal tract in the cat. *Acta physiol. scand. 59, Suppl. 214,* 1–44.

ELDRED, E., H. YELLIN, L. GADBOIS, and S. SWEENEY (1967). Bibliography on muscle receptors; their morphology, pathology and physiology. *Exp. Neurol. Suppl. 3,* 1–154.

ELLIOT, K. A. S. (1965). γ-aminobutyric acid and other inhibitory substances. *Brit. med. Bull. 21,* 70–75.

ELSBERG, C. A. (1935). The sense of smell. VIII. Olfactory fatigue. *Bull. neurol. Inst. N.Y. 4,* 479–495.

ELSBERG, C. A. (1936). The sense of smell. XII. The localization of tumors of the frontal lobe of the brain by quantitative olfactory tests. *Bull. neurol. Inst. N.Y. 4,* 535–543.

ELSBERG, C. A., E. D. BREWER, and I. LEVY (1935). The sense of smell. IV. Concerning conditions which may temporarily alter normal olfactory acuity. *Bull. neurol. Inst. N.Y. 4,* 31–34.

ELSBERG, C. A., and I. LEVY (1935). The sense of smell. I. A new and simple method of quantitative olfactometry. *Bull. neurol. Inst. N.Y. 4,* 5–19.

ELSBERG, C. A., and H. SPOTNITZ (1942). Value of quantitative olfactory tests for localization of supratentorial disease. *Arch. Neurol. Psychiat. (Chic.) 48,* 1–12.

EMMERS, R. (1964). Localization of the thalamic projection of afferents from the tongue in the cat. *Anat. Rec. 148,* 67–74.

EMMERS, R., R. M. BENJAMIN, and A. J. BLOMQUIST (1962). Thalamic localization of afferents from the tongue in albino rat. *J. comp. Neurol. 118,* 43–48.

ENGSTRÖM, H. (1958). On the double innervation of the sensory epithelia of the inner ear. *Acta oto-laryng. (Stockh.) 49,* 109–118.

ENGSTRÖM, H. (1967). The ultrastructure of the sensory cells of the cochlea. *J. Laryng. 81,* 687–715.

ENGSTRÖM, H., H. W. ADES, and A. ANDERSSON (1966). *Structural Pattern of the Organ of Corti. A Systematic Mapping of Sensory Cells and Neural Elements.* Almqvist & Wiksell, Stockholm.

ENGSTRÖM, H., H. H. LINDEMAN, and H. W. ADES (1966). Anatomical features of the auricular sensory organs. In *NASA SP-115.* Second symposium on the role of the vestibular organs in space exploration, pp. 33–44. Ames Research Center, Moffett Field, California.

ENGSTRÖM, H., and H. WERSÄLL (1958). The ultrastructural organization of the organ of Corti and of the vestibular sensory epithelia. *Exp. Cell Res., Suppl. 5,* 460–492.

ENOCH, D. M., and F. W. L. KERR (1967a). Hypothalamic vasopressor and vesicopressor pathways. I. Functional studies. *Arch. Neurol. (Chic.) 16,* 290–306.

ENOCH, D. M., and F. W. L. KERR (1967b). Hypothalamic vasopressor and vesicopressor pathways. II. Anatomic study of their course and connections. *Arch. Neurol. (Chic.) 16*, 307–320.

ERICKSON, T. C. (1945). Erotomania (nymphomania) as an expression of cortical epileptiform discharge. *Arch. Neurol. Psychiat. (Chic.) 53*, 226–230.

ERICKSON, T. C., and C. N. WOOLSEY (1951). Observations on the supplementary motor area of man. *Trans. Amer. neurol. Ass. 76*, 50–52.

ERULKAR, S. D., and M. FILLENZ (1960). Single-unit activity in the lateral geniculate body of the cat. *J. Physiol. (Lond.) 154*, 206–218.

ERVIN, F. R., and V. H. MARKS (1960). Stereotactic thalamotomy in the human. Part II. Physiologic observations on the human thalamus. *Arch. Neurol. (Chic.) 3*, 368–380.

ESCOBAR, A., E. D. SAMPEDRO, and R. S. DOW (1968). Quantitative data on the inferior olivary nucleus in man, cat and vampire bat. *J. comp. Neurol. 132*, 397–404.

ESSICK, C. R. (1912). The development of the nuclei pontis and the nucleus arcuatus in man. *Amer. J. Anat. 13*, 25–54.

EULER, C. VON (1962). On the significance of the high zinc content in the hippocampal formation. In *Physiologie de l'hippocampe*, pp. 135–145. Editions du Centre National de al Recherche Scientifique, Paris.

EULER, U. S. VON (1959). Autonomic neuroeffector transmission. In *Handbook of Physiology, Section 1, Neurophysiology, Vol. 1* (J. Field, H. W. Magoun and V. E. Hall, eds.), pp. 215–237. American Physiological Society, Washington, D.C.

EVANS, C. L. (1957). Sweating in relation to sympathetic innervation. *Brit. med. Bull. 13*, 197–201.

EVANS, E. F., H. F. ROSS, and I. C. WHITFIELD (1965). The spatial distribution of unit characteristic frequency in the primary auditory cortex of the cat. *J. Physiol. (Lond.) 179*, 238–247.

EVARTS, E. V. (1965). Relation of discharge frequency to conduction velocity in pyramidal tract neurons. *J. Neurophysiol. 28*, 216–228.

EVARTS, E. V. (1966). Pyramidal tract activity associated with conditioned hand movement in the monkey. *J. Neurophysiol. 29*, 1011–1027.

EVARTS, E. V. (1968). Relation of pyramidal tract activity to force exerted during voluntary movement. *J. Neurophysiol. 31*, 14–27.

FAABORG-ANDERSEN, K. (1957). Electromyographic investigation of intrinsic laryngeal muscles in humans. *Acta physiol. scand. 41, Suppl. 140*, 1–149.

FADIGA, E., and G. C. PUPILLI (1964). Teleceptive components of the cerebellar function. *Physiol. Rev. 44*, 432–486.

FALCK, B. (1962). Observations on the possibilities of the cellular localization of monoamines by a fluorescence method. *Acta physiol. scand. 56, Suppl. 197*, 1–25.

FALCONER, M. A. (1949). Intramedullary trigeminal tractototomy and its place in the treatment of facial pain. *J. Neurol. Neurosurg. Psychiat. 12*, 297–311.

FALCONER, M. A., E. A. SERAFETINIDES, and J. A. N. CORSELLIS (1964). Etiology and pathogenesis of temporal lobe epilepsy. *Arch. Neurol. (Chic.) 10*, 233–248.

FALCONER, M. A., and J. L. WILSON (1958). Visual field changes following anterior, temporal lobectomy, their significance in relation to "Meyer's loop" of the optic radiation. *Brain 81*, 1–14.

717

FARRELL, G., L. F. FABRE, and E. W. RAUSCHKOLB (1966). The neurohypophysis. *Ann. Rev. Physiol. 30,* 557–588.

FAVALE, E., C. LOEB, G. F. ROSSI, and G. SACCO (1961). EEG synchronization and behavioral signs of sleep following low frequency stimulation of the brain stem reticular formation. *Arch. ital. Biol. 99,* 1–22.

FAY, T. (1927). Observations and results from intracranial section of the glosso-pharyngeus and vagus nerves in man. *J. Neurol. Psychopath. 8,* 110–123.

FEINDEL, W. (1954). Anatomical overlap of motor-units. *J. comp. Neurol. 101,* 1–14.

FEINDEL, W., J. R. HINSHAW, and G. WEDDELL (1952). The pattern of motor inner-vation in mammalian striated muscle. *J. Anat. (Lond.) 86,* 35–48.

FEINSTEIN, B., B. LINDEGÅRD, E. NYMAN, and G. WOHLFART (1954). Morphologic studies of motor units in normal human muscles. *Acta anat. (Basel) 23,* 127–142.

FEREMUTSCH, K. (1955). Strukturanalyse des menschlichen Hypothalamus. *Mschr. Psychiat. Neurol. 130,* 1–85.

FEREMUTSCH, K., and K. SIMMA (1959). Beitrag zur Kenntnis der "Formatio reticularis medullae oblongatae et pontis" des Menschen. *Z. Anat. Entwickl.-Gesch. 121,* 271–291.

FERNÁNDEZ, C. (1951). The innervation of the cochlea (guinea pig). *Laryngoscope (St. Louis) 61,* 1152–1172.

FERNÁNDEZ, C., and J. M. FREDRICKSON (1964). Experimental cerebellar lesions and their effect on vestibular function. International Vestibular Symposium, Uppsala 1963. *Acta oto-laryng. (Stockh.) Suppl. 192,* 52–62.

FERNANDEZ DE MOLINA, A., and R. W. HUNSPERGER (1962). Organization of the subcortical system governing defence and flight reactions in the cat. *J. Physiol. (Lond.) 160,* 200–213.

FERRARO, A., and S. E. BARRERA (1935a). The nuclei of the posterior funiculi in *Macacus rhesus.* An anatomic and experimental investigation. *Arch. Neurol. Psychiat. (Chic.) 33,* 262–275.

FERRARO, A., and S. E. BARRERA (1935b). Posterior column fibers and their ter-mination in *Macacus rhesus. J. comp. Neurol. 62,* 507–530.

FERRARO, A., and S. E. BARRERA (1936). Lamination of the medial lemniscus in *Macacus rhesus. J. comp. Neurol. 64,* 313–324.

FETZ, E. E. (1968). Pyramidal tract effects on interneurons in the cat lumbar dorsal horn. *J. Neurophysiol. 31,* 69–80.

FEX, J. (1967). The olivocochlear feedback system. In *Sensorineural Hearing Proc-esses and Disorders.* Henry Ford Hospital International Symposium (A. B. Graham, ed.), pp. 77–86. J. & A. Churchill, London.

FILLENZ, M. (1955). Responses in the brainstem of the cat to stretch of extrinsic ocular muscles. *J. Physiol. (Lond.) 128,* 182–199.

FINK, R. P., and L. Heimer (1967). Two methods for selective silver impregnation of degenerating axons and their synaptic endings in the central nervous sys-tem. *Brain Research 4,* 369–374.

FINLEY, K. H. (1940). Angio-architecture of the hypothalamus and its peculiarities. *Res. Publ. Ass. nerv. ment. Dis. 20,* 286–309.

FISHER, C., W. R. INGRAM, W. K. HARE, and S. W. RANSON (1935). The degenera-tion of the supra-optico-hypophyseal system in diabetes insipidus. *Anat. Rec. 63,* 29–52.

References

FISHER, C. M. (1965). Pure sensory stroke involving face, arm and leg. *Neurology (Minneap.) 15,* 76–80.

FISHER, C. M. (1967). Some neuro-ophthalmological observations. *J. Neurol. Neurosurg. Psychiat. 30,* 383–392.

FISHER, C. M., and R. D. ADAMS (1956). Diphtheritic polyneuritis—A pathological study. *J. Neuropath. exp. Neurol. 15,* 243–268.

FISHER, C. M., and H. B. CURRY (1965). Pure motor hemiplegia of vascular origin. *Arch. Neurol. (Chic.) 13,* 30–44.

FITZGERALD, G., and C. S. HALLPIKE (1942). Studies in human vestibular function. I. Observations on the directional preponderance ("Nystagmusbereitschaft") of caloric nystagmus resulting from cerebral lesions. *Brain 65,* 115–137.

FITZSIMONS, J. T. (1966). The hypothalamus and drinking. *Brit. med. Bull. 22,* 232–237.

FLEISCHHAUER, K., and E. HORSTMANN (1957). Intravitale Dithizonfärbung homologer Felder der Ammonsformation von Säugern. *Z. Zellforsch. 46,* 598–609.

FLEMINGER, J. F. (1946). Discussion on cortical atrophy. *Proc. roy. Soc. Med. (London) 39,* 427–430.

FLOCK, Å. (1964). Structure of the macula utriculi with special reference to directional interplay of sensory responses as revealed by morphological polarization. *J. Cell Biol. 22,* 413–431.

FLOCK, Å., and A. J. DUVALL (1965). The ultrastructure of the kinocilium of the sensory cells in the inner ear and lateral line organs. *J. Cell Biol. 25,* 1–8.

FLOOD, S., and J. JANSEN (1961). On the cerebellar nuclei in the cat. *Acta anat. (Basel) 46,* 52–72.

FLOOD, S., and J. JANSEN (1966). The efferent fibres of the cerebellar nuclei and their distribution on the cerebellar peduncles in the cat. *Acta anat. (Basel) 63,* 137–166.

FLUUR, ERIK (1959). Influences of semicircular ducts on extraocular muscles. *Acta oto-laryng. (Stockh.) Suppl. 149,* 1–46.

FOERSTER, O. (1911). Resection of the posterior nerve roots of the spinal cord. *Lancet 2,* 76–79.

FOERSTER, O. (1929). Beiträge zur Pathophysiologie der Sehbahn und der Sehsphäre. *J. Psychol. Neurol. (Lpz.) 39,* 463–485.

FOERSTER, O. (1933). The dermatomes in man. *Brain 56,* 1–39.

FOERSTER, O. (1936a). Symptomatologie der Erkrankungen des Rückenmarks und seiner Wurzeln. In *Hdb. d. Neurol.,* Vol. 5 (Bumke and Foerster, eds.), pp. 1–403. Springer-Verlag, Berlin.

FOERSTER, O. (1936b). Motorische Felder und Bahnen. In *Hdb. d. Neurol.,* Vol. 6 (Bumke and Foerster, eds.), pp. 1–357. Springer-Verlag, Berlin.

FOERSTER, O., and O. GAGEL (1932). Die Vorderseitenstrangdurchschneidung beim Menschen. Eine klinisch-patho-physiologisch-anatomische Studie. *Z. ges. Neurol. Psychiat, 138,* 1–92.

FOERSTER, O., O. GAGEL, and W. MAHONEY (1939). Die encephalen Tumoren des verlängerten Markes, der Brücke und des Mittelhirns. *Arch. Psychiat. Nervenkr. 110,* 1–74.

FOIX, CH., and J. NICOLESCO (1925). *Anatomie cérébrale. Les noyaux gris centraux et la région mésencéphalo-sous-optique, suivi d'un appendice sur l'anatomie pathologique de la maladie de Parkinson.* Masson et Cie, Paris.

719

FOLEY, J. O., and F. DuBois (1937). Quantitative studies of the vagus nerve in the cat. I. The ratio of sensory to motor fibers. *J. comp. Neurol. 67*, 49–67.

FOLEY, J. O., and F. DuBois (1943). An experimental study of the facial nerve. *J. comp. Neurol. 79*, 79–105.

FOLTZ, E. L., and L. E. WHITE, JR. (1962). Pain "relief" by frontal cingulumotomy. *J. Neurosurg. 19*, 89–100.

FORD, F. R., and F. B. WALSH (1958). Raeder's paratrigeminal syndrome. A benign disorder, possibly a complication of migraine. *Bull. Johns Hopk. Hosp. 103*, 296–298.

FORMAN, D., and J. W. WARD (1957). Responses to electrical stimulation of caudate nucleus in cats in chronic experiments. *J. Neurophysiol. 20*, 230–244.

FOX, C. A. (1943). The stria terminals, longitudinal association bundle and pre-commissural fornix fibers in the cat. *J. comp. Neurol. 79*, 277–295.

FOX, C. A. (1949). Amygdalo-thalamic connections in *Macaca mulatta*. (Abstract). *Anat. Rec. 103*, 537.

FOX, C. A., and J. W. BARNARD (1957). A quantitative study of the Purkinje cell dendritic branchlets and their relationship to afferent fibres. *J. Anat. (Lond.) 91*, 299–313.

FOX, C. A., D. E. HILLMAN, K. A. SIEGESMUND, and C. R. DUTTA (1967). The primate cerebellar cortex: a Golgi and electron microscopic study. In *The Cerebellum, Progress in Brain Research*, Vol. 25 (C. A. Fox and R. S. Snider, eds.), pp. 174–225. Elsevier Publishing Co., Amsterdam.

FOX, C. A., D. E. HILLMAN, K. A. SIEGESMUND, and L. A. SETHER (1966). The primate globus pallidus and its feline and avian homologues: A Golgi and electron microscopic study. In *Evolution of the Forebrain. Phylogenesis and Ontogenesis of the Forebrain* (R. Hassler and H. Stephan, eds.), pp. 237–248. Georg Thieme Verlag, Stuttgart.

FOX, C. A., W. A. McKINLEY, and H. W. MAGOUN (1944). An oscillographic study of olfactory system of cats. *J. Neurophysiol. 7*, 1–16.

FOX, C. A., and J. T. SCHMITZ (1943). A Marchi study of the distribution of the anterior commissure in cat. *J. comp. Neurol. 79*, 297–314.

FOX, C. A., K. A. SIEGESMUND, and C. R. DUTTA (1964). The Purkinje cell dendritic branchlets and their relation with the parallel fibers: light and electron microscopic observations. In *Morphological and Biochemical Correlates of Neural Activity* (M. M. Cohen and R. S. Snider, eds.), pp. 112–141. Harper & Row, Publishers Inc., New York.

FOX, J. L., and J. F. KURTZKE (1966). Trauma-induced intention tremor relieved by stereotaxic thalamotomy. *Arch. Neurol. (Chic.) 15*, 247–251.

FRAZIER, C. H., and S. N. ROWE (1934). Certain observations upon localization in fifty-one verified tumors of the temporal lobe. *Res. Publ. Ass. nerv. ment. Dis. 13*, 251–258.

FREDRICKSON, J. M., U. FIGGE, P. SCHEID, and H. H. KORNHUBER (1966). Vestibular nerve projection to the cerebral cortex of the rhesus monkey. *Exp. Brain Res. 2*, 318–327.

FREDRICKSON, J. M., D. SCHWARZ, and H. H. KORNHUBER (1965). Convergence and interaction of vestibular and deep somatic afferents upon neurons in the vestibular nuclei of the cat. *Acta oto-laryng. (Stockh.) 61*, 168–186.

FREEMAN, M. A. R., and B. WYKE (1967). The innervation of the knee joint. An anatomical and histological study in the cat. *J. Anat. (Lond.) 101*, 505–532.

FREEMAN, W., and J. W. WATTS (1942). *Psychosurgery. Intelligence, Emotion and*

References

Social Behavior following Prefrontal Lobotomy for Mental Disorders. Charles C Thomas, Springfield, Illinois.

FREEMAN, W., and J. W. WATTS (1946). Pain of organic disease relieved by prefrontal lobotomy. *Proc. roy. Soc. Med. 39*, 445–447.

FREEMAN, W., and J. W. WATTS (1947). Retrograde degeneration of the thalamus following prefrontal lobotomy. *J. comp. Neurol. 86*, 65–93.

FRENCH, J. D. (1952). Brain lesions associated with prolonged unconsciousness. *Arch. Neurol. (Chic.) 68*, 722–740.

FRENCH, J. D., F. K. VON AMERONGEN, and H. W. MAGOUN (1952). An activating system in brain stem of monkey. *Arch. Neurol. Psychiat. (Chic.) 68*, 577–590.

FREZIK, J. (1963). Associative connections established by Purkinje axon collaterals between different parts of the cerebellar cortex. *Acta morph. Acad. Sci. hung. 12*, 9–14.

FRIEDE, R. L. (1959). Transport of oxidative enzymes in nerve fibers; a histochemical investigation of the regenerative cycle in neurons. *Exp. Neurol. 1*, 441–466.

FRIEDMAN, A. P., D. H. HARTER, and H. H. MERRITT (1962). Ophthalmoplegic migraine. *Arch. Neurol. (Chic.) 7*, 320–327.

FRITSCH, G., and E. HITZIG (1870). Ueber die elektrische Erregbarkeit des Grosshirns. *Arch. Anat. Physiol. Wiss. Med. 37*, 300–332.

Frontal Granular Cortex and Behavior, The (1964). (J. M. Warren and K. Akert, eds.). McGraw-Hill Book Co., New York.

FRY, W. J., R. KRUMINS, F. J. FRY, G. THOMAS, S. BORBELY, and H. ADES (1963). Origins and distributions of some efferent pathways from the mammillary nuclei of the cat. *J. comp. Neurol. 120*, 195–257.

FULTON, J. F. (1934). Forced grasping and groping in relation to the syndrome of the premotor area. *Arch. Neurol. Psychiat. (Chic.) 31*, 221–235.

FULTON, J. F., C. F. JACOBSEN, and M. A. KENNARD (1932). A note concerning the relation of the frontal lobes to posture and forced grasping in monkeys. *Brain 55*, 524–536.

FULTON, J. F., and A. D. KELLER (1932). *The Sign of Babinski. A Study of the Evolution of Cortical Dominance.* Charles C Thomas, Springfield, Illinois.

FULTON, J. F., and M. A. KENNARD (1934). A study of flaccid and spastic paralyses produced by lesions of the cerebral cortex in primates. *Res. Publ. Ass. nerv. ment. Dis. 13*, 158–210.

Functions of the Corpus Callosum (1965). Ciba Foundation Study Group, No. 20 (E. G. Ettlinger, A. V. S. de Reuck, and R. Porter, eds.). J. & A. Churchill, London.

GACEK, R. R. (1960). Efferent component of the vestibular nerve. In *Neural Mechanisms of the Auditory and Vestibular Systems* (G. L. Rasmussen and W. F. Windle, eds.), pp. 276–284. Charles C Thomas, Springfield, Illinois.

GACEK, R. R. (1961). The efferent cochlear bundle in man. *Arch. Otolaryng. 74*, 690–694.

GALAMBOS, R. (1956). Suppression of auditory nerve activity by stimulation of efferent fibers to cochlea. *J. Neurophysiol. 19*, 424–437.

GANES, T., B. R. KAADA, and R. NYBERG-HANSEN (1966). Failure to produce postural tremor by mesencephalic lesions in cats. *J. comp. Neurol. 128*, 127–132.

GARCIN, R., and J. LAPRESLE (1954). Syndrome sensitif de type thalamique et a topographie chéiro-orale par lésion localisée du thalamus. *Rev. Neurol. 90,* 124–129.

GARDNER, E. (1944). The distribution and termination of nerves in the knee joint of the cat. *J. comp. Neurol. 80,* 11–32.

GARDNER, E. (1967). Spinal cord and brain stem pathways for afferents from joints. In *Myotatic and Vestibular Mechanisms.* Ciba Foundation Symposium (A. V. D. de Reuck and J. Knight, eds.), pp. 56–76. J. & A. Churchill, Ltd., London.

GARDNER, E., and H. M. CUNEO (1945). Lateral spinothalamic tract and associated tracts in man. *Arch. Neurol. Psychiat. (Chic.) 53,* 423–430.

GAREY, L. J., E. G. JONES, and T. P. S. POWELL (1968). Interrelationships of striate and extrastriate cortex with the primary relay sites of the visual pathway. *J. Neurol. Neurosurg. Psychiat. 31,* 135–157.

GAREY, L. J., and T. P. S. POWELL (1967). The projection of the lateral geniculate nucleus upon the cortex in the cat. *Proc. roy. Soc. B 169,* 107–126.

GAREY, L. J., and T. P. S. POWELL (1968). The projection of the retina in the cat. *J. Anat. (Lond.) 102,* 189–222.

GASSEL, M. M. (1961). False localizing signs. A review of the concept and analysis of the occurrence in 250 cases of intracranial meningioma. *Arch. Neurol. (Chic.) 4,* 526–554.

GASSEL, M. M., and E. DIAMANTOPOULOS (1964). The Jendrassik maneuver. II. An analysis of the mechanism. *Neurology (Minneap.) 14,* 640–642.

GASSEL, M. M., and O. POMPEIANO (1967). Tonic and phasic changes in threshold of arousal during desynchronized sleep. *Arch. ital. Biol. 105,* 480–498.

GASSEL, M. M., and D. WILLIAMS (1963). Visual function in patients with homonymous hemianopia. Part III. The completion phenomenon; insight and attitude to the defect; and visual functional efficiency. *Brain 86,* 229–260.

GASSER, H. S. (1935). Conduction in nerves in relation to fiber types. *Res. Publ. Ass. nerv. ment. Dis. 15,* 35–56.

GASTAUT, H. (1954). The brain stem and cerebral electrogenesis in relation to consciousness. In *Brain Mechanisms and Consciousness.* A Ciba Foundation Symposium (J. F. Delafresnaye, ed.), pp. 249–279. Blackwell Scientific Publ., Oxford.

GAUTIER, C., and J. LEREBOULLET (1927). Syndrome inférieur du noyau rouge. *Rev. Neurol. 1,* 57–61.

GAZE, R. M., F. J. GILLINGHAM, S. KALYANARAMAN, R. W. PORTER, A. A. DONALDSON, and I. M. L. DONALDSON (1964). Microelectrode recordings from the human thalamus. *Brain 87,* 691–706.

GAZE, R. M., and G. GORDON (1954). The representation of cutaneous sense in the thalamus of the cat and monkey. *Quart. J. exp. Physiol. 39,* 279–304.

GAZZANIGA, M. S., J. E. BOGEN, and R. W. SPERRY (1965). Observations on visual perception after disconnexion of the cerebral hemispheres in man. *Brain 88,* 221–236.

GAZZANIGA, M. S., and R. W. SPERRY (1967). Language after section of the cerebral commissures. *Brain 90,* 131–148.

GELFAN, S., and A. F. RAPISARDA (1964). Synaptic density on spinal neurons of normal dogs and dogs with experimental hind-limb rigidity. *J. comp. Neurol. 123,* 73–96.

GEREBTZOFF, M. A. (1939). Les voies centrales de la sensibilité et du goût et leurs terminaisons thalamiques. *Cellule 48,* 91–146.

References

GERMAN, W. J., and B. S. BRODY (1940). The external geniculate bodies. Degeneration studies following occipital lobectomy. *Arch. Neurol. Psychiat. (Chic.)* *43*, 997–1003.

GERNANDT, B. (1949). Response of mammalian vestibular neurons to horizontal rotation and caloric stimulation. *J. Neurophysiol. 12*, 173–184.

GERNANDT, B. E., and S. GILMAN (1960). Interactions between vestibular, pyramidal, and cortically evoked extrapyramidal activities. *J. Neurophysiol. 23*, 516–533.

GERNANDT, B. E., M. IRANYI, and R. B. LIVINGSTON (1959). Vestibular influences on spinal mechanisms. *Exp. Neurol. 1*, 248–273.

GESCHWIND, N. (1965). Disconnexion syndromes in animals and man. *Brain 88*, 237–294.

GESCHWIND, N., and W. LEVITSKY (1968). Human brain: Left-right asymmetries in temporal speech region. *Science 161*, 186–187.

GETZ, B. (1952). The termination of spinothalamic fibres in the cat as studied by the method of terminal degeneration. *Acta. anat. (Basel) 16*, 271–290.

GETZ, B., and T. SIRNES (1949). The localization within the dorsal motor vagal nucleus. An experimental investigation. *J. comp. Neurol. 90*, 95–110.

GILLINGHAM, F. J. (1962). Small localized surgical lesion of the internal capsule in the treatment of the dyskinesias. *Confin. Neurol. (Basel) 22*, 385–392.

GILMAN, S., and D. DENNY-BROWN (1966). Disorders of movement and behaviour following dorsal column lesions. *Brain 89*, 397–418.

GILMAN, S., and J. P. VAN DER MEULEN (1966). Muscle spindle activity in dystonic and spastic monkeys. *Arch. Neurol. (Chic.) 14*, 553–563.

GJONE, R. (1965). A dual peripheral and supraspinal autonomic influence on the urinary bladder. *J. Oslo Cy Hosp. 15*, 173–182.

GLASGOW, E. F., and D. C. SINCLAIR (1962). Dissociation of thermal sensibility in procaine nerve block. *Brain 85*, 791–798.

GLEES, P. (1943). The Marchi reaction: Its use on frozen sections and its time limit. *Brain 66*, 229–232.

GLEES, P. (1944). The anatomical basis of cortico-striate connections. *J. Anat. (Lond.) 78*, 47–51.

GLEES, P. (1945). The interrelation of the strio-pallidum and the thalamus in the macaque monkey. *Brain 68*, 331–346.

GLEES, P. (1946). Terminal degeneration within the central nervous system as studied by a new silver method. *J. Neuropath. exp. Neurol. 5*, 54–59.

GLEES, P. (1952). Der Verlauf und die Endigung des Tractus spinothalamicus und der medialen Schleife, nach Beobachtungen beim Menschen und Affen. *Verh. anat. Ges. (Jena) 50*, 48–58.

GLEES, P., and W. E. LE GROS CLARK (1941). The termination of optic fibres in the lateral geniculate body of the monkey. *J. Anat. (Lond.) 75*, 295–308.

GLEES, P., J. COLE, C. W. M. WHITTY, and H. CAIRNS (1950). The effects of lesions in the cingular gyrus and adjacent areas in monkeys. *J. Neurol. Neurosurg. Psychiat. 13*, 178–190.

GLEES, P., and H. B. GRIFFITH (1952). Bilateral destruction of the hippocampus (Cornu Ammonis) in a case of dementia. *Mth. Rev. Psychiat. Neurol. 123*, 193–204.

GLEES, P., R. B. LIVINGSTON, and J. SOLER (1951). Der intraspinale Verlauf und die Endigungen der sensorischen Wurzeln in den Nucleus Gracilis und Cuneatus. *Arch. Psychiat. Nervenkr. 187*, 190–204.

GLEES, P., and P. D. WALL (1946). Fibre connections of the subthalamic region and the centro-median nucleus of the thalamus. *Brain 69*, 195–208.

GLICKSTEIN, M., R. A. KING, J. MILLER, and M. BERKLEY (1967). Cortical projections from the dorsal lateral geniculate nucleus of cats. *J. comp. Neurol. 130*, 55–76.

GLOBUS, A., and A. B. SCHEIBEL (1967a). Synaptic loci on visual cortical neurons of the rabbit: the specific afferent radiation. *Exp. Neurol. 18*, 116–131.

GLOBUS, A., and A. B. SCHEIBEL (1967b). Synaptic loci on parietal cortical neurons: termination of corpus callosum fibers. *Science 156*, 1127–1129.

GLOOR, P. (1955). Electrophysiological studies on the connections of the amygdaloid nucleus in the cat. *Electroenceph. clin. Neurophysiol. 7*, 243–264.

GLOOR, P. (1960). Amygdala. In *Handbook of Physiology*, Vol. II, Section I, Neurophysiology (J. Field, H. W. Magoun, and V. E. Hall, eds.), pp. 1395–1420. American Physiological Society, Washington, D.C.

GOLDBERG, J. M., and R. Y. MOORE (1967). Ascending projections of the lateral lemniscus in the cat and monkey. *J. comp. Neurol. 129*, 143–156.

GOLDBERG, J. M., and W. D. NEFF (1961). Frequency discrimination after bilateral section of the brachium of the inferior colliculus. *J. comp. Neurol. 116*, 265–290.

GOODMAN, D. C., R. E. HALLETT, and R. B. WELCH (1963). Patterns of localization in the cerebellar corticonuclear projections of the albino rat. *J. comp. Neurol. 121*, 51–67.

GORDON, G., and M. G. M. JUKES (1964a). Dual organization of the exteroceptive components of the cat's gracile nucleus. *J. Physiol. (Lond.) 173*, 263–290.

GORDON, G., and M. G. M. JUKES (1964b). Descending influence on the exteroceptive organizations of the cat's gracile nucleus. *J. Physiol. (Lond.) 173*, 291–319.

GORDON, G., and C. H. PAINE (1960). Functional organization in nucleus gracilis of the cat. *J. Physiol. (Lond.) 153*, 331–349.

GRANIT, R. (1950). The organization of the vertebrate retinal elements. *Ergebn. Physiol. 46*, 31–70.

GRANIT, R. (1955a). *Receptors and Sensory Perception*. Yale Univ. Press, New Haven, Connecticut.

GRANIT, R. (1955b). Centrifugal and antidromic effects on ganglion cells of retina. *J. Neurophysiol. 18*, 388–411.

GRANIT, R., H. D. HENATSCH, and G. STEG (1956). Tonic and phasic ventral horn cells differentiated by post-tetanic potentiation in cat extensors. *Acta physiol. scand. 37*, 114–126.

GRANIT, R., and B. HOLMGREN (1955). Two pathways from brain stem to gamma ventral horn cells. *Acta physiol. scand. 35*, 93–108.

GRANIT, R., B. HOLMGREN, and P. A. MERTON (1955). The two routes for excitation of muscle and their subservience to the cerebellum. *J. Physiol. (Lond.) 130*, 213–224.

GRANIT, R., C. JOB, and B. R. KAADA (1952). Activation of muscle spindles in pinna reflex. *Acta physiol. scand. 27*, 161–168.

GRANIT, R., and B. R. KAADA (1952). Influence of stimulation of central nervous structures on muscle spindles in cat. *Acta physiol. scand. 27*, 130–160.

GRANT, F. C., and L. M. WEINBERGER (1941). Experiences with intra-medullary tractotomy. I. Relief of facial pain and summary of operative results. *Arch. Surg. 42*, 681–692.

References

GRANT, G. (1962a). Spinal course and somatotopically localized termination of the spinocerebellar tracts. An experimental study in the cat. *Acta physiol. scand. 56, Suppl. 193,* 1–45.

GRANT, G. (1962b). Projection of the external cuneate nucleus onto the cerebellum in the cat: An experimental study using silver methods. *Exp. Neurol. 5,* 179–195.

GRANT, G., and H. ALDSKOGIUS (1967). Silver impregnation of degenerating dendrites, cells and axons central to axonal transection. I. A Nauta study on the hypoglossal nerve in kittens. *Exp. Brain Res. 3,* 150–162.

GRANT, G., G. ASCHAN, and L. EKVALL (1964). Nystagmus produced by localized cerebellar lesions. International Vestibular Symposium, Uppsala 1963. *Acta oto-laryng. (Stockh.) Suppl. 192,* 78–84.

GRANT, G., J. BOIVIE, and A. BRODAL (1968). The question of a cerebellar projection from the lateral cervical nucleus re-examined. *Brain Research 9,* 95–102.

GRANT, G., and O. OSCARSSON (1966). Mass discharges evoked in the olivocerebellar tract on stimulation of muscle and skin nerves. *Exp. Brain Res. 1,* 329–337.

GRANT, G., O. OSCARSSON, and I. ROSÉN (1966). Functional organization of the spinoreticulocerebellar path with identification of its spinal component. *Exp. Brain Res. 1,* 306–319.

GRANT, G., and B. REXED (1958). Dorsal spinal root afferents to Clarke's column. *Brain 81,* 567–576.

GRAY, E. G. (1959). Axo-somatic and axo-dendritic synapses of the cerebral cortex: An electron microscope study. *J. Anat. (Lond.) 93,* 420–433.

GRAY, E. G. (1961). The granule cells, mossy synapses and Purkinje spine synapses of the cerebellum: Light and electron microscope observations. *J. Anat. (Lond.) 95,* 345–356.

GRAY, E. G. (1963). Electron microscopy of presynaptic organelles of the spinal cord. *J. Anat. (Lond.) 97,* 101–106.

GRAY, E. G. (1966). Problems of interpreting the fine structure of vertebrate and invertebrate synapses. *Int. Rev. gen. exp. Zool. 2,* 139–170.

GRAY, E. G., and R. W. GUILLERY (1966). Synaptic morphology in the normal and degenerating nervous system. *Int. Rev. Cytol. 19,* 111–182.

GRAY, E. G., and L. H. HAMLYN (1962). Electron microscopy of experimental degeneration in the avian optic tectum. *J. Anat. (Lond.) 96,* 309–316.

GRAY, E. G., and V. P. WHITTAKER (1962). The isolation of nerve endings from brain: an electron-microscopic study of cell fragments derived by homogenization and centrifugation. *J. Anat. (Lond.) 96,* 79–88.

GRAY, J. A. B., and P. B. C. MATTHEWS (1951). Response of Pacinian corpuscles in the cat's toe. *J. Physiol. (Lond.) 113,* 475–482.

GREEN, J. D. (1951). The comparative anatomy of the hypophysis, with special reference to its blood supply and innervation. *Amer. J. Anat. 88,* 225–311.

GREEN, J. D. (1964). The hippocampus. *Physiol. Rev. 44,* 562–608.

GREEN, J. D., and A. A. ARDUINI (1954). Hippocampal electrical activity in arousal. *J. Neurophysiol. 17,* 533–557.

GREEN, J. D., and G. W. HARRIS (1949). Observation of the hypophysio-portal vessels of the living rat. *J. Physiol. (Lond.) 108,* 359–361.

GREVING, R. (1928). Die zentralen Anteile des vegetativen Nervensystems. *In v. Möllendorff's Handbuch der mikroskopischen Anatomie des Menschen,* IV/1, 917–1060. Springer-Verlag, Berlin.

GRILLNER, S., T. HONGO, and S. LUND (1966a). Interaction between the inhibitory pathways from the Deiters' nucleus and IA afferents to flexor motorneurones. (Abstract). *Acta physiol. scand. 68, Suppl. 277*, 61.

GRILLNER, S., T. HONGO, and S. LUND (1966b). Monosynaptic excitation of spinal α-motoneurones from the brain stem. *Experientia (Basel) 22*, 691.

GRILLO, M. A. (1966). Electron microscopy of sympathetic tissues. *Pharmacol. Rev. 18*, 387–399.

GRIM, M. (1967). Muscle spindles in the posterior cricoarytenoid muscle of the human larynx. *Folia morph. (Praha) 15*, 124–131.

GRIMBY, L. (1963a). Normal plantar response: integration of flexor and extensor reflex components. *J. Neurol. Neurosurg. Psychiat. 26*, 39–50.

GRIMBY, L. (1963b). Pathological plantar response: disturbances of the normal integration of flexor and extensor reflex components. *J. Neurol. Neurosurg. Psychiat. 26*, 314–321.

GRIMBY, L. (1965). Pathological plantar response. Part I. Flexor and extensor components in early and late reflex parts. Part II. Loss of significance of stimulus site. *J. Neurol. Neurosurg. Psychiat. 28*, 469–481.

GRIMBY, L., E. KUGELBERG, and B. LÖFSTRÖM (1966). The plantar response in narcosis. *Neurology (Minneap.) 16*, 139–144.

GROFOVÁ, I., and J. MARSALA (1959). Tvar a struktura nucleus ruber u člověka. (Form and structure of the nucleus ruber in man.) *Cs. Morfol. 8*, 215–237.

GROOT, J. DE, and G. W. HARRIS (1950). Hypothalamic control of the anterior pituitary gland and blood lymphocytes. *J. Physiol. (Lond.) 111*, 335–346.

GROWDON, J. H., W. W. CHAMBERS, and C. N. LIU (1967). An experimental study of cerebellar dyskinesia in the rhesus monkey. *Brain 90*, 603–632.

GRÜNBAUM, A. S. F., and C. S. SHERRINGTON (1902). Observations on the physiology of the cerebral cortex of some of the higher apes. *Proc. roy. Soc. B 69*, 206–209.

GRÜNBAUM, A. S. F., and C. S. SHERRINGTON (1903). Observations on the physiology of the anthropoid apes. *Proc. roy. Soc. B 72*, 152–155.

GRUNDFEST, H., and B. CAMPBELL (1942). Origin, conduction, and termination of impulses in the dorsal spino-cerebellar tracts. *J. Neurophysiol. 5*, 275–294.

GUILD, S. R. (1932). Correlations of histologic observations and the acuity of hearing. *Acta oto-laryng. (Stockh.) 17*, 207–249.

GUILD, S. R., S. J. CROWE, C. C. BUNCH, and L. M. POLVOGT (1931). Correlation of differences in the density of innervation of the organ of Corti with differences in the acuity of hearing. *Acta oto-laryng. (Stockh.) 15*, 269–308.

GUILLERY, R. W. (1956). Degeneration in the post-commissural fornix and the mammillary peduncle of the rat. *J. Anat. (Lond.) 90*, 350–370.

GUILLERY, R. W. (1957). Degeneration in the hypothalamic connexions of the albino rat. *J. Anat. (Lond.) 91*, 91–115.

GUILLERY, R. W. (1966). A study of Golgi preparations from the dorsal lateral geniculate nucleus of the adult cat. *J. comp. Neurol. 128*, 21–50.

GUILLERY, R. W., H. O. ADRIAN, C. N. WOOLSEY, and J. E. ROSE (1966). Activation of somatosensory areas I and II of cat's cerebral cortex by focal stimulation of the ventrobasal complex. In *The Thalamus* (D. P. Purpura and M. D. Yahr, eds.), pp. 197–206. Columbia Univ. Press, New York.

GUILLERY, R. W., and H. J. RALSTON (1964). Nerve fibers and terminals: electron microscopy after Nauta staining. *Science 143*, 1331–1332.

GUIOT, G., M. SACHS, E. HERTZOG, S. BRION, J. ROUGERIE, J. C. DALLOZ, and

References

F. Napoléone (1959). Stimulation électrique et lésions chirurgicales de la capsule interne. Déductions anatomiques et pysiologiques. *Neuro-chirurgie 5*, 17–36.

Guttmann, L. (1940). The distribution of disturbances of sweat secretion after extirpation of certain sympathetic cervical ganglia in man. *J. Anat. (Lond.) 74*, 537–549.

Ha, H., and F. Morin (1964). Comparative anatomical observations of the cervical nucleus, n. cervicalis lateralis, of some primates. (Abstract.) *Anat. Rec. 148*, 374.

Hagbarth, K. E., and J. Fex (1959). Centrifugal influences on single unit activity in spinal sensory paths. *J. Neurophysiol. 22*, 321–338.

Hagbarth, K. E., and D. I. B. Kerr (1954). Central influences on spinal afferent conduction. *J. Neurophysiol. 17*, 295–307.

Hagbarth, K. E., and E. Kugelberg (1958). Plasticity of the human abdominal skin reflex. *Brain 81*, 305–318.

Hagen, E. (1949/50). Neurohistologische Untersuchungen an der menschlichen Hypophyse. *Z. Anat. Entwickl.-Gesch. 114*, 640–679.

Hagen, E., H. Knoche, D. C. Sinclair, and G. Weddell (1953). The role of specialized nerve terminals in cutaneous sensibility. *Proc. roy. Soc. B 141*, 279–287.

Häggqvist, G. (1936). Analyse der Faserverteilung in einem Rückenmarkquerschnitt (Th3). *Z. mikr.-anat. Forsch. 39*, 1–34.

Häggqvist, G. (1937). Faseranalytische Studien über die Pyramidenbahn. *Acta psychiat. neurol. scand. 12*, 457–466.

Halban, H. V., and M. Infeld (1902). Zur Pathologie der Hirnschenkelhaube mit besonderer Berücksichtigung der posthemiplegischen Bevegungserscheinungen. *Arb. neurol. Inst. Univ. Wien 9*, 329–404.

Hall, E. A. (1963). Efferent connections of the basal and lateral nuclei of the amygdala in the cat. *Amer. J. Anat. 113*, 139–145.

Halstead, W. C., A. E. Walker, and P. C. Bucy (1940). Sparing and nonsparing of 'macular' vision associated with occipital lobectomy in man. *Arch. Ophthal. 24*, 948–966.

Hamberger, B., and K. A. Norberg (1965). Adrenergic synaptic terminals and nerve cells in bladder ganglia of the cat. *Int. J. Neuropharmacol. 4*, 41–45.

Hamlyn, L. H. (1962). The fine structure of the mossy fibre endings in the hippocampus of the rabbit. *J. Anat. (Lond.) 96*, 112–120.

Hamlyn, L. H. (1963). An electron microscope study of pyramidal neurons in the Ammon's horn of the rabbit. *J. Anat. (Lond.) 97*, 189–201.

Hámori, J., and J. Szentágothai (1966a). Identification under the electron microscope of climbing fibers and their synaptic contacts. *Exp. Brain Res. 1*, 65–81.

Hámori, J., and J. Szentágothai (1966b). Participation of Golgi neuron processes in the cerebellar glomeruli: An electron microscope study. *Exp. Brain Res. 2*, 35–48.

Hampson, J. L. (1949). Relationship between cat cerebral and cerebellar cortices. *J. Neurophysiol. 12*, 37–50.

Hampson, J. L., C. R. Harrison, and C. N. Woolsey (1952). Cerebro-cerebellar projections and the somatotopic localization of motor function in the cerebellum. *Res. Publ. Ass. nerv. ment. Dis. 30*, 299–316.

HANBERY, J., C. AJMONE-MARSAN, and M. DILWORTH (1954). Pathways of non-specific thalamocortical projection systems. *Electroenceph. clin. Neurophysiol.* 6, 103–118.

HAND, P. J. (1966). Lumbosacral dorsal root terminations in the nucleus gracilis of the cat. Some observations on terminal degeneration in other medullary sensory nuclei. *J. comp. Neurol. 126,* 137–156.

HAND, P., and C. N. LUI (1966). Efferent projections of the nucleus gracilis. (Abstract). *Anat. Rec. 154,* 353–354.

HANSEBOUT, R. R., and J. B. R. COSGROVE (1966). Effects of intrathecal phenol in man. *Neurology (Minneap.) 16,* 277–282.

HANSEN, K., and H. SCHLIACK (1962). *Segmentale Innervation. Ihre Bedeutung für Klinik und Praxis.* Georg Thieme Verlag, Stuttgart.

HANSTRÖM, B. (1952). Transportation of colloid from the neurosecretory hypo-thalamic centres in the brain into the blood vessels of the neural lobe of the hypophysis. *Kungl. Fysiogr. Sällsk. Lund Förh. 22,* 31–35.

HARA, T., E. FAVALE, G. F. ROSSI, and G. SACCO (1961). Responses in mesencephalic reticular formation and central gray matter evoked by somatic peripheral stimuli. *Exp. Neurol. 4,* 297–309.

HARE, W. K., H. W. MAGOUN, and S. W. RANSON (1935). Pathways for pupillary constriction. *Arch. Neurol. Psychiat. (Chic.) 34,* 1188–1194.

HARKMARK, W. (1954). The rhombic lip and its derivatives in relation to the theory of neurobiotaxis. In *Aspects of Cerebellar Anatomy* (J. Jansen and A. Brodal, eds.), pp. 264–284. Johan Grundt Tanum, Oslo.

HARLEM, O. K., and A. LÖNNUM (1957). A clinical study of the abdominal skin reflexes in newborn infants. *Arch. Dis. Childh. 32,* 127–130.

HARRINGTON, R. B., R. W. HOLLENHORST, and G. P. SAYRE (1966). Unilateral internuclear ophthalmoplegia. *Arch. Neurol. (Chic.) 15,* 29–34.

HARRIS, A. J., R. HODES, and H. W. MAGOUN (1944). The afferent path of the pupillodilator reflex in the cat. *J. Neurophysiol. 7,* 231–243.

HARRIS, G. W. (1947). The innervation and actions of the neuro-hypophysis; an investigation using the method of remote-control stimulation. *Phil. Trans. B 232,* 385–441.

HARRIS, G. W. (1948). Electrical stimulation of the hypothalamus and the mechanism of neural control of the adenohypophysis. *J. Physiol. (Lond.) 107,* 418–429.

HARRIS, G. W. (1950). Oestrous rhythm. Pseudopregnancy and the pituitary stalk in the rat. *J. Physiol. (Lond.) 111,* 347–360.

HARRIS, G. W., M. REED, and C. P. FAWCETT (1966). Hypothalamic releasing factors and the control of anterior pituitary function. *Brit. med. Bull. 22,* 266–272.

HARRISON, F., and K. B. CORBIN (1942). Oscillographic studies on the spinal tract of the fifth cranial nerve. *J. Neurophysiol. 5,* 465–482.

HARRISON, J. M., and R. IRVING (1964). Nucleus of the trapezoid body. Dual afferent innervation. *Science 143,* 473–474.

HARRISON, J. M., and R. IRVING (1965). Anterior ventral cochlear nucleus. *J. comp. Neurol. 124,* 15–21.

HARRISON, J. M., and R. IRVING (1966a). Ascending connections of the anterior ventral cochlear nucleus in the rat. *J. comp. Neurol. 126,* 51–63.

HARRISON, J. M., and R. IRVING (1966b). The organization of the posterior ventral cochlear nucleus in the rat. *J. comp. Neurol 126,* 391–401.

References

HARRISON, M. S. (1962). "Epidemic vertigo"—"vestibular neuronitis". A clinical study. *Brain* 85, 613–620.

HASSE, J., and J. P. VAN DER MEULEN (1961). Effects of supra-spinal stimulation on Renshaw cells belonging to extensor motoneurons. *J. Neurophysiol.* 24, 510–520.

HASSLER, R. (1949). Über die afferenten Bahnen und Thalamuskerne des motorischen Systems des Grosshirns. I. Mitteilung. Bindearm und Fasciculus thalamicus. II. Mitteilung. Weitere Bahnen aus Pallidum, Ruber, vestibulärem System zum Thalamus; Übersicht und Besprechung der Ergebnisse. *Arch. Psychiat. Nervenkr.* 182, 759–785, 786–818.

HASSLER, R. (1950). Projections of the cerebellum to the midbrain and the thalamus. *Dtsch. Z. Nervenheilk.* 163, 629–671.

HASSLER, R. (1956). Die zentralen Apparate der Wendebewegungen. II. Die neuronalen Apparate der vestibulären Korrekturwendungen und der Adversivbewegungen. *Arch. Psychiat. Nervenkr.* 194, 481–516.

HASSLER, R. (1959). Anatomy of the thalamus. In *Introduction to Stereotaxis with an Atlas of the Human Brain*, Vol. I (G. Schaltenbrand and P. Bailey, eds.), pp. 230–290. Grune & Stratton, New York.

HASSLER, R. (1960). Die zentralen Systeme des Schmerzes. *Acta. Neurochir. (Wien)* 8, 353–423.

HASSLER, R. (1961). Motorische und sensible Effekte umschriebener Reizungen und Ausschaltungen im menschlichen Zwischenhirn. *Dtsch. Z. Nervenheilk.* 183, 148–171.

HASSLER, R. (1964). Spezifische und unspezifische Systeme des menschlichen Zwischenhirns. In *Lectures on the Diencephalon, Progress in Brain Research*, Vol. 5 (W. Bargmann and J. P. Schadé, eds.), pp. 1–32. Elsevier Publishing Co., Amsterdam.

HASSLER, R. (1966a). Thalamic regulation of muscle tone and the speed of movements. In *The Thalamus* (D. P. Purpura and M. D. Yahr, eds.), pp. 419–436. Columbia Univ. Press, New York.

HASSLER, R. (1966b). Extrapyramidal motor areas of cat's frontal lobe: their functional and architectonic differentiation. *Int. J. Neurol. (Montevideo)* 5, 301–316.

HASSLER, R., and G. DIECKMANN (1967). Arrest reaction, delayed inhibition and unusual gaze behaviour resulting from stimulation of the putamen in awake, unrestrained cats. *Brain Research* 5, 504–507.

HASSLER, R., and K. MUHS-CLEMENT (1964). Architektonischer Aufbau des sensorimotorischen und parietalen Cortex der Katze. *J. Hirnforsch.* 6, 377–420.

HASSLER, R., and T. RIECHERT (1959). Klinische und anatomische Befunde bei stereotaktischen Schmerzoperationen im Thalamus. *Arch. Psychiat. Nervenkr.* 200, 93–122.

HAUG, F.-M. Š. (1967). Electron microscopical localization of the zinc in hippocampal mossy fibre synapses by a modified sulfide silver procedure. *Histochemie* 8, 355–368.

HAUGE, T. (1954). Catheter vertebral angiography. *Acta radiol. (Stockh.) Suppl.* 109, 1–219.

HAUGLIE-HANSSEN, E. (1968). Intrinsic neuronal organization of the vestibular nuclear complex in the cat. A Golgi study. *Ergebn. Anat. Entwickl.-Gesch.* 40, Heft 5, 1–105.

729

HAYASHI, M. (1924). Einige wichtige Tatsachen aus der ontogenetischen Entwicklung des menschlichen Kleinhirns. *Dtsch. Z. Nervenheilk. 81,* 74–82.

HAYHOW, W. R. (1958). The cytoachitecture of the lateral geniculate body in the cat in relation to the distribution of crossed and uncrossed optic fibers. *J. comp. Neurol. 110,* 1–64.

HAYMAKER, W., and B. WOODHALL (1945). *Peripheral Nerve Injuries. Principles of Diagnosis.* W. B. Saunders, Philadelphia.

HEAD, H., and G. HOLMES (1911–1912). Sensory disturbances from cerebral lesions. *Brain 34,* 102–254.

Hearing Mechanisms in Vertebrates. A Ciba Foundation Symposium (1968). (A. V. S. de Reuck and J. Knight, eds.). J. & A. Churchill, Ltd., London.

HEBB, D. A. (1945). Man's frontal lobe. A critical review. *Arch. Neurol. Psychiat. (Chic.) 54,* 10–24.

HEBB, D. A. (1954). The problem of consciousness and introspection. In *Brain Mechanisms and Consciousness.* CIOMS Symposium (J. F. Delafresnaye, ed.), pp. 402–417. Blackwell Scientific Publ., Oxford.

HEBB, D. A., and W. PENFIELD (1940). Human behaviour after extensive bilateral removal from the frontal lobes. *Arch. Neurol. Psychiat. (Chic.) 44,* 421–438.

HÉCAEN, H., and R. ANGELERGUES (1964). Localization of symptoms in aphasia. In *Disorders of Language.* Ciba Foundation Symposium (A. V. S. de Reuck and M. O'Connor, eds.), pp. 223–246. J. & A. Churchill, Ltd., London.

HÉCAEN, H., W. PENFIELD, C. BERTRAND, and R. MALMO (1956). The syndrome of apractognosia due to lesions of the minor hemisphere. *Arch. Neurol. Psychiat. (Chic.) 75,* 400–434.

HEIMER, L. (1967). Silver impregnation of terminal degeneration in some forebrain fiber systems: a comparative evaluation of current methods. *Brain Research 5,* 86–108.

HEIMER, L. (1968). Synaptic distribution of centripetal and centrifugal nerve fibres in the olfactory system of the rat. An experimental anatomical study. *J. Anat. (Lond.) 103,* 413–432.

HEIMER, L., F. F. EBNER, and W. J. H. NAUTA (1967). A note on the termination of commissural fibers in the neocortex. *Brain Research 5,* 171–177.

HEIMER, L., and P. D. WALL (1968). The dorsal root distribution to the substantia gelatinosa of the rat with a note on the distribution in the cat. *Exp. Brain Res. 6,* 89–99.

HELD, M., and F. KLEINKNECHT (1927). Die lokale Entspannung der Basilarmembran und ihre Hörlücken. *Pflügers Arch. ges. Physiol. 216,* 1–31.

HELLER, H. (1966). The hormone content of the vertebrate hypothalamo-neurohypophysial system. *Brit. med. Bull. 22,* 227–231.

HELMHOLTZ, H. L. F. (1863). Die Lehre von den Tonempfindungen als physiologische Grundlage für die Theorie der Musik. *On the Sensations of Tone* (1875). English translation of 3rd edition (A. J. Ellis, trans.). Longmans, Green, London.

HENDERSON, J. L. (1939). The congenital facial diplegia syndrome, clinical features, pathology and aetiology. *Brain 62,* 381–403.

HENNEMAN, E., and C. B. OLSON (1965). Relations between structure and function in the design of skeletal muscles. *J. Neurophysiol. 28,* 581–598.

HENNEMAN, E., G. SOMJEN, and D. O. CARPENTER (1965a). Functional significance of cell size in spinal motoneurons. *J. Neurophysiol. 28,* 560–580.

References

HENNEMAN, E., G. SOMJEN, and D. O. CARPENTER (1965b). Excitability and inhibitibility of motoneurons of different sizes. *J. Neurophysiol. 28,* 599–620.

HENRIKSSON, N. G., G. JOHANSSON, and H. ØSTLUND (1967). New techniques of otoneurological diagnosis. II. Vestibulo-spinal and postural patterns. In *Myotatic and Vestibular Mechanisms.* Ciba Foundation Symposium (A. V. D. de Reuck and J. Knight, eds.), pp. 231–237. J. & A. Churchill, Ltd., London.

HENSEL, H., and K. K. A. BOMAN (1960). Afferent impulses in cutaneous sensory nerves in human subjects. *J. Neurophysiol. 23,* 564–578.

HENSEL, H., A. IGGO, and I. WITT (1960). Quantitative study of sensitive cutaneous thermoreceptors with C afferent fibres. *J. Physiol. (Lond.) 153,* 113–126.

HERN, J. E. C., C. G. PHILLIPS, and R. PORTER (1962). Electrical thresholds of unimpaled corticospinal cells in the cat. *Quart. J. exp. Physiol. 47,* 134–140.

HERNÁNDEZ-PEÓN, R., and G. CHÁVEZ-IBARRA (1963). Sleep induced by electrical or chemical stimulation of the forebrain. *Electroenceph. clin. Neurophysiol. Suppl. 24,* 188–198.

HERNÁNDEZ-PEÓN, R., and K.-E. HAGBARTH (1955). Interaction between afferent and cortically induced reticular responses. *J. Neurophysiol. 18,* 44–55.

HERNÁNDEZ-PEÓN, R., A. LAVIN, C. ALCOCER-CUARÓN, and J. P. MARCELIN (1960). Electrical activity of the olfactory bulb during wakefulness and sleep. *Electroenceph. clin. Neurophysiol. 12,* 41–58.

HERRICK, C. J. (1933). The functions of the olfactory parts of the cerebral cortex. *Proc. nat. Acad. Sci. (Wash.) 19,* 7–14.

HESS, W. R. (1944). Das Schlafsyndrom als Folge diencephaler Reizung. *Helv. physiol. pharmacol. Acta 2,* 305–344.

HILD, W. (1954). Das morphologische, kinetische und endokrinologische Verhalten von hypothalamischem und neurohypophysärem Gewebe in vitro. *Z. Zellforsch. 40,* 257–312.

HILD, W., and G. ZETLER (1951). Über das Vorkommen der drei sogenannten "Hypophysenhinterlappenhormone" Adiuretin, Vasopressin und Oxytocin im Zwischenhirn als wahrscheinlicher Ausdruck einer neurosekretorischen Leistung der Ganglienzellen der *Nuclei supraopticus* und *paraventricularis. Experientia (Basel) 7,* 189–191.

HILD, W., and G. ZETLER (1953). Experimenteller Beweis für die Entstehung der sog. Hypophysenhinterlappenwirkstoffe im Hypothalamus. *Pflügers Arch. ges. Physiol. 257,* 169–201.

HILLARP, N.-Å. (1946). Structure of the synapse and the innervation apparatus of the autonomic nervous system. *Acta anat. (Basel) Suppl. IV,* 1–153.

HILLARP, N.-Å. (1960). Peripheral autonomic mechanisms. In *Handbook of Physiology, Section 1 Neurophysiology, Vol. II* (J. Field, H. W. Magoun, and V. E. Hall, eds.), pp. 979–1006. American Physiological Society, Washington, D.C.

HINES, M. (1937). The 'motor' cortex. *Bull. Johns Hopk. Hosp. 60,* 313–336.

HINES, M. (1944). Significance of the precentral motor cortex. In *The Precentral Motor Cortex* (P. C. Bucy, ed.), pp. 459–494. Univ. of Illinois Press, Urbana, Illinois.

HINMAN, A., and M. B. CARPENTER (1959). Efferent fiber projections of the red nucleus in the cat. *J. comp. Neurol. 113,* 61–82.

HINOJOSA, R., and J. D. ROBERTSON (1967). Ultrastructure of the spoon type synaptic endings in the nucleus vestibularis tangentialis of the chick. *J. Cell Biol. 34,* 421–430.

HINSEY, J. C., and R. A. PHILLIPS (1940). Observations upon diaphragmatic sensation. *J. Neurophysiol. 3*, 175–181.

HIRAYAMA, K., T. TSUBAKI, Y. TOYOKURA and S. OKINAYA (1962). The representation of the pyramidal tract in the internal capsule and basis pedunculi. A study based on three cases of amyotrophic lateral sclerosis. *Neurology (Minneap.) 12*, 337–342.

HOCKADAY, J. M., and C. W. M. WHITTY (1967). Patterns of referred pain in the normal subject. *Brain 90*, 481–496.

HOESSLY, G. F. (1947). Über optisch induzierte Blickbewegungen. *Helv. physiol. pharmacol. Acta 5*, 333–347.

HOFF, E. C., and H. E. HOFF (1934). Spinal termination of the projection fibres from the motor cortex of primates. *Brain 57*, 454–474.

HOFFMANN, P. (1918). Über die Beziehungen der Sehnenreflexe zur willkürlichen Bewegung und zum Tonus. *Z. Biol. 68*, 351–370.

HOFFMANN, W. (1933). Thalamussyndrom auf Grund einer kleinen Läsion. *J. Psychol. Neurol. (Lpz.) 45*, 362–374.

HOGG, I. D. (1944). The development of the nucleus dorsalis (Clarke's column). *J. comp. Neurol. 81*, 69–95.

HOLLOWAY, R. L., JR. (1968). The evolution of the primate brain: Some aspects of quantitative relations. *Brain Research 7*, 121–172.

HOLMES, G. (1917). The symptoms of acute cerebellar injuries due to gunshot injuries. *Brain 40*, 461–535.

HOLMES, G. (1938). The cerebral integration of ocular movements. *Brit. med. J. II*, 107–112.

HOLMES, G. (1939). The cerebellum of man. *Brain 62*, 1–30.

HOLMES, G., and W. T. LISTER (1916). Disturbances of vision from cerebral lesions, with special reference to the cortical representation of the macula. *Brain 39*, 34–73.

HOLMES, G. L., and W. P. MAY (1909). On the exact origin of the pyramidal tracts in man and other mammals. *Brain 32*, 1–42.

HOLMES, G., and T. G. STEWART (1908). On the connection of the inferior olives with the cerebellum in man. *Brain 31*, 125–137.

HOLMQVIST, B., A. LUNDBERG, and O. OSCARSSON (1960). Supraspinal inhibitory control of transmission to three ascending spinal pathways influenced by the flexion reflex afferents. *Arch. ital. Biol. 98*, 60–80.

HOLMQVIST, B., O. OSCARSSON, and I. ROSÉN (1963). Functional organization of the cuneocerebellar tract in the cat. *Acta physiol. scand. 58*, 216–235.

HONGO, T., and E. JANKOWSKA (1967). Effects from the sensorimotor cortex on the spinal cord in cats with transected pyramids. *Exp. Brain Res. 3*, 117–134.

HONGO, T., E. JANKOWSKA, and A. LUNDBERG (1965). Effects evoked from the rubrospinal tract in cats. *Experientia (Basel) 21*, 525–526.

HONGO, T., and Y. OKADA (1967). Cortically evoked pre- and postsynaptic inhibition of impulse transmission to the dorsal spinocerebellar tract. *Exp. Brain Res. 3*, 163–177.

HONGO, T., Y. OKADA, and M. SATO (1967). Corticofugal influences on transmission to the dorsal spinocerebellar tract from hindlimb primary afferents. *Exp. Brain Res. 3*, 135–149.

Horizons in Neuro-psychopharmacology, Progress in Brain Research, Vol. 16 (1965) (W. A. Himwich and J. P. Schadé, eds.). Elsevier Publishing Co., Amsterdam.

References

HORROBIN, D. F. (1966). The lateral cervical nucleus of the cat: an electrophysiological study. *Quart. J. exp. Physiol. 51,* 351–371.

HOUK, J., and E. HENNEMAN (1967). Responses of Golgi tendon organs to active contractions of the soleus muscle of the cat. *J. Neurophysiol. 30,* 466–481.

HOWE, H. A., and J. FLEXNER (1947). Succinic dehydrogenase activity in normal and regenerating neurons. Cited from Bodian, 1947.

HOWE, H. A., and R. C. MELLORS (1945). Cytochrome oxidase in normal and regenerating neurons. *J. exp. Med. 81,* 489–500.

HUBBARD, J. I., and O. OSCARSSON (1962). Localization of the cell bodies of the ventral spinocerebellar tract in lumbar segments of the cat. *J. comp. Neurol. 118,* 199–204.

HUBEL, D. H., and T. N. WIESEL (1961). Integrative action in the cat's lateral geniculate body. *J. Physiol. (Lond.) 155,* 385–398.

HUBEL, D. H., and T. N. WIESEL (1962). Receptive fields, binocular interaction and functional architecture in the cat's visual cortex. *J. Physiol. (Lond.) 160,* 106–154.

HUBEL, D. H., and T. N. WIESEL (1965). Receptive fields and functional architecture in two non-striate visual areas (18 and 19) of the cat. *J. Neurophysiol. 28,* 229–289.

HUBEL, D. H., and T. N. WIESEL (1968). Receptive fields and functional architecture of monkey striate cortex. *J. Physiol. (Lond.) 195,* 215–243.

HUBER, E. (1930). Evolution of facial musculature and cutaneous fields of trigeminus. *Quart. Rev. Biol. 5,* 389–437.

HUGELIN, A., M. BONVALLET, and P. DELL (1953). Topographie des projections cortico-motrices au niveau du télencéphale, du diencéphale, du tronc cérébral et du cervelet chez le chat. *Rev. Neurol. 89,* 419–425.

HUNT, C. C. (1961). On the nature of vibration receptors in the hind limb of the cat. *J. Physiol. (Lond.) 155,* 175–186.

HUNT, J. R. (1907). On herpetic inflammations of the geniculate ganglion: A new syndrome and its complications. *J. nerv. ment. Dis. 34,* 73–96.

HUNT, J. R. (1937). Geniculate neuralgia (neuralgia of the nervus facialis). *Arch. Neurol. Psychiat. (Chic.) 37,* 253–285.

HURSH, J. B. (1939). Conduction velocity and diameter of nerve fibers. *Amer. J. Physiol. 127,* 131–139.

HYDE, J. E., and R. G. EASON (1959). Characteristics of ocular movements evoked by stimulation of brainstem of cat. *J. Neurophysiol. 22,* 666–678.

HYDE, J. E., and S. G. ELIASSON (1957). Brainstem induced eye movements in cats. *J. comp. Neurol. 108,* 139–172.

HYNDMAN, O. R., and C. VON EPPS (1939). Possibility of differential section of the spino-thalamic tract: A clinical and histological study. *Arch. Surg. 38,* 1036–1053.

IGGO, A. (1962a). New specific sensory structures in hairy skin. *Acta neuroveg. (Wien) 24,* 175–180.

IGGO, A. (1962b). An electrophysiological analysis of afferent fibres in primate skin. *Acta neuroveg. (Wien) 24,* 225–240.

IGGO, A. (1966). Cutaneous receptors with a high sensitivity to mechanical displacement. In *Touch, Heat and Pain.* Ciba Foundation Symposium (A. V. S. de Reuck and J. Knight, eds.), pp. 237–256. J. & A. Churchill, Ltd., London.

ILLIS, L. (1964). Spinal cord synapses in the cat: the normal appearances by the light microscope. *Brain 87*, 543–554.

ILLIS, L. S. (1967). The motor neuron surface and spinal shock. In *Modern Trends in Neurology, 4* (D. Williams, ed.), pp. 53–68. Butterworths, London.

INGRAM, W. R. (1940). Nuclear organization and chief connections of the primate hypothalamus. *Res. Publ. Ass. nerv. ment. Dis. 20*, 195–244.

Interhemispheric Relations and Cerebral Dominance (1962). (V. B. Mountcastle, ed.). The Johns Hopkins Press, Baltimore.

International Vestibular Symposium (1964). Uppsala 1963, in memory of Robert Bárány. (A. Sjöberg, G. Aschan & J. Stahle, eds.) Almqvist & Wiksell, Uppsala. (Acta oto-laryng. Suppl. 192).

IRVING, R., and J. M. HARRISON (1967). The superior olivary complex and audition: A comparative study. *J. comp. Neurol. 130*, 77–86.

ITO, M., T. HONGO, M. YOSHIDA, Y. OKADA, and K. OBATA (1964). Antidromic and trans-synaptic activation of Deiters' neurones induced from the spinal cord. *Jap. J. Physiol. 14*, 638–658.

ITO, M., and M. YOSHIDA (1966). The origin of cerebellar-induced inhibition of Deiters neurones. I. Monosynaptic initiation of the inhibitory postsynaptic potentials. *Exp. Brain Res. 2*, 330–349.

JABBUR, S. J., and A. L. TOWE (1961). Cortical excitation of neurons in dorsal column nuclei of cat, including an analysis of pathways. *J. Neurophysiol. 24*, 499–509.

JACKSON, H. (1946). Discussion on cortical atrophy. *Proc. roy. Soc. Med. 39*, 423–427.

JACKSON, J. H., and C. E. BEEVOR (1890). Case of tumour of the right temporo-sphenoidal lobe bearing on the localisation of the sense of smell and on the interpretation of a particular variety of epilepsy. *Brain 12*, 346–357.

JACOBSEN, C. F. (1934). Influence of motor and premotor area lesions upon the retention of acquired skilled movements in monkeys and chimpanzees. *Res. Publ. Ass. nerv. ment. Dis. 13*, 225–247.

JACOBSEN, C. F. (1935). Functions of frontal association areas in primates. *Arch. Neurol, Psychiat. (Chic.) 33*, 558–569.

JAKOB, H. (1955). Zur Analyse konsekutiver Olivenschäden bei vasculär bedingten Kleinhirndefekten. *Arch. Psychiat. Nervenkr. 193*, 583–600.

JANKOWSKA, E., S. LUND, A. LUNDBERG, and O. POMPEIANO (1964). Postsynaptic inhibition in motoneurones evoked from the lower reticular formation. *Experientia (Basel) 20*, 701–702.

JANSEN, J. (1933). Experimental studies on the intrinsic fibers of the cerebellum. I. The arcuate fibers. *J. comp. Neurol. 57*, 369–400.

JANSEN, J. (1937). Experimental investigations of the associational connections of the cerebral cortex, with special reference to the conditions in the frontal lobe. *Skr. Norske Vidensk.-Akad., I. Mat.-nat. Kl. No. 1*, 1–21.

JANSEN, J. (1950). The morphogenesis of the cetacean cerebellum. *J. comp. Neurol. 93*, 341–400.

JANSEN, J. (1954). On the morphogenesis and morphology of the mammalian cerebellum. In *Aspects of Cerebellar Anatomy* (J. Jansen and A. Brodal, eds.), pp. 13–81. Johan Grundt Tanum, Oslo.

JANSEN, J., and A. BRODAL (1940). Experimental studies on the intrinsic fibers of the cerebellum. II. The corticonuclear projection. *J. comp. Neurol. 73*, 267–321.

References

JANSEN, J., and A. BRODAL (1942). Experimental studies on the intrinsic fibers of the cerebellum. III. The corticonuclear projection in the rabbit and the monkey. *Skr. Norske Vidensk.-Akad., I. Mat.-nat. Kl. No. 3,* 1–50.

JANSEN, J., and A. BRODAL (1958). Das Kleinhirn. In *Möllendorff's Handbuch der mikroskopischen Anatomie des Menschen IV/8.* Springer-Verlag, Berlin-Göttingen-Heidelberg.

JANSEN, J., and J. JANSEN JR. (1955). On the efferent fibers of the cerebellar nuclei in the cat. *J. comp. Neurol. 102,* 607–632.

JANSEN, J., and F. WALBERG (1964). Cerebellar corticonuclear projection studied experimentally with silver impregnation methods. *J. Hirnforsch. 6,* 338–354.

JANSEN, J., JR. (1957). Afferent impulses to the cerebellar hemispheres from the cerebral cortex and certain subcortical nuclei. An electroanatomical study in the cat. *Acta physiol. scand. 41, Suppl. 143,* 1–99.

JANSEN, J. K. S. (1962). Spasticity—functional aspects. *Acta neurol. scand. 38, Suppl. 3,* 41–51.

JANSEN, J. K. S., and P. B. C. MATTHEWS (1962a). The central control of the dynamic response of muscle spindle receptors. *J. Physiol. (Lond.) 161,* 357–378.

JANSEN, J. K. S., and P. B. C. MATTHEWS (1962b). The effects of fusimotor activity on the static responsiveness of primary and secondary endings of muscle spindles in the decerebrate cat. *Acta physiol. scand. 55,* 376–386.

JANSEN, J. K. S., K. NICOLAYSEN, and T. RUDJORD (1966). Discharge pattern of neurons of the dorsal spinocerebellar tract activated by static extension of primary endings of muscle spindles. *J. Neurophysiol. 29,* 1061–1086.

JANSEN, J. K. S., and T. RUDJORD (1964). On the silent period and Golgi tendon organs of the soleus muscle of the cat. *Acta physiol. scand. 62,* 364–379.

JANSEN, J. K. S., and T. RUDJORD (1965). Fusimotor activity in a flexor muscle of decerebrate cat. *Acta physiol. scand. 63,* 236–246.

JASPER, H. H. (1949). Diffuse projection systems: the integrative action of the thalamic reticular system. *Electroenceph. clin. Neurophysiol. 1,* 405–420.

JASPER, H. H., and G. BERTRAND (1966). Thalamic units involved in somatic sensation and voluntary and involuntary movements in man. In *The Thalamus* (D. P. Purpura and M. D. Yahr, eds.), pp. 365–384. Columbia Univ. Press, New York.

JASPER, H. H., and J. DROOGLEVER-FORTUYN (1946). Experimental studies on the functional anatomy of petit mal epilepsy. *Res. Publ. Ass. nerv. ment. Dis. 26,* 272–298.

JASPER, H., R. LENDE, and T. RASMUSSEN (1960). Evoked potentials from the exposed somato-sensory cortex in man. *J. nerv. ment. Dis. 130,* 526–537.

JEFFERSON, A. (1963). Trigeminal root and ganglion injections using phenol in glycerine for the relief of trigeminal neuralgia. *J. Neurol. Neurosurg. Psychiat. 26,* 345–352.

JEFFERSON, G. (1938). On the saccular aneurysms of the internal carotid artery in the cavernous sinus. *Brit. J. Surg. 26,* 267–302.

JEFFERSON, G. (1958). The reticular formation and clinical neurology. In *Reticular Formation of the Brain.* Henry Ford Hospital International Symposium (H. H. Jasper, L. D. Proctor, R. S. Knighton, and R. T. Costello, eds.), pp. 729–738. Little, Brown and Co., Boston.

JEFFERSON, G. (1960). *Selected Papers.* Pitman Medical Publishing Co., London.

JEFFERSON, M. (1952). Altered consciousness associated with brain-stem lesions. *Brain 75,* 55–67.

JENKNER, F. L. (1961). Selective anterolateral chordotomy for upper extremity pain. *Arch. Neurol. (Chic.) 4*, 660–662.

JERGE, C. R. (1963a). Organization and function of the trigeminal mesencephalic nucleus. *J. Neurophysiol. 26*, 379–392.

JERGE, C. R. (1963b). The function of the nucleus supratrigeminalis. *J. Neurophysiol. 26*, 393–402.

JERVIS, G. A. (1963). Huntington's chorea in childhood. *Arch. Neurol. (Chic.) 9*, 244–257.

JOHNSON, T. N., and C. D. CLEMENTE (1959). An experimental study of the fiber connections between the putamen, globus pallidus, ventral thalamus, and midbrain tegmentum in cat. *J. comp. Neurol. 113*, 83–101.

JONES, E. G. (1967). Pattern of cortical and thalamic connexions of the somatic sensory cortex. *Nature (Lond.) 216*, 704–705.

JONES, E. G., and T. P. S. POWELL (1968a). The ipsilateral cortical connexions of the somatic sensory areas in the cat. *Brain Research 9*, 71–94.

JONES, E. G., and T. P. S. POWELL (1968b). The commissural connexions of the somatic sensory cortex in the cat. *J. Anat. (Lond.) 103*, 433–455.

JONGKEES, L. B. W., and A. J. PHILIPSZOON (1960). Some nystagmographical methods for the investigation of the effect of drugs upon the labyrinth. The influence of cinnarazine, hyoscine, largactil and nembutal on the vestibular system. *Acta physiol. pharmacol. neerl. 9*, 240–275.

JOUVET, M. (1962). Recherches sur les structures nerveuses et les mecanismes responsables des differentes phases du sommeil physiologique. *Arch. ital. Biol. 100*, 125–206.

JOUVET, M. (1964). Étude neurophysiologique clinique des troubles de la conscience. *Acta Neurochir. (Wien) 12*, 258–269.

JOUVET, M. (1965). Paradoxical sleep—A study of its nature and mechanisms. *Progr. Brain Res. 18*, 20–62.

JOUVET, M., and D. JOUVET (1963). A study of the neurophysiological mechanisms of dreaming. *Electroenceph. clin. Neurophysiol. Suppl. 24*, 133–157.

JOYNT, R. J. (1966). Verney's concept of the osmoreceptor. *Arch. Neurol. (Chic.) 14*, 331–344.

JUNG, R. (1958). Coordination of specific and nonspecific afferent impulses at single neurons of the visual cortex. In *Reticular Formation of the Brain.* Henry Ford Hospital International Symposium. (H. H. Jasper, L. D. Proctor, R. S. Knighton, W. C. Noshay, and R. J. Costello, eds.), pp. 423–434. Little, Brown and Co., Boston.

JUNG, R., and R. HASSLER (1960). The extrapyramidal motor systems. In *Handbook of Physiology*, Section 1, Vol. II (J. Field, H. W. Magoun, and V. E. Hall, eds.), pp. 863–927. American Physiological Society, Washington, D.C.

KAADA, B. R. (1951). Somato-motor, autonomic and electrocorticographic responses to electrical stimulation of 'rhinencephalic' and other structures in primates, cat and dog.—A study of responses from the limbic, subcallosal, orbito-insular, piriform and temporal cortex, hippocampus-fornix and amygdala. *Acta physiol. scand. 23, Suppl. 83*, 1–285.

KAADA, B. (1960). Cingulate, posterior orbital, anterior insular and temporal pole cortex. In *Handbook of Physiology*, Section 1. Neurophysiology, Vol. II (J. Field, H. W. Magoun, and V. E. Hall, eds.), pp. 1345–1372. American Physiological Society, Washington, D.C.

References

KAADA, B. (1963). Pathophysiology of Parkinson tremor, rigidity and hypokinesia. *Acta neurol. scand. 39, Suppl. 4,* 39–51.

KAADA, B. (1967). Brain mechanisms related to aggressive behavior. In *Aggression and Defense. Neural Mechanisms and Social Patterns* (C. D. Clemente and D. B. Lindsley, eds.), pp. 95–216. Univ. of California Press, Berkeley.

KAADA, B. R., P. ANDERSEN, and J. JANSEN, JR. (1954). Stimulation of the amygdaloid nuclear complex in unanesthetized cats. *Neurology (Minneap.) 4,* 48–64.

KAADA, B. R., W. HARKMARK, and O. STOKKE (1961). Deep coma associated with desynchronization in EEG. *Electroenceph. clin. Neurophysiol. 13,* 785–789.

KAADA, B. R., J. JANSEN, JR., and P. ANDERSEN (1953). Stimulation of the hippocampus and medial cortical areas in unanesthetized cats. *Neurology (Minneap.) 3,* 844–857.

KAADA, B. R., E. W. RASMUSSEN, and O. KVEIM (1961). Effects of hippocampal lesions on maze learning and retention in rats. *Exp. Neurol. 3,* 333–355.

KAELBER, W. W., and C. L. MITCHELL (1967). The centrum medianum—central tegmental fasciculus complex. A stimulation, lesion and degeneration study in the cat. *Brain 90,* 83–100.

KANKI, S., and T. BAN (1952). Cortico-fugal connections of frontal lobe in man. *Med. J. Osaka Univ. 3,* 201–222.

KAPPERS, C. U. A. (1927). Three lectures on neurobiotaxis and other subjects. *Acta Psychiat. (Kbh.) 2,* 118–185.

KAPPERS, C. U. A., G. C. HUBER, and E. CROSBY (1936). *The Comparative Anatomy of the Nervous System of Vertebrates, including Man.* The Macmillan Co., New York.

KAPPERS, J. A. (1964). A survey of different opinions relating to the structure of the peripheral autonomic nervous system. *Acta Neuroveg. (Wien) 26,* 145–171.

KEEGAN, J. J., and F. D. GARRETT (1948). The segmental distribution of the cutaneous nerves in the limbs of man. *Anat. Rec. 102,* 409–437.

KEELE, C. A. (1966). Measurement of responses to chemically induced pain. In *Touch, Heat and Pain.* A Ciba Foundation Symposium (A. V. S. de Reuck and J. Knight, eds.), pp. 57–72. J. & A. Churchill, London.

KEELE, K. D. (1957). *Anatomies of Pain.* Blackwell Scientific Publ., Oxford.

KELLY, D. L., S. GOLDRING, and J. L. O'LEARY (1965). Averaged evoked somatosensory responses from exposed cortex of man. *Arch. Neurol. (Chic.) 13,* 1–9.

KENNARD, M. A. (1944). Experimental analysis of the functions of the basal ganglia in monkeys and chimpanzees. *J. Neurophysiol. 7,* 127–148.

KENNARD, M. A., S. SPENCER, and G. FOUNTAIN (1941). Hyperactivity in monkeys following lesions of the frontal lobes. *J. Neurophysiol. 4,* 512–524.

KERNELL, D. (1966). Input resistance, electrical excitability, and size of ventral horn cells in cat spinal cord. *Science 152,* 1637–1640.

KERR, D. I. B., and K.-E. HAGBARTH (1955). An investigation of olfactory centrifugal fiber system. *J. Neurophysiol. 18,* 362–374.

KERR, D. I., F. P. HAUGEN, and R. MELZACK (1955). Responses evoked in the brain stem by tooth stimulation. *Amer. J. Physiol. 183,* 253–258.

KERR, F. W. L. (1961). Structural relation of the trigeminal spinal tract to upper cervical roots and the solitary nucleus in the cat. *Exp. Neurol. 4,* 134–148.

KERR, F. W. L. (1962). Facial, vagal and glossopharyngeal nerves in the cat. Afferent connections. *Arch. Neurol. (Chic.) 6,* 264–281.

KERR, F. W. L. (1963a). The divisional organization of afferent fibres of the trigeminal nerve. *Brain 86,* 721–732.

737

KERR, F. W. L. (1963b). The etiology of trigeminal neuralgia. *Arch. Neurol. (Chic.) 8,* 15–25.

KERR, F. W. L. (1966). On the question of ascending fibers in the pyramidal tract: with observations on spinotrigeminal and spinopontine fibers. *Exp. Neurol. 14,* 77–85.

KERR, F. W. L. (1967). Function of the dorsal motor nucleus of the vagus. *Science 157,* 451–452.

KERR, F. W. L., and S. ALEXANDER (1964). Descending autonomic pathways in the spinal cord. *Arch. Neurol. (Chic.) 10,* 249–261.

KERR, F. W. L., and J. A. BROWN (1964). Pupillomotor pathways in the spinal cord. *Arch. Neurol. (Chic.) 10,* 262–270.

KERR, F. W. L., and O. W. HOLLOWELL (1964). Location of pupillomotor and accommodation fibres in the oculomotor nerve: Experimental observations on paralytic mydriasis. *J. Neurol. Neurosurg. Psychiat. 27,* 473–481.

KERR, F. W. L., and R. A. OLAFSON (1961). Trigeminal and cervical volleys: Convergence on single units in the spinal gray at C-1 and C-2. *Arch. Neurol. (Chic.) 5,* 171–178.

KILOH, L. G., and S. NEVIN (1951). Progressive dystrophy of the external ocular muscles (Ocular myopathy). *Brain 74,* 115–143.

KIMURA, R., and J. WERSÄLL, JR. (1962). Termination of the olivo-cochlear bundle to the outer hair cells of the organ of Corti in the guinea-pig. *Acta oto-laryng. (Stockh.) 55,* 11–32.

KIMMEL, D. L. (1941). Development of the afferent components of the facial, glossopharyngeal and vagus nerves in the rabbit embryo. *J. comp. Neurol. 74,* 447–471.

KIRSCHE, W. (1958). Synaptische Formationen in den Ganglia lumbalia des Truncus sympathicus vom Menschen einschliesslich Bemerkungen über den heutigen Stand der Neuronenlehre. *Z. mikr.-anat. Forsch. 64,* 707–772.

KITE, W. C., JR., R. D. WHITFIELD, and E. CAMPBELL (1957). The thoracic herniated intervertebral disc syndrome. *J. Neurosurg. 14,* 61–67.

KLEITMAN, N. (1963). *Sleep and Wakefulness,* revised and enlarged edition. The Univ. of Chicago Press, Chicago.

KLÜVER, H. (1958). "The temporal lobe syndrome" produced by bilateral ablations. In *Neurological Basis of Behaviour.* Ciba Foundation Symposium (E. E. Wolstenholme and C. M. O'Connor, eds.), pp. 175–182. J. & A. Churchill, Ltd., London.

KLÜVER, H., and P. C. BUCY (1937). Psychic blindness and other symptoms following bilateral temporal lobectomy in rhesus monkeys. *Amer. J. Physiol. 119,* 352–353.

KNIGHTON, R. S. (1950). Thalamic relay nucleus for the second somatic sensory receiving area in the cerebral cortex of the cat. *J. comp. Neurol. 92,* 183–191.

KOIKEGAMI, H. (1957). On the correlation between cellular and fibrous patterns of the human brain stem reticular formation with some cytoarchitectonic remarks on the other mammals. *Acta med. biol. (Niigata) 5,* 21–72.

KOPPANG, K. (1962). Intrathecal phenol in the treatment of spastic conditions. *Acta neurol. scand. 38, Suppl. 3,* 63–68.

KORNELIUSSEN, H. K. (1967). Cerebellar corticogenesis in Cetacea, with special reference to regional variations. *J. Hirnforsch. 9,* 151–185.

KORNELIUSSEN, H. K. (1968). On the ontogenetic development of the cerebellum

References

(nuclei, fissures, and cortex) of the rat, with special reference to regional variations in corticogenesis. *J. Hirnforsch. 10,* 379–412.

KORNELIUSSEN, H. K., and J. JANSEN (1965). On the early development and homology of the central cerebellar nuclei in Cetacea. *J. Hirnforsch. 8,* 47–56.

KORNHUBER, H. (1966). Physiologie und Klinik des zentralvestibulären Systems (Blick- und Stützmotorik). In *Hals-Nasen Ohren-Heilkunde III/3* (J. Berendes, R. Link, and F. Zöllner, eds.), pp. 2150–2351. Georg Thieme Verlag, Stuttgart.

KORNMÜLLER, A. E., and R. JANZEN (1939). Über die normalen bioelektrischen Erscheinungen des menschlichen Gehirns. *Arch. Psychiat. Nervenkr. 110,* 224–252.

KRAUTHAMER, G. M., and D. ALBE-FESSARD (1964). Electrophysiologic studies of the basal ganglia and striopallidal inhibition of non-specific afferent activity. *Neuropsychologia 2,* 73–83.

KRISTIANSEN, K. (1949). Neurological investigations of patients with acute injuries of the head. *Skr. Norske Vidensk.-Akad., I. Mat.-nat. Kl.* No. 1, 1–169.

KRISTIANSEN, K. (1964). Neurosurgical considerations on the brain mechanisms of consciousness. *Acta neurochir. (Wien) 12,* 289–314.

KROG, J. (1964). Autonomic nervous control of the cerebral blood flow in man. *J. Oslo Cy Hosp. 14,* 25–33.

KRUGER, L., and D. ALBE-FESSARD (1960). Distribution of responses to somatic afferent stimuli in the diencephalon of the cat under chloralose anesthesia. *Exp. Neurol. 2,* 442–467.

KRUGER, L., and F. MICHEL (1962a). A morphological and somatotopic analysis of single unit activity in the trigeminal sensory complex of the cat. *Exp. Neurol. 5,* 139–156.

KRUGER, L., and F. MICHEL (1962b). Reinterpretation of the representation of pain based on physiological excitation of single neurons in the trigeminal sensory complex. *Exp. Neurol. 5,* 157–178.

KRUGER, L., R. SIMINOFF, and P. WITKOVSKY (1961). Single neuron analysis of dorsal column nuclei and spinal nucleus of trigeminal in cat. *J. Neurophysiol. 24,* 333–349.

KUBIE, L. S. (1954). Psychiatric and psychoanalytic considerations of the problem of consciousness. In *Brain Mechanisms and Consciousness* (J. F. Delafresnaye, ed.), pp. 444–467. Blackwell Scientific Publ., Oxford.

KUBIK, C. S., and R. D. ADAMS (1946). Occlusion of the basilar artery.—A clinical and pathological study. *Brain 69,* 73–121.

KUGELBERG, E., K. EKLUND, and L. GRIMBY (1960). An electromyographic study of the nociceptive reflexes of the lower limb. Mechanism of the plantar responses. *Brain 83,* 394–410.

KUGELBERG, E., and K. E. HAGBARTH (1958). Spinal mechanism of the abdominal and erector spinae skin reflexes. *Brain 81,* 290–304.

KUGELBERG, E., and U. LINDBLOM (1959). The mechanism of pain in trigeminal neuralgia. *J. Neurol. Neurosurg. Psychiat. 22,* 36–43.

KUHLENBECK, H. (1954). The human diencephalon. A summary of development, structure, function and pathology. *Confin. neurol. (Basel) Suppl. 14,* 1–230.

KUHLENBECK, H. (1957). *Brain and Consciousness.* S. Karger, Basel.

KUHLENBECK, H. (1959). Further remarks on brain and consciousness: The brain-paradox and the meaning of consciousness. *Confin. neurol. (Basel)* 19, 462–485.

KUHN, R. A. (1950). Functional capacity of the isolated human cord. *Brain 73*, 1–51.

KUNC, Z. (1965). Treatment of essential neuralgia of the 9th nerve by selective tractotomy. *J. Neurosurg. 23*, 494–500.

KUNC, Z., and J. MARSALA (1962). La localisation et la terminaison des voies afférentes des nerfs IX et X dans le bulbe. *Acta neurochir. (Wien) 19*, 512–522.

KUNTZ, A. (1920). The development of the sympathetic nervous system in man. *J. comp. Neurol. 32*, 173–229.

KUNTZ, A. (1938). The structural organization of the coeliac ganglia. *J. comp. Neurol. 69*, 1–12.

KUNTZ, A. (1940). The structural organization of the inferior mesenteric ganglia. *J. comp. Neurol. 72*, 371–382.

KUNTZ, A., and D. I. FARNSWORTH (1931). Distribution of afferent fibers via the sympathetic trunks and gray communicating rami to the brachial and lumbo-sacral plexuses. *J. comp. Neurol. 53*, 389–399.

KUNTZ, A., and C. A. RICHINS (1946). Reflex pupillodilator mechanisms. An experimental analysis. *J. Neurophysiol. 9*, 1–7.

KUPFER, C. (1962). The projection of the macula in the lateral geniculate nucleus of man. *Amer. J. Ophthal. 54*, 597–609.

KUPFER, C., L. CHUMBLEY, and J. DE C. DOWNER (1967). Quantitative histology of optic nerve, optic tract and lateral geniculate nucleus of man. *J. Anat. (Lond.) 101*, 393–401.

KUSAMA, T., K. OTANI, and E. KAWANA (1966). Projections of the motor, somatic sensory, auditory and visual cortices in cats. In *Progress in Brain Research,* Vol. 21, part A (T. Tokizane and J. P. Schadé, eds.), pp. 292–322. Elsevier Publishing Co., Amsterdam.

KUYPERS, H. G. J. M. (1958a). An anatomical analysis of cortico-bulbar connexions to the pons and lower brain stem in the cat. *J. Anat. (Lond.) 92*, 198–218.

KUYPERS, H. G. J. M. (1958b). Some projections from the peri-central cortex to the pons and lower brain stem in monkey and chimpanzee. *J. comp. Neurol. 110*, 221–255.

KUYPERS, H. G. J. M. (1958c). Cortico-bulbar connexions to the pons and lower brain stem in man. An anatomical study. *Brain 81*, 364–388.

KUYPERS, H. G. J. M. (1960). Central cortical projections to motor and somato-sensory cell groups. *Brain 83*, 161–184.

KUYPERS, H. G. J. M. (1966). Discussion. In *The Thalamus* (D. P. Purpura and M. D. Yahr, eds.), pp. 122–126. Columbia Univ. Press, New York.

KUYPERS, H. G. J. M., W. R. FLEMING, and J. W. FARINHOLT (1962). Subcortico-spinal projections in the rhesus monkey. *J. comp. Neurol. 118*, 107–137.

KUYPERS, H. G. J. M., and D. G. LAWRENCE (1967). Cortical projections to the red nucleus and the brain stem in the rhesus monkey. *Brain Research 4*, 151–188.

KUYPERS, H. G. J. M., M. K. SZWARCBART, M. MISHKIN, and H. E. ROSVOLD (1965). Occipitotemporal corticocortical connections in the rhesus monkey. *Exp. Neurol. 11*, 245–262.

KUYPERS, H. G. J. M., and J. D. TUERK (1964). The distribution of the cortical

References

fibres within the nuclei cuneatus and gracilis in the cat. *J. Anat. (Lond.) 98,* 143–162.

LADPLI, R., and A. BRODAL (1968). Experimental studies of commissural and reticular formation projections from the vestibular nuclei in the cat. *Brain Research 8,* 65–96.

LANCE, J. W., P. DE GAIL, and P. D. NEILSON (1966). Tonic and phasic spinal cord mechanisms in man. *J. Neurol. Neurosurg. Psychiat. 29,* 535–544.

LANCE, J. W., R. S. SCHWAB, and E. A. PETERSON (1963). Action tremor and the cogwheel phenomenon in Parkinson's disease. *Brain 86,* 95–110.

LANDAU, W. M., and M. H. CLARE (1959). The plantar reflex in man, with special reference to some conditions where the extensor response is unexpectedly absent. *Brain 82,* 321–355.

LANDAU, W. M., and M. H. CLARE (1964). Fusimotor function. Part VI. H reflex, tendon jerk, and reinforcement in hemiplegia. *Arch. Neurol. (Chic.) 10,* 128–134.

LANDGREN, S., A. NORDWALL, and C. WENGSTRÖM (1965). The location of the thalamic relay in the spino-cervico-lemniscal path. *Acta physiol. scand. 65,* 164–175.

LANDGREN, S., C. G. PHILLIPS, and R. PORTER (1962). Cortical fields of origin of the monosynaptic pyramidal pathways to some alpha motoneurones of the baboon's hand and forearm. *J. Physiol. (Lond.) 161,* 112–125.

LANDGREN, S., and D. WOLSK (1966). A new cortical area receiving input from group I muscle afferents. *Life Sciences 5,* 75–79.

LANGFITT, T. W., K. KAMEI, G. Y. KOFF, and S. M. PEACOCK, JR. (1963). Gamma neuron control by thalamus and globus pallidus. *Arch. Neurol. (Chic.) 9,* 593–606.

LANGWORTH, E. P., and D. TAVERNER (1963). The prognosis in facial palsy. *Brain 86,* 465–480.

LANGWORTHY, O. R., and L. ORTEGA (1943). The iris. Innervation of the iris of the albino rabbit as related to its function. Theoretical discussion of abnormalities of the pupils observed in man. *Medicine (Baltimore) 22,* 287–362.

LAPIDES, J. (1958). Structure and function of the internal vesical sphincter. *J. Urol. (Baltimore) 80,* 341–353.

LARSELL, O. (1934). Morphogenesis and evolution of the cerebellum. *Arch. Neurol. Psychiat. (Chic.) 31,* 373–395.

LARSELL, O. (1937). The cerebellum. A review and interpretation. *Arch. Neurol. Psychiat. (Chic.) 38,* 580–607.

LARSELL, O. (1945). Comparative neurology and present knowledge of the cerebellum. *Bull. Minn. med. Found. 5,* 73–112.

LARSELL, O. (1952). The morphogenesis and adult pattern of the lobules and fissures of the cerebellum of the white rat. *J. comp. Neurol. 97,* 281–356.

LARSELL, O. (1953). The anterior lobe of the mammalian and the human cerebellum. *Anat. Rec. 115,* 341.

LARSELL, O. (1967). *The Comparative Anatomy and Histology of the Cerebellum from Myxinoids through Birds* (J. Jansen, ed.). Univ. of Minnesota Press, Minneapolis, Minnesota.

LARSELL, O., and R. A. FENTON (1928). The embryology and neurohistology of the sphenopalatine ganglion connections; a contribution to the study of otalgia. *Laryngoscope (St. Louis) 38,* 371–389.

LARUELLE, L. (1937). La structure de la moelle épinière en coupes longitudinales. *Rev. Neurol. 67*, 695–725.

LASHLEY, K. S. (1934). The mechanism of vision. VII. The projection of the retina upon the primary optic centers in the rat. *J. comp. Neurol. 59*, 341–373.

LASHLEY, K. S. (1941). Thalamo-cortical connections of the rat's brain. *J. comp. Neurol. 75*, 67–121.

LASHLEY, K. S., and G. CLARK (1946). The cytoarchitecture of the cerebral cortex of Ateles: A critical examination of architectonic studies. *J. comp. Neurol. 85*, 223–306.

LASSEK, A. M. (1940). The human pyramidal tract. II. A numerical investigation of the Betz cells of the motor area. *Arch. Neurol. Psychiat. (Chic.) 44*, 718–724.

LASSEK, A. M. (1941). The human pyramidal tract. III. Magnitude of the large cells of the motor area (area 4). *Arch. Neurol. Psychiat. (Chic.) 45*, 964–972.

LASSEK, A. M. (1942a). The pyramidal tract. The effect of pre- and postcentral cortical lesions on the fiber components of the pyramids in monkey. *J. nerv. ment. Dis. 95*, 721–729.

LASSEK, A. M. (1942b). The human pyramidal tract. IV. A study of the mature, myelinated fibers of the pyramid. *J. comp. Neurol. 76*, 217–225.

LASSEK, A. M. (1944). The human pyramidal tract. X. The Babinski sign and destruction of the pyramidal tract. *Arch. Neurol. Psychiat. (Chic.) 52*, 484–494.

LASSEK, A. M. (1945). The human pyramidal tract. XI. Correlations of the Babinski sign and the pyramidal syndrome. *Arch. Neurol. Psychiat. (Chic.) 53*, 375–377.

LASSEK, A. M., and G. L. RASMUSSEN (1939). The human pyramidal tract. A fiber and numerical analysis. *Arch. Neurol. Psychiat. (Chic.) 42*, 872–876.

LASSEK, A. M., and M. D. WHEATLEY (1945). The pyramidal tract. An enumeration of the large motor cells of area 4 and the axons in the pyramids of chimpanzee. *J. comp. Neurol. 82*, 299–302.

LATIES, A. M., and J. M. SPRAGUE (1966). The projection of optic fibers to the visual centers in the cat. *J. comp. Neurol. 127*, 35–70.

LAURSEN, A. M. (1963). Corpus striatum. *Acta physiol. scand. 59, Suppl. 211*, 1–106.

LAURSEN, A. M., and M. WIESENDANGER (1967). The effect of pyramidal lesions on response latency in cats. *Brain Research 5*, 207–220.

LAVELLE, A., and F. W. LAVELLE (1958). Neuronal swelling and chromatolysis as influenced by the state of cell development. *Amer. J. Anat. 102*, 219–241.

LAVELLE, A., and F. W. LAVELLE (1959). Neuronal reaction to injury during development. Severance of the facial nerve *in utero. Exp. Neurol. 1*, 82–95.

LAVELLE, A., C.-N. LIU, and F. W. LAVELLE (1954). Acid phosphatase activity as related to nucleic acid sites in the nerve cell. *Anat. Rec. 119*, 305–323.

LAWN, A. M. (1966). The localization, in the nucleus ambiguus of the rabbit, of the cells of origin of motor nerve fibers in the glossopharyngeal nerve and various branches of the vagus nerve by means of retrograde degeneration. *J. comp. Neurol. 127*, 293–305.

LAWRENCE, D. G., and H. G. J. M. KUYPERS (1968a). The functional organization of the motor system in the monkey. I. The effects of bilateral pyramidal lesions. *Brain 91*, 1–14.

References

LAWRENCE, D. G., and H. G. J. M. KUYPERS (1968b). The functional organization of the motor system in the monkey. II. The effects of lesions of the descending brain-stem pathways. *Brain 91*, 15–36.

LE BEAU, J., M. DONDEY, and D. ALBE-FESSARD (1962). Détermination de la fonction de certaines structures cérébrales profondes par refroidissement localisé et réversible. (Principles de la méthode, premières applications animales et humaines). *Rev. Neurol. 107*, 485–499.

LE BEAU, J., and A. PETRIE (1953). A comparison of the personality changes after (1) prefrontal selective surgery for the relief of intractable pain and for the treatment of mental cases; (2) cingulectomy and topectomy. *J. ment. Sci. 99*, 53–61.

LEES, F., and L. A. LIVERSEDGE (1962). Descending ocular myopathy. *Brain 85*, 701–710.

LEKSELL, L. (1945). The action potential and excitatory effects of the small ventral root fibres to skeletal muscle. *Acta physiol. scand. 10, Suppl. 31*, 1–84.

LELE, P. P., and G. WEDDELL (1956). The relationship between neurohistology and corneal sensibility. *Brain 79*, 119–154.

LELE, P. P., G. WEDDELL, and C. WILLIAMS (1954). The relationship between heat transfer, skin temperature and cutaneous sensibility. *J. Physiol. (Lond.) 126*, 206–234.

LEONTOVICH, T. A., and G. P. ZHUKOVA (1963). The specificity of the neuronal structure and topography of the reticular formation in the brain and spinal cord of carnivora. *J. comp. Neurol. 121*, 347–379.

LEVIN, P. M. (1936). The efferent fibers of the frontal lobe of the monkey, macaca mulatta. *J. comp. Neurol. 63*, 369–419.

LEVIN, P. M., and F. K. BRADFORD (1938). The exact origin of the cortico-spinal tract in the monkey. *J. comp. Neurol. 68*, 411–422.

LEVITT, M., M. CARRERAS, C. N. LIU, and W. W. CHAMBERS (1964). Pyramidal and extrapyramidal modulation of somatosensory acitvity in gracile and cuneate nuclei. *Arch. ital. Biol. 102*, 197–229.

LEWIN, R. J., G. V. DILLARD, and R. W. PORTER (1967). Extrapyramidal inhibition of the urinary bladder. *Brain Research 4*, 301–307.

LEWIN, W. (1961). Observations on selective leucotomy. *J. Neurol. Neurosurg. Psychiat. 24*, 37–44.

LEWIN, W., and C. G. PHILLIPS (1952). Observations on partial removal of the post-central gyrus for pain. *J. Neurol. Neurosurg. Psychiat. 15*, 143–147.

LEWIS, D., and W. E. DANDY (1930). The course of the nerve fibers transmitting sensation of taste. *Arch. Surg. 21*, 249–288.

LEWIS, R., and G. S. BRINDLEY (1965). The extrapyramidal cortical motor map. *Brain 88*, 397–406.

LEWIS, T. (1942). *Pain.* The Macmillan Co., New York.

LEWIS, T., and J. H. KELLGREN (1939). Observations relating to referred pain, visceromotor reflexes and other associated phenomena. *Clin. Sci. 4*, 47–71.

LEWY, F. H., and H. KOBRAK (1936). The neural projection of the cochlear spirals on the primary acoustic centers. *Arch. Neurol. Psychiat. (Chic.) 35*, 839–852.

LEYTON, A. S. F., and C. S. SHERRINGTON (1917). Observations on the excitable cortex of the chimpanzee, orang-utan, and gorilla. *Quart. J. exp. Physiol. 11*, 135–222.

LIBET, B., W. W. ALBERTS, E. W. WRIGHT, JR., and B. FEINSTEIN (1967). Responses of human somatosensory cortex to stimuli below threshold for conscious sensation. *Science 158,* 1597–1600.

LIDDELL, E. G. T., and C. G. PHILLIPS (1944). Pyramidal section in the cat. *Brain 67,* 1–9.

LIDDELL, E. G. T., and C. G. PHILLIPS (1950). Thresholds of cortical representation. *Brain 73,* 125–140.

LINDBLOM, U. F., and J. O. OTTOSSON (1956). Bulbar influence on spinal cord dorsum potentials and ventral root reflexes. *Acta physiol. scand. 35,* 203–214.

LINDBLOM, U. F., and J. O. OTTOSSON (1957). Influence of pyramidal stimulation upon the relay of coarse cutaneous afferents in the dorsal horn. *Acta physiol. scand. 38,* 309–318.

LINDGREN, I., and H. OLIVECRONA (1947). Surgical treatment of angina pectoris. *J. Neurosurg. 4,* 19–39.

LINDSLEY, D. B., L. H. SCHREINER, W. B. KNOWLES, and H. W. MAGOUN (1950). Behavioral and EEG changes following chronic brain stem lesions in the cat. *Electroenceph. clin. Neurophysiol. 2,* 483–498.

LIST, C. F., and M. M. PEET (1939). Sweat secretion in man. V. Disturbances of sweat secretion with lesions of the pons, medulla and cervical portion of the cord. *Arch. Neurol. Psychiat. (Chic.) 42,* 1098–1127.

LIST, C. F., and J. R. WILLIAMS (1957). Pathogenesis of trigeminal neuralgia. A review. *Arch. Neurol. Psychiat. (Chic.) 77,* 36–43.

LIU, C-N. (1956). Afferent nerves to Clarke's and the lateral cuneate nuclei in the cat. *Arch. Neurol. Psychiat. (Chic.) 75,* 67–77.

LIU, C-N., and W. W. CHAMBERS (1958). Intraspinal sprouting of dorsal root axons. *Arch. Neurol. Psychiat. (Chic.) 79,* 46–61.

LIU, C-N., and W. W. CHAMBERS (1964). An experimental study of the corticospinal system in the monkey (*Macaca mulatta*). The spinal pathways and preterminal distribution of degenerating fibers following discrete lesions of the pre- and postcentral gyri and bulbar pyramid. *J. comp. Neurol. 123,* 257–284.

LLINAS, R., and C. A. TERZUOLO (1964). Mechanisms of supraspinal actions upon cord activities. Reticular inhibitory mechanisms on alpha-extensor motoneurons. *J. Neurophysiol. 27,* 579–591.

LLOYD, D. P. C. (1941). The spinal mechanism of the pyramidal system in cats. *J. Neurophysiol. 4,* 525–546.

LOCKE, S. (1960). The projection of the medial pulvinar of the macaque. *J. comp. Neurol. 115,* 155–167.

LOCKE, S. (1961). The projection of the magnocellular medial geniculate body. *J. comp. Neurol. 116,* 179–193.

LOCKE, S. (1967). Thalamic connections to insular and opercular cortex of monkey. *J. comp. Neurol. 129,* 219–240.

LOCKE, S., J. B. ANGEVINE, JR., and P. I. YAKOVLEV (1964). Limbic nuclei of thalamus and connections of limbic cortex. VI. Thalamocortical projection of lateral dorsal nucleus in cats and monkeys. *Arch. Neurol. (Chic.) 11,* 1–12.

LOEB, C., and G. POGGIO (1953). Electroencephalograms in a case with pontomesencephalic haemorrhage. *Electroenceph. clin. Neurophysiol. 5,* 295–296.

LOHMAN, A. H. M. (1963). The anterior olfactory lobe of the guinea pig. A descriptive and experimental anatomical study. *Acta. anat. (Basel) 53, Suppl. 49,* 1–109.

LOHMAN, A. H. M., and G. M. MENTINK (1968). The lateral olfactory tract, the anterior commissure and the cells of the olfactory bulb. *Brain Research 12,* 396–413.

LONG, D. M., A. S. LEONARD, S. N. CHOU, and L. A. FRENCH (1962). Hypothalamus and gastric ulceration. I. Gastric effects of hypothalamic lesions. *Arch. Neurol. (Chic.) 7,* 167–175.

LONG, D. M., A. S. LEONARD, J. STORY, and L. A. FRENCH (1962). Hypothalamus and gastric ulceration. II. Production of gastrointestinal ulceration by chronic hypothalamic stimulation. *Arch. Neurol. (Chic.) 7,* 167–183.

LORENTE DE NÓ, R. (1933a). Anatomy of the eighth nerve. I. The central projection of the nerve endings of the internal ear. *Laryngoscope (St. Louis) 43,* 1–38.

LORENTE DE NÓ, R. (1933b). Anatomy of the eighth nerve. III. General plan of structure of the primary cochlear nuclei. *Laryngoscope (St. Louis) 43,* 327–350.

LORENTE DE NÓ, R. (1933c). Studies on the structure of the cerebral cortex. I. The area entorhinalis. *J. Psychol. Neurol. (Lpz.) 45,* 381–438.

LORENTE DE NÓ, R. (1934). Studies on the structure of the cerebral cortex. II. Continuation of the study of the Amnonic system. *J. Psychol. Neurol. (Lpz.) 46,* 117–177.

LORENTE DE NÓ, R. (1949). Cerebral cortex: architecture, intracortical connections, motor projections. In Fulton's *Physiology of the Nervous System,* 3rd ed., pp. 288–312. Oxford Univ. Press, New York.

LOWENSTEIN, O. (1966). The functional significance of the ultrastructure of the vestibular end organs. In *NASA SP-115.* Second symposium on the role of the vestibular organs in space exploration, pp. 73–87. Ames Research Center, Moffett Field, California.

LOWENSTEIN, O. (1967). Functional aspects of vestibular structure. In *Myotatic and Vestibular Mechanisms,* Ciba Foundation Symposium (A. V. D. de Reuck and J. Knight, eds.), pp. 121–128. J. & A. Churchill, Ltd., London.

LÖWENSTEIN, O., and A. SAND (1940). The mechanism of the semicircular canal. A study of the responses of single-fibre preparations to angular accelerations and to rotation at constant speed. *Proc. roy. Soc. B 129,* 256–275.

LUCAS KEENE, M. F. (1961). Muscle spindles in the human laryngeal muscles. *J. Anat. (Lond.) 95,* 25–29.

LUND, R. D., and K. E. WEBSTER (1967a). Thalamic afferents from the dorsal column nuclei. An experimental anatomical study in the rat. *J. comp. Neurol. 130,* 301–312.

LUND, R. D., and K. E. WEBSTER (1967b). Thalamic afferents from the spinal cord and trigeminal nuclei. An experimental anatomical study in the rat. *J. comp. Neurol. 130,* 313–327.

LUND, R. D., and L. E. WESTRUM (1966). Neurofibrils and the Nauta method. *Science 151,* 1397–1399.

LUND, S., and O. POMPEIANO (1965). Descending pathways with monosynaptic action on motoneurones. *Experientia (Basel) 21,* 602–603.

LUNDBERG, A. (1966). Integration in the reflex pathway. In *Nobel Symposium I: Muscular Afferents and Motor Control* (R. Granit, ed.), pp. 275–305. Almqvist & Wiksell, Stockholm; John Wiley & Sons, New York.

LUNDBERG, A. (1967). The supraspinal control of transmission in spinal reflex pathways. In *Recent Advances in Clinical Neurophysiology* (L. Widén, ed.), *Electroenceph. clin. Neurophysiol. Suppl. 25,* 35–46.

LUNDBERG, A., U. NORSELL, and P. VOORHOEVE (1962). Pyramidal effects on lumbo-sacral interneurones activated by somatic afferents. *Acta physiol. scand.* *56*, 220–229.

LUNDBERG, A., and O. OSCARSSON (1960). Functional organization of the dorsal spino-cerebellar tract in the cat. VII. Identification of units by antidromic activation from the cerebellar cortex with recognition of five functional subdivisions. *Acta physiol. scand. 50*, 356–374.

LUNDBERG, A., and P. VOORHOEVE (1962). Effects from the pyramidal tract on spinal reflex arcs. *Acta physiol. scand. 56*, 201–219.

LUNDBERG, P. O. (1957). A study of neurosecretory and related phenomena in the hypothalamus and pituitary of man. *Acta morph. neerl.-scand. 1*, 256–285.

LUNDBERG, P. O. (1960). Cortico-hypothalamic connexions in the rabbit. An experimental neuro-anatomical study. *Acta physiol. scand. 49, Suppl. 171*, 1–80.

LUNDERVOLD, A., T. HAUGE, and AA. C. LØKEN (1956). Unusual EEG in unconscious patient with brain stem atrophy. *Electroenceph. clin. Neurophysiol. 8*, 665–670.

LØKEN, AA. C., and A. BRODAL (1969). A somatotopical pattern in the lateral vestibular nucleus in man. In preparation.

MABUCHI, M., and T. KUSAMA (1966). The corticorubral projection in the cat. *Brain Research 2*, 254–273.

MACCHI, G., F. ANGELERI, and G. GUAZZI (1959). Thalamo-cortical connections of the first and second somatic sensory areas in the cat. *J. comp. Neurol. 111*, 387–405.

MACHNE, X., and J. P. SEGUNDO (1956). Unitary responses to afferent volleys in amygdaloid complex. *J. Neurophysiol. 19*, 232–240.

McCANN, S. M., A. P. S. DHARIWAL, and J. C. PORTER (1968). Regulation of the adenohypophysis. *Ann. Rev. Physiol. 30*, 589–640.

McCOUCH, G. P., J. D. DEERING, and T. H. LING (1951). Location of receptors for tonic neck reflexes. *J. Neurophysiol. 14*, 191–195.

McCOUCH, G. P., C-N. LIU, and W. W. CHAMBERS (1966). Descending tracts and spinal shock in the monkey (*Macaca mulatta*). *Brain 89*, 359–376.

McCULLOCH, W. S. (1944). Cortico-cortical connections. In *The Precentral Motor Cortex* (P. C. Bucy, ed.), pp. 211–242. Univ. of Illinois Press, Urbana, Illinois.

McILWAIN, J. T., and P. BUSER (1968). Receptive fields of single cells in the cat's superior colliculus. *Exp. Brain Res. 5*, 314–325.

McINTYRE, A. K. (1962). Cortical projection of impulses in the interosseus nerve of the cat's hind limb. *J. Physiol. (Lond.) 163,* 46–60.

McINTYRE, A. K., M. E. HOLMAN, and J. L. VEALE (1967). Cortical responses to impulses from single Pacinian corpuscles in the cat's hind limb. *Exp. Brain Res. 4*, 243–255.

MACKAY, D. M. (1967). The human brain. *Science Journal 3*, 43–47.

MACKEY, E. A., D. SPIRO, and J. WIENER (1964). A study of chromatolysis in dorsal root ganglia at the cellular level. *J. Neuropath. exp. Neurol. 23*, 508–526.

McKINLEY, W. A., and H. W. MAGOUN (1942). The bulbar projection of the trigeminal nerve. *Amer. J. Physiol. 137*, 217–224.

McKISSOCK, W., and K. W. E. PAINE (1958). Primary tumours of the thalamus. *Brain 81*, 41–63.

References

McLardy, T. (1950). Thalamic projections to frontal cortex in man. *J. Neurol. Neurosurg. Psychiat. 13*, 198–202.

McLardy, T. (1955a). Observations on the fornix of the monkey. I. Cell studies. *J. comp. Neurol. 103*, 305–326.

McLardy, T. (1955b). Observations on the fornix of the monkey. II. Fiber studies. *J. comp. Neurol. 103*, 327–344.

MacLean, J. B., and H. Leffman (1967). Supraspinal control of Renshaw cells. *Exp. Neurol. 18*, 94–104.

McLeod, J. G., and S. H. Wray (1967). Conduction velocity and fibre diameter of the median and ulnar nerves of the baboon. *J. Neurol. Neurosurg. Psychiat. 30*, 240–247.

McMahan, U. J. (1967). Fine structure of synapses in the dorsal nucleus of the lateral geniculate body of normal and blinded rats. *Z. Zellforsch. 76*, 116–146.

McMasters, R. E., A. H. Weiss, and M. B. Carpenter (1966). Vestibular projections to the nuclei of the extraocular muscles. Degeneration resulting from discrete partial lesions of the vestibular nuclei in the monkey. *Amer. J. Anat. 118*, 163–194.

Maffei, L., and O. Pompeiano (1962a). Cerebellar control of flexor motoneurons. An analysis of the postural responses to stimulation of the paramedian lobule in the decerebrate cat. *Arch. ital. Biol. 100*, 476–509.

Maffei, L., and O. Pompeiano (1962b). Effects of stimulation of the mesencephalic tegmentum following interruption of the rubrospinal tract. *Arch. ital. Biol. 100*, 510–525.

Magladery, J. W., and R. D. Teasdall (1961). Corneal reflexes. An electromyographic study in man. *Arch. Neurol. (Chic.) 5*, 269–274.

Magnes, J., G. Moruzzi, and O. Pompeiano (1961). Synchronization of the EEG produced by low-frequency electrical stimulation of the region of the solitary tract. *Arch. ital. Biol. 99*, 33–67.

Magni, F., R. Melzack, G. Moruzzi, and C. J. Smith (1959). Direct pyramidal influences on the dorsal-column nuclei. *Arch. ital. Biol. 97*, 357–377.

Magni, F., F. Moruzzi, G. F. Rossi, and Z. Zanchetti (1959). EEG arousal following inactivation of the lower brain stem by selective injection of barbiturate into the vertebral circulation. *Arch. ital. Biol. 97*, 33–46.

Magni, F., and W. D. Willis (1963). Identification of reticular formation neurons by intracellular recording. *Arch. ital. Biol. 101*, 681–702.

Magni, F., and W. D. Willis (1964a). Cortical control of brain stem reticular neurons. *Arch. ital. Biol. 102*, 418–433.

Magni, F., and W. D. Willis (1964b). Subcortical and peripheral control of brain stem reticular neurones. *Arch. ital. Biol. 102*, 434–448.

Magoun, H. W., and W. A. McKinley (1942). The termination of ascending trigeminal and spinal tracts in the thalamus of the cat. *Amer. J. Physiol. 137*, 409–416.

Magoun, H. W., and S. W. Ranson (1935). The afferent path of the light reflex. A review of the literature. *Arch. Ophthal. 13*, 862–874.

Magoun, H. W., and S. W. Ranson (1939). Retrograde degeneration of the supraoptic nuclei after section of the infundibular stalk in the monkey. *Anat. Rec. 75*, 107–124.

Magoun, H. W., and R. Rhines (1946). An inhibitory mechanism in the bulbar reticular formation. *J. Neurophysiol. 9*, 165–171.

MAKOUS, W., S. NORD, B. OAKLEY, and C. PFAFFMANN (1962). The gustatory relay in the medulla. In *Olfaction and Taste*. Proceedings First International Symposium, Wenner-Gren Center 1962 (Y. Zotterman, ed.), pp. 381–393. Pergamon Press, Oxford.

MALAMUD, N. (1966). The epileptogenic focus in temporal lobe epilepsy from a pathological standpoint. *Arch. Neurol. (Chic.) 14,* 190–195.

MALIS, L. I., K. H. PRIBRAM, and L. KRUGER (1953). Action potentials in motor cortex evoked by peripheral nerve stimulation. *J. Neurophysiol. 16,* 161–167.

MANCIA, M., J. D. GREEN, and R. VON BAUMGARTEN (1962). Reticular control of single neurons in the olfactory bulb. *Arch. ital. Biol. 100,* 463–475.

MANNI, E. (1950). Localizzazioni cerebellari corticali nella cavia. Nota 2a: Effetti di lesioni della "parti vestibolari" del cerveletto. *Arch. Fisiol. 50,* 1–14.

MARCHIAFAVA, P. L. (1968). Activities of the central nervous system: motor. *Ann. Rev. Physiol. 30,* 359–400.

MARIE, P., C. FOIX, and T. ALAJOUANINE (1922). De l'atrophie cérébelleuse tardive à predominance corticale. *Rev. Neurol. 38,* 849–885, 1082–1111.

MARIE, P., and G. GUILLAIN (1903). Lésion ancienne du noyau rouge. Dégénérations secondaires. *Nouv. Iconogr. Salpêt. 16,* 80–83.

MARIN, O. S. M., J. B. ANGEVINE, JR., and S. LOCKE (1962). Topographical organization of the lateral segment of the basis pedunculi in man. *J. comp. Neurol. 118,* 165–183.

MARIN-PADILLA, M. (1967). Number and distribution of the apical dendritic spines of the layer V pyramidal cells in man. *J. comp. Neurol. 131.* 475–489.

MARIN-PADILLA, M. (1968). Cortical axo-spinodentritic synapses in man: a Golgi study. *Brain Research 8,* 196–200.

MARK, V. H., F. R. ERVIN, and T. P. HACKETT (1960). Clinical aspects of stereotactic thalamotomy. Part I. The treatment of severe pain. *Arch. Neurol. (Chic.) 3,* 351–367.

MARK, V. H., F. R. ERVIN, and P. I. YAKOVLEV (1963). Stereotactic thalamotomy. III. The verification of anatomical lesion sites in the human thalamus. *Arch. Neurol. (Chic.) 8,* 528–538.

MARKEE, J. E., C. H. SAWYER, and W. H. HOLLINSHEAD (1946). Activation of the anterior hypophysis by electrical stimulation in the rabbit. *Endocrinology 38,* 345–357.

MARKHAM, C. H., W. J. BROWN, and R. W. RAND (1966). Stereotaxic lesions in Parkinson's disease. Clinicopathological correlations. *Arch. Neurol. (Chic.) 15,* 480–497.

MARKHAM, C. H., and R. W. RAND (1963). Stereotactic surgery in Parkinson's disease. *Arch. Neurol. (Chic.) 8,* 621–631.

MARQUARDSEN, J., and B. HARVALD (1964). The electroencephalogram in acute vascular lesions of the brain stem and the cerebellum. *Acta neurol. scand. 40,* 58–68.

MARSHALL, J. (1951). Sensory disturbances in cortical wounds with special reference to pain. *J. Neurol. Neurosurg. Psychiat. 14,* 187–204.

MARTIN, J. P. (1967). Role of the vestibular system in the control of posture and movement in man. In *Myotatic, Kinesthetic and Vestibular Mechanisms*. Ciba Foundation Symposium (A. V. S. de Reuck and J. Knight, eds.), pp. 92–96. J. & A. Churchill, Ltd., London.

MARTIN, J. P., and J. R. MCCAUL (1959). Acute herniballismus treated by ventrolateral thalamolysis. *Brain 82,* 104–108.

748

References

MARTINEZ, A. (1955). Some efferent connexions of the human frontal lobe. *J. Neurosurg. 12*, 18–25.

MARTINEZ, A. (1961). Fiber connections of the globus pallidus in man. *J. comp. Neurol. 117*, 37–41.

MARTINEZ, S. N., C. BERTRAND, and C. BOTANA-LOPEZ (1967). Motor fiber distribution within the cerebral peduncle. *Confin. neurol. (Basel) 29*, 117–122.

MASCITTI, T. A., and S. N. ORTEGA (1966). Efferent connections of the olfactory bulb in the cat. An experimental study with silver impregnation methods. *J. comp. Neurol. 127*, 121–136.

MASSION, J. (1967). The mammalian red nucleus. *Physiol. Rev. 47*, 383–436.

MASSOPUST, L. C. JR., and H. J. DAIGLE (1960). Cortical projection of the medial and spinal vestibular nuclei in the cat. *Exp. Neurol. 2*, 179–185.

MASTERTON, B., J. A. JANE, and I. T. DIAMOND (1967). Role of brainstem auditory structures in sound localization. I. Trapezoid body, superior olive, and lateral lemniscus. *J. Neurophysiol. 30*, 341–359.

MASTERTON, R. B., J. A. JANE, and I. T. DIAMOND (1968). Role of brain-stem auditory structures in sound localization. II: Inferior colliculus and its brachium. *J. Neurophysiol. 31*, 96–108.

MATTHEWS, B. H. C. (1933). Nerve endings in mammalian muscle. *J. Physiol. (Lond.) 78*, 1–53.

MATTHEWS, M. R., W. M. COWAN, and T. P. S. POWELL (1960). Transneuronal cell degeneration in the lateral geniculate nucleus of the macaque monkey. *J. Anat. (Lond.) 94*, 145–169.

MATTHEWS, M. R., and T. P. S. POWELL (1962). Some observations on transneuronal cell degeneration in the olfactory bulb of the rabbit. *J. Anat. (Lond.) 96*, 89–102.

MATTHEWS, P. B. C. (1962). The differentiation of two types of fusimotor fibre by their effects on the dynamic response of muscle spindle primary endings. *Quart. J. exp. Physiol. 47*, 324–33.

MATTHEWS, P. B. C. (1964). Muscle spindles and their motor control. *Physiol. Rev. 44*, 219–288.

MATZKE, H. A. (1951). The course of the fibers arising from the nucleus gracilis and cuneatus of the cat. *J. comp. Neurol. 94*, 439–452.

MEESSEN, H., and J. OLSZEWSKI (1949). *A Cytoarchitectonic Atlas of the Rhombencephalon of the Rabbit.* S. Karger, Basel.

MEHLER, W. R. (1962). The anatomy of the so-called "pain tract" in man: An analysis of the course and distribution of the ascending fibers of the fasciculus anterolateralis. In *Basic Research in Paraplegia* (J. D. French and R. W. Porter, eds.), pp. 26–55. Charles C Thomas, Springfield, Illinois.

MEHLER, W. R. (1966a). Some observations on secondary ascending afferent systems in the central nervous system. In *Pain* (R. S. Knighton and P. R. Dumke, eds.), pp. 11–32. Little, Brown and Co., Inc., Boston.

MEHLER, W. R. (1966b). Further notes on the centre médian, nucleus of Luys. In *The Thalamus* (D. P. Purpura and M. D. Yahr, eds.), pp. 109–127. Columbia Univ. Press, New York.

MEHLER, W. R., M. E. FEFERMAN, and W. J. H. NAUTA (1960). Ascending axon degeneration following anterolateral cordotomy. An experimental study in the monkey. *Brain 83*, 718–750.

MEIKLE, T. H., JR., and J. M. SPRAGUE (1964). The neural organization of the visual pathways in the cat. *Int. Rev. Neurobiol. 6*, 149–189.

749

MELLGREN, S. I., and T. W. BLACKSTAD (1967). Oxidative enzymes (tetrazolium reductase) in the hippocampal region of the rat. Distribution and relation to architectonics. *Z. Zellforsch. 78,* 167–207.

MELTZER, G. E., R. S. HUNT, and W. M. LANDAU (1963). Fusimotor function. Part III. The spastic monkey. *Arch. Neurol. (Chic.) 9,* 133–136.

MELZACK, R., and F. P. HAUGEN (1957). Responses evoked at the cortex by tooth stimulation. *Amer. J. Physiol. 190,* 570–574.

MELZACK, R., and P. D. WALL (1962). On the nature of cutaneous sensory mechanisms. *Brain 83,* 331–356.

MELZACK, R., and P. D. WALL (1965). Pain mechanisms: A new theory. *Science 150,* 971–979.

MERRILLEES, N. C. R., S. SUNDERLAND, and W. HAYHOW (1950). Neuromuscular spindles in the extraocular muscles in man. *Anat. Rec. 108,* 23–30.

METTLER, F. A. (1935). Corticofugal fiber connections of the cortex of *Macaca mulatta.* The occipital region. *J. comp. Neurol. 61,* 221–256. The frontal region. Ibid. 509–542. The parietal region. Ibid. *62,* 263–292. The temporal region. Ibid. *63,* 25–48.

METTLER, F. A. (1942). Relation between pyramidal and extrapyramidal function. *Res. Publ. Ass. nerv. ment. Dis. 21,* 150–227.

METTLER, F. A. (1944). Physiologic consequences and anatomic degenerations following lesions of the primate brain-stem: plantar and patellar reflexes. *J. comp. Neurol. 80,* 69–148.

METTLER, F. A. (1945). Fiber connections of the corpus striatum of the monkey and baboon. *J. comp. Neurol. 82,* 169–204.

METTLER, F. A. (1964). Substantia nigra and parkinsonism. *Arch. Neurol. (Chic.) 11,* 529–542.

METTLER, F. A. (1966). Experimentally produced tremor. Temporal factors in its development and disappearance in the monkey. *Arch. Neurol. (Chic.) 15,* 241–246.

METTLER, F. A., H. W. ADES, E. LIPMAN, and E. A. CULLER (1939). The extrapyramidal system. An experimental demonstration of function. *Arch. Neurol. Psychiat. (Chic.) 41,* 984–995.

METTLER, F. A., and A. J. LUBIN (1942). Termination of the brachium pontis. *J. comp. Neurol. 77,* 391–397.

METTLER, F. A., and G. M. STERN (1962). Somatotopic localization in rhesus subthalamic nucleus. *Arch. Neurol. (Chic.) 7,* 328–329.

MEYER, A. (1957). Hippocampal lesions in epilepsy. In *Modern Trends in Neurology* (D. Williams, ed.), pp. 301–306. Butterworths, London.

MEYER, A., and E. BECK (1945). Neuropathological problems arising from prefrontal leucotomy. *J. ment. Sci. 91,* 411–422.

MEYER, A., and E. BECK (1954). *Prefrontal Leucotomy and Related Operations: Anatomical Aspects of Success and Failure.* William Ramsay Henderson Trust Lecture. Oliver and Boyd, Edinburgh—London.

MEYER, J. S., and R. M. HERNDON (1962). Bilateral infarction of the pyramidal tracts in man. *Neurology (Minneap.) 12,* 637–642.

MEYER, M. (1949). A study of efferent connexions of the frontal lobe in the human brain after leucotomy. *Brain 72,* 265–296.

MEYER, M., and A. C. ALLISON (1949). An experimental investigation of the connexions of the olfactory tracts in the monkey. *J. Neurol. Neurosurg. Psychiat. 12,* 274–286.

References

MEYERS, R. (1953). The extrapyramidal system. An inquiry into the validity of the concept. *Neurology (Minneap.) 3,* 627–655.

MEYERS, R. (1958). Historical background and personal experiences in the surgical relief of hyperkinesia and hypertonus. In *Pathogenesis and Treatment of Parkinsonism* (W. S. Fields, ed.), pp. 229–270. Charles C Thomas, Springfield, Illinois.

MINCKLER, J. (1940). The morphology of the nerve terminals of the human spinal cord as seen in block silver preparations, with estimates of the total number per cell. *Anat. Rec. 77,* 9–25.

MINCKLER, J., R. M. KLEMME, and D. MINCKLER (1944). The course of efferent fibers from the human premotor cortex. *J. comp. Neurol. 81,* 259–277.

MIRSKY, A. F., H. E. ROSVOLD, and K. H. PRIBRAM (1957). Effects of cingulectomy on social behavior in monkeys. *J. Neurophysiol. 20,* 588–601.

MISKOLCZY, D. (1931). Ueber die Endigungsweise der spinocerebellaren Bahnen. *Z. Anat. Entwickl.-Gesch. 96,* 537–542.

MISKOLCZY, D. (1934). Die Endigungsweise der olivo-cerebellaren Faserung. *Arch. Psychiat. Nervenkr. 102,* 197–201.

MITCHELL, G. A. G. (1953). *Anatomy of the Autonomic Nervous System.* E. and S. Livingstone Ltd., Edinburgh.

MITCHELL, G. A. G., and R. WARWICK (1955). The dorsal vagal nucleus. *Acta anat. (Basel) 25,* 371–395.

MIZUNO, N. (1966). An experimental study of the spino-olivary fibers in the rabbit and the cat. *J. comp. Neurol. 127,* 267–291.

MOATAMED, F. (1966). Cell frequencies in the human inferior olivary nuclear complex. *J. comp. Neurol. 128,* 109–116.

MOLLARET, B., and M. GOULON (1959). Le coma dépassé. *Rev. Neurol. 101,* 3–15.

MONRAD-KROHN, G. H. (1927). Clinical neurology of the facial nerve. *Trans. Amer. neurol. Ass.,* pp. 190–193.

MONRAD-KROHN, G. H. (1939). On facial dissociation. *Acta psychiat. (Kbh). 14,* 557–566. (See also *Brain 47,* 1924.)

MONRAD-KROHN, G. H. (in cooperation with S. Refsum) (1964). *The Clinical Examination of the Nervous System,* 12th ed. H. K. Lewis, London.

MONRO, P. A. G. (1959). *Sympathectomy. An Anatomical and Physiological Study with Clinical Applications.* Oxford Univ. Press, London-New York-Toronto.

MOORE, R. Y., and J. M. GOLDBERG (1963). Ascending projections of the inferior colliculus in the cat. *J. comp. Neurol. 121,* 109–136.

MOORE, R. Y., and J. M. GOLDBERG (1966). Projections of the inferior colliculus in the monkey. *Exp. Neurol. 14,* 429–438.

MOREST, D. K. (1964). The neuronal architecture of the medial geniculate body of the cat. *J. Anat. (Lond.) 98,* 611–630.

MOREST, D. K. (1965a). The laminar structure of the medial geniculate body of the cat. *J. Anat. (Lond.) 99,* 143–160.

MOREST, D. K. (1965b). The lateral tegmental system of the midbrain and the medial geniculate body: study with Golgi and Nauta methods in cat. *J. Anat. (Lond.) 99,* 611–634.

MOREST, D. K. (1967). Experimental study of the projections of the nucleus of the tractus solitarius and the area postrema in the cat. *J. comp. Neurol. 130,* 277–300.

MORILLO, A., and D. BAYLOR (1963). Electrophysiological investigation of lemniscal and paraleminsical input to the midbrain reticular formation. *Electroenceph. clin. Neurophysiol. 15,* 455–464.

MORIN, F., and J. V. CATALANO (1955). Central connections of a cervical nucleus (nucleus cervicalis lateralis of the cat). *J. comp. Neurol. 103,* 17–32.

MORIN, F., D. T. KENNEDY, and E. GARDNER (1966). Spinal afferents to the lateral reticular nucleus. I. An histological study. *J. comp. Neurol. 126,* 511–522.

MORIN, F., S. T. KITAI, H. PORTNOY, and C. DEMIRJIAN (1963). Afferent projections to the lateral cervical nucleus: a microelectrode study. *Amer. J. Physiol. 204,* 667–672.

MORIN, F., H. G. SCHWARTZ, and J. L. O'LEARY (1951). Experimental study of the spinothalamic and related tracts. *Acta psychiat. neurol. scand. 26,* 371–396.

MORISON, R. S., and E. W. DEMPSEY (1942). A study of thalamo-cortical relations. *Amer. J. Physiol. 135,* 281–292.

MORTIMER, E. M., and K. AKERT (1961). Cortical control and representation of fusimotor neurons. *Amer. J. phys. Med. 40,* 228–248.

MORUZZI, G. (1940). Palaeocerebellar inhibition of vasomotor and respiratory carotid sinus reflexes. *J. Neurophysiol. 3,* 20–32.

MORUZZI, G. (1963). Active processes in the brain stem during sleep. *Harvey Lect. 58,* 233–297. Academic Press, New York.

MORUZZI, G., and H. W. MAGOUN (1949). Brain stem reticular formation and activation of the EEG. *Electroenceph. clin. Neurophysiol. 1,* 455–473.

MORUZZI, G., and O. POMPEIANO (1956). Crossed fastigial influence on decerebrate rigidity. *J. comp. Neurol. 106,* 371–392.

MOUNTCASTLE, V. B. (1957). Modality and topographic properties of single neurons of cat's somatic sensory cortex. *J. Neurophysiol. 20,* 408–434.

MOUNTCASTLE, V. B., M. R. COVIAN, and C. R. HARRISON (1952). The central representation of some forms of deep sensibility. *Ass. Res. nerv. Dis. Proc. 30,* 339–370.

MOUNTCASTLE, V., and E. HENNEMAN (1949). Pattern of tactile representation in thalamus of cat. *J. Neurophysiol. 12,* 85–100.

MOUNTCASTLE, V. B., and E. HENNEMAN (1952). The representation of tactile sensibility in the thalamus of the monkey. *J. comp. Neurol. 97,* 409–440.

MOUNTCASTLE, V. B., G. F. POGGIO, and G. WERNER (1963). The relation of thalamic cell response to peripheral stimuli varied over an intensive continuum. *J. Neurophysiol. 26,* 807–834.

MOUNTCASTLE, V. B., and T. P. S. POWELL (1959a). Central nervous mechanisms subserving position sense and kinesthesis. *Bull. Johns Hopk. Hosp. 105,* 173–200.

MOUNTCASTLE, V. B., and T. P. S. POWELL (1959b). Neural mechanisms subserving cutaneous sensibility, with special reference to the role of afferent inhibition in sensory perception and discrimination. *Bull. Johns Hopk. Hosp. 105,* 201–232.

MOUSHEGIAN, G., A. L. RUPERT, and T. L. LANGFORD (1967). Stimulus coding by medial superior olivary neurons. *J. Neurophysiol. 30,* 1239–1261.

MUGNAINI, E., and F. WALBERG (1967). An experimental electron microscopical study on the mode of termination of cerebellar corticovestibular fibres in the cat lateral vestibular nucleus (Deiters' nucleus). *Exp. Brain Res. 4,* 212–236.

MUGNAINI, E., F. WALBERG, and A. BRODAL (1967). Mode of termination of primary vestibular fibres in the lateral vestibular nucleus. An experimental electron microscopical study in the cat. *Exp. Brain Res. 4,* 187–211.

References

MULLAN, S., and W. PENFIELD (1959). Illusions of comparative interpretation and emotion. *Arch. Neurol. Psychiat. (Chic.) 81*, 269–284.

MÜLLER, R., and G. WOHLFART (1947). Om tumörer i corpus pineale (Pineal tumours). *Nord. Med. 33*, 15–21.

MURRAY, M. (1966). Degeneration of some intralaminar thalamic nuclei after cortical removals in the cat. *J. comp. Neurol. 127*, 341–367.

Muscular Afferents and Motor Control (1966). Proceedings of the First Nobel Symposium, Stockholm 1965 (R. Granit, ed.). Almqvist and Wiksell, Stockholm; John Wiley and Sons, New York.

MYERS, R. E. (1956). Function of corpus callosum in interocular transfer. *Brain 79*, 358–363.

MYERS, R. E. (1959). Localization of function in the corpus callosum. Visual gnostic transfer. *Arch. Neurol. (Chic.) 1*, 74–77.

MYERS, R. E. (1962). Commissural connections between occipital lobes of the monkey. *J. comp. Neurol. 118;* 1–16.

MYERS, R. E. (1965). Phylogenetic studies of commissural connexions. In *Functions of the Corpus Callosum*. Ciba Foundation Study Group, No. 20 (E. G. Ettlinger, A. V. S. de Reuck, and R. Porter, eds.), pp. 138–142. J. & A. Churchill, Ltd., London.

MYERS, R. E., and C. O. HENSON (1960). Role of corpus callosum in transfer of tactuokinesthetic learning in chimpanzee. *Arch. Neurol. (Chic.) 3*, 404–409.

Myotatic, Kinesthetic and Vestibular Mechanisms. Ciba Foundation Symposium (1967). (A. V. D. de Reuck and J. Knight, eds.). J. & A. Churchill, Ltd., London.

NANSEN, F. (1886). The structure and combination of the histological elements of the central nervous system. *Bergen Museums Årsberetn.*

NARABAYASHI, H., T. NAGAO, Y. SAITO, M. YOSHIDA, and M. NAGAHATA (1963). Stereotaxic amygdalotomy for behavior disorders. *Arch. Neurol. (Chic.) 9*, 1–16.

NARKIEWICZ, O., and S. BRUTKOWSKI (1967). The organization of projections from the thalamic mediodorsal nucleus to the prefrontal cortex of the dog. *J. comp. Neurol. 129*, 361–374.

NATHAN, P. W. (1956a). Reference of sensation at the spinal level. *J. Neurol. Neurosurg. Psychiat. 19*, 88–100.

NATHAN, P. W. (1956b). Awareness of bladder filling with divided sensory tract. *J. Neurol. Neurosurg. Psychiat. 19*, 101–105.

NATHAN, P. W. (1963). Results of antero-lateral cordotomy for pain in cancer. *J. Neurol. Neurosurg. Psychiat. 26*, 353–362.

NATHAN, P. W., and T. A. SEARS (1960). Effects of phenol on nervous conduction. *J. Physiol. (Lond.) 150*, 565–580.

NATHAN, P. W., T. A. SEARS, and M. C. SMITH (1965). Effects of phenol solutions on the nerve roots of the cat: An electrophysiological and histological study. *J. Neurol. Sci. 2*, 7–29.

NATHAN, P. W., and M. C. SMITH (1950). Normal mentality associated with a maldeveloped "rhinencephalon." *J. Neurol. Neurosurg. Psychiat. 13*, 191–197.

NATHAN, P. W., and M. C. SMITH (1951). The centripetal pathway from the bladder and urethra within the spinal cord. *J. Neurol. Neurosurg. Psychiat. 14*, 262–280.

NATHAN, P. W., and M. C. SMITH (1955a). Long descending tracts in man. I. Review of present knowledge. *Brain 78*, 248–303.

NATHAN, P. W., and M. C. SMITH (1955b). The Babinski response: A review and new observations. *J. Neurol. Neurosurg. Psychiat. 18,* 250–259.

NATHAN, P. W., and M. C. SMITH (1958). The centrifugal pathway for micturition within the spinal cord. *J. Neurol. Neurosurg. Psychiat. 21,* 177–189.

NATHAN, P. W., and M. C. SMITH (1959). Fasciculi proprii of the spinal cord in man: Review of present knowledge. *Brain 82,* 610–668.

Nature of Sleep, The. Ciba Foundation Symposium (1961). (G. E. W. Wolstenholme and M. O'Connor, eds.). J. & A. Churchill, Ltd., London.

NAUTA, W. J. H. (1946). Hypothalamic regulation of sleep in rats. An experimental study. *J. Neurophysiol. 9,* 285–314.

NAUTA, W. J. H. (1956). An experimental study of the fornix in the rat. *J. comp. Neurol. 104,* 247–272.

NAUTA, W. J. H. (1957). Silver impregnation of degenerating axons. In *New Research Techniques of Neuroanatomy* (W. F. Windle, ed.), pp. 17–26. Charles C Thomas, Springfield, Illinois.

NAUTA, W. J. H. (1958). Hippocampal projections and related neural pathways to the mid-brain in the cat. *Brain 81,* 319–340.

NAUTA, W. J. H. (1961). Fibre degeneration following lesions of the amygdaloid complex in the monkey. *J. Anat. (Lond.) 95,* 515–531.

NAUTA, W. J. H. (1962). Neural associations of the amygdaloid complex in the monkey. *Brain 85,* 505–520.

NAUTA, W. J. H. (1964). Some efferent connections of the prefrontal cortex in the monkey. In *The Frontal Granular Cortex and Behavior* (J. M. Warren and K. Akert, eds.), pp. 397–407. McGraw-Hill Book Co., New York.

NAUTA, W. J. H., and V. M. BUCHER (1954). Efferent connections of the striate cortex in the albino rat. *J. comp. Neurol. 100,* 257–286.

NAUTA, W. J. H., and P. A. GYGAX (1954). Silver impregnation of degenerating axons in the central nervous system. A modified technic. *Stain Technol. 29,* 91–93.

NAUTA, W. J. H., and H. G. J. M. KUYPERS (1958). Some ascending pathways in the brain stem reticular formation. In *Reticular Formation of the Brain.* Henry Ford Hospital Symposium (H. H. Jasper and L. D. Proctor, eds.), pp. 3–30. Little, Brown and Co., Boston.

NAUTA, W. J. H., and W. R. MEHLER (1966). Projections of the lentiform nucleus in the monkey. *Brain Research 1,* 3–42.

NAUTA, W. J. H., and D. G. WHITLOCK (1954). An anatomical analysis of the nonspecific thalamic projection system. In *Brain Mechanisms and Consciousness* (J. F. Delafresnaye, ed.), pp. 81–104. Blackwell Scientific Publ., Oxford.

NEFF, W. D., J. F. FISHER, I. T. DIAMOND, and M. YELA (1956). Role of auditory cortex in discrimination requiring localization of sound in space. *J. Neurophysiol. 19,* 500–512.

Nervous Control of the Heart (1965). (W. C. Randall, ed.). The Williams & Wilkins Co., Baltimore.

NEUBÜRGER, K. (1937). Über die nichtalkoholische Wernickesche Krankheit, insbesondere über ihr Vorkommen beim Krebsleiden. *Virchows Arch. path. Anat. 298,* 68–86.

Neural Mechanisms of the Auditory and Vestibular Systems (1960). (G. L. Rasmussen and W. Windle, eds.). Charles C Thomas, Springfield, Illinois.

Neurogenic Bladder, The (1966). (E. Pedersen, ed.). *Acta neurol. scand. 42,* Suppl. 20, 1–186. (Proc. Third Scand. Symp. Multiple Sclerosis, Aarhus 1965).

References

Neurological Aspects of Auditory and Vestibular Disorders (1964). (W. S. Fields and B. R. Alford, eds.). Charles C Thomas, Springfield, Illinois.

Neurological Basis of Behavior. Ciba Foundation Symposium (1958). (E. E. W. Wolstenholme and C. M. O'Connor, eds.). J. & A. Churchill, Ltd., London.

Neurophysiologie und Psychophysik des visuellen Systems (1961). Symposium Freiburg 1960 (R. Jung and H. Kornhuber, eds.) Springer-Verlag, Berlin.

NICOLAISSEN, B., and A. BRODAL (1959). Chronic progressive external ophthalmoplegia. *Arch. Ophthal. 61*, 202–210.

NIELSEN, J. M. (1946). *Agnosia, Apraxia, Aphasia*. Their Value in Cerebral Localization, 2nd. ed. P. B. Hoeber, Inc., New York.

NISSL, F. (1892). Über die Veränderungen der Ganglienzellen am Facialiskern des Kaninchens nach Ausreissung der Nerven. *Allg. Z. Psychiat. 48*, 197–198.

NISSL, F. (1908). Experimentalergebnisse zur Frage der Hirnrindenschichtung. *Mschr. Psychiat. Neurol. 23*, 186–188.

NOORDENBOS, W. (1959). *Pain. Problems Pertaining to the Transmission of Nerve Impulses which give Rise to Pain*. Elsevier Publishing Co., Amsterdam.

NORBERG, K. A. (1967). Transmitter histochemistry of the sympathetic adrenergic nervous system. *Brain Research 5*, 125–170.

NORBERG, K. A., and L. OLSON (1965). Adrenergic innervation of the salivary glands in the rat. *Z. Zellforsch. 68*, 183–189.

NORRSELL, U., and P. VOORHOEVE (1962). Tactile pathways from the hindlimb to the cerebral cortex in cat. *Acta physiol. scand. 54*, 9–17.

NYBERG-HANSEN, R. (1964a). Origin and termination of fibers from the vestibular nuclei descending in the medial longitudinal fasciculus. An experimental study with silver impregnation methods in the cat. *J. comp. Neurol. 122*, 355–367.

NYBERG-HANSEN, R. (1964b). The location and termination of tectospinal fibers in the cat. *Exp. Neurol. 9*, 212–227.

NYBERG-HANSEN, R. (1965a). Sites and mode of termination of reticulospinal fibers in the cat. An experimental study with silver impregnation methods. *J. comp. Neurol. 124*, 71–100.

NYBERG-HANSEN, R. (1965b). Anatomical demonstration of gamma motoneurons in the cat's spinal cord. *Exp. Neurol. 13*, 71–81.

NYBERG-HANSEN, R. (1966a). Functional organization of descending supraspinal fibre systems to the spinal cord. Anatomical observations and physiological correlations. *Ergebn. Anat. Entwickl.-Gesch. 39*, Heft 2, 1–48.

NYBERG-HANSEN, R. (1966b). Sites of termination of interstitiospinal fibers in the cat. An experimental study with silver impregnation methods. *Arch. ital. Biol. 104*, 98–111.

NYBERG-HANSEN, R. (1966c). Innervation and nervous control of the urinary bladder. *Acta neurol. scand. 42, Suppl. 20*, 7–24.

NYBERG-HANSEN, R. (1969). Corticospinal fibres from the medial aspect of the cerebral hemisphere in the cat. An experimental study with the Nauta method. *Exp. Brain Res. 7*, 120–132.

NYBERG-HANSEN, R., and A. BRODAL (1963). Sites of termination of corticospinal fibers in the cat. An experimental study with silver impregnation methods. *J. comp. Neurol. 120*, 369–391.

NYBERG-HANSEN, R., and A. BRODAL (1964). Sites and mode of termination of rubrospinal fibres in the cat. An experimental study with silver impregnation methods. *J. Anat. (Lond.) 98*, 235–253.

NYBERG-HANSEN, R., and T. MASCITTI (1964). Sites and mode of termination of fibers of the vestibulospinal tract in the cat. An experimental study with silver impregnation methods. *J. comp. Neurol. 122,* 369–387.

NYBERG-HANSEN, R., and E. RINVIK (1963). Some comments on the pyramidal tract, with special reference to its individual variations in man. *Acta neurol. scand. 39,* 1–30.

NYBY, O., and J. JANSEN (1951). An experimental investigation of the cortico-pontine projection in *Macaca mulatta. Skr. Norske Vidensk.-Akad., I. Mat.-nat. Kl. No. 3,* 1–47.

NYLÉN, C. O. (1950). Positional nystagmus. A review and further prospects. *J. Laryng. 64,* 295–318.

NYQUIST, B., S. REFSUM, and A. TORKILDSEN (1939). Det infraclinoide carotis interna-aneurysme—hemicrania ophthalmoplegica. *Nord. Med. 3,* 2325–2335.

NØRHOLM, T., and I. TYGSTRUP (1960). Correlation between the clinical effect of stereotactic operations and brain-autopsy findings. *Acta neurol. scand. 39, Suppl. 4,* 196–203.

O'CONNOR, W. J. (1948). Atrophy of the supraoptic and paraventricular nuclei after interruption of the pituitary stalk in dogs. *Quart. J. exp. Physiol. 34,* 29–42.

Oculomotor System, The (1964). (M. B. Bender, ed.). Harper & Row, Publishers, New York—Evanston—London.

OGAWA, T., and S. MITOMO (1938). Eine experimentell-anatomische Studie über zwei merkwürdige Faserbahnen im Hirnstamm des Hundes: Tractus mesen-cephalo-olivaris medialis (Economo et Karplus) und Tractus tecto-cerebellaris. *Jap. J. med. Sci., Trans. I. Anat. 7,* 77–94.

OGURA, J. H., and R. L. LAM (1953). Anatomical and physiological correlations on stimulating the human superior laryngeal nerve. *Laryngoscope (St. Louis) 63,* 947–959.

OHYE, C., K. KUBOTA, T. HONGO, T. NAGAO, and H. NARABAYASHI (1964). Ventro-lateral and subventrolateral thalamic stimulation. *Arch. Neurol. (Chic.) 11,* 427–434.

OJEMANN, G. A., P. FEDIO, and J. M. VAN BUREN (1968). Anomia from pulvinar and subcortical parietal stimulation. *Brain 91,* 99–116.

O'LEARY, J. L. (1940). A structural analysis of the lateral geniculate nucleus of the cat. *J. comp. Neurol. 73,* 405–430.

O'LEARY, J. (1941). Structure of the area striata of the cat. *J. comp. Neurol. 75,* 131–164.

Olfaction and Taste. Wenner-Gren Center International Symposium Series, Vol. 1 (1963). (Y. Zotterman, ed.). Pergamon Press, Oxford—London—New York —Paris.

Olfaction and Taste 2. Wenner-Gren Center International Symposium Series, Vol. 8 (1967). (T. Hayashi, ed.). Pergamon Press, Oxford—London—Edinburgh —New York—Toronto—Sidney—Paris—Braunschweig.

OLIVECRONA, HANS (1957). Paraventricular nucleus and pituitary gland. *Acta physiol. scand. 40, Suppl. 136,* 1–178.

OLIVECRONA, HERBERT (1942). Tractotomy for relief of trigeminal neuralgia. *Arch. Neurol. Psychiat. (Chic.) 47,* 544–564.

OLIVER, L. C. (1952). The supranuclear arc of the corneal reflex. *Acta psychiat. scand. 27,* 329–333.

756

References

OLSZEWSKI, J. (1950). On the anatomical and functional organization of the spinal trigeminal nucleus. *J. comp. Neurol. 92*, 401–413.

OLSZEWSKI, J. (1952). *The Thalamus of the Macaca Mulatta. An Atlas for Use with the Stereotaxic Instrument.* S. Karger, Basel—New York.

OLSZEWSKI, J. (1954). The cytoarchitecture of the human reticular formation. In *Brain Mechanisms and Consciousness* (J. F. Delafresnaye, ed.), pp. 54–80. Blackwell Scientific Publ., Oxford.

OLSZEWSKI, J., and D. BAXTER (1954). *Cytoarchitecture of the Human Brain Stem.* S. Karger, New York—Basel.

ORBACH, J., and K. L. CHOW (1959). Differential effects of resections of somatic areas I and II in monkeys. *J. Neurophysiol. 22*, 195–203.

ORIOLI, F. L., and F. A. METTLER (1956). The rubro-spinal tract in *Macaca mulatta. J. comp. Neurol. 106*, 299–318.

ORTMANN, R. (1951). Über experimentelle Veränderungen der Morphologie des Hypophysenzwischenhirnsystems und die Beziehung der sog. "Gomorisubstanz" zum Adiuretin. *Z. Zellforsch. 36*, 92–140.

ORTMANN, R. (1960). Neurosecretion. In *Handbook of Physiology, Section 1: Neurophysiology,* Vol. II. (J. Field, H. W. Magoun, and V. E. Hall, eds.), pp. 1039–1065. Amer. Physiol. Soc., Washington, D.C.

OSCARSSON, O. (1965). Functional organization of the spino- and cuneocerebellar tracts. *Physiol. Rev. 45*, 495–522.

OSCARSSON, O. (1967). Termination and functional organization of a dorsal spino-olivocerebellar path. *Brain Research 5*, 531–534.

OSCARSSON, O., and I. ROSÉN (1963). Cerebral projection of group I afferents in fore-limb muscle nerves of cat. *Experientia (Basel) 19*, 206–207.

OSCARSSON, O., and I. ROSÉN (1966a). Short-latency projections to the cat's cerebral cortex from skin and muscle afferents in the contralateral forelimb. *J. Physiol. (Lond.) 182*, 164–184.

OSCARSSON, O., and I. ROSÉN (1966b). Response characteristics of reticulocerebellar neurones activated from spinal afferents. *Exp. Brain Res. 1*, 320–328.

OSCARSSON, O., and N. UDDENBERG (1964). Identification of a spinocerebellar tract activated from forelimb afferents in the cat. *Acta physiol. scand. 62*, 125–136.

OSCARSSON, O., and N. UDDENBERG (1966). Somatotopic termination of spino-olivocerebellar path. *Brain Research 3*, 204–207.

OSEN, K. K. (1969a). The cytoarchitecture of the cochlear nuclei in the cat. *J. comp. Neurol.* (In press.)

OSEN, K. K. (1969b). The intrinsic organization of the cochlear nuclei in the cat. *Acta oto-laryng. (Stockh.) Suppl.* (In press.)

OSEN, K. K. (1969c). The projection of the cochlear nuclei on the inferior colliculi in the cat. (In preparation.)

OSEN, K. K., and J. JANSEN (1965). The cochlear nuclei in the common porpoise, *Phocaena phocaena. J. comp. Neurol. 125*, 223–257.

O'STEEN, W. K., and G. M. VAUGHAN (1968). Radioactivity in the optic pathway and hypothalamus of the rat after intraocular injection of tritiated 5-hydroxytryptophan. *Brain Research 8*, 209–212.

OSTERTAG, B. (1936). *Einteilung und Charakteristik der Hirngewächse.* G. Fischer, Jena.

OTSUKA, R., and R. HASSLER (1962). Über Aufbau und Gliederung der corticalen Sehsphäre bei der Katze. *Arch. Psychiat. Z. ges. Neurol. 203*, 212–234.

757

Pain. Res. Publ. Ass. Res. nerv. Dis., Vol. 23 (1943). (H. G. Wolff, H. S. Gasser, and J. C. Hinsey, eds.). The Williams & Wilkins Co., Baltimore.

PAKKENBERG, H. (1966). The number of nerve cells in the cerebral cortex of man. *J. comp. Neurol. 128,* 17–20.

PALAY, L. (1955). An electron microscope study of the neurohypophysis in normal, hydrated and dehydrated rats. (Abstract.) *Anat. Rec. 121,* 348.

PALAY, S. L. (1957). The fine structure of the neurohypophysis. In *Ultrastructure and Cellular Chemistry of Neural Tissue* (H. Waelsch, ed.), pp. 31–44. Paul B. Hoeber, Inc., New York.

PANDYA, D. N., and L. A. VIGNOLO (1968). Interhemispheric neocortical projections of somatosensory areas I and II in the rhesus monkey. *Brain Research 7,* 300–303.

PANNESE, E. (1963). Investigations on the ultrastructural changes of the spinal ganglion neurons in the course of axon regeneration and cell hypertrophy. I. Changes during axon regeneration. *Z. Zellforsch. 60,* 711–740.

PAPEZ, J. W. (1937). A proposed mechanism of emotion. *Arch. Neurol. Psychiat. (Chic.) 38,* 725–743.

PAPPAS, G. D., E. B. COHEN, and D. P. PURPURA (1966). Fine structure and nonsynaptic neuronal relations in the thalamus of the cat. In *The Thalamus* (D. P. Purpura and M. D. Yahr, eds.), pp. 47–71. Columbia Univ. Press, New York—London.

PASS, I. J. (1933). Anatomic and functional relationship of the nucleus dorsalis (Clarke's column) and of the dorsal spinocerebellar tract (Flechsig's). *Arch. Neurol. Psychiat. (Chic.) 30,* 1025–1045.

PATTON, H. D., T. C. RUCH, and A. E. WALKER (1944). Experimental hypogeusia from Horsley-Clarke lesions of the thalamus in *Macaca mulatta. J. Neurophysiol. 7,* 171–184.

PAULSEN, K. (1958). Über Vorkommen und Zahl von Muskelspindeln in inneren Kehlkopfmuskeln des Menschen (M. cricoarytaenoideus dorsalis, M. cricothyreoideus). *Z. Zellforsch. 48,* 349–355.

PEARCE, G. W. (1960). Some cortical projections to the midbrain reticular formation. In *Structure and Function of the Cerebral Cortex* (D. B. Tower and J. P. Schadé, eds.), pp. 131–137. Elsevier Publishing Co., Amsterdam—London—New York—Princeton.

PEARSON, A. A. (1938). The spinal accessory nerve in human embryos. *J. comp. Neurol. 68,* 243–266.

PEARSON, A. A. (1939). The hypoglossal nerve in human embryos. *J. comp. Neurol. 71,* 21–39.

PEARSON, A. A. (1944). The oculomotor nucleus in the human fetus. *J. comp. Neurol. 80,* 47–68.

PEARSON, A. A. (1945). Observations on the root of the facial nerve in human fetuses. (Abstract.) *Anat. Rec. 91,* 294–295.

PEARSON, A. A. (1949a). The development and connections of the mesencephalic root of the trigeminal nerve in man. *J. comp. Neurol. 90,* 1–46.

PEARSON, A. A. (1949b). Further observations on the mesencephalic root of the trigeminal nerve. *J. comp. Neurol. 91,* 147–194.

PEARSON, A. A. (1952). Role of gelatinous substance of spinal cord in conduction of pain. *Arch. Neurol. Psychiat. (Chic.) 68,* 515–529.

PEDERSEN, E. (1959). Epidemic vertigo. Clinical picture, epidemiology and relation to encephalitis. *Brain 82,* 566–580.

References

PEDERSEN, E., and V. GRYNDERUP (1966). Clinical pharmacology of the neurogenic bladder. *Acta neurol. scand. 42, Suppl. 20,* 111–120.

PEDERSEN, E., and P. JUUL-JENSEN (1965). Treatment of spasticity by subarachnoid phenolglycerin. *Neurology 15,* 256–262.

PEELE, T. L. (1942). Cytoarchitecture of individual parietal areas in the monkey (*Macaca mulatta*) and the distribution of the efferent fibers. *J. comp. Neurol. 77,* 693–737.

PEITERSEN, E. (1965). *Vestibulo-spinale reflexer. Kliniske og eksperimentelle undersøgelser ved hjælp af steppingtesten.* Munksgaard, København.

PENFIELD, W. (1958). Centrencephalic integrating system. *Brain 81,* 231–234.

PENFIELD, W. G., and E. BOLDREY (1937). Somatic motor and sensory representation in the cerebral cortex of man as studied by electrical stimulation. *Brain 60,* 389–443.

PENFIELD, W., and T. C. ERICKSON (1941). *Epilepsy and Cerebral Localization. A Study of the Mechanism, Treatment and Prevention of Epileptic Seizures.* Charles C Thomas, Springfield, Illinois.

PENFIELD, W., and M. E. FAULK, JR. (1955). The insula. Further observations on its function. *Brain 78,* 445–470.

PENFIELD, W., and H. JASPER (1954). *Epilepsy and the Functional Anatomy of the Human Brain.* Little, Brown and Company, Boston.

PENFIELD, W., and K. KRISTIANSEN (1951). *Epileptic Seizure Patterns.* Charles C Thomas, Springfield, Illinois.

PENFIELD, W., and B. MILNER (1958). Memory deficit produced by bilateral lesions in the hippocampal zone. *Arch. Neurol. Psychiat. (Chic.) 79,* 475–497.

PENFIELD, W., and P. PEROT (1963). The brain's record of auditory and visual experience. A final summary and discussion. *Brain 86,* 595–696.

PENFIELD, W., and T. RASMUSSEN (1950). *The Cerebral Cortex of Man.* Macmillan, New York.

PENFIELD, W., and L. ROBERTS (1959). *Speech and Brain Mechanisms.* Princeton Univ. Press, Princeton.

PENFIELD, W., and K. WELCH (1951). The supplementary motor area of the cerebral cortex. A clinical and experimental study. *Arch. Neurol. Psychiat. (Chic.) 66,* 289–317.

PERL, E. R., and D. G. WHITLOCK (1961). Somatic stimuli exciting spinothalamic projections to thalamic neurons in cat and monkey. *Exp. Neurol. 3,* 256–296.

PERL, E. R., D. G. WHITLOCK, and J. R. GENTRY (1962). Cutaneous projection to second-order neurons of the dorsal column system. *J. Neurophysiol. 25,* 337–358.

PERLMAN, H. B. (1960). The place of the middle ear muscle reflex in auditory research. *Arch. Otolaryng. 72,* 201–206.

PERRIA, L., G. ROSADINI, and G. F. ROSSI (1961). Determination of side of cerebral dominance with amobarbital. *Arch. Neurol. (Chic.) 4,* 172–181.

PETERS, A., and S. L. PALAY (1966). The morphology of laminae A and A₁ of the dorsal nucleus of the lateral geniculate body of the cat. *J. Anat. (Lond.) 100,* 451–486.

PETERSÉN, I., S. KOLLBERG, and K.-G. DHUNÉR (1961). The effect of the intravenous injection of succinylcholine on micturition. An electromyographic study. *Brit. J. Urol. 33,* 392–396.

PETERSÉN, I., I. STENER, U. SELLDÉN, and S. KOLLBERG (1962). Investigation of urethral sphincter in women with simultaneous electromyography and micturition urethro-cystography. *Acta neurol. scand. 38, Suppl. 3,* 145–151.

PETERSON, B. W. (1967). Effect of tilting on the activity of neurons in the vestibular nuclei of the cat. *Brain Research 6,* 606–609.

PETRÉN, K. (1910). Ueber die Bahnen der Sensibilität im Rückenmarke, besonders nach den Fällen von Stichverletzung studiert. *Arch. Psychiat. 47,* 495–557.

PETROVICKY, P. (1966). A comparative study of the reticular formation of the guinea pig. *J. comp. Neurol. 128,* 85–108.

PFAFFMANN, C. (1939). Afferent impulses from the teeth due to pressure and noxious stimulation. *J. Physiol. (Lond.) 97,* 207–219.

PFEIFER, R. A. (1920). Myelogenetisch-anatomische Untersuchungen über das kortikale Ende der Hörleitung. *Abh. math.-physik. Kl. Sächs. Akad. Wiss.,* Vol. *37,* No. II, 1–54.

PFEIFER, R. A. (1925). Myelogenetisch-anatomische Untersuchungen über den zentralen Abschnitt der Sehleitung. *Monogr. Gesamtgeb. Neurol. Psychiat.,* Heft *43,* 1–149.

PFEIFER, R. A. (1936). Pathologie der Hörstrahlung und der corticalen Hörsphäre. In *Handbuch der Neurologie* (Bumke-Foerster, eds.), Vol. *6,* pp. 533–626. Berlin.

PFEIFER, R. A. (1940). *Die angioarchitektonische areale Gliederung der Grosshirnrinde.* Georg Thieme, Leipzig.

PHILLIPS, C. G. (1967). Corticomotoneuronal organization. Projection from the arm area of the Baboon's motor cortex. *Arch. Neurol. (Chic.) 17,* 188–195.

Physiological Basis of Mental Activity, The (1963). (R. Hernández-Peón, ed.). *Electroenceph. clin. Neurophysiol. Suppl. 24.* Elsevier Publishing Co., Amsterdam—London—New York.

PICK, J., and D. SHEEHAN (1946). Sympathetic rami in man. *J. Anat. (Lond.) 80,* 12–20.

PIERCY, M. (1967). Studies of the neurological basis of intellectual functions. Clinical studies. In *Modern Trends in Neurology,* Vol. 4 (D. Williams, ed.), pp. 106–124. Butterworths, London.

PITTS, R. F. (1940). The respiratory center and its descending pathways. *J. comp. Neurol. 72,* 605–625.

PITTS, R. F., H. W. MAGOUN, and S. W. RANSON (1939). Localization of the medullary respiratory centers in the cat. *Amer. J. Physiol. 126,* 673–688.

Pituitary Gland, The, Vols. 1–3 (1966). (G. W. Harris and B. T. Donovan, eds.). Butterworths, London.

POGGIO, G. F., and V. B. MOUNTCASTLE (1960). A study of the functional contributions of the lemniscal and spinothalamic systems to somatic sensibility. *Bull. Johns Hopk. Hosp. 106,* 266–316.

POGGIO, G. F., and V. B. MOUNTCASTLE (1963). The functional properties of ventrobasal thalamic neurons studied in unanesthetized monkeys. *J. Neurophysiol. 26,* 775–806.

POIRIER, L. J. (1960). Experimental and histological study of midbrain dyskinesias. *J. Neurophysiol. 23,* 534–551.

POIRIER, L. J., and G. BOUVIER (1966). The red nucleus and its efferent nervous pathways in the monkey. *J. comp. Neurol. 128,* 223–244.

POLÁCEK, P. (1966). Receptors of the joints. Their structure, variability and classification. *Acta Fac. med. Univ. Brun. 23,* 1–107 + 60 Plates.

POLJAK, S. (1924). Die Struktureigentümlichkeiten des Rückenmarkes bei den

References

Chiropteren. Zugleich ein Beitrag zu der Frage über die spinalen Zentren des Sympathicus. *Z. Anat. Entwickl.-Gesch. 74*, 509–576.

POLLACK, S. L. (1960). The grasp response in the neonate. Its characteristics and interaction with the tonic neck reflex. *Arch. Neurol. (Chic.) 3*, 574–588.

POLLOCK, M., and R. W. HORNABROOK (1966). The prevalence, natural history and dementia of Parkinson's disease. *Brain 89*, 429–448.

POLYAK, S. (1927a). Über den allgemeinen Bauplan des Gehörsystems und über seine Bedeutung für die Physiologie, für die Klinik, und für die Psychologie. *Z. Neurol. 110*, 1–49.

POLYAK, S. (1927b). An experimental study of the association, callosal and projection fibers of the cerebral cortex of the cat. *J. comp. Neurol. 44*, 197–258.

POLYAK, S. (1932). *The Main Afferent Fiber Systems of the Cerebral Cortex in Primates. Univ. Calif. Publ. Anat.*, Vol. 2. Berkeley.

POLYAK, S. (1933). A contribution to the cerebral representation of the retina. *J. comp. Neurol. 57*, 541–617.

POLYAK, S. (1936). Minute structure of the retina in monkeys and in apes. *Arch. Ophthal. 15*, 477–519.

POLYAK, S. (1941). *The Retina. The Anatomy and Histology of the Retina in Man, Ape and Monkey, including the Consideration of Visual Functions, the History of Physiological Optics, and the Laboratory Technique.* Univ. of Chicago Press, Chicago, Illinois.

POLYAK, S. (1957). *The Vertebrate Visual System* (H. Klüver, ed.). Univ. of Chicago Press, Chicago, Illinois.

POMPEIANO, O. (1957). Analisi degli effetti della stimolazione elettrica del nucleo rosso nel Gatto decerebrato. *Rend. Acc. naz. Lincei, Cl. Sci. fis., mat. nat. 22*, 100–103.

POMPEIANO, O. (1959). Organizzazione somatotopica delle risposte flessorie alla stimolazione elettrica del nucleo interposito nel Gatto decerebrato. *Arch. Sci. biol. (Bologna) 43*, 163–176.

POMPEIANO, O. (1960). Organizzazione somatotopica delle risposte posturali alla stimolazione elettrica del nucleo di Deiters nel Gatto decerebrato. *Arch. Sci. biol. (Bologna) 44*, 497–511.

POMPEIANO, O. (1962). Somatotopic organization of the postural responses to stimulation and destruction of the caudal part of the fastigial nucleus. *Arch. ital. Biol. 100*, 259–271.

POMPEIANO, O. (1967). Functional organization of the cerebellar projections to the spinal cord. In *The Cerebellum. Progress in Brain Research*, Vol. 25. (J. P. Schadé, ed.), pp. 282–321. Elsevier Publishing Co., Amsterdam—London—New York.

POMPEIANO, O., and A. BRODAL (1957a). The origin of vestibulospinal fibres in the cat. An experimental-anatomical study, with comments on the descending medial longitudinal fasciculus. *Arch. ital. Biol. 95*, 166–195.

POMPEIANO, O., and A. BRODAL (1957b). Spino-vestibular fibers in the cat. *J. comp. Neurol. 108*, 353–382.

POMPEIANO, O., and A. BRODAL (1957c). Experimental demonstration of a somatotopical origin of rubrospinal fibers in the cat. *J. comp. Neurol. 108*, 225–252.

POMPEIANO, O., and E. COTTI (1959). Analisi microelettrodica delle proiezioni cerebello-deitersiane. *Arch. Sci. biol. (Bologna) 43*, 57–101.

POMPEIANO, O., and A. R. MORRISON (1966). Vestibular influences during sleep. III. Dissociation of the tonic and phasic inhibition of spinal reflexes during desynchronized sleep following vestibular lesions. *Arch. ital. Biol. 104,* 231–246.

POMPEIANO, O., and J. E. SWETT (1962a). EEG and behavioral manifestations of sleep induced by cutaneous nerve stimulation in normal cats. *Arch. ital. Biol. 100,* 311–342.

POMPEIANO, O., and J. E. SWETT (1962b). Identification of cutaneous and muscular afferent fibers producing EEG synchronization or arousal in normal cats. *Arch. ital. Biol. 100,* 343–380.

POMPEIANO, O., and J. E. SWETT (1963). Actions of graded cutaneous and muscular afferent volleys on brain stem units in the decerebrate, cerebellectomized cat. *Arch. ital. Biol. 101,* 552–582.

POMPEIANO, O., and F. WALBERG (1957). Descending connections to the vestibular nuclei. An experimental study in the cat. *J. comp. Neurol. 108,* 465–502.

POPA, G. T., and U. FIELDING (1930). A portal circulation from the pituitary to the hypothalamic region. *J. Anat. (Lond.) 65,* 88–91.

POPE, A. (1967). Microchemical architecture of human isocortex. *Arch. Neurol. (Chic.) 16,* 351–356.

POPE, A., H. H. HESS, and E. LEWIN (1964). Studies on the microchemical pathology of human cerebral cortex. In *Morphological and Biochemical Correlates of Neural Activity* (M. M. Cohen and R. S. Snider, eds.), pp. 98–111. Hoeber Medical Division, Harper & Row, Publ., New York.

PORTER, R. W. (1953). Hypothalamic involvement in the pituitary-adrenocortical response to stress stimuli. *Amer. J. Physiol. 172,* 515–519.

PORTUGAL, J. R., and M. BROCK (1962). On the pathogenesis of the Dandy-Walker-Brodal syndrome. *Zbl. Neurochir. 23,* 80–97.

POWELL, T. P. S. (1952). Residual neurons in the human thalamus following hemidecortication. *Brain 75,* 571–584.

POWELL, T. P. S., and W. M. COWAN (1954). The origin of the mamillothalamic tract in the rat. *J. Anat. (Lond.) 88,* 489–497.

POWELL, T. P. S., and W. M. COWAN (1956). A study of thalamo-striate relations in the monkey. *Brain 79,* 364–390.

POWELL, T. P. S., and W. M. COWAN (1963). Centrifugal fibres in the lateral olfactory tract. *Nature 199,* 1296–1297.

POWELL, T. P. S., and W. M. COWAN (1964). A note on retrograde fibre degeneration. *J. Anat. (Lond.) 98,* 579–585.

POWELL, T. P. S., W. M. COWAN, and G. RAISMAN (1963). Olfactory relationships of the diencephalon. *Nature 199,* 710–712.

POWELL, T. P. S., W. M. COWAN, and G. RAISMAN (1965). The central olfactory connexions. *J. Anat. (Lond.) 99,* 791–813.

POWELL, T. P. S., and S. D. ERULKAR (1962). Transneuronal cell degeneration in the auditory relay nuclei of the cat. *J. Anat. (Lond.) 96,* 249–268.

POWELL, T. P. S., R. W. GUILLERY, and W. M. COWAN (1957). A quantitative study of the fornix-mamillo-thalamic system. *J. Anat. (Lond.) 91,* 419–437.

POWELL, T. P. S., and V. B. MOUNTCASTLE (1959a). The cytoarchitecture of the postcentral gyrus of the monkey macaca mulatta. *Bull. Johns Hopk. Hosp. 106,* 108–131.

POWELL, T. P. S., and V. B. MOUNTCASTLE (1959b). Some aspects of the functional organization of the postcentral gyrus of the monkey: a correlation of findings obtained in a single unit analysis with cytoarchitecture. *Bull. Johns Hopk. Hosp. 105,* 133–162.

References

Precentral Motor Cortex, The (1944). (P. C. Bucy, ed.). Univ. of Illinois Press, Urbana, Illinois.

PRECHT, W., and H. SHIMAZU (1965). Functional connections of tonic and kinetic vestibular neurons with primary vestibular afferents. *J. Neurophysiol. 28,* 1014–1028.

PRESTIGE, M. C. (1966). Initial collaterals of motor axons within the spinal cord of the cat. *J. comp. Neurol. 126,* 123–136.

PRESTON, J. B., and D. G. WHITLOCK (1961). Intracellular potentials recorded from motoneurons following precentral gyrus stimulation in primate. *J. Neurophysiol. 24,* 91–100.

PRIBRAM, K. H., K. L. CHOW, and J. SEMMES (1953). Limit and organization of the cortical projection from the medial thalamic nucleus in monkey. *J. comp. Neurol. 98,* 433–448.

PRICE, J. L. (1968). The termination of centrifugal fibres in the olfactory bulb. *Brain Research 7,* 483–486.

PROVINS, K. A. (1958). The effect of peripheral nerve block on the appreciation and execution of finger movements. *J. Physiol. (Lond.) 143,* 55–67.

PUBOLS, B. H., JR. (1968). Retrograde degeneration study of somatic sensory thalamocortical connections in brain of *Virginia opossum. Brain Research 7,* 232–251.

PUBOLS, B. H., JR., W. I. WELKER, and C. I. JOHNSON, JR. (1965). Somatic sensory representation of forelimb in dorsal root fibers of raccoon, coatimundi, and cat. *J. Neurophysiol. 28,* 312–341.

PURVES, H. D. (1966). Cytology of the adenohypophysis. In *The Pituitary Gland,* Vol. 1 (G. W. Harris and B. T. Donovan, eds.), pp. 147–232. Butterworths, London.

PUTNAM, T. J. (1926). Studies on the central visual system. IV. The details of the organization of the geniculo-striate system in man. *Arch. Neurol. Psychiat. (Chic.) 16,* 683–707.

PUTNAM, T. J., and S. LIEBMAN (1942). Cortical representation of the macula lutea with special reference to the theory of bilateral representation. *Arch. Ophthal. 28,* 415–443.

PUTNAM, T. J., and I. K. PUTNAM (1926). Studies on the central visual system. I. The anatomic projection of the retinal quadrants on the striate cortex of the rabbit. *Arch. Neurol. Psychiat. (Chic.) 16,* 1–20.

RAAF, J., and J. W. KERNOHAN (1944). Relation of abnormal collections of cells in posterior medullary velum of cerebellum to origin of medulloblastoma. *Arch. Neurol. Psychiat. (Chic.) 52,* 163–169.

RAEDER, J. G. (1924). Paratrigeminal paralysis of the oculopupillary sympathetic. *Brain 47,* 149–158.

RAISMAN, G. (1966a). The connexions of the septum. *Brain 89,* 317–348.

RAISMAN, G. (1966b). Neural connections of the hypothalamus. *Brit. med. Bull. 22,* 197–201.

RAISMAN, G., W. M. COWAN, and T. P. S. POWELL (1965). The extrinsic afferent, commissural and association fibres of the hippocampus. *Brain 88,* 963–996.

RAISMAN, G., W. M. COWAN, and T. P. S. POWELL (1966). An experimental analysis of the efferent projection of the hippocampus. *Brain 89,* 83–108.

RAKIC, P., and P. I. YAKOVLEV (1968). Development of the corpus callosum and cavum septi in man. *J. comp. Neurol. 132,* 45–72.

RALL, W., G. M. SHEPHERD, T. S. REESE, and M. W. BRIGHTMAN (1966). Dendrodendritic synaptic pathway for inhibition in the olfactory bulb. *Exp. Neurol. 14,* 44–56.

RALSTON, H. J. (1965). The organization of the substantia gelatinosa Rolandi in the cat lumbosacral cord. *Z. Zellforsch. 67,* 1–23.

RAMÓN-MOLINER, E., and W. J. H. NAUTA (1966). The isodendritic core of the brain stem. *J. comp. Neurol. 126,* 311–335.

RANSON, S. W. (1943). *The Anatomy of the Nervous System.* 7th ed. W. B. Saunders Co., Philadelphia—London.

RANSON, S. W., and P. R. BILLINGSLEY (1918). The superior cervical ganglion and the cervical portion of the sympathetic trunk. *J. comp. Neurol. 29,* 313–358.

RANSON, S. W., H. K. DAVENPORT, and E. A. DOLES (1932). Intramedullary course of the dorsal root fibers of the first three cervical nerves. *J. comp. Neurol. 54,* 1–12.

RANSON, S. W., W. H. DROEGEMUELLER, H. K. DAVENPORT, and C. FISHER (1935). Number, size and myelination of the sensory fibers in the cerebrospinal nerves. *Res. Publ. Ass. nerv. ment. Dis. 15,* 3–28.

RANSON, S. W., and H. W. MAGOUN (1933). The central path of the pupilloconstriction reflex in response to light. *Arch. Neurol. Psychiat. (Chic.) 30,* 1193–1202.

RANSON, S. W., S. W. RANSON, JR., and M. RANSON (1941). Fiber connections of corpus striatum as seen in Marchi preparations. *Arch. Neurol. Psychiat. (Chic.) 46,* 230–249.

RASMUSSEN, A. T. (1932). *The Principal Nervous Pathways.* The Macmillan Co., New York—London.

RASMUSSEN, A. T. (1938). The proportions of the various subdivisions of the normal adult human hypophysis cerebri and the relative number of the different types of cells in pars distalis, with biometric evaluation of age and sex differences and special consideration of basophilic invasion into the infundibular process. *Res. Publ. Ass. nerv. ment. Dis. 17,* 118–150.

RASMUSSEN, A. T. (1940a). Studies of the VIIIth cranial nerve of man. *Laryngoscope (St. Louis) 50,* 67–83.

RASMUSSEN, A. T. (1940b). Effects of hypophysectomy and hypophysial stalk resection on the hypothalamic nuclei of animals and man. *Res. Publ. Ass. nerv. ment. Dis. 20,* 245–269.

RASMUSSEN, A. T., and W. T. PEYTON (1948). The course and termination of the medial lemniscus in man. *J. comp. Neurol. 88,* 411–424.

RASMUSSEN, G. L. (1946). The olivary peduncle and other fiber projections of the superior olivary complex. *J. comp. Neurol. 84,* 141–220.

RASMUSSEN, G. L. (1953). Further observations of the efferent cochlear bundle. *J. comp. Neurol. 99,* 61–74.

RASMUSSEN, G. L. (1957). Selective silver impregnation of synaptic endings. In *New Research Techniques of Neuroanatomy* (W. F. Windle, ed.), pp. 27–39. Charles C Thomas, Springfield, Illinois.

RASMUSSEN, G. L. (1960). Efferent fibers of the cochlear nerve and cochlear nucleus. In *Neural Mechanisms of the Auditory and Vestibular Systems* (G. L. Rasmussen and W. Windle, eds.), pp. 105–115. Charles C Thomas, Springfield, Illinois.

RASMUSSEN, G. L. (1961). Distribution of fibers originating from the inferior colliculus. (Abstract.) *Anat. Rec. 139,* 266.

References

RASMUSSEN, G. L. (1964). Anatomic relationships of the ascending and descending auditory systems. In *Neurological Aspects of Auditory and Vestibular Disorders*. (W. S. Fields and B. R. Alford, eds.), pp. 5–23. Charles C Thomas, Springfield, Illinois.

RASMUSSEN, G. L. (1967). Efferent connections of the cochlear nerve. In *Sensorineural Hearing Processes and Disorders*. Henry Ford Hospital International Symposium (A. B. Graham, ed.), pp. 61–75. Little, Brown and Co., Boston.

RASMUSSEN, G. L., R. R. GACEK, E. P. MCCRANE, and C. C. BAKER (1960). Model of cochlear nucleus (cat) displaying its afferent and efferent connections. (Abstract.) *Anat. Rec. 136,* 344.

RAYMOND, F., and R. CESTAN (1902). Sur un cas de papillome épithélioïde du noyau rouge. Contribution à l'étude des fonctions du noyau rouge. *Arch. Neurol. (Paris) Sér. 2, 14,* 81–100.

REICHERT, F. L. (1934). Neuralgias of the glossopharyngeal nerve. With particular reference to the sensory, gustatory and secretory functions of the nerve. *Arch. Neurol. Psychiat. (Chic.) 32,* 1030–1037.

Reticular Formation of the Brain (1958). (H. H. Jasper, L. D. Proctor, R. S. Knighton, W. C. Noshay, and R. T. Costello, eds.). Henry Ford Hospital International Symposium. Little, Brown and Co., Boston—Toronto.

REUBEN, R. N., and C. GONZALEZ (1964). Ocular electromyography in brain stem dysfunction. *Arch. Neurol. (Chic.) 11,* 265–272.

REXED, B. (1944). Contributions to the knowledge of the post-natal development of the peripheral nervous system in man. *Acta psychiat. (Kbh.) Suppl. 33,* 1–206.

REXED, B. (1952). The cytoarchitectonic organization of the spinal cord in the cat. *J. comp. Neurol. 96,* 415–495.

REXED, B. (1954). A cytoarchitectonic atlas of the spinal cord in the cat. *J. comp. Neurol. 100,* 297–379.

REXED, B., and A. BRODAL (1951). The nucleus cervicalis lateralis. A spinocerebellar relay nucleus. *J. Neurophysiol. 14,* 399–407.

REXED, B., and G. STRØM (1952). Afferent nervous connexions of the lateral cervical nucleus. *Acta physiol. scand. 25,* 219–229.

REXED, B., and K. G. WENNERSTRÖM (1959). Arachnoidal proliferation and cystic formation in the spinal nerveroot pouches of man. *J. Neurosurg. 16,* 73–84.

Rhinencephalon and Related Structures, The. Progress in Brain Research, Vol. 3. (1963). (W. Bargmann and J. P. Schadé, eds.). Elsevier Publishing Co., Amsterdam—London—New York.

RHINES, R., and H. W. MAGOUN (1946). Brain stem facilitation of cortical motor response. *J. Neurophysiol. 9,* 219–229.

RHOTON, A. L., J. L. O'LEARY, and J. P. FERGUSON (1966). The trigeminal, facial, vagal and glossopharyngeal nerves in the monkey. *Arch. Neurol. (Chic.) 14,* 530–540.

RICHARDS, R. L. (1967). Causalgia. A centennial review. *Arch. Neurol. (Chic.) 16,* 339–350.

RICHARDSON, K. C. (1958). Electronmicroscopic observations on Auerbach's plexus in the rabbit, with special reference to the problem of smooth muscle innervation. *Amer. J. Anat. 103,* 99–135.

RICHARDSON, K. C. (1962). The fine structure of autonomic nerve endings in smooth muscle of the rat vas deferens. *J. Anat. (Lond.) 96,* 427–442.

RICHARDSON, K. C. (1964). The fine structure of the albino rabbit iris with special reference to the identification of adrenergic and cholinergic nerves and nerve endings in its intrinsic muscles. *Amer. J. Anat. 114,* 173–205.

RICHTER, C. P., and M. HINES (1934). The production of the 'grasp reflex' in adult macaques by experimental frontal lobe lesions. *Res. Publ. Ass. nerv. ment. Dis. 13,* 211–224.

RICHTER, C. P., and B. G. WOODRUFF (1945). Lumbar sympathetic dermatomes in man determined by the electrical skin resistance method. *J. Neurophysiol. 8,* 323–338.

RIES, E. A., and O. R. LANGWORTHY (1937). A study of the surface structure of the brain of the whale (*Balaenoptera physalus* and *Physeter catadon*). *J. comp. Neurol. 68,* 1–47.

RINNE, U. K. (1966). Ultrastructure of the median eminence of the rat. *Z. Zellforsch. 74,* 98–122.

RINVIK, E. (1965). The corticorubral projection in the cat. Further observations. *Exp. Neurol. 12,* 278–291.

RINVIK, E. (1966). The cortico-nigral projection in the cat. An experimental study with silver impregnation methods. *J. comp. Neurol. 126,* 241–254.

RINVIK, E. (1968a). The corticothalamic projection from the pericruciate and coronal gyri in the cat. An experimental study with silver-impregnation methods. *Brain Research 10,* 79–119.

RINVIK, E. (1968b). The corticothalamic projection from the second somatosensory cortical area in the cat. An experimental study with silver impregnation methods. *Exp. Brain Res. 5,* 153–172.

RINVIK, E. (1968c). The corticothalamic projection from the gyrus proreus and the medial wall of the rostral hemisphere in the cat. An experimental study with silver impregnation methods. *Exp. Brain Res. 5,* 129–152.

RINVIK, E., and F. WALBERG (1963). Demonstration of a somatotopically arranged cortico-rubral projection in the cat. An experimental study with silver methods. *J. comp. Neurol. 120,* 393–407.

ROBERTS, T. D. M. (1967). *Neurophysiology of Postural Mechanisms.* Butterworths, London.

ROBERTS, T. S., and K. AKERT (1963). Insular and opercular cortex and its thalamic projection in *Macaca mulatta. Schweiz. Arch. Neurol. Neurochir. Psychiat. 92,* 1–43.

ROGERS, D. C., and G. BURNSTOCK (1966). The interstitial cell and its place in the concept of the autonomic ground plexus. *J. comp. Neurol. 126,* 255–284.

ROMANES, G. J. (1953). The motor cell groupings of the spinal cord. In *The Spinal Cord.* Ciba Symposium. (J. L. Malcolm, J. A. B. Gray, and G. E. Wolstenholme, eds.), pp. 24–42. J. & A. Churchill Ltd., London.

ROOFE, P. G. (1940). Innervation of annulus fibrosus and posterior longitudinal ligament. *Arch. Neurol. Psychiat.* (*Chic.*) *44,* 100–103.

ROSADINI, G., and G. F. ROSSI (1967). On the suggested cerebral dominance for consciousness. *Brain 90,* 101–112.

ROSE, J. E. (1949). The cellular structure of the auditory region of the cat. *J. comp. Neurol. 91,* 409–439.

ROSE, J. E. (1952). The cortical connections of the reticular complex of the thalamus. *Res. Publ. Ass. nerv. ment. Dis. 30,* 454–479.

ROSE, J. E., R. GALAMBOS, and J. R. HUGHES (1959). Microelectrode studies of the cochlear nuclei of the cat. *Bull. Johns Hopk. Hosp. 104,* 211–251.

ROSE, J. E., D. D. GREENWOOD, J. M. GOLDBERG, and J. E. HIND (1963). Some discharge characteristics of single neurons in the inferior colliculus of the cat. I. Tonotopical organization, relation of spike counts to tone intensity, and firing patterns of single elements. *J. Neurophysiol. 26*, 294–320.

ROSE, J. E., and L. I. MALIS (1965a). Geniculo-striate connections in the rabbit. I. Retrograde changes in the dorsal lateral geniculate body after destruction of cells in various layers of the striate region. *J. comp. Neurol. 125*, 95–120.

ROSE, J. E., and L. I. MALIS (1965b). Geniculo-striate connections in the rabbit. II. Cytoarchitectonic structure of the striate region and of the dorsal lateral geniculate body; organization of the geniculo-striate projections. *J. comp. Neurol. 125*, 121–140.

ROSE, J. E., and V. B. MOUNTCASTLE (1952). The thalamic tactile region in rabbit and cat. *J. comp. Neurol. 97*, 441–489.

ROSE, J. E., and C. N. WOOLSEY (1948). The orbitofrontal cortex and its connections with the mediodorsal nucleus in rabbit, sheep and cat. *Res. Publ. Ass. nerv. ment. Dis. 27*, 210–232.

ROSE, J. E., and C. N. WOOLSEY (1949a). Organization of the mammalian thalamus and its relationships to the cerebral cortex. *Electroenceph. clin. Neurophysiol. 1*, 391–403.

ROSE, J. E., and C. N. WOOLSEY (1949b). The relations of thalamic connections, cellular structure and evocable electrical activity in the auditory region of the cat. *J. comp. Neurol. 91*, 441–466.

ROSE, M. (1935). Cytoarchitektonik und Myeloarchitektonik der Grosshirnrinde. In *Handbuch der Neurologie* (Bumke-Foerster, eds.), Vol. 1, pp. 588–778. Julius Springer, Berlin.

ROSS, A. T., and W. E. DEMYER (1966). Isolated syndrome of the medial longitudinal fasciculus in man. *Arch. Neurol. (Chic.) 15*, 203–205.

ROSSI, G., and G. CORTESINA (1965). The "efferent cochlear and vestibular system" in *Lepus cuniculus* L. *Acta anat. 60*, 362–381.

ROSSI, G. F. (1964). A hypothesis on the neural basis of consciousness. *Acta neurochir. 12*, 187–197.

ROSSI, G. F. (1965). Brain stem facilitating influences on EEG synchronization. Experimental findings and observations in man. *Acta neurochir. 13*, 257–288.

ROSSI, G. F., and A. BRODAL (1956a). Corticofugal fibres to the brain stem reticular formation. An experimental study in the cat. *J. Anat. (Lond.) 90*, 42–62.

ROSSI, G. F., and A. BRODAL (1956b). Spinal afferents to the trigeminal sensory nuclei and the nucleus of the solitary tract. *Confin. neurol. (Basel) 16*, 321–332.

ROSSI, G. F., and A. BRODAL (1957). Terminal distribution of spinoreticular fibers in the cat. *Arch. Neurol. Psychiat. (Chic.) 78*, 439–453.

ROSSI, G. F., and A. ZANCHETTI (1957). The brain stem reticular formation. *Arch. ital. Biol. 95*, 199–435.

ROTHMAN, S. (1960). Pathophysiology of itch sensation. In *Cutaneous Innervation* (W. Montagna, ed.), pp. 189–200. Pergamon Press, Oxford—London—New York—Paris.

ROWBOTHAM, G. F. (1939). Observations on the effect of trigeminal denervation. *Brain 62*, 364–380.

RUCH, T. C. (1960). Central control of the bladder. In *Handbook of Physiology. Section 1: Neurophysiology, Vol. II*. (J. Field, H. W. Magoun, and V. E. Hall, eds.), pp. 1207–1223. Amer. Physiol. Soc., Washington, D.C.

RUCH, T. C., J. F. FULTON, and W. J. GERMAN (1938). Sensory discrimination in monkey, chimpanzee and man after lesions of the parietal lobe. *Arch. Neurol. Psychiat. (Chic.) 39*, 919–938.

RUCH, T. C., and H. A. SHENKIN (1943). The relation of area 13 on orbital surface of frontal lobes to hyperactivity and hyperphagia in monkeys. *J. Neurophysiol. 6*, 349–360.

RUSHWORTH, G. (1960). Spasticity and rigidity: an experimental study and review. *J. Neurol. Neurosurg. Psychiat. 23*, 99–118.

RUSKA, H., and C. RUSKA (1961). Licht- und Elektronenmikroskopie des peripheren neurovegetativen Systems im Hinblick auf die Funktion. *Dtsch. med. Wschr. 86*, 1697–1701; 1770–1772.

RUSSELL, I. S., and S. OCHS (1963). Localization of a memory trace in one cortical hemisphere and transfer to the other hemisphere. *Brain 86*, 37–54.

RUSSELL, J. R., and W. DeMEYER (1961). The quantitative cortical origin of pyramidal axons of Macaca rhesus. *Neurology 11*, 96–108.

RYLANDER, G. (1939). Personality changes after operations on the frontal lobes. A clinical study of 32 cases. *Acta psychiat. scand. Suppl. 20*, 1–327.

SADJADPOUR, K., and A. BRODAL (1968). The vestibular nuclei in man. A morphological study in the light of experimental findings in the cat. *J. Hirnforsch. 10*, 299–323.

SALA, O. (1965). The efferent vestibular system. Electrophysiological research. *Acta oto-laryng. (Stockh.) Suppl. 197*, 1–34.

SALMOIRAGHI, C. C., and F. A. STEINER (1963). Acetylcholine sensitivity of cat's medullary neurons. *J. Neurophysiol. 26*, 581–597.

SAMUEL, E. P. (1952). The autonomic and somatic innervation of the articular capsule. *Anat. Rec. 113*, 53–70.

SANCHEZ-LONGO, L. P., and F. M. FORSTER (1958). Clinical significance of impairment of sound localization. *Neurology 8*, 119–125.

SANDO, I. (1965). The anatomical interrelationships of the cochlear nerve fibers. *Acta oto-laryng. (Stockh.) 59*, 417–436.

SANFORD, H. S., and H. L. BAIR (1939). Visual disturbances associated with tumours of the temporal lobe. *Arch. Neurol. Psychiat. (Chic.) 42*, 21–43.

SASAKI, K., A. NAMIKAWA, and S. HASHIRAMOTO (1960). The effect of midbrain stimulation upon alpha motoneurons in lumbar spinal cord of the cat. *Jap. J. Physiol. 10*, 303–316.

SAUERLAND, E. K., Y. NAKAMURA, and C. D. CLEMENTE (1967). The role of the lower brain stem in cortically induced inhibition of somatic reflexes in the cat. *Brain Research 6*, 164–180.

SCALIA, F. (1966). Some olfactory pathways in the rabbit brain. *J. comp. Neurol. 126*, 285–310.

SCHARLOCK, D. P., W. D. NEFF, and N. L. STROMINGER (1965). Discrimination of tone duration after bilateral ablation of cortical auditory areas. *J. Neurophysiol. 28*, 673–681.

SCHARRER, E., and R. GAUPP (1933). Neuere Befunde am Nucleus supraopticus und Nucleus paraventricularis des Menschen. *Z. ges. Neurol. Psychiat. 148*, 766–772.

SCHARRER, E., and B. SCHARRER (1954). Neurosekretion. In v. Möllendorff's *Handbuch der mikroskopischen Anatomie des Menschen*, Bd. VI/5, pp. 953–1066. Springer, Berlin-Göttingen-Heidelberg.

SCHEIBEL, M. E., and A. B. SCHEIBEL (1954). Observations on the intracortical relations of the climbing fibers of the cerebellum. A Golgi study. *J. comp. Neurol. 101,* 733–764.

SCHEIBEL, M. E., and A. B. SCHEIBEL (1955). The inferior olive. A Golgi study. *J. comp. Neurol. 102,* 77–132.

SCHEIBEL, M. E., and A. B. SCHEIBEL (1958). Structural substrates for integrative patterns in the brain stem reticular core. In *Reticular Formation of the Brain* (Henry Ford Hosp. Symposium), (H. H. Jasper, L. D. Proctor et al., eds.) pp. 31–55. Little, Brown & Co., Boston.

SCHEIBEL, M. E., and A. B. SCHEIBEL (1965). Periodic sensory nonresponsiveness in reticular neurons. *Arch. ital. Biol. 103,* 300–316.

SCHEIBEL, M. E., and A. B. SCHEIBEL (1966a). Spinal motorneurons, interneurons and Renshaw cells. A Golgi study. *Arch. ital. Biol. 104,* 328–353.

SCHEIBEL, M. E., and A. B. SCHEIBEL (1966b). Terminal axonal patterns in cat spinal cord. I. The lateral corticospinal tract. *Brain Research 2,* 333–350.

SCHEIBEL, M. E., and A. B. SCHEIBEL (1966c). The organization of the ventral anterior nucleus of the thalamus. A Golgi study. *Brain Research 1,* 250–268.

SCHEIBEL, M. E., and A. B. SCHEIBEL (1966d). The organization of the nucleus reticularis thalami: A Golgi study. *Brain Research 1,* 43–62.

SCHEIBEL, M. E., and A. B. SCHEIBEL (1966e). Patterns of organization in specific and nonspecific thalamic fields. In *The Thalamus* (D. P. Purpura and M. D. Yahr, eds.), pp. 13–46. Columbia Univ. Press, New York—London.

SCHEIBEL, M. E., and A. B. SCHEIBEL (1967). Structural organization of nonspecific thalamic nuclei and their projection toward cortex. *Brain Research 6,* 60–94.

SCHEIBEL, M. E., and A. B. SCHEIBEL (1968). Terminal axonal patterns in cat spinal cord. II. The dorsal horn. *Brain Research 9,* 32–58.

SCHEIBEL, M., A. SCHEIBEL, A. MOLLICA, and G. MORUZZI (1955). Convergence and interaction of afferent impulses on single units of reticular formation. *J. Neurophysiol. 18,* 309–331.

SCHEIBEL, M., A. SCHEIBEL, F. WALBERG, and A. BRODAL (1956). Areal distribution of axonal and dendritic patterns in inferior olive. *J. comp. Neurol. 106,* 21–49.

SCHILDKRAUT, J. J., and S. S. KETY (1967). Biogenic amines and emotion. *Science 156,* 21–30.

SCHIMERT, J. S. (1939). Das Verhalten der Hinterwurzelkollateralen im Rückenmark. *Z. Anat. Entwickl. Gesch. 109,* 665–687.

SCHIMERT, J. S. (1941). Die Endigungsweise des Tractus vestibulospinalis. *Z. Anat. Entwickl. Gesch. 108,* 761–767.

SCHOLTEN, J. M. (1946). *De Plaats van den Paraflocculus in het Geheel der Cerebellaire Correlaties.* Acad. Proefschr., N. V. Noord-Hollandsche Uitgevers Maatschappij, Amsterdam.

SCHUKNECHT, H. F. (1960). Neuroanatomical correlates of auditory sensitivity and pitch discrimination in the cat. In *Neural Mechanisms of the Auditory and Vestibular Systems* (G. L. Rasmussen and W. F. Windle, eds.), pp. 76–90. Charles C Thomas, Springfield, Illinois.

SCHULZE, M. L. (1955–56). Die absolute und relative Zahl der Muskelspindeln in den kurzen Daumenmuskeln des Menschen. *Anat. Anz. 102,* 290–291.

SCHUMACHER, P. (1940). Zur Prognose der Fazialislähmung bei Poliomyelitis. *Münch. med. Wschr. 87,* 591–593.

SCHWARTZ, H. G., and J. L. O'LEARY (1941). Section of the spinothalamic tract in the medulla with observations on the pathway for pain. *Surgery 9,* 183–193.

SCHWARTZ, H. G., G. E. ROULHAC, R. L. LAM, and J. O'LEARY (1951). Organization of the fasciculus solitarius in man. *J. comp. Neurol. 94,* 221–237.

SCHWARTZ, H. G., and G. WEDDELL (1938). Observations on the pathways transmitting the sensation of taste. *Brain 61,* 99–115.

SCHWARZ, G. A., and L. J. BARROWS (1960). Hemiballism without involvement of Luys' body. *Arch. Neurol. (Chic.) 2,* 420–434.

SCHWARZ, G. A., and C-N. LIU (1954). Chronic progressive external ophthalmoplegia. *Arch. Neurol. Psychiat. (Chic.) 71,* 31–53.

SCOLLO-LAVIZZARI, G., and K. AKERT (1963). Cortical area 8 and its thalamic projection in *Macaca mulatta. J. comp. Neurol. 121,* 259–270.

SCOTT, B. L., and D. C. PEASE (1959). Electron microscopy of the salivary and lacrimal glands of the rat. *Amer. J. Anat. 104,* 115–161.

SCOVILLE, W. B., and B. MILNER (1957). Loss of recent memory after bilateral hippocampal lesions. *J. Neurol. Neurosurg. Psychiat. 20,* 11–21.

Second Symposium on the Role of the Vestibular Organs in Space Exploration (1966). NASA SP-115, Ames Research Center, Moffett Field, California.

Selective Partial Ablation of the Frontal Cortex (1949). (F. A. Mettler, ed.). Paul B. Hoeber, Inc., New York.

SEM-JACOBSEN, C. W., M. C. PETERSEN, H. W. DODGE, Q. D. JACKS, J. A. LAZARTE, and C. B. HOLMAN (1956). Electric activity of the olfactory bulb in man. *Amer. J. med. Sci. 232,* 243–251.

SEMMES, J., and M. MISHKIN (1965). Somatosensory loss in monkeys after ipsilateral cortical ablation. *J. Neurophysiol. 28,* 473–486.

Sensorineural Hearing Processes and Disorders. (Henry Ford Hosp. Symp.) (1967). (A. B. Graham, ed.). J. & A. Churchill Ltd., London.

SERAFETINIDES, E. A., R. D. HOARE, and M. V. DRIVER (1965). Intracarotid sodium amylobarbitone and cerebral dominance for speech and consciousness. *Brain 88,* 107–130.

SEYFFARTH, H. (1940). The behaviour of motor units in voluntary contraction. *Norske Vid.-Akad. Avh. I, Math.-Nat. Kl.* No. 4, and *Acta Psychiat. scand. 16,* 79–109 and 261–278 (1941).

SEYFFARTH, H., and D. DENNY-BROWN (1948). The grasp reflex and the instinctive grasp reaction. *Brain 71,* 109–183.

SHANGER, S., and M. B. BENDER (1959). Oculomotor responses on vestibular stimulation of monkeys with lesions of the brain stem. *Brain 82,* 669–682.

SHARRARD, W. J. W. (1955). The distribution of the permanent paralysis in the lower limb in poliomyelitis. *J. Bone Jt. Surg. 37,* 540–558.

SHEEHAN, D. (1941). Spinal autonomic outflows in man and monkey. *J. comp. Neurol. 75,* 341–370.

SHEEHAN, D., and J. PICK (1943). The rami communicantes in the rhesus monkey. *J. Anat. (Lond.) 77,* 125–139.

SHELDEN, C. H., R. H. PUNDENZ, D. B. FRESHWATER, and B. L. CRUE (1955). Compression rather than decompression for trigeminal neuralgia. *J. Neurosurg. 12,* 123–126.

SHENKIN, H. A., and F. H. LEWEY (1944). Taste aura preceding convulsions in a lesion of the parietal operculum. *J. nerv. ment. Dis. 100,* 352–354.

770

References

SHEPPARD, R. N., and N. H. WADIA (1956). Atypical features in acoustic neuroma. *Brain 79*, 282–318.

SHEPS, J. G. (1945). The nuclear configuration and cortical connections of the human thalamus. *J. comp. Neurol. 83*, 1–56.

SHIMAZU, H., T. HONGO, and K. KUBOTA (1962). Two types of central influences on gamma motor system. *J. Neurophysiol. 25*, 309–323.

SHIMAZU, H., T. HONGO, K. KUBOTA, and H. NARABAYASHI (1962). Rigidity and spasticity in man. Electromyographic analysis with reference to the role of the globus pallidus. *Arch. Neurol. (Chic.) 6*, 10–17.

SHIMAZU, H., and W. PRECHT (1965). Tonic and kinetic responses of cat's vestibular neurons to horizontal angular acceleration. *J. Neurophysiol. 28*, 991–1013.

SHIMAZU, H., and W. PRECHT (1966). Inhibition of central vestibular neurons from the contralateral labyrinth and its mediating pathway. *J. Neurophysiol. 29*, 467–492.

SHOLL, D. A. (1953). Dendritic organization in the neurons of the visual and motor cortices of the cat. *J. Anat. (Lond.) 87*, 387–406.

SHOLL, D. A. (1955). The organization of the visual cortex in the cat. *J. Anat. (Lond.) 89*, 33–46.

SHOLL, D. A. (1956). *The Organization of the Cerebral Cortex*. Methuen & Co. Ltd., London, and John Wiley and Sons Inc., New York.

SHUTE, C. C. D., and P. R. LEWIS (1966). Cholinergic and monoaminergic pathways in the hypothalamus. *Brit. med. Bull. 22*, 221–226.

SIEGFRIED, J., F. R. ERVIN, Y. MIYAZAKI, and V. H. MARK (1962). Localized cooling of the central nervous system. I. Neurophysiological studies in experimental animals. *J. Neurosurg. 19*, 840–852.

SILVERMAN, S. M., P. S. BERGMAN, and M. B. BENDER (1961). The dynamics of transient cerebral blindness. Report of nine episodes following vertebral angiography. *Arch. Neurol. (Chic.) 4*, 333–348.

SIMPSON, D. A. (1952a). The projection of the pulvinar to the temporal lobe. *J. Anat. (Lond.) 86*, 20–28.

SIMPSON, D. A. (1952b). The efferent fibres of the hippocampus in the monkey. *J. Neurol. Neurosurg. Psychiat. 15*, 79–92.

SINCLAIR, D. (1967). *Cutaneous Sensation*. Oxford University Press, London—New York—Toronto.

SINCLAIR, D. C., and B. A. R. STOKES (1964). The production and characteristics of "second pain." *Brain 87*, 609–618.

SINCLAIR, D. C., G. WEDDELL, and W. H. FEINDEL (1948). Referred pain and associated phenomena. *Brain 71*, 184–211.

SINCLAIR, D. C., G. WEDDELL, and E. ZANDER (1952). The relationship of cutaneous sensibility to neurohistology in the human pinna. *J. Anat. (Lond.) 86*, 402–411.

SINGLETON, M. C., and T. L. PEELE (1965). Distribution of optic fibers in the cat. *J. comp. Neurol. 125*, 303–328.

SIQUEIRA, E. B. (1965). The temporo-pulvinar connections in the rhesus monkey. *Arch. Neurol. (Chic.) 13*, 321–330.

SJÖBERG, A. (1943). Något om centrala och perifera läsioner av nionde och tionde hjärnnerverna. *Nord. Med. 19*, 1398–1402.

SJÖQVIST, O. (1938). Studies on the pain conduction in the trigeminal nerve. *Acta psychiat. scand. Suppl. 17*, 1–139.

SJÖSTRAND, F. (1961). Electron microscopy of the retina. In *The Structure of the Eye* (G. K. Smelser, ed.), pp. 1–28. Academic Press, New York—London.

SKINNER, J. E., and D. B. LINDSLEY (1967). Electrophysiological and behavioral effects of blockade of the nonspecific thalamocortical system. *Brain Research* 6, 95–118.

SKOGLUND, S. (1956). Anatomical and physiological studies of knee joint innervation in the cat. *Acta physiol. scand. 36, Suppl. 124*, 1–101.

SLAUCK, A. (1921). Beiträge zur Kenntnis der Muskelpathologie. *Z. Neurol. 71*, 352–356.

Sleep Mechanisms. Progress in Brain Research, Vol. 18 (1965). (K. Akert, C. Bally, and J. P. Schadé, eds.). Elsevier Publishing Co., Amsterdam—London—New York.

SLOAN, N., and H. JASPER (1950). The identity of spreading depression and "suppression." *Electroenceph. clin. Neurophysiol. 2*, 59–78.

SLOPER, J. C. (1966). Hypothalamic neurosecretion. *Brit. med. Bull. 22*, 209–215.

SMITH, C. A., and G. L. RASMUSSEN (1963). Recent observations of the olivocochlear bundle. *Ann. Otol. (St. Louis) 72*, 489–506.

SMITH, C. A., and F. S. SJÖSTRAND (1961). Structure of the nerve endings on the external hair cells of the guinea pig cochlea as studied by serial sections. *J. Ultrastruct. Res. 5*, 523–556.

SMITH, K. U., and A. J. AKELAITIS (1942). Studies on the corpus callosum. I. Laterality in behavior and bilateral motor organization in man before and after section of the corpus callosum. *Arch. Neurol. Psychiat. (Chic.) 47*, 519–543.

SMITH, M. C. (1951). The use of Marchi staining in the later stages of human tract degeneration. *J. Neurol. Neurosurg. Psychiat. 14*, 222–225.

SMITH, M. C. (1956a). Observations on the extended use of the Marchi method. *J. Neurol. Neurosurg. Psychiat. 19*, 67–73.

SMITH, M. C. (1956b). The recognition and prevention of artefacts of the Marchi method. *J. Neurol. Neurosurg. Psychiat. 19*, 74–83.

SMITH, M. C. (1957). The anatomy of the spino-cerebellar fibers in man. 1. The course of the fibers in the spinal cord and brain stem. *J. comp. Neurol. 108*, 285–352.

SMITH, M. C. (1960). Nerve fibre degeneration in the brain in amyotrophic lateral sclerosis. *J. Neurol. Neurosurg. Psychiat. 23*, 269–282.

SMITH, M. C. (1961). The anatomy of the spino-cerebellar fibers in man. II. The distribution of the fibers in the cerebellum. *J. comp. Neurol. 117*, 329–354.

SMITH, M. C. (1962). Location of stereotactic lesions confirmed at necropsy. *Brit. med. J. 1*, 900–906.

SMITH, M. C. (1967). Stereotactic operations for Parkinson's disease—Anatomical observations. In *Modern Trends in Neurology* (D. Williams, ed.), pp. 21–52. Butterworths, London.

SMITH, M. C., S. J. STRICH, and P. SHARP (1956). The value of the Marchi method for staining tissue stored in formalin for prolonged periods. *J. Neurol. Neurosurg. Psychiat. 19*, 62–64.

SMITH, W. K. (1944a). The frontal eye fields. In *The Precentral Motor Cortex* (Paul C. Bucy, ed.), pp. 307–342. Univ. of Illinois Press, Urbana, Illinois.

SMITH, W. K. (1944b). The results of ablation of the cingular region of the cerebral cortex. *Fed. Proc. 3*, 42.

SMYTH, G. E. (1939). The systematization and central connections of the spinal

References

tract and nucleus of the trigeminal nerve. A clinical and pathological study. *Brain 62*, 41–87.

SNIDER, R. S. (1936). Alterations which occur in mossy terminals of the cerebellum, following transection of the brachium pontis. *J. comp. Neurol. 64*, 417–431.

SNIDER, R. S. (1940). Morphology of the cerebellar nuclei in the rabbit and the cat. *J. comp. Neurol. 72*, 399–415.

SNIDER, R. S. (1945). Electro-anatomical studies on a tecto-cerebellar pathway. (Abstract.) *Anat. Rec. 91*, 299.

SNIDER, R. S. (1950). Recent contributions to the anatomy and physiology of the cerebellum. *Arch. Neurol. Psychiat. (Chic.) 64*, 196–219.

SNIDER, R. S., and E. ELDRED (1948). Cerebral projections to the tactile, auditory and visual areas of the cerebellum. (Abstract.) *Anat. Rec. 100*, 714.

SNIDER, R., and E. ELDRED (1951). Electro-anatomical studies on cerebro-cerebellar connections in the cat. *J. comp. Neurol. 95*, 1–16.

SNIDER, R. S., and E. ELDRED (1952). Cerebro-cerebellar relationships in the monkey. *J. Neurophysiol. 15*, 27–40.

SNIDER, R. S., and A. STOWELL (1942). Evidence of a representation of tactile sensibility in the cerebellum of the cat. *Fed. Proc. 1*, 82–83.

SNIDER, R. S., and A. STOWELL (1944). Receiving areas of the tactile, auditory and visual systems in the cerebellum. *J. Neurophysiol. 7*, 331–357.

SNIDER, R. S., and N. WETZEL (1965). Electroencephalographic changes by stimulation of the cerebellum of man. *Electroenceph. clin. Neurophysiol. 18*, 176–183.

SOFFIN, G., M. FELDMAN, and M. B. BENDER (1968). Alterations of sensory levels in vascular lesions of lateral medulla. *Arch. Neurol. (Chic.) 18*, 178–190.

SOMJEN, G., D. O. CARPENTER, and E. HENNEMAN (1965). Responses of motoneurons of different sizes of graded stimulation of supraspinal centres of the brain. *J. Neurophysiol. 28*, 958–965.

SOUSA-PINTO, A., and A. BRODAL (1969). Demonstration of a somatotopical pattern in the cortico-olivary projection in the cat. An experimental-anatomical study. *Exp. Brain Res. 8* (in press).

SPALDING, J. M. K. (1952a). Wounds of the visual pathway. Part I: The visual radiation. *J. Neurol. Neurosurg. Psychiat. 15*, 99–109.

SPALDING, J. M. K. (1952b). Wounds of the visual pathway. Part II: The striate cortex. *J. Neurol. Neurosurg. Psychiat. 15*, 169–183.

SPERRY, R. W. (1966). Brain bisection and mechanisms of consciousness. In *Brain and Conscious Experience* (J. C. Eccles, ed.), pp. 298–308. Springer-Verlag, Berlin—Heidelberg—New York.

SPIEGEL, E. A., and E. G. SZEKELY (1961). Prolonged stimulation of the head of the caudate nucleus. *Arch. Neurol. (Chic.) 4*, 55–65.

SPIEGEL, E. A., H. T. WYCIS, M. MARKS, and A. J. LEE (1947). Stereotaxic apparatus for operations on the human brain. *Science 106*, 349–350.

SPILLER, W. G., and C. H. FRAZIER (1901). The division of the sensory root of the trigeminus for the relief of tic douloureux; an experimental, pathological and clinical study, with a preliminary report of one surgically successful case. *Philad. med. J. 8*, 1039–1049.

SPOENDLIN, H. H. (1964). Organization of the sensory hairs in the gravity receptors in utricle and saccule of the squirrel monkey. *Z. Zellforsch. 62*, 701–716.

SPOENDLIN, H. (1965). Strukturelle Eigenschaften der vestibulären Rezeptoren. *Schweiz. Arch. Neurol. Psychiat. 96*, 219–230.

SPOENDLIN, H. (1966). *The Organization of the Cochlear Receptor.* Advances in Oto-Rhino-Laryngology, Vol. 13 (L. Rüedi, ed.). S. Karger, Basel—New York.

SPRAGUE, J. M. (1958). The distribution of dorsal root fibres on motor cells in the lumbosacral spinal cord of the cat, and the site of excitatory and inhibitory terminals in monosynaptic pathways. *Proc. roy. Soc. B 149,* 534–556.

SPRAGUE, J. M., and W. W. CHAMBERS (1954). Control of posture by reticular formation and cerebellum in the intact, anesthetized and unanesthetized and in the decerebrated cat. *Amer. J. Physiol. 176,* 52–64.

SPRAGUE, J. M., and H. HA (1964). The terminal fields of dorsal root fibers in the lumbosacral cord of the cat, and the dendritic organization of the motor nuclei. In *Organization of the Spinal Cord* (J. C. Eccles and J. P. Schadé, eds.), pp. 120–152. Elsevier Publishing Co., Amsterdam—London—New York.

SPRAGUE, J. M., M. LEVITT, K. ROBSON, C. N. LIU, E. STELLAR, and W. W. CHAMBERS (1963). A neuroanatomical and behavioral analysis of the syndromes resulting from midbrain lemniscal and reticular lesions in the cat. *Arch. ital. Biol. 101,* 225–295.

SPRAGUE, J. M., and T. H. MEIKLE (1965). The role of the superior colliculus in visually guided behavior. *Exp. Neurol. 11,* 115–146.

SPRAGUE, J. M., L. H. SCHREINER, D. B. LINDSLEY, and H. W. MAGOUN (1948). Reticulo-spinal influences on stretch reflexes. *J. Neurophysiol. 11,* 501–508.

SPURLING, R. G., and E. G. GRANTHAM (1940). Neurologic picture of herniations of the nucleus pulposus in the lower part of the lumbar region. *Arch. Surg. 40,* 375–388.

STAHL, M. (1963). Elektronenmikroskopische Untersuchungen über die vegetative Innervation der Bauchspeicheldrüse. *Z. mikr.-anat. Forsch. 70,* 62–102.

STANFIELD, J. P. (1960). The blood supply of the human pituitary gland. *J. Anat. (Lond.) 94,* 257–273.

STARZL, T. E., and D. G. WHITLOCK (1952). Diffuse thalamic projection system in monkey. *J. Neurophysiol. 15,* 449–468.

STEG, G. (1966). Efferent muscle control in rigidity. In *Muscular afferents and Motor Control.* Proceedings 1st Nobel Symposium, Stockholm 1965 (R. Granit, ed.), pp. 437–443. Almqvist & Wiksell, Stockholm; John Wiley & Sons, New York—London—Sidney.

STEIN, B. M., and M. B. CARPENTER (1967). Central projections of portions of the vestibular ganglia innervating specific parts of the labyrinth in the rhesus monkey. *Amer. J. Anat. 120,* 281–318.

STEINHAUSEN, W. (1931). Über den Nachweis der Bewegungen der Cupula in der intakten Bogengangampulle des Labyrinthes bei der natürlichen rotatorischen und calorischen Reizung. *Pflügers Arch. ges. Physiol. 228,* 322–328.

STEPHAN, H., and O. J. ANDY (1962). The septum (A comparative study on its size in insectivores and primates). *J. Hirnforsch. 5,* 229–244.

STEPIEN, L. S., J. P. CORDEAU, and T. RASMUSSEN (1960). The effect of temporal lobe and hippocampal lesions on auditory and visual recent memory in monkeys. *Brain 83,* 470–489.

STERLING, P., and H. G. J. M. KUYPERS (1967a). Anatomical organization of the brachial spinal cord of the cat. I. The distribution of dorsal root fibers. *Brain Research 4,* 1–15.

STERLING, P., and H. G. J. M. KUYPERS (1967b). Anatomical organization of the

References

brachial spinal cord of the cat. II. The motoneuron plexus. *Brain Research 4,* 16–32.

STERN, G. (1966). The effects of lesions in the substantia nigra. *Brain 89,* 449–478.

STERN, J., and A. WARD, JR. (1960). Inhibition of the muscle spindle discharge by ventrolateral thalamic stimulation. Its relation to Parkinsonism. *Arch. Neurol. (Chic.) 3,* 193–204.

STERN, K. (1938). Note on the nucleus ruber magnocellularis and its efferent pathway in man. *Brain 61,* 284–289.

STEVENS, J. R., C. KIM, and P. D. MACLEAN (1961). Stimulation of caudate nucleus. Behavioral effects of chemical and electrical excitation. *Arch. Neurol. (Chic.) 4,* 47–65.

STEWART, D. H., JR., C. J. SCIBETTA, and R. B. KING (1967). Presynaptic inhibition in the trigeminal relay nuclei. *J. Neurophysiol. 30,* 135–153.

STEWART, R. M. (1939). Arhinencephaly. *J. Neurol. Psychiat. 2,* 303–312.

STEWART, W. A., and R. B. KING (1963). Fiber projections from the nucleus caudalis of the spinal trigeminal nucleus. *J. comp. Neurol. 121,* 271–286.

STIBBE, E. P. (1939). Surgical anatomy of the subtentorial angle with special reference to the acoustic and trigeminal nerves. *Lancet ii,* 859–862.

STONE, J., and S. M. HANSEN (1966). The projection of the cat's retina on the lateral geniculate nucleus. *J. comp. Neurol. 126,* 601–624.

STOOKEY, B., and J. RANSOHOFF (1959). *Trigeminal Neuralgia. Its History and Treatment.* Charles C Thomas, Springfield, Illinois.

STOPFORD, J. S. B. (1922). The nerve supply of the interphalangeal and metacarpophalangeal joints. *J. Anat. (Lond.) 56,* 1–11.

STORM MATHISEN, J., and T. W. BLACKSTAD (1964). Cholinesterase in the hippocampal region. Distribution and relation to architectonics and afferent systems. *Acta anat. 56,* 216–253.

STOTLER, W. A. (1949). The projection of the cochlear nerve on the acoustic relay nuclei of the medulla. (Abstract.) *Anat. Rec. 103,* 561.

STOTLER, W. A. (1953). An experimental study of the cells and connections of the superior olivary complex of the cat. *J. comp. Neurol. 98,* 401–432.

STROMINGER, N. L., and M. B. CARPENTER (1965). Effects of lesions in the substantia nigra upon subthalamic dyskinesia in the monkey. *Neurology 15,* 587–594.

STRONG, O. S., and A. ELWYN (1943). *Human Neuroanatomy.* The Williams and Wilkins Co., Baltimore.

Structure and Function of the Limbic System (1967). Progress in Brain Research, Vol. 27 (W. R. Adey and T. Tokizane, eds.). Elsevier Publishing Co., Amsterdam—London—New York.

STÜRUP, G. K., and E. A. CARMICHAEL (1935). Pain: The peripheral pathway. *Brain 58,* 216–219.

SULLIVAN, P. R., J. KUTEN, M. S. ATKINSON, J. B. ANGEVINE, and P. I. YAKOVLEV (1958). Cell count in the lateral geniculate nucleus of man. *Neurology 8,* 566–567.

SUMMER, D. (1964). Post-traumatic anosmia. *Brain 87,* 107–120.

SUNDERLAND, S. (1940). The projection of the cerebral cortex on the pons and cerebellum in the macaque monkey. *J. Anat. (Lond.) 74,* 201–226.

SUNDERLAND, S. (1948). Neurovascular relations and anomalies at the base of the brain. *J. Neurol. Neurosurg. Psychiat. 11,* 243–257.

SUNDERLAND, S., and K. C. BRADLEY (1953). Disturbances of oculomotor function accompanying extradural haemorrhage. *J. Neurol. Neurosurg. Psychiat. 16,* 35–46.

SUNDERLAND, S., and D. F. COSSAR (1953). The structure of the facial nerve. *Anat. Rec. 116,* 147–165.

SUNDERLAND, S., and E. S. R. HUGHES (1946). The pupillo-constrictor pathway and the nerves to the ocular muscles in man. *Brain 69,* 301–309.

SUNDERLAND, S., and J. O. LAVARACK (1953). The branching of nerve fibres. *Acta anat. 17,* 46–61.

SUNDERLAND, S., and W. E. SWANEY (1952). The intraneural topography of the recurrent laryngeal nerve in man. *Anat. Rec. 114,* 411–426.

SUZUKI, J.-I., and B. COHEN (1964). Head, eye, body and limb movements from semicircular canal nerves. *Exp. Neurol. 10,* 393–405.

SWANSON, A. G., G. C. BUCHAN, and E. C. ALVORD, JR. (1965). Anatomic changes in congenital insensitivity to pain. *Arch. Neurol. (Chic.) 12,* 12–18.

SWETT, J. E., and E. ELDRED (1960). Distribution and numbers of stretch receptors in medial gastrocnemius and soleus muscles of the cat. *Anat. Rec. 137,* 453–460.

SWETT, W. H., V. H. MARK, and H. HAMLIN (1960). Radiofrequency lesions in the central nervous system of man and cat. *J. Neurosurg. 17,* 213–225.

SZABO, J. (1962). Topical distribution of the striatal efferents in the monkey. *Exp. Neurol. 5,* 21–36.

SZABO, T., and M. DUSSARDIER (1964). Les noyaux d'origine du nerf vague chez le mouton. *Z. Zellforsch. 63,* 247–276.

SZENTÁGOTHAI, J. (1942a). Die innere Gliederung des Oculomotoriuskernes. *Arch. Psychiat. Nervenkr. 115,* 127–135.

SZENTÁGOTHAI, J. (1942b). Die zentrale Leitungsbahn des Lichtreflexes der Pupillen. *Arch. Psychiat. Nervenkr. 115,* 136–156.

SZENTÁGOTHAI, J. (1943a). Die Lokalisation der Kehlkopfmuskulatur in den Vaguskernen. *Z. Anat. Entwickl. Gesch. 112,* 704–710.

SZENTÁGOTHAI, J. (1943b). Die zentrale Innervation der Augenbewegungen. *Arch. Psychiat. Nervenkr. 116,* 721–760.

SZENTÁGOTHAI, J. (1948). Anatomical considerations of monosynaptic reflex arcs. *J. Neurophysiol. 11,* 445–454.

SZENTÁGOTHI, J. (1949). Functional representation in the motor trigeminal nucleus. *J. comp. Neurol. 90,* 111–120.

SZENTÁGOTHAI, J. (1951). Short propriospinal neurons and intrinsic connections of the spinal gray matter. *Acta morph. Acad. Sci. hung. 1,* 81–94.

SZENTÁGOTHAI, J. (1952a). *Die Rolle der einzelnen Labyrinthrezeptoren bei der Orientation von Augen und Kopf im Raume.* Akadémiai Kiado, Budapest.

SZENTÁGOTHAI, J. (1952b). The general visceral efferent column of the brain stem. *Acta morph. Acad. Sci. hung. 2,* 313–328.

SZENTÁGOTHAI, J. (1958). The anatomical basis of synaptic transmission of excitation and inhibition in motoneurons. *Acta morph. Acad. Sci. hung. 8,* 287–309.

SZENTÁGOTHAI, J. (1961). Somatotopic arrangement of synapses of primary sensory neurones in Clarke's column. *Acta morph. Acad. Sci. hung. 10,* 307–311.

SZENTÁGOTHAI, J. (1964a). Neuronal and synaptic arrangement in the substantia gelatinosa Rolandi. *J. comp. Neurol. 122,* 219–239.

SZENTÁGOTHAI, J. (1964b). Pathways and synaptic articulation patterns connecting vestibular receptors and oculomotor nuclei. In *The Oculomotor System*

776

References

(Morris B. Bender, ed.), pp. 205–223. Hoeber Medical Division, Harper & Row, New York.

SZENTÁGOTHAI, J. (1964c). The structure of the autonomic interneuronal synapse. *Acta neuroveg. (Wien) 26*, 338–359.

SZENTÁGOTHAI, J. (1965a). Complex synapses. In *Aus der Werkstatt der Anatomen* (W. Bargmann, ed.), pp. 147–167. Georg Thieme Verlag, Stuttgart.

SZENTÁGOTHAI, J. (1965b). The use of degeneration methods in the investigation of short neuronal connexions. In *Degeneration Patterns in the Nervous System. Progress in Brain Research*, Vol. 14 (M. Singer and J. P. Schadé, eds.), pp. 1–32. Elsevier Publishing Co., Amsterdam—London—New York.

SZENTÁGOTHAI, J. (1967). Synaptic architecture of the spinal motoneuron pool. In *Recent Advances in Clinical Neurophysiology*. Electroenceph. clin. Neurophysiol., Suppl. 25 (L. Widén, ed.), pp. 4–19. Elsevier Publishing Co., Amsterdam.

SZENTÁGOTHAI, J., and A. ALBERT (1955). The synaptology of Clarke's column. *Acta morph. Acad. Sci. hung. 5*, 43–51.

SZENTÁGOTHAI, J., A. DONHOFFER, and K. RAJKOVITS (1954). Die Lokalisation der Cholinesterase in der interneuronalen Synapse. *Acta histochem. (Jena) 1*, 272–281.

SZENTÁGOTHAI, J., B. FLERKÓ, B. MESS, and B. HALÁSZ (1968). *Hypothalamic Control of the Anterior Pituitary*, 2nd ed. Akadémiai Kiadó, Budapest.

SZENTÁGOTHAI, J., J. HÁMORI, and T. TÖMBÖL (1966). Degeneration and electron microscope analysis of the synaptic glomeruli in the lateral geniculate body. *Exp. Brain. Res. 2*, 283–301.

SZENTÁGOTHAI, J., and K. RAJKOVITS (1958). Der Hirnnervenanteil der Pyramidenbahn und der prämotorische Apparat motorischer Hirnnervenkerne. *Arch. Psychiat. Nervenkr. 197*, 335–354.

SZENTÁGOTHAI, J., and K. RAJKOVITS (1959). Über den Ursprung der Kletterfasern des Kleinhirns. *Z. Anat. Entwickl. Gesch. 121*, 130–141.

SZENTÁGOTHAI-SCHIMERT, J. (1941a). Die Endigungsweise der absteigenden Rückenmarksbahnen. *Z. Anat. Entwickl. Gesch. 111*, 322–330.

SZENTÁGOTHAI-SCHIMERT, J. (1941b). Die Bedeutung des Faserkalibers und der Markscheidendicke im Zentralnervensystem. *Z. Anat. Entwickl. Gesch. 111*, 201–223.

TAARNHØJ, P. (1952). Decompression of the trigeminal root and the posterior part of the ganglion as treatment in trigeminal neuralgia. Preliminary communication. *J. Neurosurg. 9*, 288–290.

TABER, E. (1961). The cytoarchitecture of the brain stem of the cat. I. Brain stem nuclei of cat. *J. comp. Neurol. 116*, 27–70.

TABER, E., A. BRODAL, and F. WALBERG (1960). The raphe nuclei of the brain stem in the cat. I. Normal topography and cytoarchitecture and general discussion. *J. comp. Neurol. 114*, 161–187.

TANDON, P. N., and K. KRISTIANSEN (1966). Clinico-pathological observations on brain stem dysfunction in cranio-cerebral injuries. Proc. IIIrd Int. Congr. Neurol. Surg., Copenhagen, 1965. *Excerpta med. Int. Congr. Ser. 110*, 126–129.

TAREN, J. A., and E. A. KAHN (1962). Anatomic pathways related to pain in face and neck. *J. Neurosurg. 19*, 116–119.

TARKHAN, A. A. (1934). The innervation of the extrinsic ocular muscles. *J. Anat. (Lond.) 68*, 293–313.

777

TARLOV, E. C., and R. Y. MOORE (1966). The tecto-thalamic connections in the brain of the rabbit. *J. comp. Neurol. 126,* 403–422.

TAVERNER, D. (1955). Bell's palsy. A clinical and electromyographic study. *Brain 78,* 209–228.

TAXI, J. (1965). Contribution a l'étude des connexions des neurones moteurs du système nerveux autonome. *Ann. Sci. nat. Zool. 7,* 413–674.

TEASDALL, R. D., and J. W. MAGLADERY (1959). Superficial abdominal reflexes in man. *Arch. Neurol. Psychiat. (Chic.) 81,* 28–36.

TEASDALL, R. D., and M. L. SEARS (1960). Ocular myopathy. Clinical and electromyographic considerations. *Arch. Neurol. (Chic.) 2,* 281–292.

TERKILDSEN, K. (1960). Acoustic reflexes of the human musculus tensor tympani. *Acta. oto-laryng. (Stockh.) Suppl. 158,* 230–238.

TERZIAN, H., and G. D. ORE (1955). Syndrome of Klüver-Bucy reproduced in man by bilateral removal of the temporal lobes. *Neurology 5,* 373–380.

TERZUOLO, C. A., and R. LLINÁS (1966). Distribution of synaptic inputs in the spinal motoneurone and its functional significance. In *Muscular Afferents and Motor Control.* Proceedings 1st Nobel Symposium, Stockholm (R. Granit, ed.), pp. 373–384. Almqvist & Wiksell, Stockholm; John Wiley & Sons, New York—London—Sidney.

TESTA, C. (1964). Functional implications of the morphology of spinal ventral horn neurons of the cat. *J. comp. Neurol. 123,* 425–444.

THACH, W. T., JR. (1967). Somatosensory receptive fields of single units in cat cerebellar cortex. *J. Neurophysiol. 30,* 675–696.

THAGE, O. (1964). The myotomes L2—S2 in man. *Acta neurol. scand. 41, Suppl. 13,* 241–243.

THAGE, O. (1965). Underekstremiteternes segmentale motoriske innervation belyst ved rodstimulation. *Nord. Med. 73,* 298–299.

Thalamus, The (1966). (D. P. Purpura and M. D. Yahr, eds.). Columbia Univ. Press, New York—London.

THOMAS, D. M., R. P. KAUFMAN, J. M. SPRAGUE, and W. W. CHAMBERS (1956). Experimental studies of the vermal cerebellar projections in the brain stem of the cat (fastigiobulbar tract). *J. Anat. (Lond.) 90,* 371–385.

THOMPSON, R., S. K. LANGER, and I. RICH (1964). Lesions of the limbic system and short-term memory in albino rats. *Brain 87,* 537–542.

TORVIK, A. (1956a). Transneuronal changes in the inferior olive and pontine nuclei in kittens. *J. Neuropath. exp. Neurol. 15,* 119–145.

TORVIK, A. (1956b). Afferent connections to the sensory trigeminal nuclei, the nucleus of the solitary tract and adjacent structures. An experimental study in the rat. *J. comp. Neurol. 106,* 51–142.

TORVIK, A. (1957a). The ascending fibers from the main trigeminal sensory nucleus. An experimental study in the cat. *Amer. J. Anat. 100,* 1–16.

TORVIK, A. (1957b). The spinal projection from the nucleus of the solitary tract. An experimental study in the cat. *J. Anat. (Lond.) 91,* 314–322.

Torvik, A. (1957c). Die Lokalisation des "Speichelzentrums" bei der Katze. *Z. mikrosk.-anat. Forsch. 63,* 317–326.

TORVIK, A. (1959). Sensory, motor, and reflex changes in two cases of intractable pain after stereotactic mesencephalic tractotomy. *J. Neurol. Neurosurg. Psychiat. 22,* 299–305.

TORVIK, A., and A. BRODAL (1954). The cerebellar projection of the peri-hypo-

References

glossal nuclei (nucleus intercalatus, nucleus praepositus hypoglossi and nucleus of Roller) in the cat. *J. Neuropath. exp. Neurol. 13,* 515–527.

TORVIK, A., and A. BRODAL (1957). The origin of reticulospinal fibers in the cat. An experimental study. *Anat. Rec. 128,* 113–137.

Touch, Heat and Pain. Ciba Foundation Symposium (1966). (A. V. S. de Reuck and J. Knight, eds.). J. & A. Churchill Ltd., London.

TOWE, A. L., and S. J. JABBUR (1961). Cortical inhibition of neurons in dorsal column nuclei of cat. *J. Neurophysiol. 24,* 488–498.

TOWER, S. S. (1940). Pyramidal lesions in the monkey. *Brain 63,* 36–90.

TOWER, S. S. (1944). The pyramidal tract. Definition and structure. In *The Precentral Motor Cortex* (P. C. Bucy, ed.), pp. 151–172. Univ. of Illinois Press, Urbana, Illinois.

TOWER, S., D. BODIAN, and H. HOWE (1941). Isolation of intrinsic and motor mechanism of the monkey's spinal cord. *J. Neurophysiol. 4,* 388–397.

TRAVIS, A. M. (1955). Neurological deficiencies following supplementary motor area lesions in *Macaca mulatta. Brain 78,* 174–198.

TROTTER, W., and H. M. DAVIES (1909). Experimental studies in the innervation of the skin. *J. Physiol. (Lond.) 38,* 134–246.

TSUCHITANI, C., and J. C. BOUDREAU (1966). Single unit analysis of cat superior olive S segment with tonal stimuli. *J. Neurophysiol. 29,* 684–697.

TSUKAHARA, N., and K. KOSAKA (1968). The mode of cerebral excitation of red nucleus neurons. *Exp. Brain Res. 5,* 102–117.

TSUKAHARA, N., K. TOYAMA, and K. KOSAKA (1964). Intracellulary recorded responses of red nucleus neurones during antidromic and orthodromic activation. *Experientia (Basel) 20,* 632.

TSUKAHARA, N., K. TOYAMA, and K. KOSAKA (1967). Electrical activity of red nucleus neurones investigated with intracellular microelectrodes. *Exp. Brain Res. 4,* 18–33.

TUNTURI, A. R. (1950). Physiological determination of the arrangement of the afferent connections to the middle ectosylvian auditory area in the dog. *Amer. J. Physiol. 162,* 489–502.

TÜRCK, L. (1851). Über secundäre Erkrankung einzelner Rückenmarkstränge und ihrer Fortsetzung zum Gehirne. *S. B. Akad. Wiss. Wien 6,* 288. (Cited from Nathan and Smith, 1955a.)

TÖMBÖL, T. (1966–67). Short neurons and their synaptic relations in the specific thalamic nuclei. *Brain Research 3,* 307–326.

UDDENBERG, N. (1968). Differential localization in dorsal funiculus of fibres originating from different receptors. *Exp. Brain Res. 4,* 367–376.

UNO, M., K. KUBOTA, C. OHYE, T. NAGAO, and H. NARABAYASHI (1967). Topographical arrangement between thalamic ventro-lateral nucleus and precentral motor cortex in man. *Electroenceph. clin. Neurophysiol. 22,* 437–443.

UNTERHARNSCHEIDT, F., D. JACHNIK, and H. GÖTT (1968). *Der Balkenmangel. Monographien aus dem Gesamtgebiete der Neurologie und Psychiatrie.* Heft *128,* pp. 1–232. Springer-Verlag, Berlin—Heidelberg—New York.

URSIN, H. (1965). Effect of amygdaloid lesions on avoidance behavior and visual discrimination in cats. *Exp. Neurol. 11,* 298–317.

URSIN, H., and B. R. KAADA (1960). Functional localization within the amygdaloid complex in the cat. *Electroenceph. clin. Neurophysiol. 12,* 1–20.

779

Ustvedt, H. J. (1937). Über die Untersuchung der musikalischen Funktionen bei Patienten mit Gehirnleiden, besonders bei Patienten mit Aphasie. *Acta med. scand., Suppl. 86,* 1–737.

Uvnäs, B. (1960). Central cardiovascular control. In *Handbook of Physiology. Section 1: Neurophysiology, Vol. II* (J. Field, H. W. Magoun, and V. E. Hall, eds.), pp. 1131–1162. Amer. Physiol. Soc., Washington, D.C.

Vachananda, B. (1959). The major spinal afferent systems to the cerebellum and the cerebellar corticonuclear connections in *Macaca mulatta. J. comp. Neurol. 112,* 303–351.

Valenstein, E. S., and W. J. H. Nauta (1959). A comparison of the distribution of the fornix system in the rat, guinea pig, cat, and monkey. *J. comp. Neurol. 113,* 337–363.

Valsø, J. (1936). Die Hypophyse des Blauwals (*Balaenoptera sibbaldii*). Makroskopische und mikroskopische Anatomie. *Z. Anat. Entwickl.-Gesch. 105,* 713–719.

Valverde, F. (1961a). Reticular formation of the pons and medulla oblongata. A Golgi study. *J. comp. Neurol. 116,* 71–100.

Valverde, F. (1961b). A new type of cell in the lateral reticular formation of the brain stem. *J. comp. Neurol. 117,* 189–195.

Valverde, F. (1962). Reticular formation of the albino rat's brain stem; cytoarchitecture and corticofugal connections. *J. comp. Neurol. 119,* 25–53.

Valverde, F. (1963). Amygdaloid projection field. In *The Rhinencephalon and Related Structures.* Progress in Brain Research, Vol. 3 (W. Bargmann and J. P. Schadé, eds.), pp. 20–30. Elsevier Publishing Co., Amsterdam—London—New York.

Valverde, F. (1965). *Studies on the Piriform Lobe.* Harvard Univ. Press, Cambridge, Massachusetts.

Valverde, F. (1966). The pyramidal tract in rodents. A study of its relations with the posterior column nuclei, dorsolateral reticular formation of the medulla oblongata, and cervical spinal cord (Golgi and electron microscopic observations). *Z. Zellforsch. 71,* 297–363.

Valverde, F. (1967). Apical dendritic spines of the visual cortex and light deprivation in the mouse. *Exp. Brain Res. 3,* 337–353.

Valverde, F. (1968). Structural changes in the area striata of the mouse after enucleation. *Exp. Brain Res. 5,* 274–292.

Verney, E. B. (1947). The antidiuretic hormone and the factors which determine its release. *Proc. roy. Soc. B. 135,* 25–106.

Victor, M., R. D. Adams, and E. L. Mancall (1959). A restricted form of cerebellar cortical degeneration occurring in alcoholic patients. *Arch. Neurol. (Chic.) 1,* 579–688.

Victor, M., J. B. Angevine, E. L. Mancall, and C. M. Fisher (1961). Memory loss with lesions of hippocampal formation. *Arch. Neurol. (Chic.) 5,* 244–263.

Vogt, C., and O. Vogt (1919). Allgemeinere Ergebnisse unserer Hirnforschung. *J. Psychol. Neurol. (Lpz.) 25,* 279–462.

Vogt, C., and O. Vogt (1920). Zur Lehre der Erkrankungen des striären Systems. *J. Psychol. Neurol. (Lpz.) 25, Ergänzungsheft 3,* 627–846.

Vonderahe, A. R. (1940). Changes in the hypothalamus in organic disease. *Res. Publ. Ass. nerv. ment. Dis. 20,* 689–712.

Voneida, T. J. (1960). An experimental study of the course and destination of

References

fibers arising in the head of the caudate nucleus in the cat and monkey. *J. comp. Neurol. 115*, 75–87.

Voogd, J. (1964). *The Cerebellum of the Cat. Structure and Fibre Connexions.* Proefschr. Van Gorcum & Co. N.V., Assen.

Voss, H. (1956). Zahl und Anordnung der Muskelspindeln in den oberen Zungenbeinmuskeln, im M. trapezius und M. latissimus dorsi. *Anat. Anz. 103*, 443–446.

Vraa-Jensen, G. (1942). *The Motor Nucleus of the Facial Nerve.* Munksgaard, Copenhagen.

Wachs, H., and B. Boshes (1961). Tremor studies in normals and in Parkinsonism. *Arch. Neurol. (Chic.) 4*, 66–82.

Wada, J., and T. Rasmussen (1960). Intracarotid injection of sodium amytal for the lateralization of cerebral speech dominance: Experimental and clinical observations. *J. Neurosurg. 17*, 266–282.

Wagman, I. H. (1964). Eye movements induced by electrical stimulation of cerebrum in monkeys and their relationship to bodily movements. In *The Oculomotor System* (M. B. Bender, ed.), pp. 18–39. Hoeber, New York.

Walberg, F. (1952). The lateral reticular nucleus of the medulla oblongata in mammals. A comparative-anatomical study. *J. comp. Neurol. 96*, 283–344.

Walberg, F. (1956). Descending connections to the inferior olive. An experimental study in the cat. *J. comp. Neurol. 104*, 77–174.

Walberg, F. (1957a). Corticofugal fibres to the nuclei of the dorsal columns. An experimental study in the cat. *Brain 80*, 273–287.

Walberg, F. (1957b). Do the motor nuclei of the cranial nerves receive corticofugal fibres? An experimental study in the cat. *Brain 80*, 597–605.

Walberg, F. (1960). Further studies on the descending connections to the inferior olive. Reticulo-olivary fibers: an experimental study in the cat. *J. comp. Neurol. 114*, 79–87.

Walberg, F. (1964). The early changes in degenerating boutons and the problem of argyrophilia. Light and electron microscopic observations. *J. comp. Neurol. 122*, 113–137.

Walberg, F. (1965a). An electron microscopic study of terminal degeneration in the inferior olive of the cat. *J. comp. Neurol. 125*, 205–222.

Walberg, F. (1965b). Axoaxonic contacts in the cuneate nucleus, probable basis for presynaptic depolarization. *Exp. Neurol. 13*, 218–231.

Walberg, F. (1966). The fine structure of the cuneate nucleus in normal cats and following interruption of afferent fibres. An electron microscopical study with particular reference to findings made in Glees and Nauta sections. *Exp. Brain Res. 2*, 107–128.

Walberg, F., D. Bowsher, and A. Brodal (1958). The termination of primary vestibular fibers in the vestibular nuclei in the cat. An experimental study with silver methods. *J. comp. Neurol. 110*, 391–419.

Walberg, F., and A. Brodal (1953a). Pyramidal tract fibers from temporal and occipital lobes. An experimental study in the cat. *Brain 76*, 491–508.

Walberg, F., and A. Brodal (1953b). Spino-pontine fibers in the cat. An experimental study. *J. comp. Neurol. 99*, 251–288.

Walberg, F., and J. Jansen (1961). Cerebellar corticovestibular fibers in the cat. *Exp. Neurol. 3*, 32–52.

Walberg, F., and J. Jansen (1964). Cerebellar corticonuclear projection studied experimentally with silver impregnation methods. *J. Hirnforsch. 6*, 338–354.

WALBERG, F., and O. POMPEIANO (1960). Fastigiofugal fibers to the lateral reticular nucleus: An experimental study in the cat. *Exp. Neurol. 2*, 40–53.

WALBERG, F., O. POMPEIANO, A. BRODAL, and J. JANSEN (1962). The fastigio-vestibular projection in the cat. An experimental study with silver impregnation methods. *J. comp. Neurol. 118*, 49–76.

WALBERG, F., O. POMPEIANO, L. E. WESTRUM, and E. HAUGLIE-HANSSEN (1962). Fastigioreticular fibers in cat. An experimental study with silver methods. *J. comp. Neurol. 119*, 187–199.

WALKER, A. E. (1934). The thalamic projection to the central gyri in *Macacus rhesus*. *J. comp. Neurol. 60*, 161–184.

WALKER, A. E. (1936). An experimental study of the thalamocortical projection of the macaque monkey. *J. comp. Neurol. 64*, 1–39.

WALKER, A. E. (1937). Experimental anatomical studies of the topical localization within the thalamus of the chimpanzee. *Proc. kon. ned. Akad. Wet. 40*, 198–206.

WALKER, A. E. (1938a). The thalamus of the chimpanzee. I. Terminations of the somatic afferent systems. *Confin. neurol. (Basel) 1*, 99–127.

WALKER, A. E. (1938b). The thalamus of the chimpanzee. IV. Thalamic projections to the cerebral cortex. *J. Anat. (Lond.) 73*, 37–93.

WALKER, A. E. (1938c). *The Primate Thalamus*. Univ. of Chicago Press, Illinois.

WALKER, A. E. (1939). The origin, course and terminations of the secondary pathways of the trigeminal nerve in primates. *J. comp. Neurol. 71*, 59–89.

WALKER, A. E. (1940a). The spinothalamic tract in man. *Arch. Neurol. Psychiat. (Chic.) 43*, 284–298.

WALKER, A. E. (1940b). The medial thalamic nucleus. A comparative anatomical, physiological and clinical study of the nucleus medialis dorsalis thalami. *J. comp. Neurol. 73*, 87–115.

WALKER, A. E. (1942a). Somatotopic localization of spinothalamic and secondary trigeminal tracts in mesencephalon. *Arch. Neurol. Psychiat. (Chic.) 48*, 884–889.

WALKER, A. E. (1942b). Relief of pain by mesencephalic tractotomy. *Arch. Neurol. Psychiat. (Chic.) 48*, 865–880.

WALKER, A. E. (1943). Central representation of pain. In *Pain. Res. Publ. Ass. nerv. ment. Dis.*, Vol. 23. (H. G. Wolff, H. S. Gasser, and J. C. Hinsey, eds.), pp. 63–85. The Williams and Wilkins Co., Baltimore.

WALKER, A. E., and E. H. BOTTERELL (1937). The syndrome of the superior cerebellar peduncle in the monkey. *Brain 60*, 329–353.

WALKER, A. E., and J. F. FULTON (1938). The thalamus of the chimpanzee. III. Methathalamus. Normal structure and cortical connections. *Brain 61*, 250–268.

WALKER, A. E., and H. RICHTER (1966). Section of the cerebral peduncle in the monkey. *Arch. Neurol. (Chic.) 14*, 231–240.

WALKER, A. E., and T. A. WEAVER, JR. (1940). Ocular movements from the occipital lobe in the monkey. *J. Neurophysiol. 3*, 353–357.

WALKER, A. E., and T. A. WEAVER, JR. (1942). The topical organization and termination of the fibers of the posterior columns in *Macaca mulatta*. *J. comp. Neurol. 76*, 145–158.

WALL, P. D. (1960). Cord cells responding to touch, damage, and temperature of skin. *J. Neurophysiol. 23*, 197–210.

References

WALL, P. D. (1967). The laminar organization of dorsal horn and effects of descending impulses. *J. Physiol. (Lond.) 188*, 403–423.

WALL, P. D., and J. R. CRONLY-DILLON (1960). Pain, itch and vibration. *Arch. Neurol. (Chic.) 2*, 365–375.

WALL, P. D., and A. TAUB (1962). Four aspects of the trigeminal nucleus and a paradox. *J. Neurophysiol. 25*, 110–126.

WALLGREN, A. (1929). Zur Aetiologie der 'rheumatischen' Facialisparese im Kindesalter. *Acta med. scand. 71*, 21–28.

WALSH, E. G. (1957). An investigation of sound localization in patients with neurological abnormalities. *Brain 80*, 222–250.

WALSHE, F. (1956). The Babinski plantar response, its forms and its physiological and pathological significance. *Brain 79*, 529–556.

WALSHE, F. M. R. (1924). Observations on the nature of the muscular rigidity of paralysis agitans and its relationship to tremor. *Brain 47*, 159–177.

WALSHE, F. M. R. (1942a). The anatomy and physiology of cutaneous sensibility: A critical review. *Brain 65*, 48–114.

WALSHE, F. M. R. (1942b). The giant cells of Betz, the motor cortex and the pyramidal tract: A critical review. *Brain 65*, 409–461.

WALSHE, F. M. R. (1943). On the mode of representation of movements in the motor cortex, with special reference to "convulsions beginning unilaterally" (Jackson). *Brain 66*, 104–139.

WALTER, R. D., R. W. RAND, P. H. CRANDALL, C. H. MARKHAM, and W. R. ADEY (1963). Depth electrode studies of thalamus and basal ganglia. Results in movement disorders in man. *Arch. Neurol. (Chic.) 8*, 388–397.

WANG, G. H. (1964). *The Neural Control of Sweating.* Univ. of Wisconsin Press, Madison.

WANG, S. C., and S. W. RANSON (1939). Autonomic responses to electrical stimulation of the lower brain stem. *J. comp. Neurol. 71*, 437–455.

WARD, A. A., JR. (1948). The cingular gyrus: area 24. *J. Neurophysiol. 11*, 13–23.

WARR, W. B. (1966). Fiber degeneration following lesions in the anterior ventral cochlear nucleus of the cat. *Exp. Neurol. 14*, 453–474.

WARTENBERG, R. (1954). Cerebellar signs. *J. Amer. med. Ass. 156*, 102–105.

WARWICK, R. (1953). Representation of the extra-ocular muscles in the oculomotor nuclei of the monkey. *J. comp. Neurol. 98*, 449–503.

WARWICK, R. (1954). The ocular parasympathetic nerve supply and its mesencephalic sources. *J. Anat. (Lond.) 88*, 71–93.

WARWICK, R. (1955). The so-called nucleus of convergence. *Brain 78*, 92–114.

WEAVER, R., W. M. LANDAU, and J. F. HIGGINS (1963). Fusimotor function. Part II. Evidence of fusimotor depression in human spinal shock. *Arch. Neurol. (Chic.) 9*, 127–132.

WEAVER, T. A., JR., and A. E. WALKER (1941). Topical arrangement within the spinothalamic tract of the monkey. *Arch. Neurol. Psychiat. (Chic.) 46*, 877–883.

WEBSTER, K. E. (1961). Cortico-striate interrelations in the albino rat. *J. Anat. (Lond.) 95*, 532–544.

WEBSTER, K. E. (1965). The cortico-striatal projection in the cat. *J. Anat. (Lond.) 99*, 329–337.

WEDDELL, G. (1941a). The multiple innervation of sensory spots in the skin. *J. Anat. (Lond.) 75*, 441–446.

783

WEDDELL, G. (1941b). The pattern of cutaneous innervation in relation to cutaneous sensibility. *J. Anat. (Lond.) 75*, 346–368.

WEDDELL, G., B. FEINSTEIN, and R. E. PATTLE (1944). The electrical activity of voluntary muscle in man under normal and pathological conditions. *Brain 67*, 178–257.

WEDDELL, G., J. A. HARPMAN, D. G. LAMBLEY, and L. YOUNG (1940). The innervation of the musculature of the tongue. *J. Anat. (Lond.) 74*, 255–267.

WEINBERGER, L. N., and F. C. GRANT (1942). Experiences with intramedullary tractotomy. III. Studies in sensation. *Arch. Neurol. Psychiat. (Chic.) 48*, 355–381.

WEINBERGER, N. M., M. VELASCO, and D. B. LINDSLEY (1965). Effects of lesions upon thalamically induced electrocortical desynchronization and recruiting. *Electroenceph. clin. Neurophysiol. 18*, 369–377.

WEINSTEIN, E. A., and M. B. BENDER (1941). Pupillodilator reactions to sciatic and diencephalic stimulation. A comparative study in cat and monkey. *J. Neurophysiol. 4*, 44–50.

WEINSTEIN, E. A., M. COLE, M. S. MITCHELL, and O. G. LYERLY (1964). Anosognosia and aphasia. *Arch. Neurol. (Chic.) 10*, 376–386.

WEINSTEIN, S., J. SEMMES, L. GHENT, and H.-L. TEUBER (1958). Roughness discrimination after penetrating brain injury in man: Analysis according to locus of lesion. *J. comp. physiol. Psychol. 51*, 269–275.

WEISENBURG, T., and K. E. MCBRIDE (1935). *Aphasia. A Clinical and Psychological Study.* Commonwealth Fund, New York.

WEISSCHEDEL, E. (1937). Die zentrale Haubenbahn und ihre Bedeutung für das extra-pyramidal-motorische System. *Arch. Psychiat. Nervenkr. 107*, 443–579.

WELCH, W. K., and M. A. KENNARD (1944). Relation of cerebral cortex to spasticity and flaccidity. *J. Neurophysiol. 7*, 255–268.

WELKER, W. I., R. M. BENJAMIN, R. C. MILLES, and C. N. WOOLSEY (1957). Motor effects of stimulation of cerebral cortex of squirrel monkey (*Saimiri sciureus*). *J. Neurophysiol. 20*, 347–364.

WELKER, W. I., and J. I. JOHNSON, JR. (1965). Correlation between nuclear morphology and somatotopic organization in ventro-basal complex of the raccoon's thalamus. *J. Anat. (Lond.) 99*, 761–790.

WELKER, W. I., and S. SEIDENSTEIN (1959). Somatic sensory representation in the cerebral cortex of the racoon (*Procyon lotor*). *J. comp. Neurol. 111*, 469–502.

WENDT, R., and D. ALBE-FESSARD (1962). Sensory responses of the amygdala with special reference to somatic afferent pathways. In *Physiologie de l'hippocampe*, pp. 171–200. Ed. Centre National de la Recherche Scientifique, Paris.

WERSÄLL, J. (1956). Studies on the structure and innervation of the sensory epithelium of the cristae ampullares in the guinea pig. A light and electron microscopic investigation. *Acta oto-laryng. (Stockh.), Suppl. 126*, 1–85.

WERSÄLL, J., L. GLEISNER, and P.-G. LUNDQUIST (1967). Ultrastructure of the vestibular end organs. In *Myotatic and Vestibular Mechanisms.* Ciba Foundation Symposium. (A. V. D. de Reuck and J. Knight, eds.), pp. 105–116. J. & A. Churchill Ltd., London.

WERSÄLL, J., and P.-G. LUNDQUIST (1966). Morphological polarization of the mechanoreceptors of the vestibular and acoustic system. In *NASA SP-115: Second symposium on the role of the vestibular organs in space exploration.* Ames Research Center, Moffett Field, California, pp. 57–71.

References

WESTON, J. K. (1939). Notes on the comparative anatomy of the sensory areas of the vertebrate inner ear. *J. comp. Neurol. 70*, 355–394.

WESTRUM, L. E., and T. W. BLACKSTAD (1962). An electron microscopic study of the stratum radiatum of the rat hippocampus (regio superior, CA 1) with particular emphasis on synaptology. *J. comp. Neurol. 119*, 281–309.

WHITE, J. C., and R. H. SMITHWICK (1942). *The Autonomic Nervous System. Anatomy, Physiology, and Surgical Application*, 2nd ed., Henry Kimpton, London.

WHITE, J. C., and W. H. SWEET (1955). *Pain. Its Mechanisms and Neurosurgical Control*. Charles C Thomas, Springfield, Illinois.

WHITE, L. E., JR. (1959). Ipsilateral afferents to the hippocampal formation in the albino rat. I. Cingulum projections. *J. comp. Neurol. 113*, 1–42.

WHITE, L. E., JR. (1965a). Olfactory bulb projections of the rat. *Anat. Rec. 152*, 465–479.

WHITE, L. E., JR. (1965b). A morphological concept of the limbic lobe. *Int. Rev. Neurobiol. 8*, 1–34.

WHITE, L. E., JR., W. M. NELSON, and E. L. FOLTZ (1960). Cingulum fasciculus study by evoked potentials. *Exp. Neurology 2*, 406–421.

WHITFIELD, I. C. (1967). *The Auditory Pathway*. Edward Arnold (Publishers) Ltd., London.

WHITFIELD, I. C., and E. F. EVANS (1965). Responses of auditory cortical neurons to changing frequency. *J. Neurophysiol. 28*, 655–672.

WHITLOCK, D. G. (1952). A neurohistological and neurophysiological study of afferent fiber tracts and receptive areas of the avian cerebellum. *J. comp. Neurol. 97*, 567–636.

WHITLOCK, D. G., and W. J. H. NAUTA (1956). Subcortical projections from the temporal neocortex in *Macaca mulatta*. *J. comp. Neurol. 106*, 183–212.

WHITLOCK, D. G., and E. R. PERL (1961). Thalamic projections of spinothalamic pathways in monkey. *Exp. Neurol. 3*, 240–255.

WHITTERIDGE, D. (1960). Central control of eye movements. In *Handbook of Physiology. Section 1: Neurophysiology*, Vol. II (J. Field, H. W. Magoun, and V. E. Hall, eds.), pp. 1089–1109. Amer. Physiol. Soc., Washington, D.C.

WHITTIER, J. R. (1947). Ballism and the subthalamic nucleus (nucleus hypothalamicus; corpus Luysi). Review of the literature and study of thirty cases. *Arch. Neurol. Psychiat. (Chic.) 58*, 672–692.

WHITTIER, J. R., and F. A. METTLER (1949). Studies on the subthalamus of the rhesus monkey. I. Anatomy and fiber connections of the subthalamic nucleus of Luys. *J. comp. Neurol. 90*, 281–317.

WHITTY, C. W. M., and W. LEWIN (1960). A Korsakoff syndrome in the post-cingulectomy confusional state. *Brain 83*, 648–653.

WIDÉN, L., and C. AJMONE MARSAN (1961). Action of afferent and corticofugal impulses on single elements in the dorsal lateral geniculate nucleus. In *Neurophysiologie und Psychophysik des visuellen Systems* (R. Jung and H. Kornhuber, eds.), pp. 125–132. Springer-Verlag, Berlin—Göttingen—Heidelberg.

WIESEL, T. N., and D. H. HUBEL (1965). Extent of recovery from the effects of visual deprivation in kittens. *J. Neurophysiol. 28*, 1060–1072.

WIESMAN, G. G., D. S. JONES, and W. C. RANDALL (1966). Sympathetic outflows from cervical spinal cord in the dog. *Science 152*, 381–382.

WILLIAMS, D. (1965). The thalamus and epilepsy. *Brain 88*, 539–556.

785

WILLIAMS, M., and J. PENNYBACKER (1954). Memory disturbances in third ventricle tumours. *J. Neurol. Neurosurg. Psychiat. 17,* 115–123.

WILLIAMS, T. H. (1967). Electron microscopic evidence for an autonomic interneuron. *Nature 214,* 309–310.

WILLIS, W. D., and J. C. WILLIS (1966). Properties of interneurons in the ventral spinal cord. *Arch. ital. Biol. 104,* 354–386.

WILSON, M. E., and B. G. CRAGG (1967). Projections from the lateral geniculate nucleus in the cat and monkey. *J. Anat. (Lond.) 101,* 677–692.

WILSON, V. J., M. KATO, B. W. PETERSON, and R. M. WYLIE (1967). A single-unit analysis of the organization of Deiters' nucleus. *J. Neurophysiol. 30,* 603–619.

WILSON, V. J., M. KATO, R. C. THOMAS, and B. W. PETERSON (1966). Excitation of lateral vestibular neurons by peripheral afferent fibers. *J. Neurophysiol. 29,* 508–529.

WINDLE, W. F. (1926). Non-bifurcating nerve fibers of the trigeminal nerve. *J. comp. Neurol. 40,* 229–240.

WINDLE, W. F. (1931). The sensory component of the spinal accessory nerve. *J. comp. Neurol. 53,* 115–127.

WINTER, D. L. (1965). N. gracilis of cat. Functional organization and corticofugal effects. *J. Neurophysiol. 28,* 48–70.

WOHLFAHRT, S. (1932). Die vordere Zentralwindung bei Pyramidenbahnläsionen verschiedener Art. *Acta med. scand., Suppl. 46,* 1–234.

WOHLFAHRT, S., and G. WOHLFART (1935). Mikroskopische Untersuchungen an progressiven Muskelatrophien. *Acta med. scand., Suppl. 63,* 1–137.

WOHLFART, G., and K. G. HENRIKSSON (1960). Observations on the distribution, number and innervation of Golgi musculo-tendinous organs. *Acta anat. 41,* 192–204.

WOLF, G., and J. SUTIN (1966). Fiber degeneration after lateral hypothalamic lesions in the rat. *J. comp. Neurol. 127,* 137–155.

WOLF, G. A., JR. (1941). The ratio of preganglionic neurons to postganglionic neurons in the visceral nervous system. *J. comp. Neurol. 75,* 235–243.

WOLSTENCROFT, J. H. (1964). Reticulospinal neurones. *J. Physiol. (Lond.) 174,* 91–108.

WOODBURNE, R. T. (1936). A phylogenetic consideration of the primary and secondary centers and connections of the trigeminal complex in a series of vertebrates. *J. comp. Neurol. 65,* 403–502.

WOODBURNE, R. T. (1939). Certain phylogenetic anatomical relations of localizing significance for the mammalian nervous system. *J. comp. Neurol. 71,* 215–257.

WOODBURNE, R. T., E. C. CROSBY, and R. E. McCOTTER (1946). The mammalian midbrain and isthmus regions. Part II. The fiber connections. A. The relations of the tegmentum of the midbrain with the basal ganglia in *Macaca mulatta. J. comp. Neurol. 85,* 67–92.

WOOLLARD, H. H. (1935). Observations on the termination of cutaneous nerves. *Brain 58,* 352–367.

WOOLLARD, H. H., and J. H. HARPMAN (1939). The cortical projection of the medial geniculate body. *J. Neurol. Psychiat. 2,* 35–44.

WOOLLARD, H. H., and J. A. HARPMAN (1940). The connexions of the inferior colliculus and of the dorsal nucleus of the lateral lemniscus. *J. Anat. (Lond.) 74,* 441–458.

References

WOOLLARD, H. H., G. WEDDELL, and J. A. HARPMAN (1940). Observations on the neurohistological basis of cutaneous pain. *J. Anat.* (*Lond.*) *74*, 413–440.

WOOLSEY, C. N. (1947). Patterns of sensory representation in the cerebral cortex. *Fed. Proc. 6*, 437–441.

WOOLSEY, C. N. (1958). Organization of somatic sensory and motor areas of the cerebral cortex. In *Biological and Biochemical Bases of Behavior* (H. F. Harlow and C. N. Woolsey, eds.), pp. 63–81. Univ. Wisconsin Press, Madison.

WOOLSEY, C. N. (1960). Organization of cortical auditory system: A review and a synthesis. In *Neural Mechanisms of the Auditory and Vestibular Systems* (G. L. Rasmussen and W. F. Windle, eds.), pp. 165–180. Charles C Thomas, Springfield, Illinois.

WOOLSEY, C. N. (1964). Cortical localization as defined by evoked potential and electrical stimulation studies. In *Cerebral Localization and Organization* (G. Schaltenbrand and C. N. Woolsey, eds.), pp. 17–32. Univ. Wisconsin Press, Madison.

WOOLSEY, C. N., and D. FAIRMAN (1946). Contralateral, ipsilateral, and bilateral representation of cutaneous receptors in somatic areas I and II of the cerebral cortex of pig, sheep, and other mammals. *Surgery 19*, 684–702.

WOOLSEY, C. N., W. H. MARSHALL, and P. BARD (1942). Representation of cutaneous tactile sensibility in the cerebral cortex of the monkey as indicated by evoked potentials. *Bull. Johns Hopk. Hosp. 70*, 399–441.

WOOLSEY, C. N., W. H. MARSHALL, and P. BARD (1943). Note on the organization of the tactile sensory area of the cerebral cortex of the chimpanzee. *J. Neurophysiol. 6*, 287–291.

WOOLSEY, C. N., P. H. SETTLAGE, D. R. MEYER, W. SPENCER, T. P. HAMUY, and A. M. TRAVIS (1952). Patterns of localization in precentral and "supplementary" motor areas and their relation to the concept of a premotor area. *Res. Publ. Ass. nerv. ment. Dis. 30*, 238–264.

WOOLSEY, C. N., and E. M. WALZL (1942). Topical projection of nerve fibers from local regions of the cochlea to the cerebral cortex of the cat. *Bull. Johns Hopk. Hosp. 71*, 315–344.

WRETE, M. (1930). Morphogenetische und anatomische Untersuchungen über die Rami communicantes der Spinalnerven beim Menschen. *Uppsala Läk.-Fören. Förh. 35*, 219–380.

WRETE, M. (1935). Die Entwicklung der intermediären Ganglien beim Menschen. *Morph. Jb. 75*, 229–268.

WYKE, B. D. (1947). Clinical physiology of the cerebellum. *Med. J. Aust. 2/18*, 533–540.

WYKE, B. D. (1967). The neurology of joints. Arris and Gale Lecture. *Ann. roy. Coll. Surg. Engl. 41*, 25–50.

XUEREB, G. P., M. M. L. PRICHARD, and P. M. DANIEL (1954a). The arterial supply and venous drainage of the human hypophysis cerebri. *Quart. J. exp. Physiol. 39*, 199–217.

XUEREB, G. P., M. M. L. PRICHARD, and P. M. DANIEL (1954b). The hypophysial portal system of vessels in man. *Quart. J. exp. Physiol. 39*, 219–230.

YAKOVLEV, P. I., S. LOCKE, D. Y. KOSKOFF, and R. A. PATTON (1960). Limbic nuclei of thalamus and connections of limbic cortex. I. Organization of the projections of the anterior group of nuclei and of the midline nuclei of the thalamus to the anterior cingulate gyrus and hippocampal rudiment in the monkey. *Arch. Neurol. (Chic.) 3,* 621–641.

YEE, J., F. HARRISON, and K. B. CORBIN (1939). The sensory innervation of the spinal accessory and tongue musculature in the rabbit. *J. comp. Neurol. 70,* 305–314.

YOSS, R. E. (1952). Studies of the spinal cord. Part I. Topographic localization within the dorsal spino-cerebellar tract in *Macaca mulatta. J. comp. Neurol. 97,* 5–20.

YOSS, R. E. (1953). Studies of the spinal cord. Part II. Topographic localization within the ventral spino-cerebellar tract in the macaque. *J. comp. Neurol. 99,* 613–638.

ZANDER OLSEN, P., and E. DIAMANTOPOULOS (1967). Excitability of spinal motor neurons in normal subjects and patients with spasticity, Parkinsonian rigidity, and cerebellar hypotonia. *J. Neurol. Neurosurg. Psychiat. 30,* 325–331.

ZANGWILL, O. L. (1960). *Cerebral Dominance and its Relation to Psychological Function.* William Ramsay Henderson Trust Lecture. Oliver and Boyd, Edinburgh—London.

ZENTAY, PAUL J. (1937). Motor disorders of the central nervous system and their significance for speech. Part I. Cerebral and cerebellar dysarthrias. *Laryngoscope (St. Louis) 47,* 147–156.

ZERVAS, N. T., F. A. HORNER, and K. S. PICKREN (1967). The treatment of dyskinesia by stereotaxic dendatectomy. *Conf. neurol. (Basel) 29,* 93–100.

ZILSTORFF-PEDERSEN, K. (1964). Determinations and variations of olfactory thresholds. *Arch. Otolaryng. 79,* 412–417.

ZIMMERMAN, H. M. (1940). Temperature disturbances and the hypothalamus. *Res. Publ. Ass. nerv. ment. Dis. 20,* 824–840.

ZOTTERMAN, Y. (1959). The peripheral nervous mechanism of pain: A brief review. In *Pain and Itch. Nervous Mechanisms.* Ciba Foundation Study Group no. 1 (G. E. Wolstenholme and M. O'Connor, eds.), pp. 13–24. J. & A. Churchill Ltd., London.

Index

Index

Body (*continued*)
 pontobulbar, 280
 trapezoid, 494
Body scheme, 674 ff.
Bolk's theory of cerebellar localization, 268
Bouton, terminal, 9
 degeneration of, 17 ff.
Brachial plexus, *see* Plexus
Brachium
 conjunctivum, 287
  lesions of, 296
 pontis, 279
 quadrigeminal, inferior, 497
Brodmann's cytoarchitectural map, 643
Brown-Séquard syndrome, 203, 207
Bulbar palsy, chronic, 361, 373, 408
Bundle, olivocochlear (*see also* Nerve, cochlear), 490, 492, 496 n., 501

Capillaries, changes in caliber, 609, 612
Capsula, externa, 180
 extrema, 180
 interna, 157
  lesions (*see also* Hemiplegia), 207 ff.
Carbon monoxide poisoning, lesions of basal ganglia, 218
Carotid sinus, *see* Sinus
Cauda equina, lesions of, 631
Caudate nucleus, *see* Nucleus
Causalgia, 638
Celiac ganglion, *see* Ganglion
 plexus, *see* Plexus
"Center" (Centers, Centrum)
 autonomic, integrative, 597 ff.
 cardiovascular, medulla, 325
  hypothalamus, 597
 ciliospinale, 582, 614
 ejaculation, 622
 erection, 622
 gaze, 441, 456
 of reticular formation, *see* Reticular formation
 sleep, 338
 thirst, 587
 waking, 338
Central gray matter of spinal cord, lesions of, 101 ff.
"Centrencephalic system," 348
Cerebellum (cerebellar), 255 ff.
 affections in man, 299
  diagnosis of, 300
 compensation in lesions of, 302
 connections, 264 ff.
  afferent fibers, 268 ff.

efferent fibers, 283 ff.
cortex, 258 ff., 297
 physiology, 262 ff.
experiments, 291 ff.
functional considerations, 291 ff.
glomerulus, 262
lesions of
 in animals, 291 ff.
 in man, 299 ff.
localization, 268
nuclei, 264 ff.
nystagmus, *see* Nystagmus
phylogenesis, 255
somatotopical localization, 268 ff., 294
subdivisions, 256
 longitudinal zones, 265, 293 ff.
symptoms, 290 ff.
 in acoustic nerve tumors, 301
 in lesions of brachium conjunctivum, 296; frontal lobe, 302
syndromes, 298
Cerebral cortex, 640 ff.
 afferents, "specific" and "non-specific," 331, 653, 658
 agranular, 645
 angioarchitecture, 646
 area, areas, in general, 640 ff.
  acoustic, 498 ff.; functional aspects, 499, 502 ff., 507
  association, 649
  autonomic, 602
  entorhinal, 513, 518, 526
  "extrapyramidal," 191
  gustatory, *see* Taste
  motor, 190 ff.; primary, first (MsI, SmI), 191 ff., functional aspects, 192 ff., 229 ff., lesions, 207 ff., 231 ff.; secondary (SmII), 77, 85 ff., 191, functional aspects, 85, 199; supplementary, 86, 167, 191, 197, functional aspects, 197 ff.
  olfactory, 516
  orbitofrontal, 335, 662, 664, 665
  sensorimotor, 77, 191
  somatosensory, 75 ff., 85 ff.; first (SmI), 75 ff., functional aspects, 79 ff.; second (SmII), 77, 85 ff., 191, functional aspects, 85, 199
  striate, *see* Cerebral cortex, area, visual
  supplementary motor, *see* Cerebral cortex, area, motor
  vestibular, 387
  visual (17, 18, 19), 463, 467, 473 ff.

Index

Index

Pain (*continued*)
  thalamic, 113
  treatment, by chordotomy, *see* Chordotomy
    leucotomy, 655
  visceral, 622 ff.
Paleocerebellum, 257
Paleocortex, 511
Paleostriatum, 182
Pallidohypothalamic fibers, *see* Tract
Pallidum, 181 ff.
  experiments on, 244
  fiber connections, 186 ff.
  lesions, 217
Paraflocculus, 257
Paralysis agitans, 216 ff., 228
  surgical treatment, 248 ff.
Paralysis (Paresis), of bladder, 621, 630 ff.
  of extrinsic eye muscles, 111, 449 ff.
    in herpes zoster, 427
  facial, central, 408
    congenital, 408
    in herpes zoster oticus, 411
    in lesions of pons, 111
    peripheral, 405 ff.
  flaccid, 143, 211.
  of laryngeal muscles, 370
  in lesions of motor cortex, 207 ff.
    peripheral motor neurones, 143 ff.
    transverse lesions of spinal cord, 204
  of masticatory muscles, 423 ff.
    in herpes zoster, 427
  of mimetic muscles, 405 ff.
  oculomotor, external (*see also* Nerve, oculomotor), 450 ff.
    internal, 450, 452
  postparoxysmal, 209 n.
  spastic, *see* Spasticity
  of tongue, peripheral, 359
    supranuclear, 360
  of trapezius and sternoclei toid, 362
  of velum palati, 369, 372
    postdiphtheritic, 372
Paraplegia in flexion, spastic, 205
Parastriate area, *see* Visual areas
Parasympathetic system (*see also* Autonomic and Fibers), 547 ff.
  cranial division, 550 ff.
    ganglia and fibers, 560 ff.
  innervation of organs (table), 616
  sacral division, 550 ff.
    ganglia and fibers, 561 ff.
Paraventricular nucleus, *see* Nucleus

Paresis, *see* Paralysis
Paresthesias
  in lesions of dorsal roots, 94
    medulla oblongata, 110
    sensory cortex, 115
  in protrusion of intervertebral disc, 94
Parkinsonism, atherosclerotic, 218
  luetic, 218
  postencephalitic, 217
Parkinson's disease, *see* Paralysis agitans
Past pointing in cerebellar disease, 291
  in vestibular tests, 393, 394
Pathway, *see* Tract, Olfactory system, Optic system, etc.
Peduncle, cerebral, arrangement of fibers, 158
  transection of, 233 ff.
Pelvic nerve, *see* Nerve
Periaqueductal gray, 523, 581
Petrosal ganglion, *see* Ganglion
Phenol, intrathecal injections of, 95, 228
Pick's disease, 663
Piloarrection (*see also* Innervation, autonomic)
  from hypothalamus, 599
Piriform lobe, *see* Lobe
Pituicytes, 584 n., 588.
Pituitary body, *see* Hypophysis
Plexus (plexuses), autonomic, 560, 571
  brachial, 145
    lesions, autonomic disturbances, 611, 633; motor disturbances, 145 ff.; sensory disturbances, 51
    palsy, 147
  cardiac, 556
  enteric, 561
  gastric, 561
  hepatic, 561
  hypogastric, 556
    resection of, 636
  lumbosacral, lesions, motor disturbances, 148
  myenteric, 561
  pudendal, 562
  submucosus, 561
Polioencephalitis hemorrhagica superior, 530
Poliomyelitis, 143, 454
  affection of ambiguus nucleus, 372
    facial nucleus, 408
    hypoglossal nucleus, 359
    motor ventral horn cells, 143
    oculomotor nucleus, 454
    reticular formation, 345
  changes in muscles, 121

8 0 1

Index

Sensibility (*continued*)
in lesions of anterolateral funiculi,
103 ff.
dorsal funiculi, 105 ff.
dorsal horns, 101
dorsal roots, 94 ff.
medulla oblongata, pons, mesencephalon, 109 ff.
sensory cortex, 113 ff.
thalamus, 112
deep, 38 ff.
in lesions of dorsal funiculi, 107;
medial lemniscus, 109; sensory
cortex, 113; thalamus, 112
discriminattive, *see* Discriminative
epicritic, 41
exteroceptive, 31
muscular, *see* Sensibility, deep, and
proprioceptive
pain, *see* Pain
proprioceptive (*see also* Sensibility,
deep), 31, 38 ff., 125 ff.
dorsal funiculi, 55
of extrinsic eye muscles, 434
of face, 399, 420
impulses to cerebellum, 272 ff.
of larynx, 368
of tongue, 358
protopathic, 41
stereognostic, 108, 114
temperature, *see* Temperature
vascular, 627
vibratory, 38
in lesions of dorsal funiculi, 107;
medial lemniscus, 110; sensory
cortex, 114
visceral, 622 ff.
Sensitization, in autonomically denervated organs, 567 ff., 611
in denervated muscles, 145
Sensory, cortical areas, *see* Cerebral
cortex, areas
impulses, central control, 57, 62, 201,
355, 419, 471 n., 501, 514
modalities, 31 ff.
spots, cutaneous, 35
Septum, septal region, 523, 525, 533,
580, 581
Sham rage, 600
Sinus, carotid, 366
Sleep, 335 ff.
"centers," 338, 600
disturbances, 628
REM phases, 337, 341
theories on mechanism, 338 ff.
Smell, sense of (*see also* Olfactory system), 510, 539

examination of, 540
impairment of, in lesions, 541 ff.
Somatotopical arrangement (of fibers or
nerve cells)
ambiguus nucleus, 363
cerebellum, 268 ff., 294
dorsal funiculi, 55
facial nucleus, 399
hypoglossal nucleus, 356
lateral thalamic nucleus, 69, 79, 288
lateral vestibular nucleus, 172, 383
medial lemniscus, 58
motoneurons, 119 ff.
motor areas, 192 ff.
oculomotor nucleus, 431
pyramidal tract, 157 ff.
red nucleus, 166
somatosensory areas, 79 ff.
spinothalamic tract, 61
ventral horn of spinal cord, 119 ff.
Spasticity (*see also* Muscular hypertonus), 211, 225 ff.
in capsular hemiplegias, 211
in transverse lesions of spinal cord,
205
"Specific" cortical afferents, 331, 653,
658
"Specific" thalamic nuclei, *see* Nuclei,
thalamic
Speech, disorders of, 291, 668 ff.
Sphenopalatine ganglion, *see* Ganglion
Spinal cord
lesions, 203 ff.
organization, 44 ff., 200 ff.
supraspinal influences, 200 ff.
Spinal shock, 203 ff.
Spines, dendritic, 12
Spinocerebellar tracts, *see* Tract
Spinocerebellum, 257
lesions, 293
Spiral ganglion, *see* Ganglion
Splanchnic nerve, *see* Nerve
Status marmoratus, 220
Stepping test, 390
Stereognosis, *see* Sensibility, stereognos-
tic
Stratum, external sagittal, 472
Stretch reflex, 131 ff.
Stria (Striae), acoustic, 494
longitudinal, 522
medullaris, 533
olfactory, 514
terminalis, 533, 534
Striate area, *see* Cerebral cortex, area,
visual
Striatum (*see also* Corpus striatum),
180 ff.